CLINICAL ATLAS OF

HYPERTENSION

John D Swales MA, MD, FRCP
Professor of Medicine
Leicester University Medical School
Leicester, UK

Peter S Sever MB, BChir, PhD, MRCP
Professor of Clinical Pharmacology and Therapeutics
St Mary's Hospital Medical School
London, UK

Sir W Stanley Peart MD, FRCP, FRS
Master, The Hunterian Institute
Royal College of Surgeons of England
London, UK

Published in association with
Clinical Communications Inc.

Gower Medical Publishing

LONDON • NEW YORK

Distributed in USA and Canada by:
Raven Press Ltd.
1185 Avenue of the Americas
New York
New York 10036
USA

Distributed in the rest of the world by:
Gower Medical Publishing
Middlesex House
34–42 Cleveland Street
London W1P 5FB
UK

Project editor: Stephen McGrath

Design: Mark Willey

Line Artists: Marion Tasker, Lee Smith, David McElwaine, Mai Ling Wong, Jenni Miller, Sue Tyler

Paste-up: Richard Prime, Clare Gillmore, Olgun Hassan, Ruth Miles

Index: Nina Boyd

ISBN 1-56375-637-4

Originated in Hong Kong by Bright Arts

Text set in Palatino; captions and figures set in Futura

Produced by Imago. Reprinted in Singapore in 1992

Preface

The present work is a completely rewritten and expanded version of 'Hypertension Illustrated' which was first published in 1984. The success of that work indicated the need for a book on Hypertension which emphasized the clinical aspects of the condition by means of top quality graphical and photographic illustration. Indeed, it became commonplace for the authors, when attending clinical meetings in many parts of the world, to see the familiar illustrations used as a basic for lectures and seminars on the clinical and scientific basis of hypertension. Inevitably in a field which is changing so rapidly many of our illustrations and text appear dated or have been superseded. We know more about basic mechanisms, about drugs and even our understanding of epidemiology has grown over the last few years. A new edition was long overdue. We can but hope that this will be as successful a tool for teaching and learning as our first edition. Our only sorrow in setting out on this task is the loss of our co-author, Robert Tarazi. His unique clinical and scientific expertise has produced a lasting contribution to our understanding of hypertension. We have greatly missed his gentle but incisive comments and dedicate this edition to his memory.

W S Peart P S Sever J D Swales

Contents

CHAPTER 4

Pathological Consequences of Hypertension

CHAPTER 5

Known Causes of Hypertension

CHAPTER 6

Clinical Subgroups

CHAPTER 7

History and Examination

CHAPTER 8

Investigation of the Patient

CHAPTER 9

Drug Treatment

CHAPTER 10

Treatment

CHAPTER 1

Epidemiology and Natural History

INTRODUCTION

Although many aspects of the physiology of hypertension remain mysterious, it is nevertheless true to say that there is a greater body of knowledge about the natural history of hypertension than about any other common disorder. There are two reasons for this. Firstly, the indirect measurement of blood pressure is a painless and straightforward technique, learnt and performed by all doctors and nurses. Secondly, the importance of hypertension was recognized at an early stage by insurance companies, who meticulously compiled blood pressure data from millions of people. These studies have made it possible to define the life expectancy associated with a particular systolic or diastolic pressure with some precision.

Because of the numbers involved in the insurance companies' studies, the errors introduced in taking blood pressure only once in an ambulant patient were relatively insignificant. However, the technique and circumstances of blood pressure measurement become of prime importance when assessing an individual hypertensive patient; in this situation single casual readings provide insufficient information.

MEASUREMENT

Direct measurement of blood pressure, obtained by cannulating a large artery in several species of mammal, was first carried out by Stephen Hales (Fig. 1.1), who reported his results in 1733. The need to open an artery precluded the use of this technique in human patients; the presence of hypertension could only be inferred from the evidence of pathological changes such as left ventricular hypertrophy. In 1855 Vierordt suggested that a non-invasive technique could be developed which measured the pressure needed to occlude arterial pulsation in a limb. In an attempt to achieve carefully regulated pressures at the brachial or radial arteries, Vierordt initially used counterweights; these proved unsatisfactory and a period of experimentation followed. Marey (1860) developed a sphygmographic method which, with further modifications devised particularly by Mahomed and Dudgeon, was used throughout the remainder of the 19th century (Fig. 1.2). Early measurements of systolic blood pressure were extremely unreliable but Mahomed, using his modification of Marey's sphygmograph, was able to report the presence of high blood pressure even in the absence of renal disease (which had up to that time been considered a *sine qua non* for elevated pressure). While it is now of historical interest only, the sphygmograph provided the basis for the recognition of essential hypertension as a distinct disease entity.

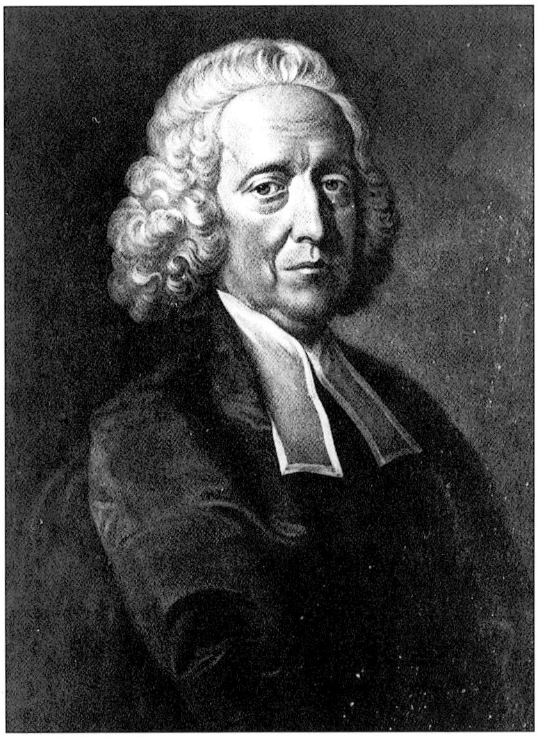

Fig. 1.1 Rev. Stephen Hales, 1677–1761.

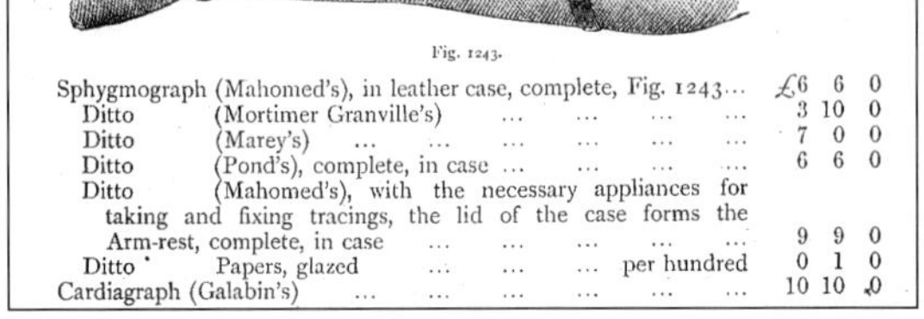

Fig. 1.2 The modified Marey Sphygmograph.

The measurement of diastolic pressure remained a major problem until Nikolai Korotkoff (Fig. 1.3) described his auscultatory method in 1905. Korotkoff was a Russian military surgeon who had published a thesis on arteriovenous fistulae occurring as a result of war injuries. His interest in arterial bruits led him to apply a stethoscope to a patient's upper arm just below an inflated sphygmographic cuff, while the latter slowly deflated. To quote:

'At first there are no sounds whatsoever. As the mercury in the manometer drops to a certain height there appear the first short or faint tones, the appearance of which indicates that part of the pulse wave of the blood stream has passed under the sleeve. Consequently the reading of the manometer when the first sound appears corresponds to the maximum blood pressure; with a further fall of mercury in the manometer there are heard systolic pressure murmurs which become again sounds (secondary). Finally all the sounds disappear. The time of disappearance of the sounds indicated the free passage or flow of the blood stream. In other words at the moment of disappearance or fading out of the sounds the minimum blood pressure in the artery surpasses pressure in the sleeve. Consequently the reading of the manometer at this time corresponds to the minimum blood pressure'.

Manual measurement of blood pressure in the clinic still rests firmly on the auscultation of the Korotkoff sounds, and is likely to do so for the foreseeable future.

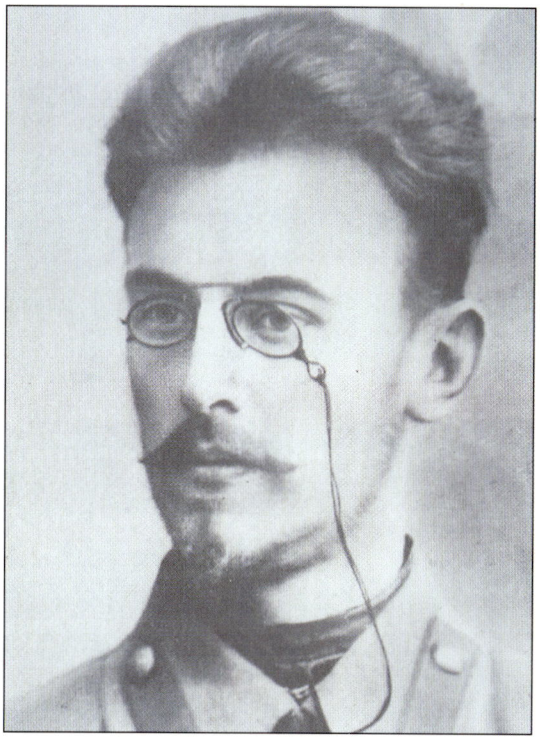

Fig. 1.3 N.S. Korotkoff, 1874–1920.

Blood Pressure Variability

An individual's blood pressure frequently changes from one measurement to the next. Such variations within individuals can arise in two ways (Fig. 1.4). Firstly, there may be differences in the

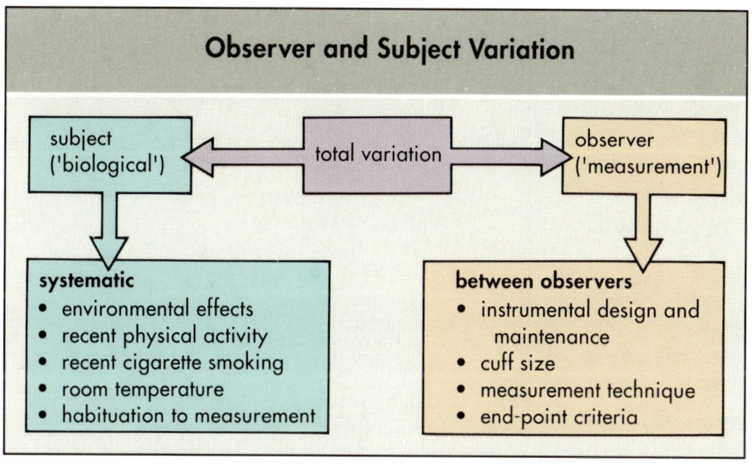

Fig. 1.4 When blood pressure is measured in the same individual on two occasions the observed value may be different. Such variations may be due to factors influencing blood pressure or to differences in measurement.

way in which blood pressure is recorded (observer variation). Secondly, the patient's blood pressure may actually be different, as a result of spontaneous changes or environmental influences (subject or biological variability).

Observer variation

The technique of blood pressure measurement is described elsewhere (see chapter 8). Observer variation in the reported values can result from differences in technique or faults in the instrument employed. Differences due to observer technique may therefore summate with instrument error.

For an accurate measurement of blood pressure, the cuff should be inflated to about 30mmHg above the point at which the radial pulse disappears. Failure to do this may result in artefactually low systolic blood pressures, particularly where there is a silent interval (the first Korotkoff sounds are heard, disappear and then reappear again with deflation of the cuff). Too rapid deflation of the cuff (at a rate in excess of the recommended 2–3mmHg per second over the critical points) may also produce erroneously low readings for systolic and diastolic blood pressures. If the deflation of the cuff is too prolonged, or if the cuff is reinflated, sustained venous occlusion of the forearm occurs with an increase in local blood volume. This alters the level at which the Korotkoff sounds appear.

Observer bias may also contribute to variability in blood pressure values. Thus, observers can show digit preference, which leads to a preponderance of values ending in 0 or 5mmHg (Fig. 1.5). Equally important is the influence exerted by an arbitrary cut-off point. For example, if a decision has been made to treat any patient whose diastolic blood pressure is 100mmHg or more, this may well influence the selection of values when blood pressure approaches that figure. Such observer bias can be avoided by the use of special instruments, the two most widely used being the Hawksley Random Zero sphygmomanometer and the London School of Hygiene and Tropical Medicine sphygmomanometer (Fig.1.6). In the former the mercury zero is altered in a random fashion; the operator does not know the extent of its displacement until after the reading has been obtained. The latter is a more elaborate instrument with a cuff which is inflated by means of a gas cylinder and deflated through a constant escape valve. The observer records the point at which the Korotkoff sounds appear and disappear without knowledge of the blood pressures they represent. Both of these instruments are used extensively in clinical trials but are too cumbersome for routine clinical use.

The selection of different criteria for recording diastolic blood pressure may also cause interobserver variability. Some clinicians take the point of muffling of Korotkoff sounds (Phase IV) as a diastolic pressure, while others take the point of disappearance (Phase V). Although Korotkoff's original paper suggested that these two phases are nearly identical, this is not the case; the difference between the two end-points may account for a discrepancy of between 3 and 10mmHg in the

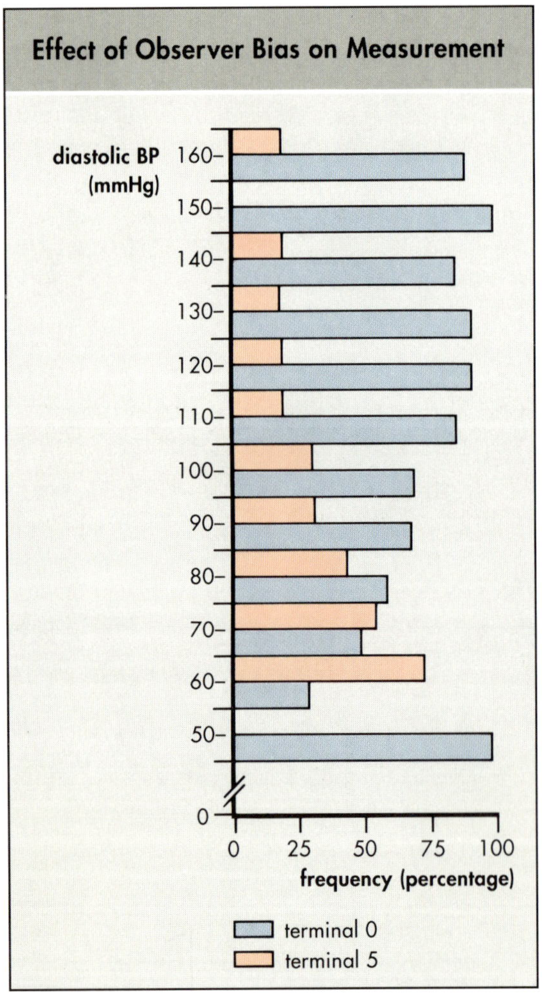

Fig. 1.5 Effect of observer bias on measured blood pressure. Clinicians tend to record blood pressure values ending in a zero with increasing frequency as observed blood pressure increases.

observed diastolic pressure, although on average it is about 4mmHg (Fig 1.7). Phase V provides a more reproducible value, and since the insurance data upon which much of our understanding of the epidemiology of hypertension is based also use Phase V, it is probably preferable. The majority of the large multicentre studies on treatment of hypertension have employed Phase V diastolic measurements. However, patients are occasionally encountered in whom the Korotkoff sounds can be heard down to zero manometric pressure (this constitutes a particular problem in pregnant women). Under these circumstances there is no alternative to the use of Phase IV.

The Hawksley and Rose Sphygmomanometers

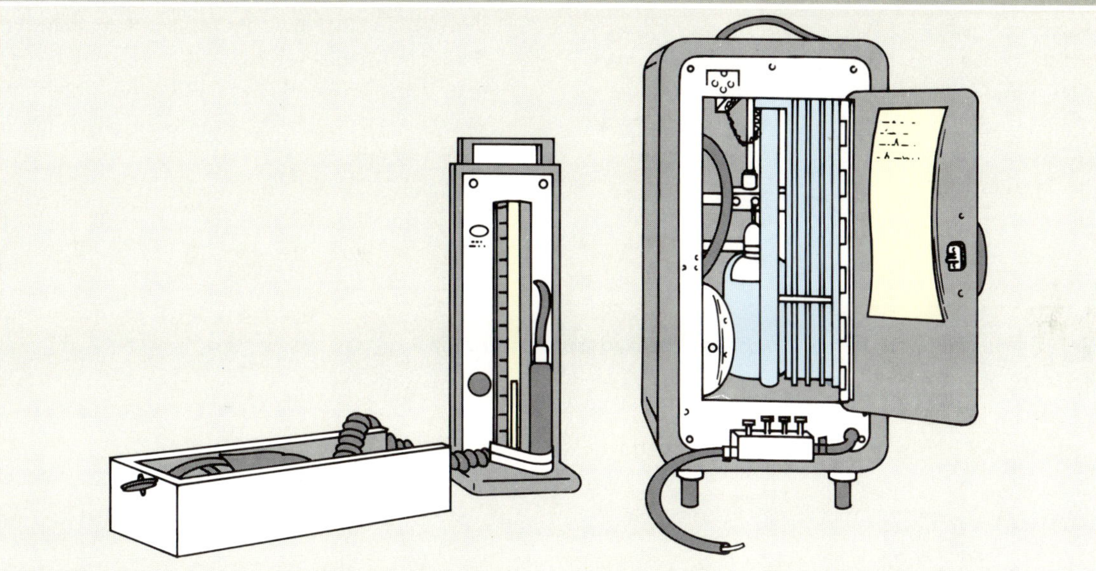

Fig. 1.6 Two types of 'blind' sphygmomanometers. On the left, the Hawksley random zero, in which the position of the zero is altered by the manipulation of the screw to left of the scale, giving a value which is unknown to the observer until the end of the measurement. On the right is the Rose (London School of Hygiene and Tropical Medicine) sphygmomanometer, in which the cuff is inflated and deflated semi-automatically. The mercury in each column is stopped by pressing a button, and the values for systolic and diastolic pressure are read subsequently.

The Korotkoff Sounds

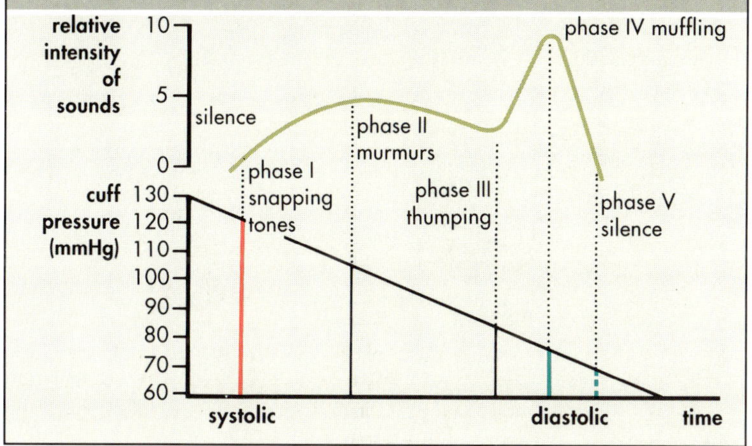

Fig. 1.7 Use of the Korotkoff sounds in the measurement of blood pressure. The point of appearance of the sounds provides a good measure of systolic blood pressure. Diastolic blood pressure may be taken either at the point of sudden muffling of sounds (Phase IV), or at their disappearance (Phase V). There is a difference of 5–10mmHg between these two phases.

While mercury manometers are normally reliable instruments, they can on occasion be the source of significant errors (Fig 1.8):

- If the doctor's eye is not level with the mercury meniscus there may be an error due to parallax.
- The instrument may not be placed in a strictly vertical position.
- Dirt in the escape valve may cause irregular deflation of the cuff.
- Aneroid instruments lose accuracy over time, usually leading to underestimation of blood pressure.
- The manometer, whether aneroid or mercury, may not be zeroed before the cuff is inflated.
- Inappropriate cuff size is responsible for important errors in blood pressure measurement in obese subjects and subjects of small stature, for example children (see chapter 6). If too short a bladder is used, pressure within the cuff is not fully transmitted to the artery and blood pressure is therefore overestimated. The cuff length should, for that reason, be at least 80% of the bladder's circumference. Likewise, too narrow a bladder leads to overestimation of blood pressure, although this is not a common problem. The width of the cuff should be at least 40% of the arm's circumference, and in children over five years of age the bladder should be at least 8cm wide.
- If the arm is not at the level of the mid-sternum blood pressure can be significantly over- or underestimated.

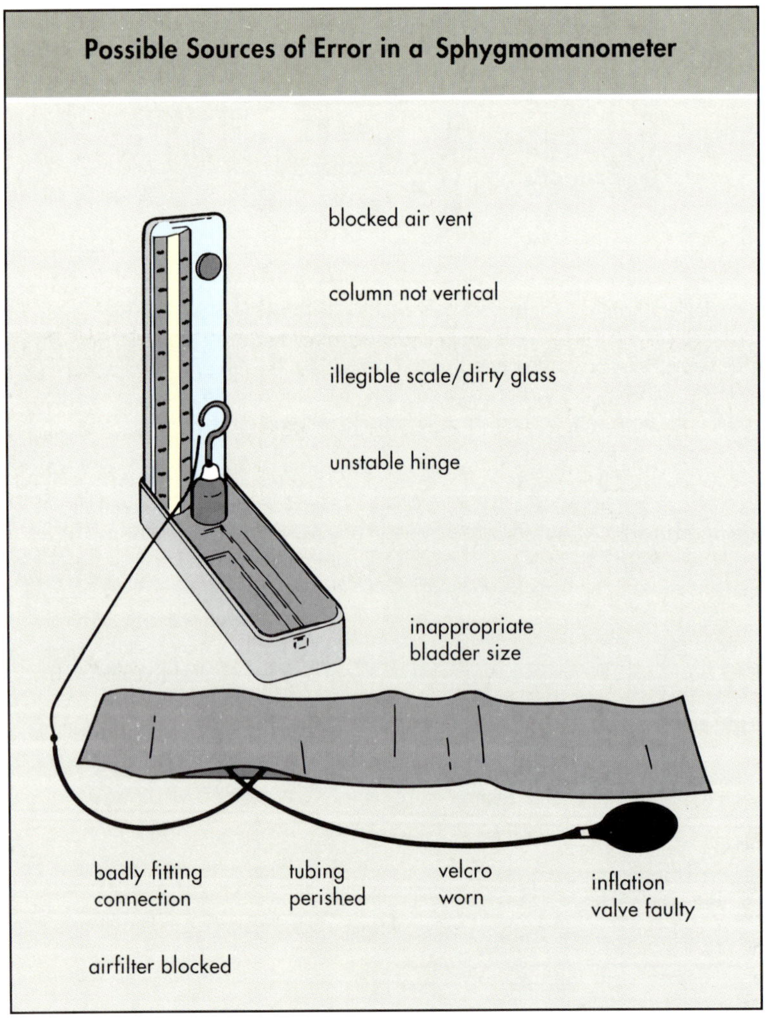

Fig. 1.8 Possible sources of error in a sphygmomanometer.

Subject Variability

Blood pressure shows a regular diurnal variation. Minimal values are observed in the early hours of the morning, during sleep, and maximal values a little later, on getting up. Superimposed upon this regular variability are transient changes in blood pressure provoked by environmental factors, which may substantially affect casual blood pressure measurements observed in the clinic.

The most important factor is the emotional response of the patient to the environment. If he is attending a hospital clinic for the first time, is brought into contact with new faces and is unfamiliar with the measuring procedure, it is likely that a higher blood pressure will be recorded than would be the case if the patient were attending a family doctor who had frequently measured his blood pressure before. Continuous intra-arterial ambulatory monitoring has made evaluation of the pressor response to psychological stress much more precise. This has shown that the appearance of a doctor in a patient's room can have a major pressor effect, creating an artefact known as 'white coat hypertension' (Fig 1.9). In one study, the blood pressure of hypertensive patients was elevated by an average of 27/15mmHg in this way. Furthermore, the extent of the pressor effect varied unpredictably between individual subjects.

As these results make clear, evaluation of a patient using a single blood pressure measurement may lead to an erroneous diagnosis of

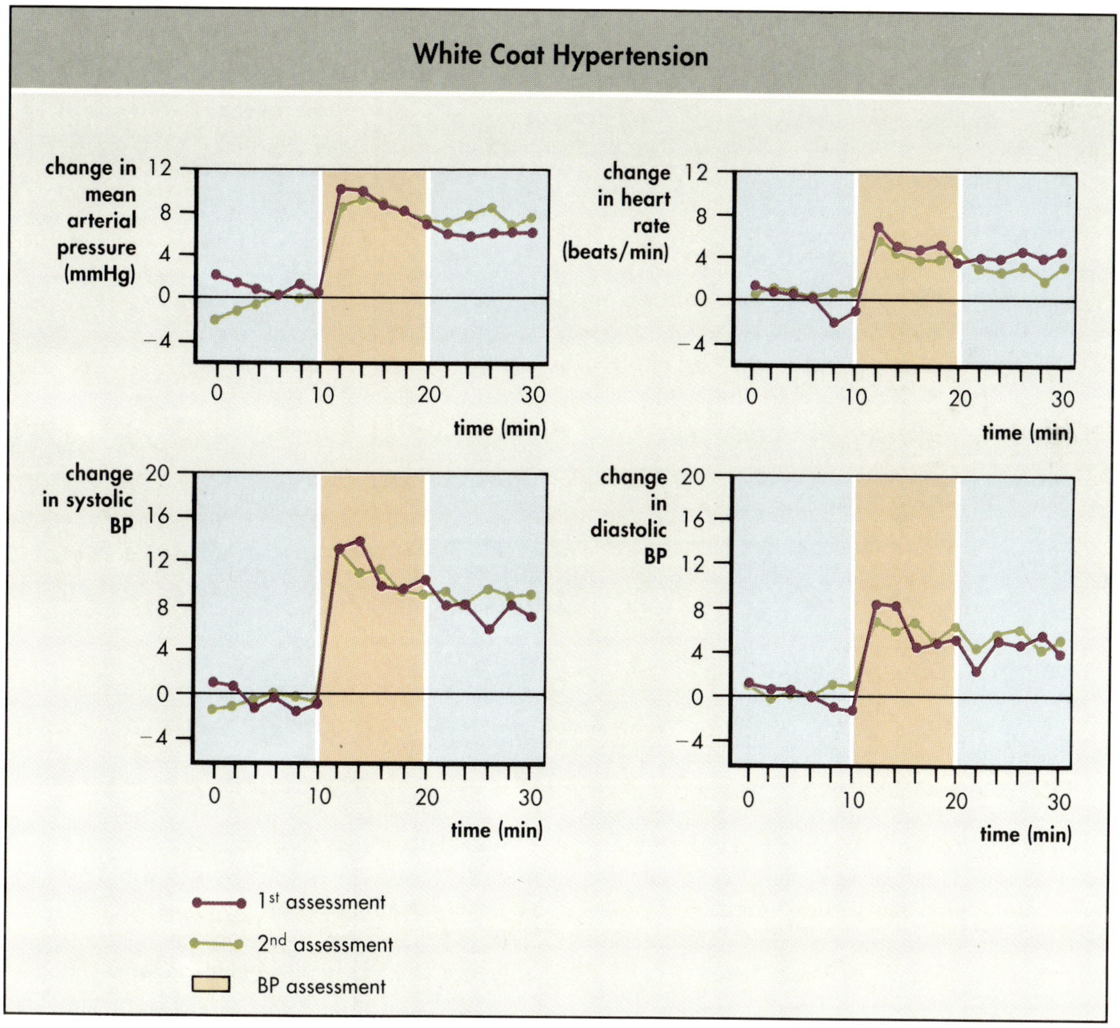

Fig. 1.9 White coat hypertension. In this experiment patients were visited twice by the same doctor. Each visit had the same, unmistakable effect, raising systolic and diastolic blood pressure. [Modified from Mancia *et al.* (1983) *Lancet*, **ii**, 695–698.]

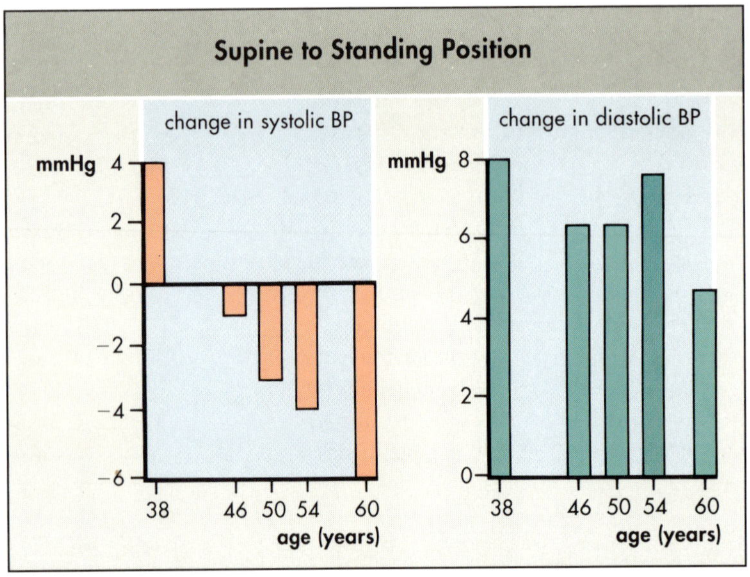

Fig. 1.10 Change in blood pressure produced by moving from the supine to the standing position. Systolic blood pressure falls and diastolic blood pressure rises. The fall in systolic blood pressure is greater in the higher age groups. This is probably due to a reduction in baroreceptor sensitivity (see chapter 2).

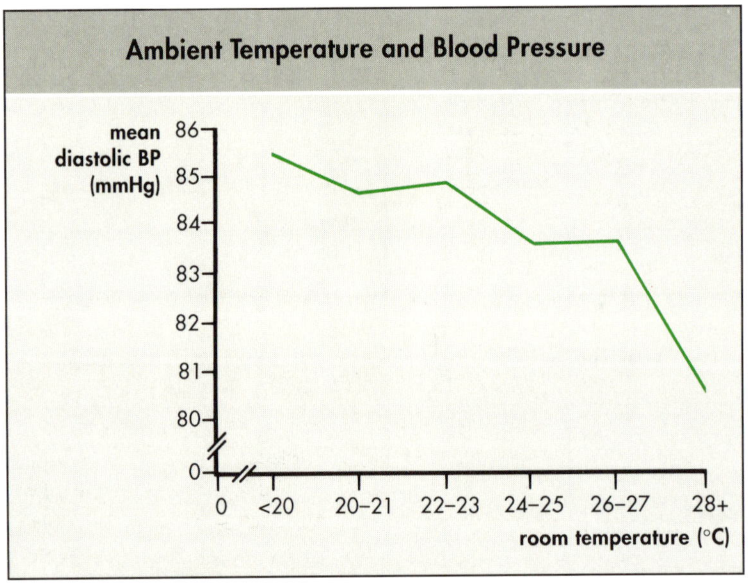

Fig 1.11 Effect of ambient temperature upon diastolic blood pressure. Blood pressures are lower in a warm environment.

hypertension and subsequent, pointless treatment.

Posture and ambient temperature may influence blood pressure (Figs 1.10 & 1.11); measurements taken in a cold room are slightly higher than those taken at room temperature. Differences in ambient temperature probably account for the seasonal variation in blood pressure, the highest levels being recorded during the winter period.

Recent cigarette smoking causes a slight increase in blood pressure as a result of sympathetic nervous system overactivity and catecholamine release, although it is not associated with a sustained elevation.

The effect of exercise is more complex. During exercise systolic blood pressure is elevated; afterwards it falls acutely (Fig. 1.12). Repetitive chronic exercise (training) has a sustained lowering action on blood pressure (see chapter 10).

The fact that so many environmental factors may influence an individual's blood pressure emphasizes both the importance of standardizing the environment as far as possible, and the need for repeated casual measurements before making clinical decisions about patient management.

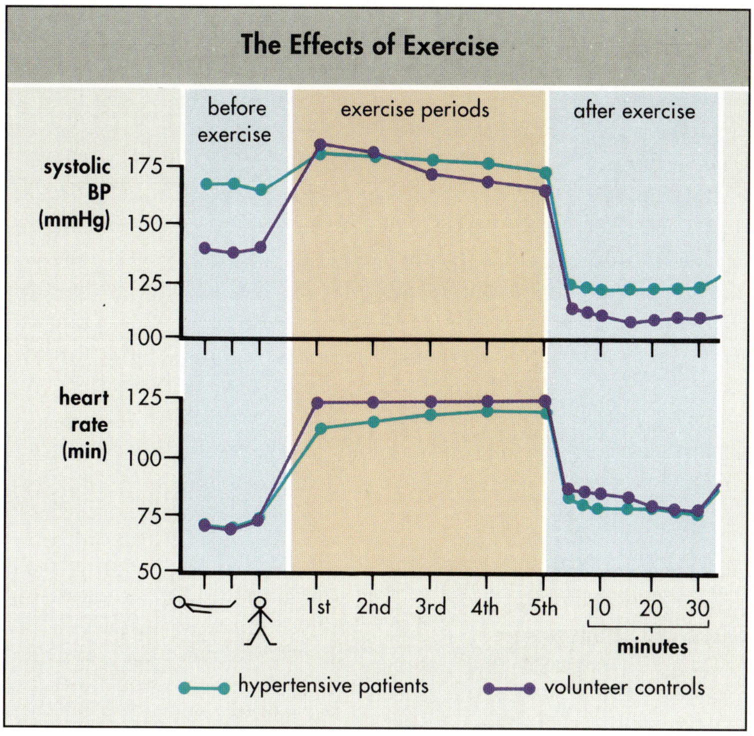

Fig. 1.12 The effects of exercise upon heart rate and systolic blood pressure. Note the sharp fall in systolic pressure immediately after the exercise period. [Modified from Wilcox *et al.* (1982) *BMJ*, **285**, 768.]

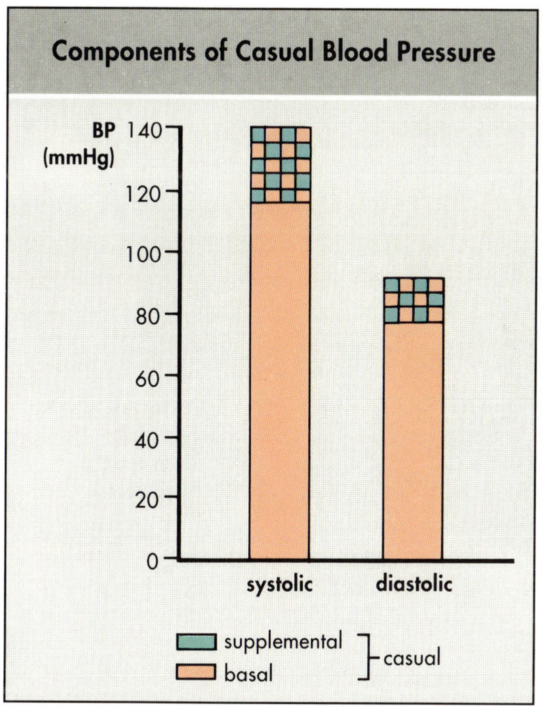

Fig. 1.13 The casual blood pressure can be regarded as having two components. The basal pressure is observed when external stimuli are minimized. Under normal conditions the observed (casual) blood pressure is higher than this, and the difference between the two is referred to as the supplemental pressure.

Basal and Casual Pressures

Smirk and co-workers have identified two components of the casual blood pressure, namely the basal and supplemental pressures (Fig. 1.13). The basal blood pressure is recorded after the effects of external stimuli have been minimized in the following way. Patients sleep overnight in a quiet single room under barbiturate sedation. They are then habituated to the procedure by repeated half minute measurements over a period of ten to fifteen minutes. The values obtained under these circumstances are of course substantially lower than casual blood pressures. The difference between the two is termed supplemental blood pressure. Follow-up of hypertensive subjects indicates that morbidity and mortality are more closely related to basal than to casual blood pressure. However, the routine measurement of basal blood pressure is clearly not feasible, bearing in mind the time required for such an assessment. Although actuarial, epidemiological and clinical trial data are almost entirely based upon casual blood pressure measurements, it seems likely that under carefully standardized basal conditions a better estimate of prognosis would be obtained.

Regression to the Mean

Blood pressure measured in a single hypertensive individual over a period of time shows a tendency to move towards the population mean, despite the absence of any treatment. This is particularly well demonstrated in the placebo treated groups in large clinical trials. This fall in blood pressure represents a habituation to the measuring procedure (Fig 1.14). It is not seen when pressures are measured using continuous intra-arterial ambulatory recording techniques. Regression to the mean could also be the result of a statistical phenomenon. Statistically speaking, a single high observed value is more likely to be an overmeasurement than a genuinely high reading. A blood pressure observed to be high on one occasion, therefore, is more likely to be lower the next time it is measured (Fig. 1.15).

Labile Blood Pressure

Even when precautions are taken to standardize the conditions of blood pressure measurement, the standard deviation of repeated blood pressure measurements taken from the same individual averages 8–10mmHg. Thus, the 95% range is approximately 30–40mmHg. Such blood pressure lability can be expressed in terms of the range of blood pressures over a period of time, as a simple range or as a standard deviation (Fig. 1.16). This is related to blood pressure level and is therefore

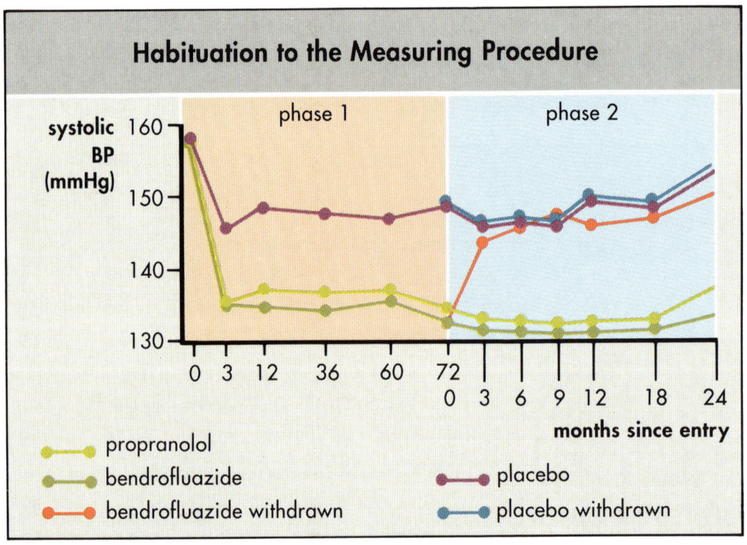

Fig. 1.14 Habituation to the measuring procedure produces a drop in blood pressure, as can be seen here. Note also that where treatment was withdrawn (in phase 2), blood pressure rose to join that of subjects in the placebo group. [Modified from MRC Trial Group (1986) *BMJ*, **293**, 990.]

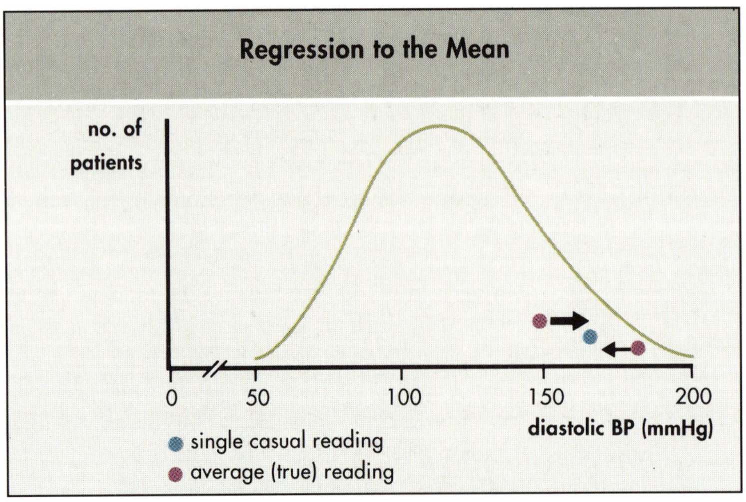

Fig. 1.15 Regression to the mean. A single high blood pressure reading is more likely to be an overestimate of a lower 'true' blood pressure.

greater in hypertension. However, variability can also be expressed as a coefficient of variation (standard deviation of blood pressure divided by the mean); this value is independent of absolute blood pressure. When it is expressed as a coefficient of variation, hypertensive patients (as a group) show no greater variability than normotensive individuals.

It has been suggested that 'labile hypertension' represents an initial phase in the development of later 'fixed hypertension'. There are two reasons why this view is probably incorrect. Firstly, as has been explained above, when variability is expressed as a coefficient of variation it shows no increase in the early stages of hypertension. Secondly, 'labile hypertension' may be an artefact. It is usually defined as a series of blood pressures which lie either above or below an arbitrarily defined level (for example 160/95mmHg) on successive occasions. According to this criterion, although labile hypertensives may sometimes have a 'normal' blood pressure, they will inevitably tend to have higher blood pressures than normotensive controls (Fig 1.17). They are therefore more likely to develop 'true' hypertension. There is no doubt that certain patients, such as those with phaeochromocytoma or impaired baroreceptor function, have excessively variable blood pressure. However, there is little justification for identifying a subset of essential hypertensives as suffering from 'labile hypertension'.

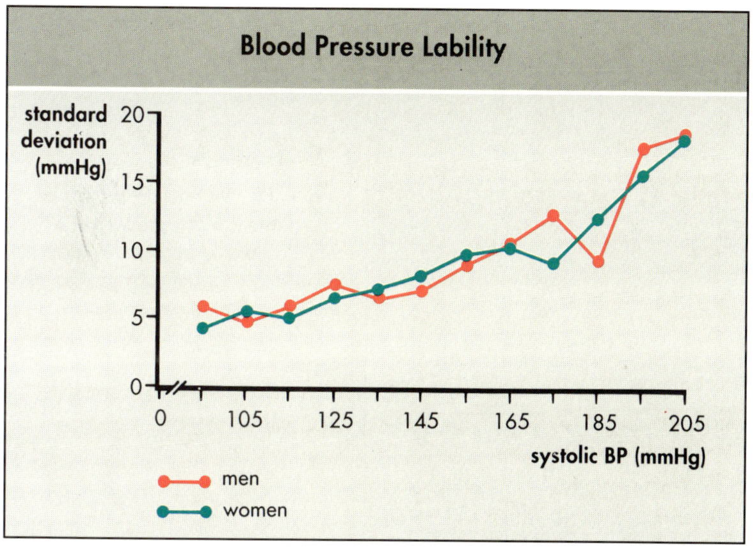

Fig. 1.16 Increasing lability of systolic blood pressure, expressed in terms of the average standard deviation: Framingham Study. [Modified from Kannel (1980) Epidemiology of Arterial Blood Pressure. The Hague: Martinus Nijhoff.]

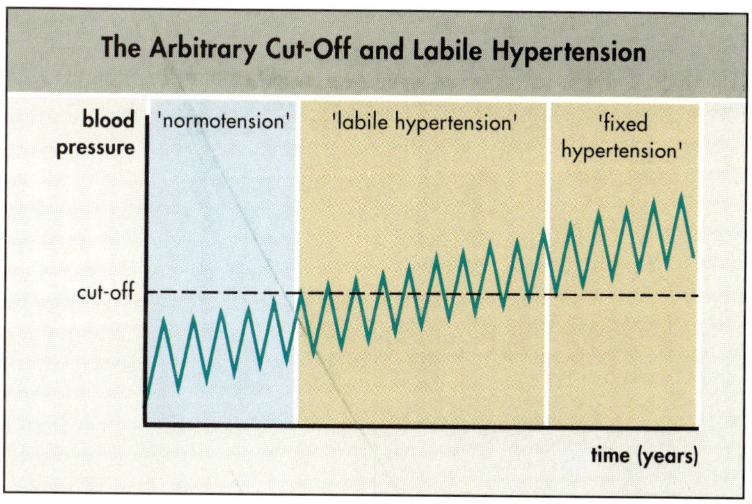

Fig. 1.17 The blood pressure of this hypothetical individual shows a long term rise with short term fluctuations. The use of an arbitrary cut-off here leads to the creation of an artefactual, labile hypertension.

NORMAL BLOOD PRESSURE AND HYPERTENSION

Blood pressure in the general population has a smooth unimodal distribution which is skewed to the right, particularly for systolic blood pressure (Fig. 1.18). Thus there is no natural dividing line between hypertensive and normotensive subjects. The suggestion that distribution curves conceal a group of subjects with the distinct disorder of essential hypertension was the subject of a vigorous debate between Platt and Pickering in the 1950s and 1960s. Platt described separate higher peaks of blood pressure giving rise to a bimodal (or perhaps trimodal) distribution. It is now clear that this appearance was an artefact attributable to a relatively small sample size and observer bias in favour of blood pressures ending in 0 or 5mmHg. Nonetheless, it is now generally accepted that the distribution curves do include subsets of individuals genetically predisposed to hypertension. A bimodal distribution is not observed because blood pressure is multifactorial, influenced by a number of factors both genetic and environmental. It is the summation and possible interaction of these factors which gives rise to an individual's blood pressure on any particular occasion. The effect of this multiplicity of factors is to 'iron out' multimodality of blood pressure, so that relatively smooth distribution curves are found if the sample size is adequate. It is important to bear in mind that analyses of blood pressure distribution curves in developed nations are based upon data that were compiled before widespread treatment of hypertension was implemented. Therapeutic lowering of blood pressure in the higher blood pressure groups will of course influence the shape of distribution curves.

Since there is no natural dividing line between high and normal blood pressures, any attempt to define hypertension is necessarily arbitrary. The most widely used criterion is that set by the World

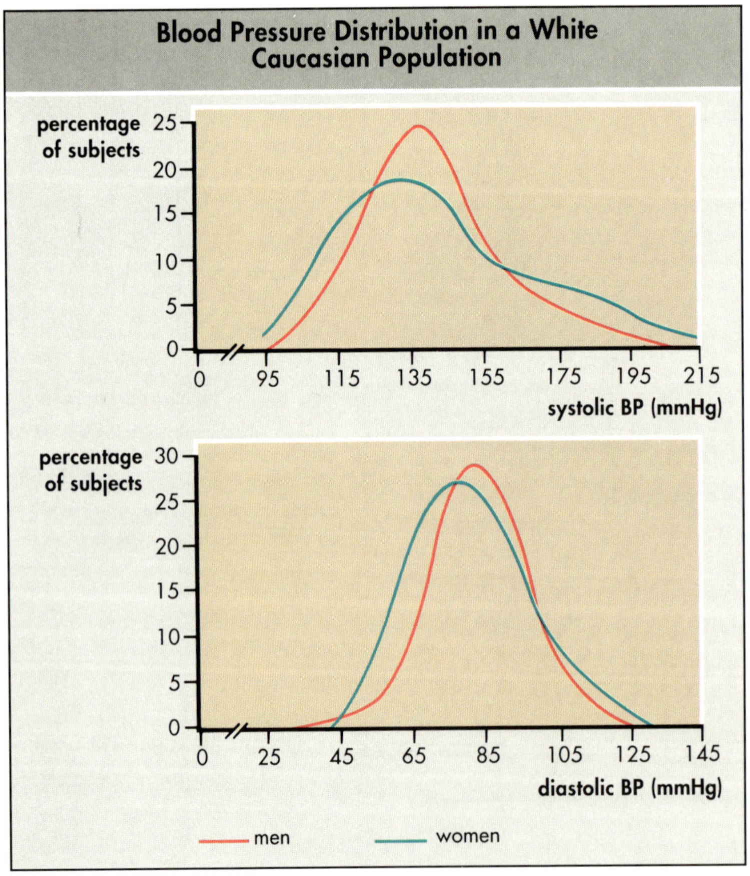

Fig 1.18 Distribution of systolic and diastolic blood pressure in a white caucasian population. There is no evidence for bimodality, although there is a slight skew to the right which is more marked with systolic pressure.

Health Organization, whereby an individual with a blood pressure of 160/95mmHg or above (Korotkoff phase V) is regarded as being hypertensive. Such cut-off points can assume medico–legal importance when used as diagnostic criteria for hypertension or as a threshold for treatment. The trend towards treatment of lower levels of blood pressure probably makes a diastolic pressure of 90mmHg a more reasonable empirical figure. Although the cut-off point selected is simply a matter of convenience, having no particular biological significance, it has a massive effect upon the apparent prevalence of hypertension (Fig. 1.19). It is important to remember that figures for the prevalence of hypertension are meaningless unless the criteria for hypertension and the conditions of measurement are stated.

The exclusion of patients with secondary hypertension in large-scale surveys is well-nigh impossible to achieve. In fact this has no significant effect upon blood pressure distribution, since the numbers are so small in relation to primary (essential) hypertension.

THE RISKS OF HYPERTENSION

Our knowledge of the effect of elevated blood pressure upon prognosis is based upon two types of evidence. Life insurance statistics have provided data upon life expectancy in large populations, and longitudinal investigations (such as the Framingham Study, see below) have supplied data not only upon mortality but also upon the incidence of specific diseases. The numbers recruited in longitudinal studies are of course very much smaller than those included in life insurance data and so, although the breadth of information is much greater, the power to detect weak relationships is much lower.

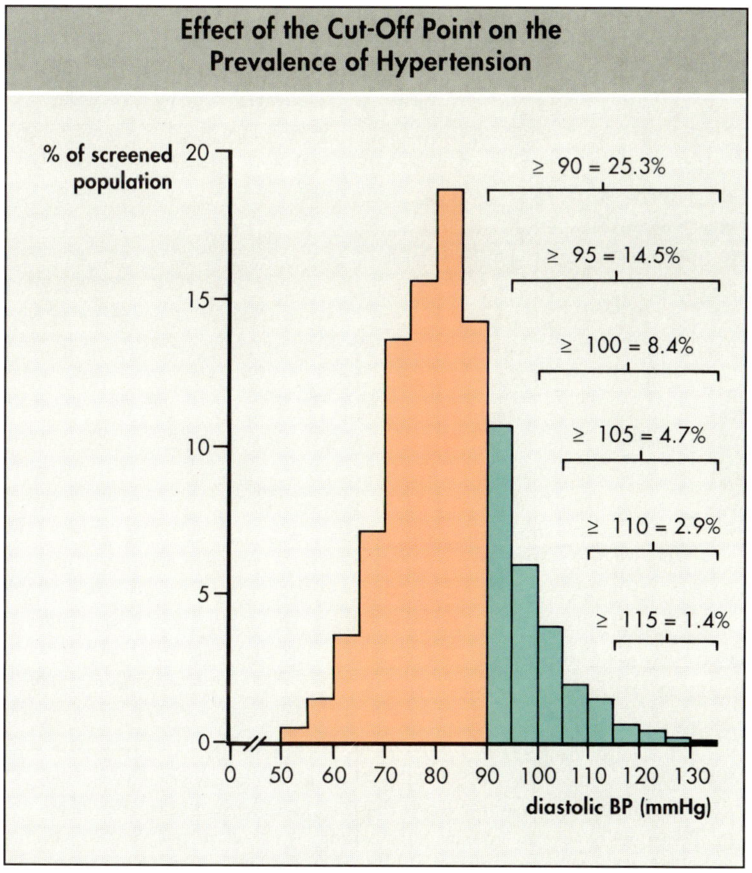

Fig. 1.19 Frequency distribution of diastolic blood pressures, and the effect of the cut-off point on the prevalence of hypertension. [Modified from HDFP-Cooperative (1977) *Circ Res*, **40**, I-106–I-109.]

The actuarial data indicate that life expectancy falls progressively with increasing blood pressure (Fig. 1.20). Furthermore, the risks of hypertension apply equally to systolic and diastolic pressures so that for any given systolic pressure life expectancy diminishes as diastolic pressure increases, and vice versa (Fig. 1.21). Just as there is no discrete dividing line between hypertensive and normotensive blood pressures, so there is no dividing line between those blood pressures which are harmful and those which are not. Lower than average pressures are associated with better than average life expectancy (Fig. 1.22). Hypertension cannot therefore be defined by simply considering subjects at risk either of dying or developing cardiovascular disease as a result of high blood pressure.

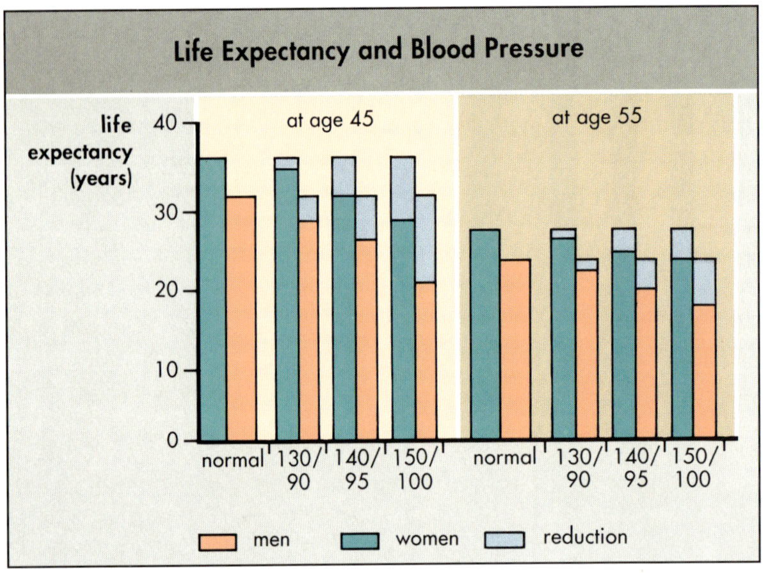

Fig. 1.20 Reduction in life expectancy produced by mild blood pressure elevation.

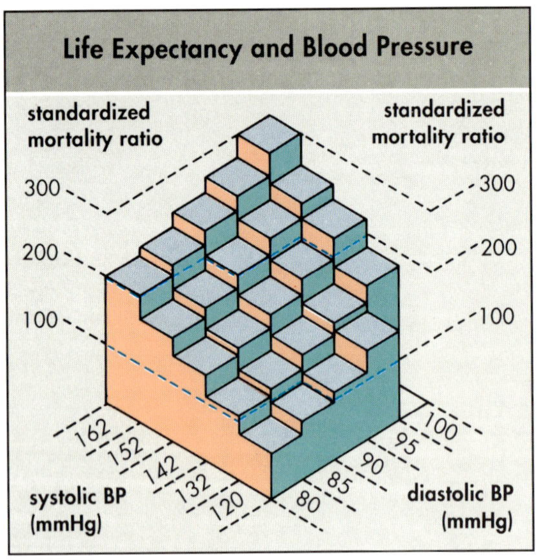

Fig. 1.21 Standardised mortality ratios in a healthy population. An increase in risk is observed with an elevation of both systolic and diastolic blood pressures independently. Risk increases progressively with increasing blood pressure with no evidence for a threshold. [Modified from The Society of Actuaries (1959) *Build and Blood Pressure Study*, **1**. Chicago: Society of Actuaries.]

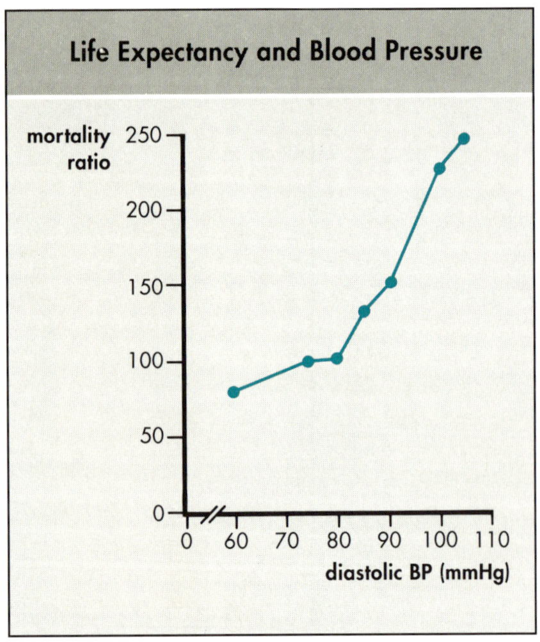

Fig. 1.22 Mortality ratio as a function of diastolic blood pressure. Lower diastolic blood pressures are associated with a better than average life expectancy. (For source see Fig. 1.21.)

Hypertensive Morbidity

The risks associated with hypertension are due to cerebrovascular, cardiovascular, peripheral vascular and renal disease (Fig. 1.23). Just as with overall mortality, specific morbidity and mortality from these different causes is associated equally with either systolic or diastolic blood pressure. The most valuable study to date of the specific consequences of hypertension has been the long term prospective survey carried out in the town of Framingham in Massachusetts on a sample of over 5,000 individuals. This was originally set up in 1949 with the objective of identifying factorr related to the development of cardiovascular disease and stroke and used a random sample of men and women aged between 30 and 62. In this study, the findings on the cerebrovascular and cardiovascular risks of hypertension proved to be unequivocal. In both men and women blood pressure was the most reliable factor for predicting a subsequent stroke (atherothrombotic brain infarction). Hypertension (defined as a blood pressure of 160/95mmHg or above) was associated with a 5 to 30-fold increase in the risk of stroke, depending upon the subject's age and sex (Fig. 1.24).

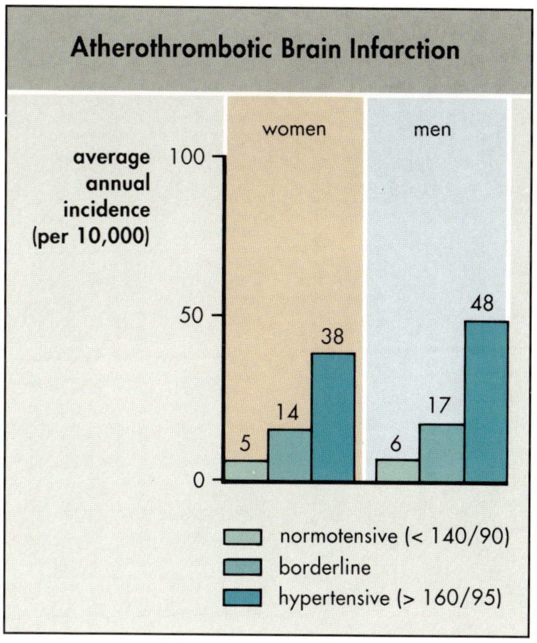

Fig. 1.24 Risk of atherothrombotic brain infarction according to hypertensive status. Follow-up to the Framingham study. [Modified from Kannel & Sorlie (1975) *Epidemiology and Control of Hypertension*. New York: Stratton.]

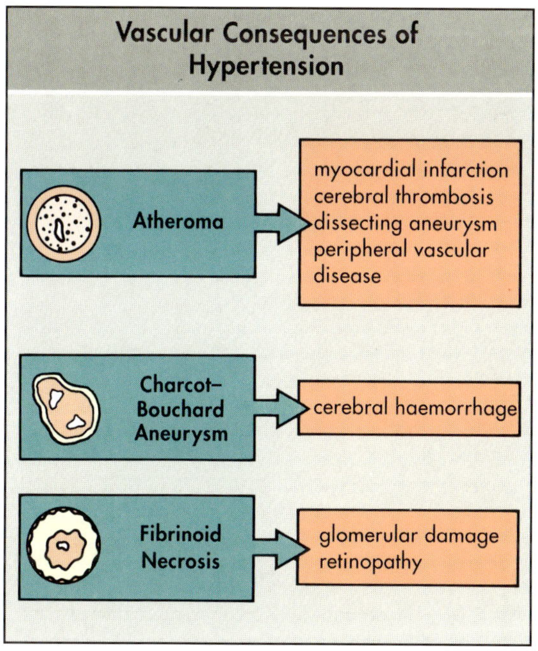

Fig. 1.23 The major vascular consequences of hypertension producing clinical sequelae are atheroma, Charcot–Bouchard aneurysms and fibrinoid necroses.

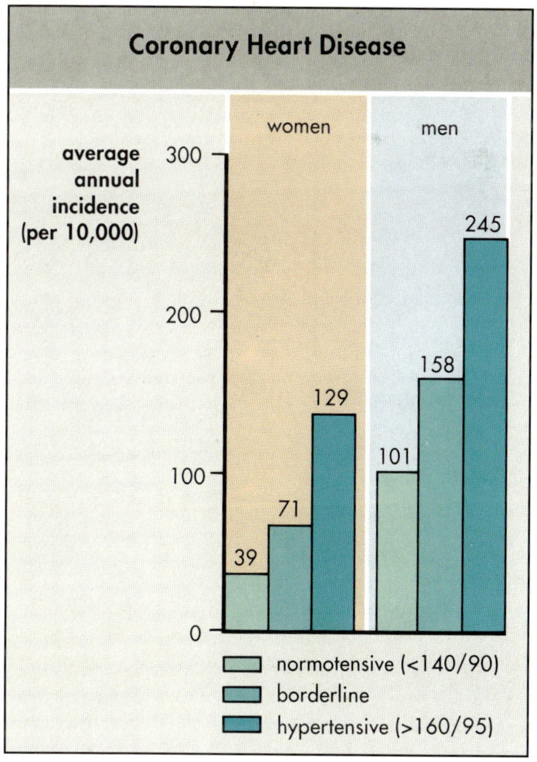

Fig. 1.25 Risk of coronary heart disease according to hypertensive status. (For source see Fig. 1.24.)

The Framingham Study also demonstrated that hypertension was a risk factor for coronary artery disease, congestive cardiac failure, intermittent claudication and various other forms of cardiovascular morbidity (Figs 1.25, 1.26 & 1.27). The relationship between blood pressure and ischaemic heart disease was weaker than the relationship between blood pressure and stroke. In summary, hypertensive patients were seven times as likely to develop a stroke, four times as likely to develop congestive heart failure, three times as likely to develop coronary heart disease and twice as likely to develop peripheral arterial disease as normotensive individuals. The risk of developing major cardiovascular disease increased by approximately 30% for each 10mmHg rise in blood pressure in men and women of all ages. The Framingham study also confirmed the importance of systolic blood pressure as an independent risk factor (Figs 1.28 & 1.29).

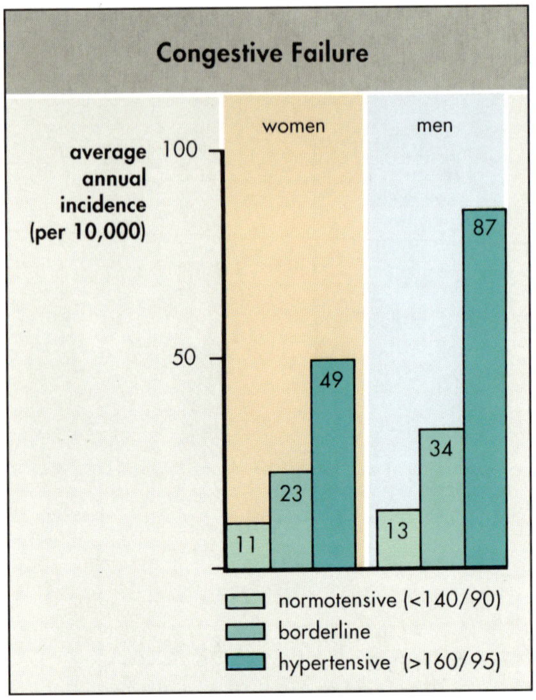

Fig. 1.26 Risk of congestive failure according to hypertensive status. (For source see Fig. 1.24.)

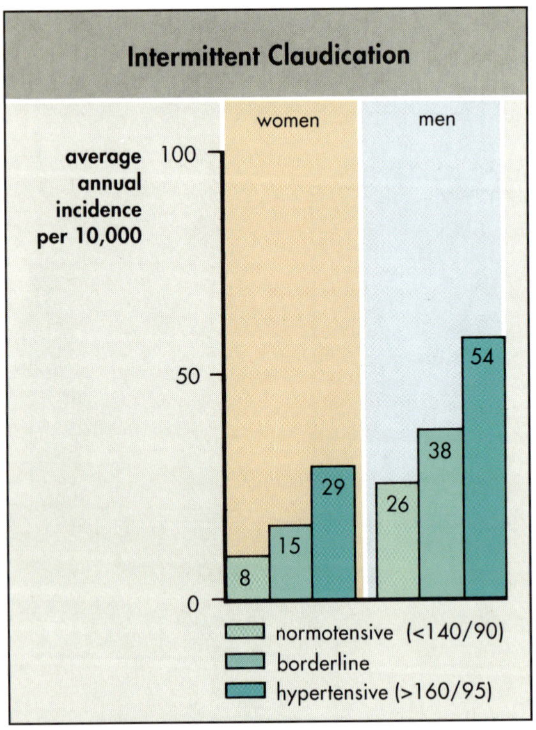

Fig. 1.27 Risk of intermittent claudication according to hypertensive status. (For source see Fig. 1.24.)

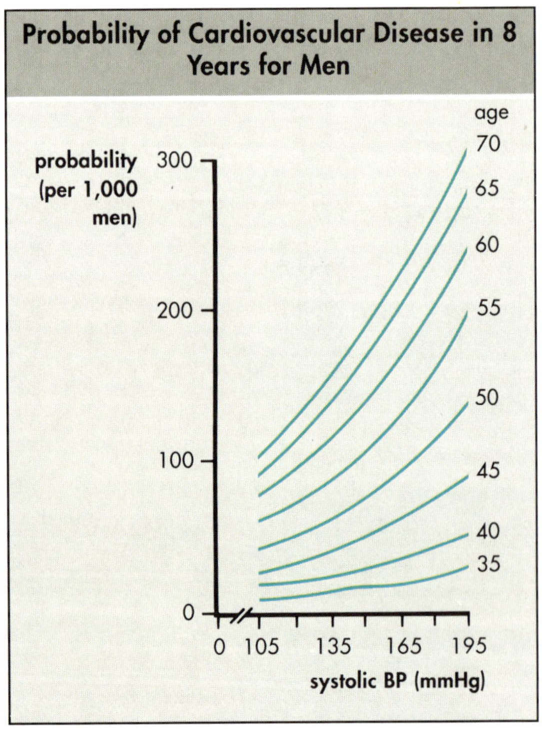

Fig. 1.28 The probability of cardiovascular disease increases with increasing systolic blood pressure. This relationship is most marked in the older age groups. [Modified from Kannel (1975) *Hypertension – In Nature and Treatment*. Horsham, England: CIBA.]

The reasons for the difference in the risk carried by a hypertensive individual for a stroke or a heart attack is unknown. It may in part be related to differences in the pathology of the underlying condition; blood pressure may be more closely related to cerebral haemorrhage than to atheromatous complications. Perhaps related to this explanation is the fact that other risk factors (such as smoking and hypercholesterolaemia) are much more closely related to coronary heart disease than to stroke. It may be of relevance that although the risk of stroke is substantially reduced by antihypertensive (drug) treatment, such an approach has little effect upon the risk of myocardial infarction (see Figs 1.30 & 1.31 & chapter 10).

Renal failure is now a much less common cause of death in hypertension. For this reason there is no adequate epidemiological information on the association between blood pressure and renal failure. It seems likely however that the incidence of

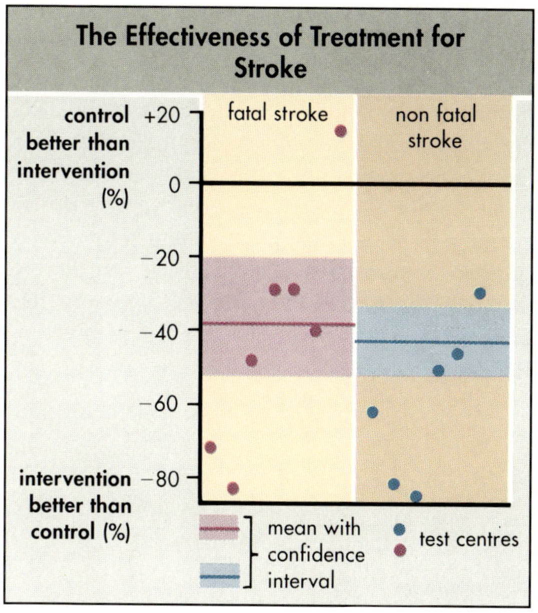

Fig. 1.30 Estimates of the relative difference in fatal and non-fatal stroke between study (intervention) and control groups, showing drug intervention to be an effective strategy. [Modified from MacMahon *et al.*, *Prog Cardiovasc Dis*, **29**, Suppl: 99–118.]

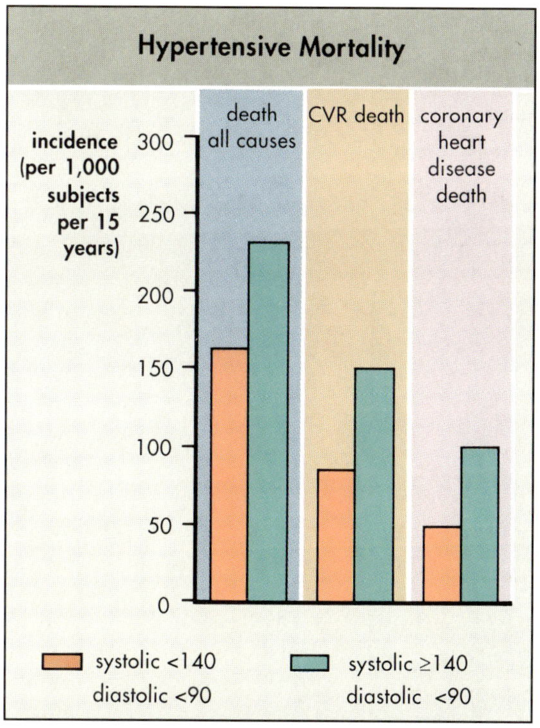

Fig. 1.29 Deaths from both cardiovascular–renal causes (CVR) and coronary heart disease are greater in patients with an elevated systolic level, even when diastolic pressure levels are normal. [Modified from Stamler *et al.* (1975) *J Chronic Dis*, **28**, 527–548.]

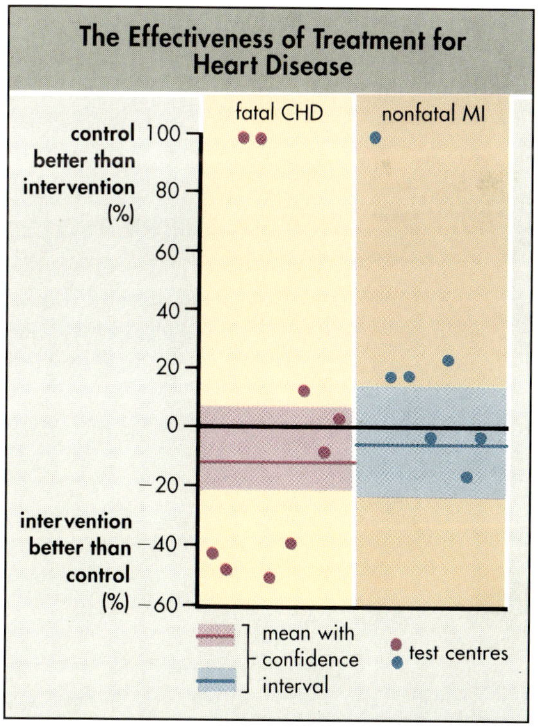

Fig. 1.31 Estimates of the relative diference in fatal CHD and non-fatal MI between study (intervention) and control groups. Drug intervention is less effective here than it is against stroke. (For source see Fig. 1.30.)

renal failure in hypertension has declined with the development of effective antihypertensive therapy. When blood pressure has been controlled for a period of time the risk of developing clinically significant renal failure falls dramatically. As a result, the majority of patients who now die of renal failure secondary to hypertension do so within a short period of presentation, before blood pressure control has allowed renal function to improve (Fig. 1.32). Where blood pressure has been controlled for some time, the risk of developing renal failure is dramatically reduced. In the majority of cases where renal failure and hypertension are associated, renal disease is the cause of hypertension rather than a manifestation of it. Since atheroma of the main renal arteries, which leads to renal failure, may be improved by surgery or balloon angioplasty, the possibility of renovascular disease should always be considered in patients with hypertension and renal failure.

In North America, Western Europe, Australia and Japan, mortality due to stroke has fallen steadily since around 1960 (Fig. 1.33). This decline accelerated in the early 1970s (over the same peri-

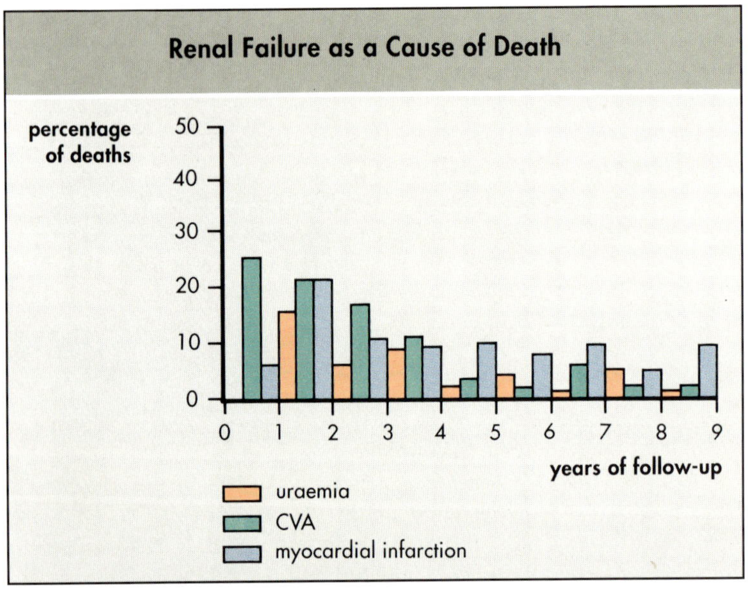

Fig. 1.32 Most deaths from renal failure in patients with essential hypertension attending a hypertension clinic occur within one year of presentation. With prolonged control of blood pressure, renal failure becomes much less important as a cause of death. [Modified from Breckenridge *et al.* (1970) *Q J Med*, **1**, 411–429.]

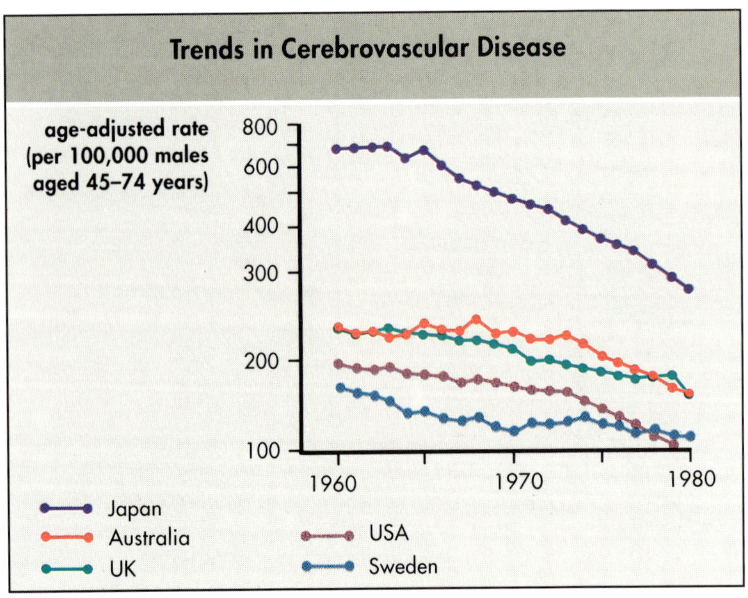

Fig. 1.33 Trends in cerebrovascular disease, 1959–1981, showing a general decline in mortality in five developed nations. (Modified from WHO data.)

od, mortality due to stroke in Eastern Europe substantially increased). The explanation for this downturn in stroke mortality is uncertain. The initial decline is unlikely to have been due to detection and treatment of hypertension, since such treatment was not widely practised at that time. It does however seem probable that effective blood pressure control techniques have been at least partly responsible for the more recently observed decline in stroke mortality. Evidence from Japan suggests that the decline is in cerebral haemorrhage rather than cerebral infarction (Fig. 1.34). These trends are only detectable when age-specific rates are analysed, that is when statistics are corrected for the steadily increasing proportion of elderly people in the population (Fig. 1.35). In the UK, for instance, the overall number of stroke deaths increased until 1970, due to population growth and ageing. Since 1970 the absolute number of deaths has fallen by about 1% each year; the age-adjusted value of course exceeds this figure. An accelerating decline in death from cardiovascular disease (myocardial infarction and stroke) has been well documented in the USA (Fig. 1.36).

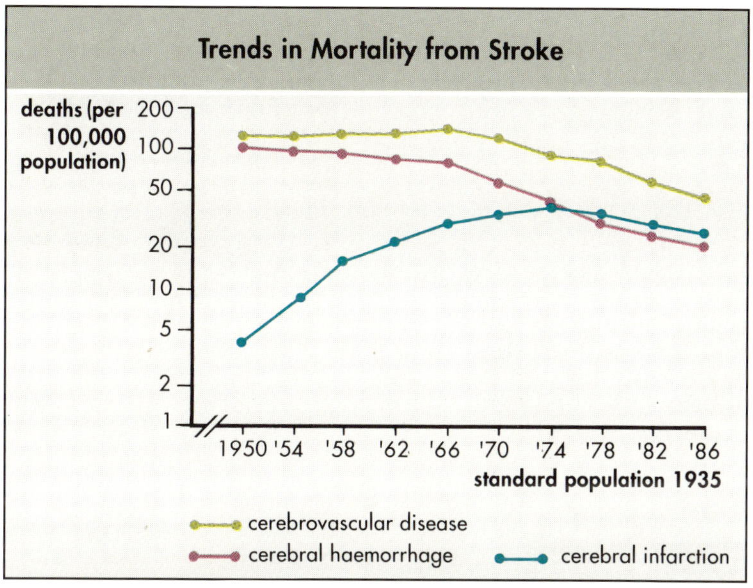

Fig. 1.34 In Japan, there has been a general decline in male mortality from intracerebral haemorrhage and stroke, while cerebral infarction has increased. [Modified from Omae & Ueda (1988) *J Hypertension*, **6**, 343–349.]

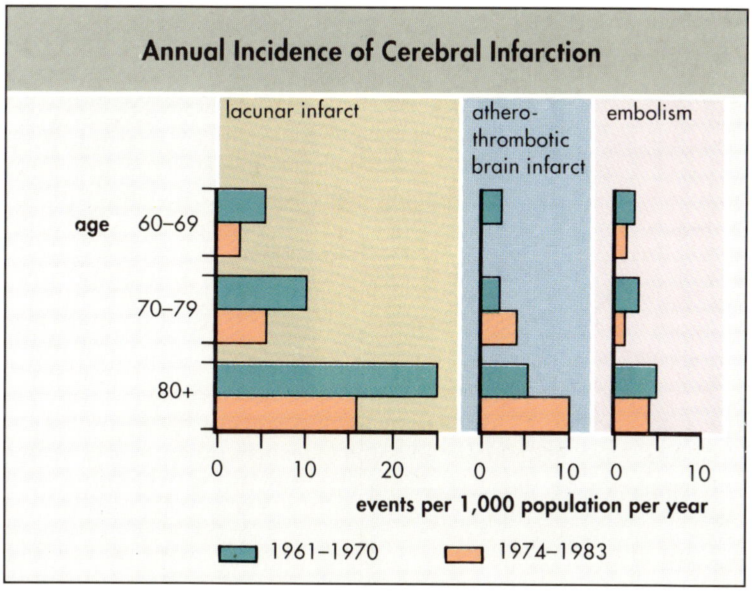

Fig. 1.35 Age-adjusted comparison of cerebral infarction (by type) in the Japanese. (For source see Fig. 1.34.)

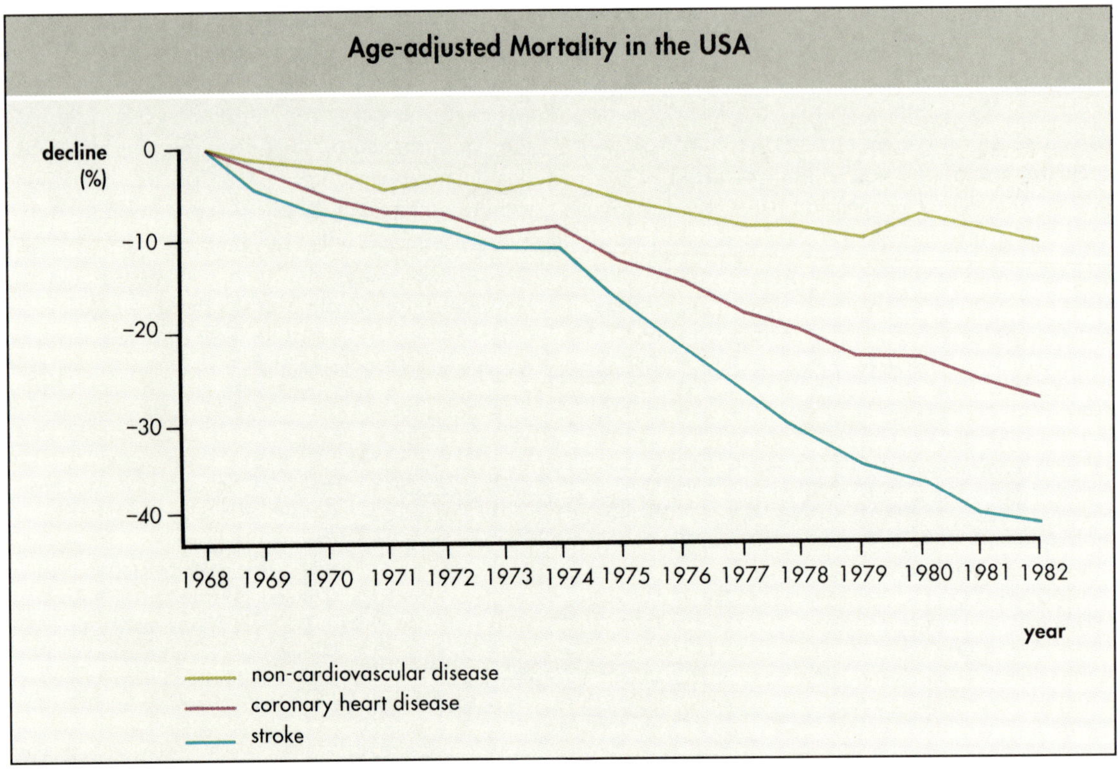

Fig. 1.36 Mortality due to stroke and to coronary heart disease declined in the USA between 1968 and 1982. [Modified from Moser & Gifford (1985) *J Hypertension*, **3**, 445.]

Here too, better control of blood pressure may be a contributory factor. A similar trend has been seen in the UK over the past decade.

Other Risk Factors and Hypertension

The Framingham Study also examined the importance of other risk factors. The results clearly indicated that these were additive in their effect. The degree of risk at any one blood pressure level varied according to the presence or absence of other known risk factors, such as hyperlipidaemia, glucose intolerance, cigarette smoking or the presence of left ventricular hypertrophy on the ECG (the latter is now emerging as a particularly strong predictor of subsequent mortality quite independently of its association with hypertension). The highest risk is therefore borne by individuals who carry all these risk factors in addition to hypertension. Defining high and low-risk hypertensive patients in this way can demonstrate a dramatic effect upon outlook (Fig. 1.37). In the Medical Research Council (MRC) Study of treatment of mild hypertension it was calculated that high risk patients were sixty times more likely to suffer a stroke than were low-risk patients. The difference in incidence of cardiovascular disease in smokers as opposed to non-smokers exceeded the reduction in cardiovascular disease produced by treatment (Fig 1.38). This further underlines the importance of examining other risk factors in the hypertensive patient.

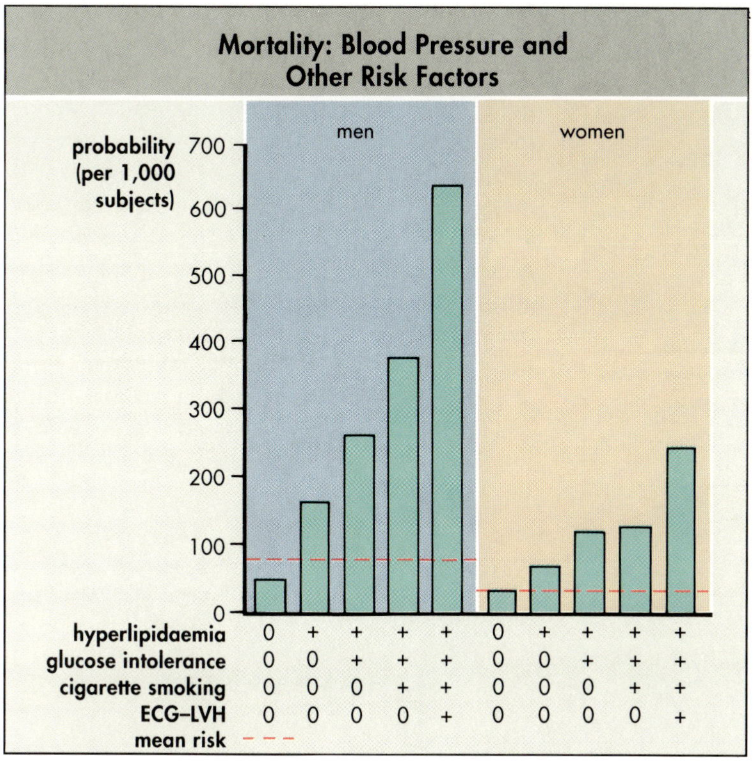

Fig. 1.37 An increased risk of cardiovascular disease is conferred by factors other than blood pressure. An additive effect can be seen here. [Modified from Kannel & Kreger (1981) in *Blood Pressure Measurement and Systemic Hypertension*. Edited by Arntzenius *et al.* Medical World Publishing.]

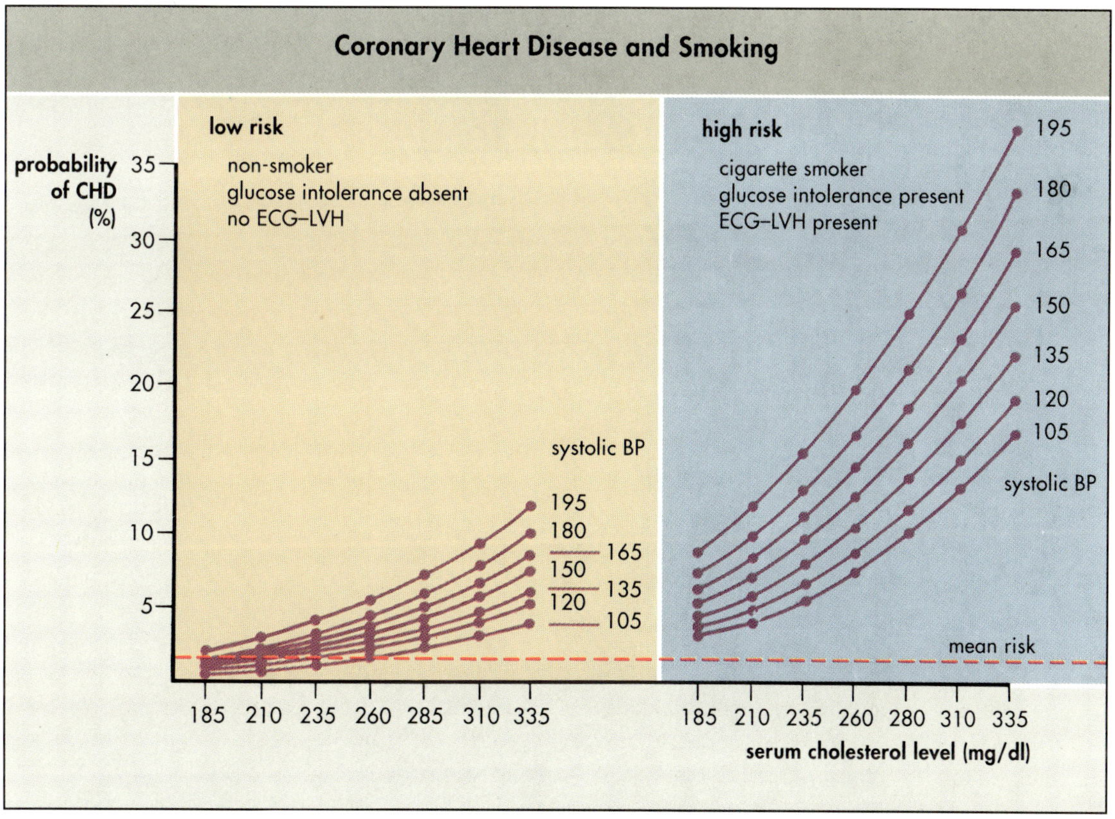

Fig. 1.38 The risk of developing coronary heart disease is significantly greater in smokers. (For source see Fig. 1.37.)

Individual and Population Risks

Strokes do occur in normotensive as well as in hypertensive individuals. We can therefore divide the risk to which a hypertensive patient is exposed into two components (Fig. 1.39). Firstly, there is the excess risk which is borne in comparison with a normotensive individual. This component is generally referred to as the hypertension attributable risk. The remaining risk is explained by other genetic and environmental factors, known and unknown. From the individual's point of view the important feature is the total (absolute) risk to which he or she is exposed (Fig. 1.40). Risk can, however, also be expressed as a relative risk

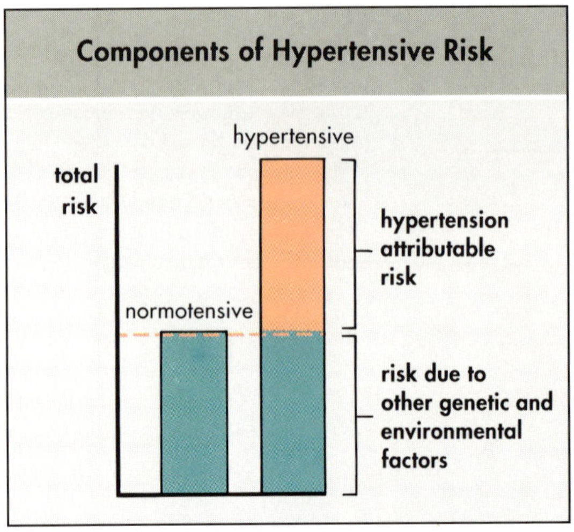

Fig. 1.39 The two components of hypertensive risk.

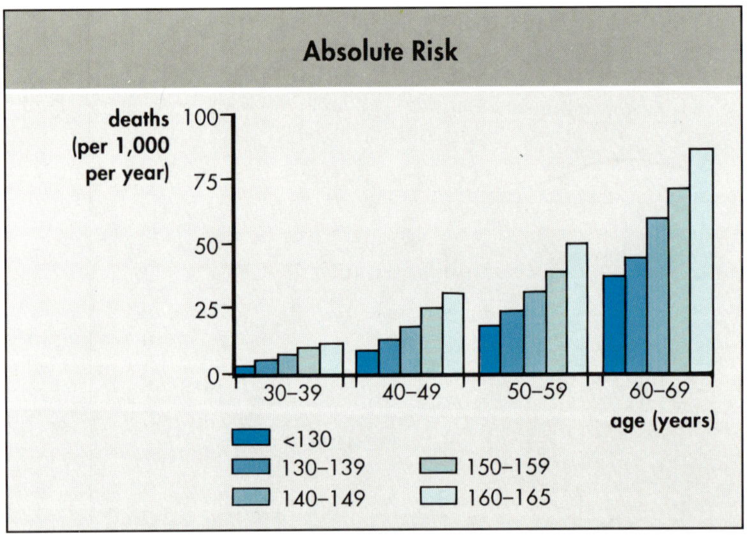

Fig. 1.40 The absolute risk of death due to hypertension. [Modified from Rose (1980) in *The Hypertensive Patient.* Edited by Marshall & Barritt. London: Pitman Medical.)

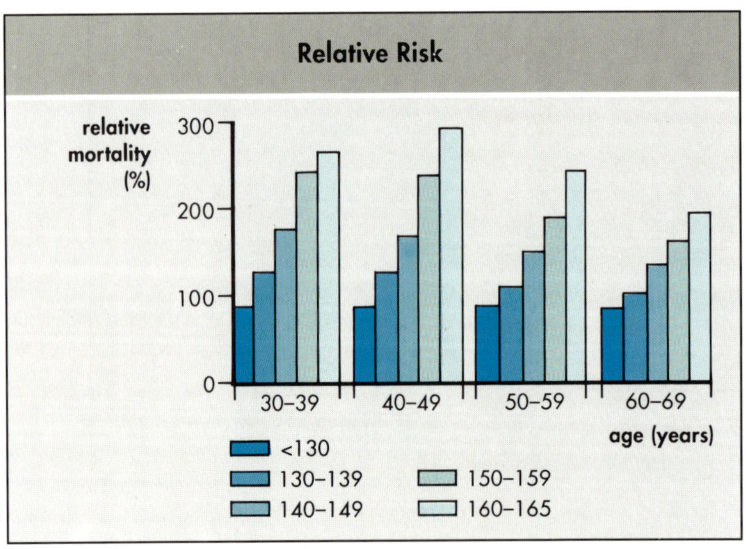

Fig. 1.41 The same data displayed in Fig. 1.40, expressed as relative risk.

(Fig. 1.41). Thus, a hypertensive individual may be twice as likely to suffer a stroke within a year compared to other individuals in the population. Reducing this risk, for example from one in 5,000 to one in 10,000, may be unimportant from an individual patient's point of view. However, since stroke is a common condition, halving the number of cases may be extremely important for the population as a whole. It is possible to calculate from the Framingham data how many strokes would be predicted if the entire population risk were reduced to that of the lowest blood pressure class. Under these circumstances the number of strokes would be roughly 40% of the present total. Thus, in this particular population, the hypertension attributable risk is about 60%. The bell-shaped nature of the blood pressure distribution curve means that milder degrees of hypertension are much more prevalent than severe hypertension, which is in fact a comparative rarity. It therefore follows that a very large number of people are exposed to a small absolute risk, and a very small number of people are exposed to a high absolute risk (Fig 1.42). It is possible to calculate the number of strokes which can be attributed to any particular blood pressure level in a population by multiplying the prevalence of that degree of hypertension by the risk attributable to it. When this is done it becomes clear that it is mild hypertension that gives rise to the majority of hypertension-attributable strokes; the less common, moderate or severe (higher risk) hypertension causes only a minority of the total number of strokes. It has been calculated that more than 60% of the cardiovascular complications attributable to elevated diastolic blood pressure result from exposure to sustained diastolic blood pressures below 95mmHg and 45% of such complications occur at diastolic blood pressures below 90mmHg (Fig. 1.43). The pattern is essentially similar with systolic hypertension, with more than 50% of complications occurring below the WHO cut-off of 160mmHg.

Population and Absolute Risk

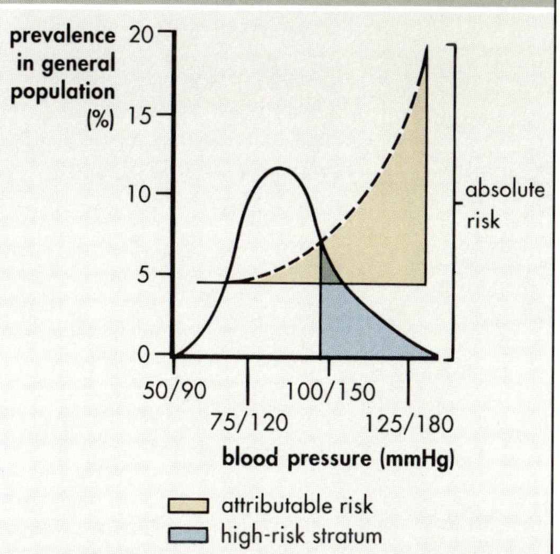

Fig. 1.42 When the curves for risk and for blood pressure distribution are superimposed, it can be seen that the number of people exposed to a high absolute risk is relatively small. [Modified from Whelton (1984) *J Hypertension*, **2**, 6.]

Blood Pressure and Mortality in the USA

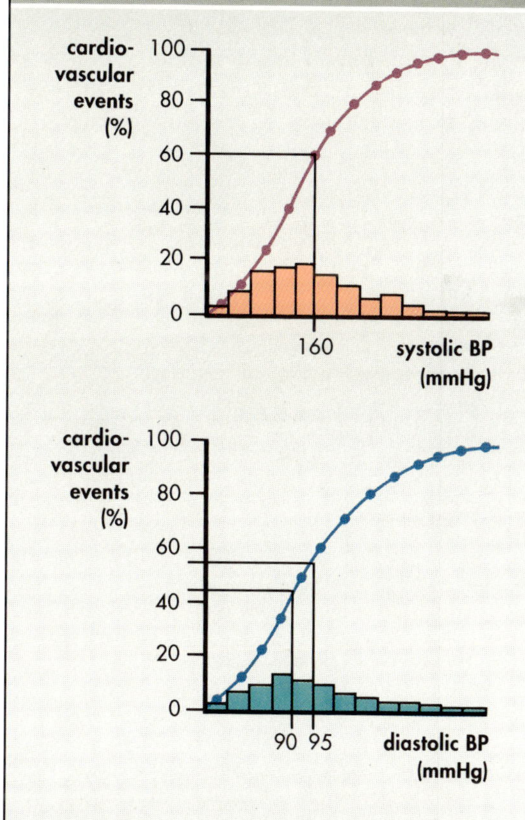

Fig. 1.43 An analysis of the number of events attributable to blood pressure in the USA. More than 60% of cardiovascular disease attributable to blood pressure occurs below the WHO cut-off point of 160mmHg systolic or 95mmHg diastolic. (For source see Fig. 1.42.)

There are consequently two strategies for the treatment of hypertension. A high-risk treatment strategy selects those patients with severe hypertension. This is extremely important for the individual patient and will have a degree of impact upon the incidence of stroke, but not as great as might be expected from a strategy directed at the whole population. The MRC trial estimated that about two-thirds of all strokes in middle-aged, mild hypertensives are preventable by pharmacological control of blood pressure. If one extrapolates these findings to the general population, effective treatment of diastolic pressures of 95mmHg or above (mean of three readings or more) may reduce the total burden of strokes by 40% at the very most. Bearing in mind the difficulties of universal detection and effective treatment, the realistic effects of pursuing a high risk treatment strategy must be considerably lower than this.

It is clearly not feasible to recommend drug treatment for all low risk individuals whose blood pressure nevertheless lies above the population mean. For this reason the identification of potentially reversible, hypertension-associated environmental factors has assumed great importance.

DETERMINANTS OF BLOOD PRESSURE

When blood pressure is measured in unselected populations it is found to be associated with certain defined factors. The best recognised are:

- age and sex;
- heredity;
- race;
- body mass;
- alcohol consumption.

Other factors such as diet and stress are more controversial and will be discussed in chapter 3.

Age and Sex

Blood pressure rises both in childhood (see chapter 6) and in adult life in Western populations (Fig. 1.44). Systolic pressure in females rises throughout adult life at a uniform rate which is slightly higher than that in males. As a consequence of this, female systolic pressure, initially the lower of the two, overtakes that of males at about the age of 50. The rise in diastolic blood pressure is more gradual in both males and females. After the age of 60, diastolic blood pressure in both sexes tends to fall;

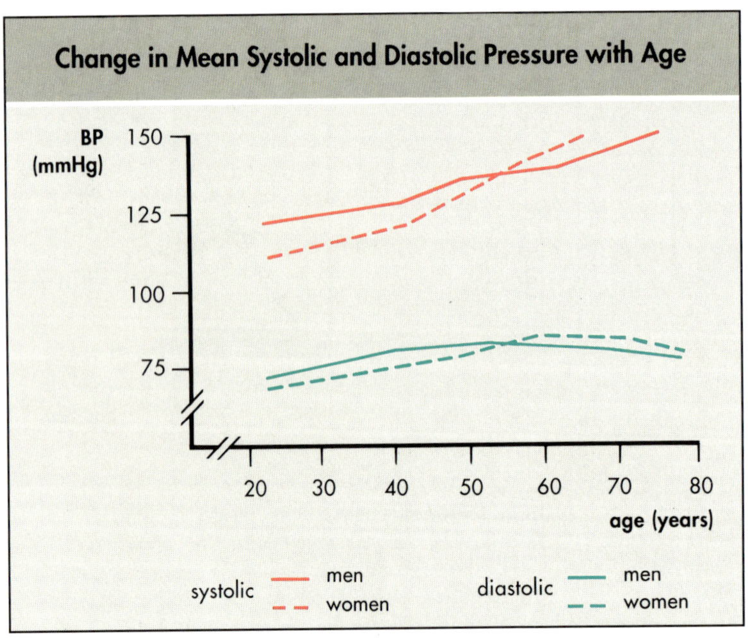

Fig. 1.44 Mean systolic pressure rises with age in both sexes. [Modified from Acheson (1973) *Int J Epidemiol*, **2**, 293–301.]

pulse pressure (the difference between diastolic and systolic pressures) tends to rise as a consequence. The reasons for this fall in diastolic blood pressure are uncertain. One contributory factor is probably selective mortality; a smaller proportion of subjects with high diastolic blood pressures survive and so tend to be under-represented in the higher age groups. Nevertheless, some longitudinal studies have also shown a fall in blood pressure, suggesting that there are underlying physiological causes. The elevation in systolic blood pressure and consequent increased pulse pressure is largely attributable to loss of elasticity in the aorta and large arteries (the Windkessel vessels; see chapter 6).

This rise in blood pressure with age is not observed in many non-Western cultures, in which blood pressure distribution curves are shifted to the left (Figs 1.45 & 1.46). This is not due to genetic differences; immigrants from so-called low

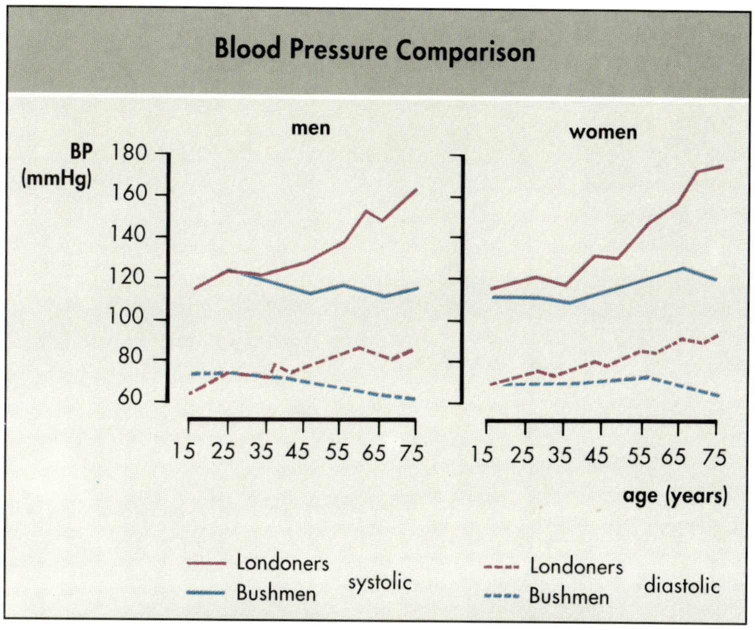

Fig. 1.45 Blood pressure shows no increase with age in certain primitive peoples.

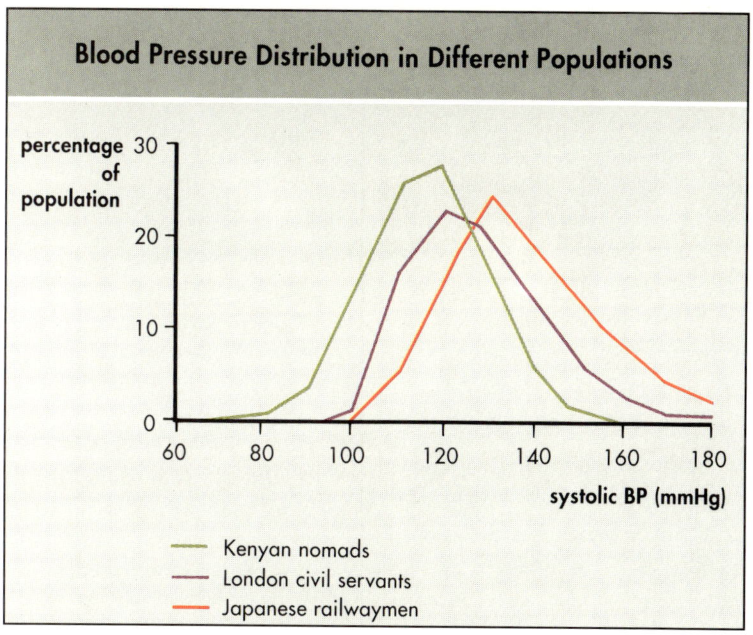

Fig. 1.46 Blood pressure distribution in three different populations. Although mean blood pressures were higher in the Japanese railwaymen, the shape of the distribution curve is preserved, indicating a difference throughout the population. There is no evidence therefore for the presence of differing proportions of hypertensive subjects between these racial groups.

pressure cultures into a Western-style culture have been shown to assume the blood pressure pattern of the surrounding population (Fig. 1.47). Possible explanations are discussed in chapter 3.

When blood pressures are measured at prolonged intervals in the same individual they tend to remain in the same position in the overall distribution so that, for instance, a subject with a high blood pressure tends to remain in the top percentiles subsequently (Fig. 1.48). This phenomenon has been referred to as tracking. It is seen in both children (see chapter 6) and adults, although it is stronger in the latter. This means that, since blood pressure increases with age, hypertension at a later age will be predicted by high pressures when young.

Another observation which has been made in longitudinal studies is that the rate of change of blood pressure with age is proportional to the absolute level of blood pressure. Thus, individuals with the highest blood pressures in their group show the greatest increase in blood pressure with ageing. This phenomenon, known as 'horse racing' (Fig. 1.49), has not been detected in children.

A third phenomenon has also been described in longitudinal studies. This is the tendency for pressure which is high or low to revert to a more 'normal' level on later examination. This tendency,

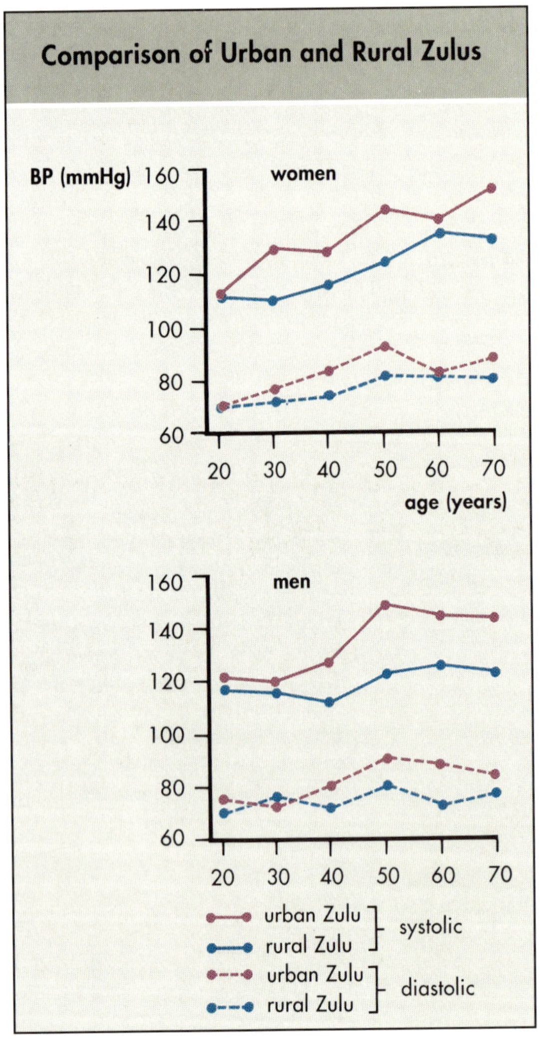

Fig. 1.47 When urban Zulus migrate to an urban environment, a rise in blood pressure with age can be observed.

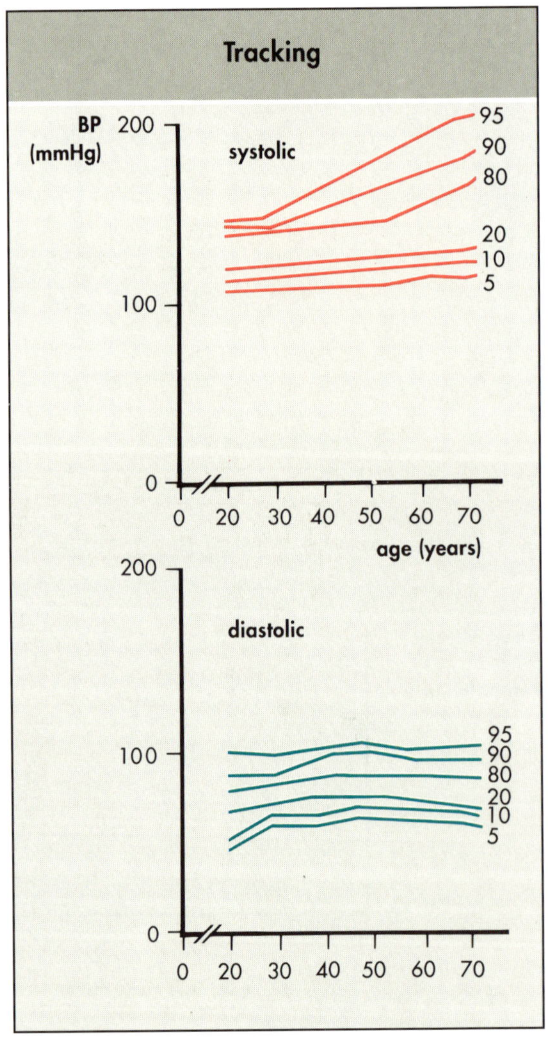

Fig. 1.48 Upper and lower percentile blood pressures for a population. Patients followed longitudinally tend to remain in the same percentile with increasing age.

which was first reported in US Army officers in 1934, has been named the Jenss phenomenon after its discoverer. This was originally attributed to homeostatic mechanisms (which would tend to bring blood pressure back to normal) but it is clear that regression to the mean (see above) would produce a similar effect. However, it has been claimed that when regression to the mean is taken into consideration, the Jenss phenomenon can still be demonstrated.

The three phenomena described above are summarized in Fig. 1.50.

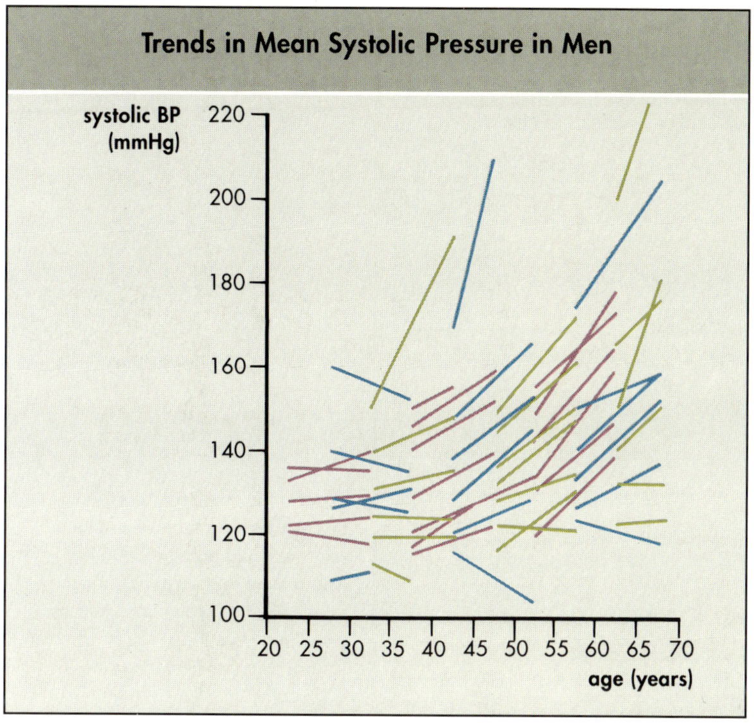

Fig. 1.49 These data, from a survey in Wales, demonstrate horse racing. [Modified from Miall & Chinn (1973) *Clin Sci*, **45**, 23s–33s.]

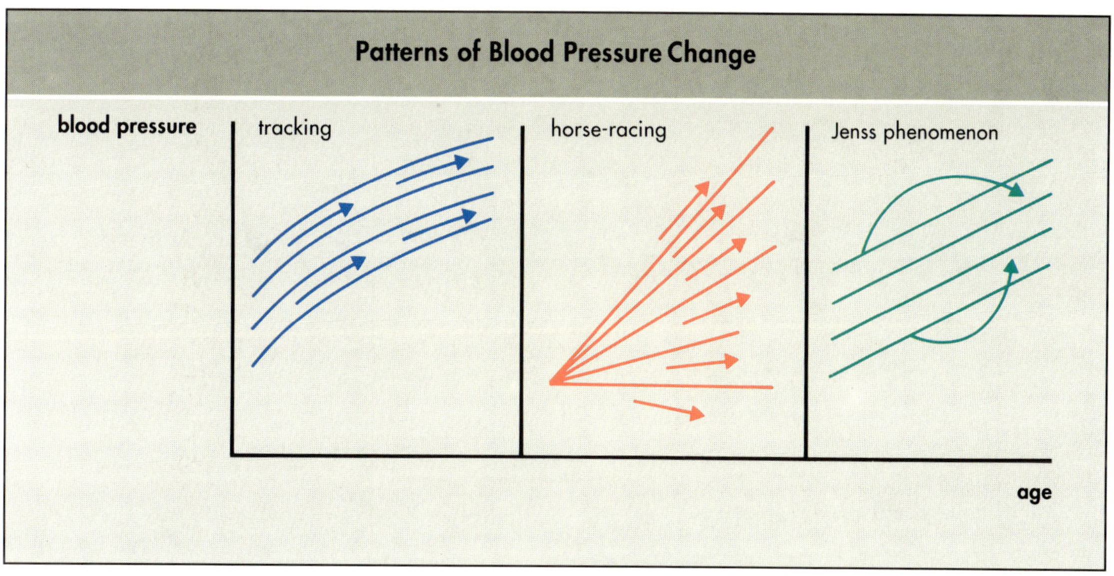

Fig. 1.50 Patterns of blood pressure change with time. (a) Tracking; (b) horse racing; (c) the Jenss phenomenon. [Modified from Hofman (1984) *J Hypertension*, **2**, 323–328.]

Heredity

Platt's original view that blood pressure was transmitted as a dominant monogenic trait is now no longer accepted, since it has not been possible to demonstrate that the offspring of one hypertensive parent fall into two distinct hypertensive and normotensive populations, one with and one without the proposed hypertension gene. There is, however, strong evidence for genetic factors in essential hypertension. When blood pressures are compared between blood relatives, significant cor-

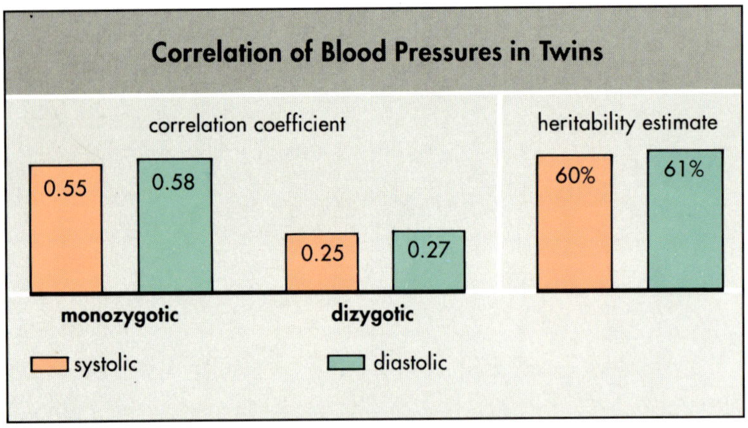

Fig. 1.51 Blood pressures are more highly correlated in monozygotic than dizygotic twins.

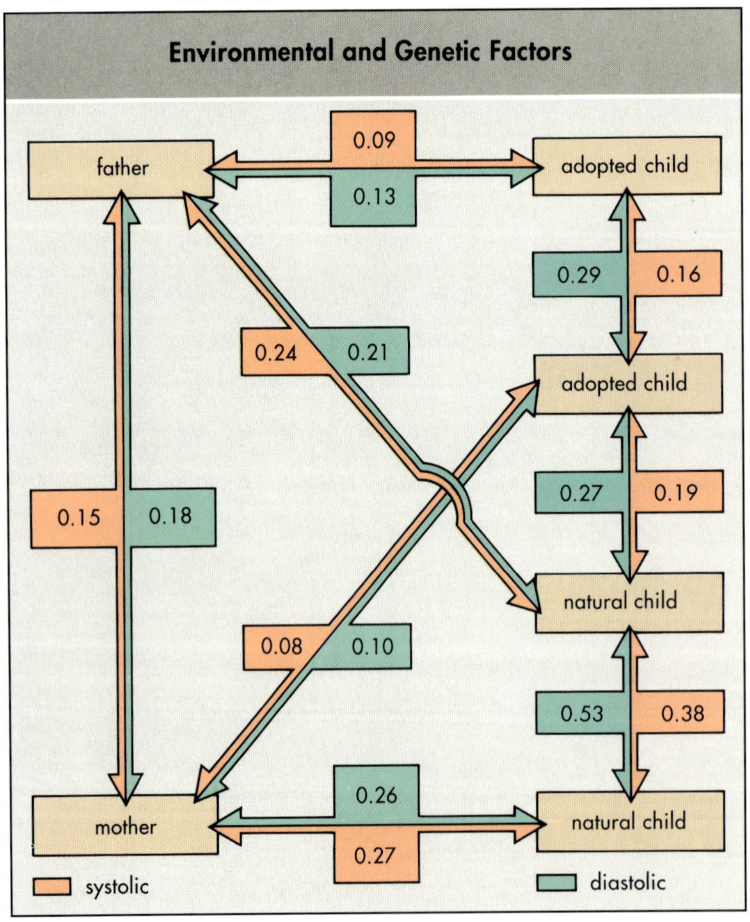

Fig. 1.52 The Montreal Twin Study: Correlation between blood relatives and non-blood relatives indicate the relative importance of genetic and environmental factors. [Modified from Mongeau *et al.* (1986) *Clin Exp Hypertens* (A), **8**, 653–660.]

relations can be demonstrated which are greatest for monozygotic twins and least for non-twin siblings (Fig. 1.51).

A weak relationship between the blood pressures of spouses has also been demonstrated. This could be the result of two factors. Firstly, there is a greater sharing of environmental factors and secondly, there is a tendency for constitutionally similar people to marry ('assortive mating').

It is possible to estimate the relative roles of environmental and genetic factors by comparing the blood pressure of monozygotic twins, dizygotic twins and spouses. A factor which has to be considered is the variability of blood pressure measurement, even when carried out under standardized conditions in the same individual. Thus a separate measurement of errors introduced by this phenomenon must be made. On the basis of the data obtained from several studies, Feinleib *et al.* have estimated the relative contribution of genetic and environmental factors in human hypertension (Fig. 1.52). The figures obtained, although only an approximation, emphasize the importance of genetic factors. This assessment should be regarded with caution. There is a tendency, for instance, for monozygotic twins to share a large number of environmental factors compared with dizygotic twins, who are dissimilar in many ways. This may result in an overestimation of the genetic component. The relative importance of genetic and inherited factors was assessed in the Montreal study (Fig. 1.52).

The genetic factor can also be assessed by comparing blood pressure in first degree relatives of hypertensive patients. Allowance has to be made for age, which will vary in the groups being compared. This has been achieved by allocating a score based upon the relationship of the observed blood pressure to that of the healthy population of the same age. Allocating scores in this way, it has been possible to demonstrate similarity of blood pressure in first degree relatives across the entire pressure range (Fig. 1.53). For instance, in a population study carried out in South Wales there was a highly significant correlation between the diastolic blood pressure of first degree relatives. This correlation held true for first degree relatives not only of hypertensives, but also of individuals whose blood pressure was lower than the population mean. These findings are particularly striking in view of the fact that single measurements of blood pressure inevitably impose substantial random errors which dilute any true resemblance. Allowing for this, for every 1mmHg by which diastolic blood pressure of the propositors exceeded the expected level for someone of that age, the first degree relative's blood pressure was 0.4mmHg higher. This calculation, of course, takes no account of the possible contribution of shared environment.

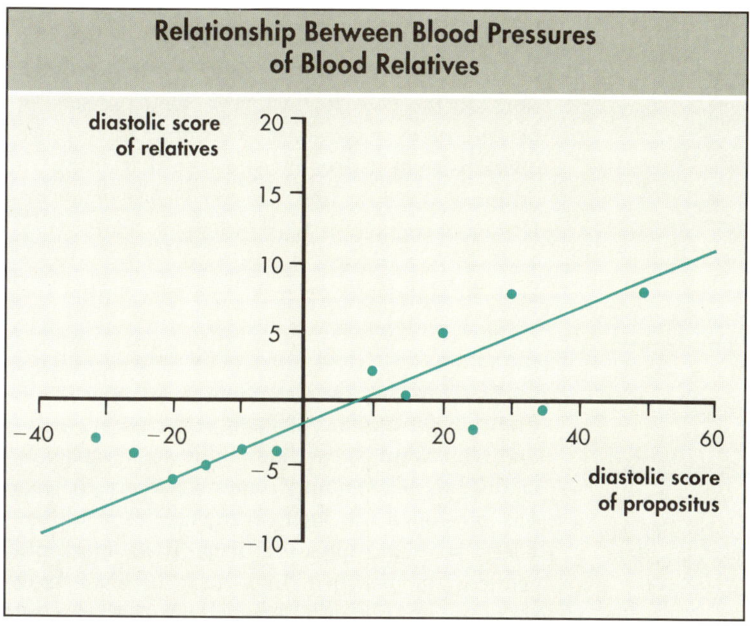

Fig. 1.53 Relationship between the blood pressures of blood relatives. The diastolic values (adjusted for age and sex) are closely correlated, suggesting a genetic component in blood pressure.

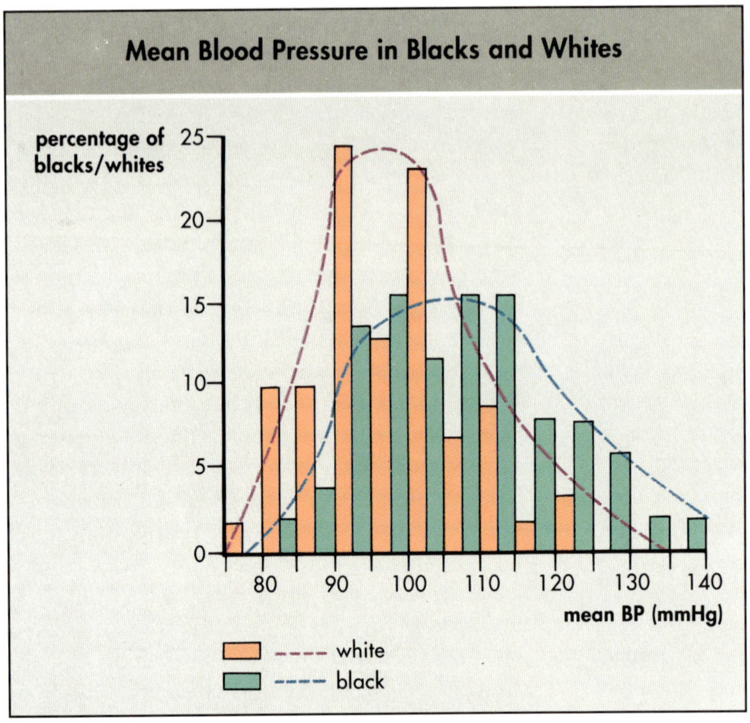

Fig. 1.54 Distribution of mean blood pressure in age-matched black and white factory workers in the USA. Although there is no difference in the shape of the distribution curves, blacks show a definite shift to the right.

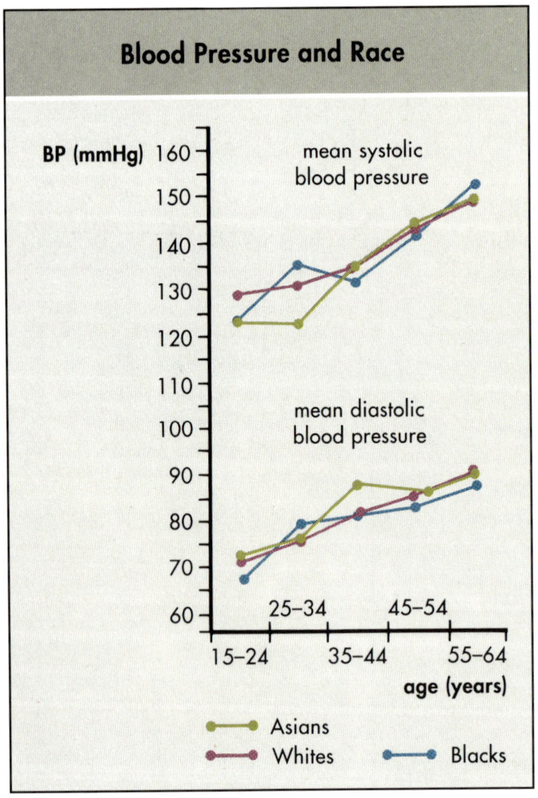

Fig. 1.55 A study in Birmingham showed little difference between the blood pressures of West Indian, white and Asian men. [Modified from Cruikshank *et al.* (1985) *J Hypertension*, **3**, 367.]

Race

It has already been pointed out that there are substantial differences in both blood pressure and the rise in blood pressure with age in geographically dispersed populations. However, there are also racial variations in blood pressure within populations. In the USA for instance, blood pressure in blacks rises more rapidly from adolescence onwards than it does in whites so that, using an arbitrary dividing line, the prevalence of hypertension is higher in blacks than in whites (Fig. 1.54). In fact, diastolic blood pressure is, on average, 5–10mmHg higher in both black men and women. Differences are also somewhat greater in the southern states of America than they are in the north. How far these variations are genetic in origin is uncertain. Differences between blacks and whites in body weight and in socio-economic status may play an important role; where analysis has controlled for such divergence, racial differences in blood pressure have been markedly reduced or abolished. In a study of black West Indians working in a Birmingham (UK) factory

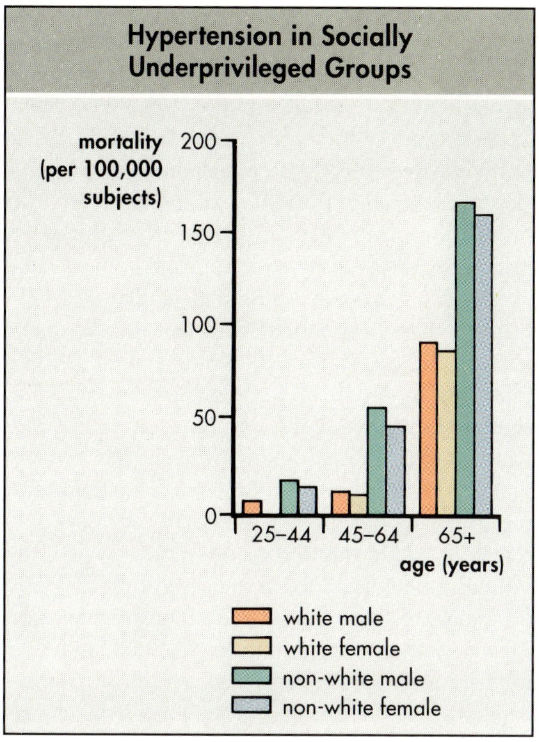

Fig. 1.56 Mortality from hypertensive disease in black and white subjects belonging to different age groups. Older blacks have a significantly higher mortality.

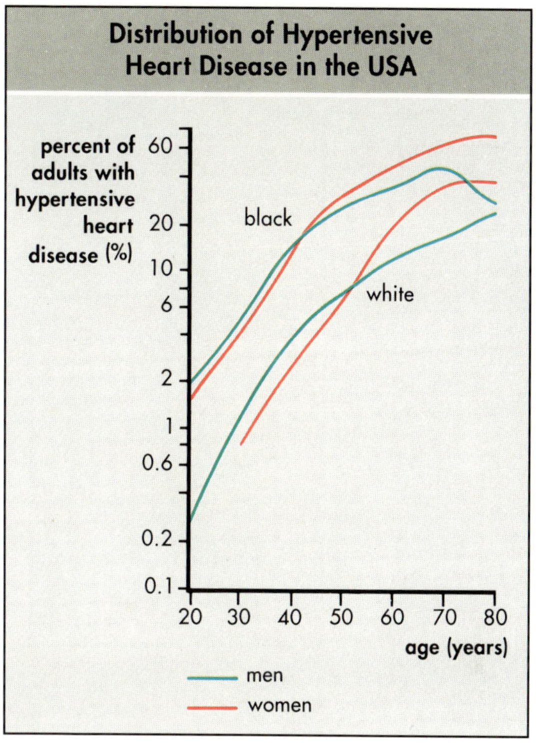

Fig. 1.57 Distribution of hypertensive heart disease in the USA by age, race and sex. (Modified from the National Health Survey, 1960–1962.)

there was no difference in blood pressure compared with either whites or Asians of similar social background (Fig. 1.55). The implication that there were no genetic differences in blood pressure between blacks and the white controls was further examined by studying blood pressure in the population from which they were derived, in this case black West Indians. Blood pressures amongst blacks in Jamaica were found to be similar to those observed in British white controls.

Although mortality attributable to hypertension is elevated in the black American population (Figs 1.56 & 1.57), it is still uncertain whether black American individuals carry a higher risk for a given blood pressure level. Even if the risk were greater, social factors could account for it, since less advantaged socio-economic groups would be less likely to have their hypertension diagnosed and adequately treated. Given that American blacks form a relatively large percentage of the lower socio-economic groups, hypertension in the black population may therefore be less likely to be diagnosed and treated when compared to American whites (Fig. 1.58).

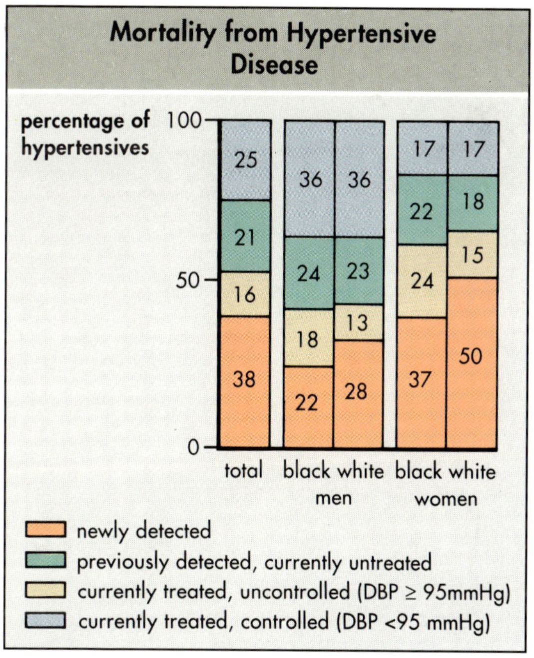

Fig. 1.58 Socially under-privileged groups show a higher prevalence of undiagnosed or uncontrolled hypertension. the most highly privileged whites are much more likely to have adequately treated hypertension when populations are surveyed.

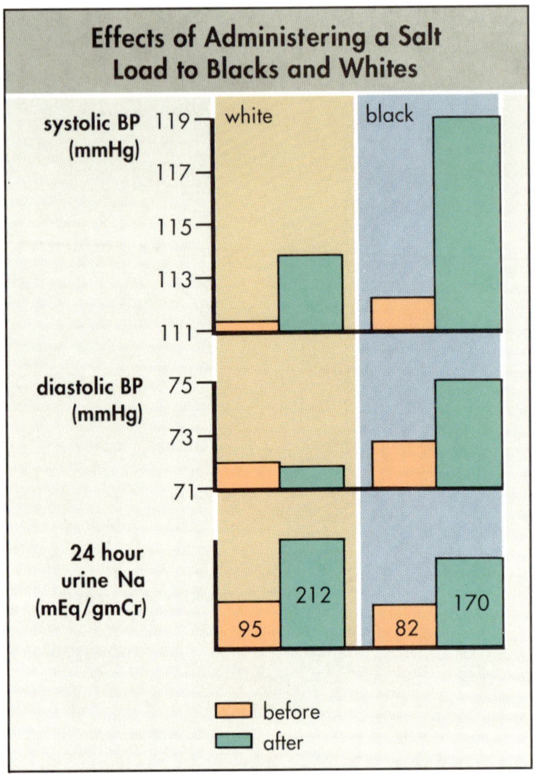

Fig. 1.59 Racial differences in the efects of administering a salt load in blacks and whites. The blacks show an increased pressor response and retain slightly more of the sodium, as shown by the urinary excretion of sodium before and after a total daily intake of 458mEq.

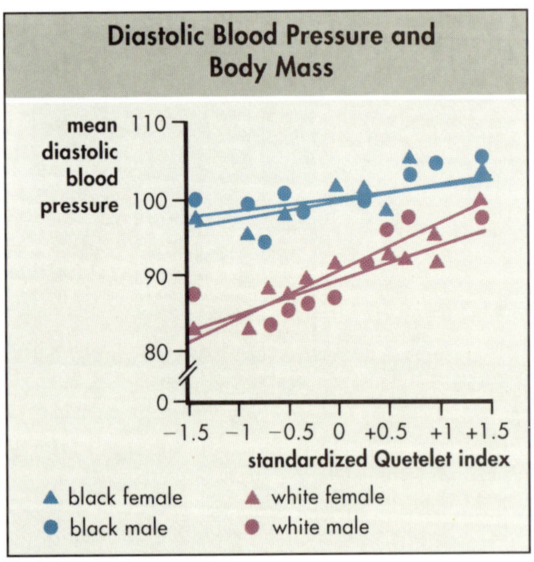

Fig. 1.60 When diastolic blood pressure is plotted against a standardized Quetelet (body mass) index, a clear relationship between the two can be seen. [Modified from Tyroler *et al.* (1975) in *Epidemiology and Control of Hypertension*. Edited by Paul, O. New York: Stratton.]

There is, however, some indirect evidence for an underlying genetic factor in hypertension amongst blacks. Low plasma renin levels are more common in blacks than in whites and likewise 'low renin hypertension' is more often seen in blacks. Black normotensive subjects excrete sodium loads more slowly than white normotensives (Fig. 1.59). The normal increase in urinary kallikrein produced by salt depletion is also less pronounced in black subjects. On the basis of these and similar observations it has been suggested that blacks have evolved a particularly avid form of renal sodium retention in order to protect their extracellular fluid volume against the consequences of salt and water deprivation in a hot climate. The penalty which has been paid for this is an increased susceptibility to the pressor effects of excessive salt retention. This penalty is manifest only when individuals are exposed to an increase in dietary salt, occurring, for example, as a result of urbanization. This hypothesis remains quite speculative at the moment and there is no evidence for fluid volume expansion in black hypertensive or normotensive subjects. Nevertheless, the hypothesis does emphasise how intertwined genetic and environmental factors may be. Differences in blood pressure responses to therapeutic agents may also reflect genetic factors. For example, blacks show enhanced hypotensive responses to diuretics and a poorer response to beta blockers and ACE inhibitors. This may be attributable to the lower plasma renin in black subjects.

Body Mass

There is a consistent relationship between body mass and blood pressure which is independent of other factors such as race and age (Fig. 1.60). This correlation extends throughout the normal and hypertensive range and is not wholly attributable to cuff artefact (using too small a cuff on a large arm), although the latter probably does cause overestimation of the relationship in poorly controlled surveys, such as those based upon insurance examination.

The nature of the relationship between obesity and hypertension is uncertain. Metabolic abnormalities have been descibed in essential hypertension which may give rise to obesity; for example, hypertensive subjects are relatively resistant to the hypoglycaemic effect of insulin infusion (see below). In the Framingham Study, normotensive fat people were more likely to become hypertensive and thin hypertensives were more likely to become fat. Untreated hypertensive patients tend as a group to be heavier than normotensive age-matched controls. A further, unexplained anomaly is that the risk of cardiovascular death among hypertensive subjects is higher in the thin than in the overweight. Although in poorly controlled studies cuff artefact could have lead to an overestimation of blood pressure in obese individuals, this finding has also been reported where cuff artefact has been carefully avoided (Fig. 1.61).

The connection between weight and blood pressure is confirmed by analysis of the effect of

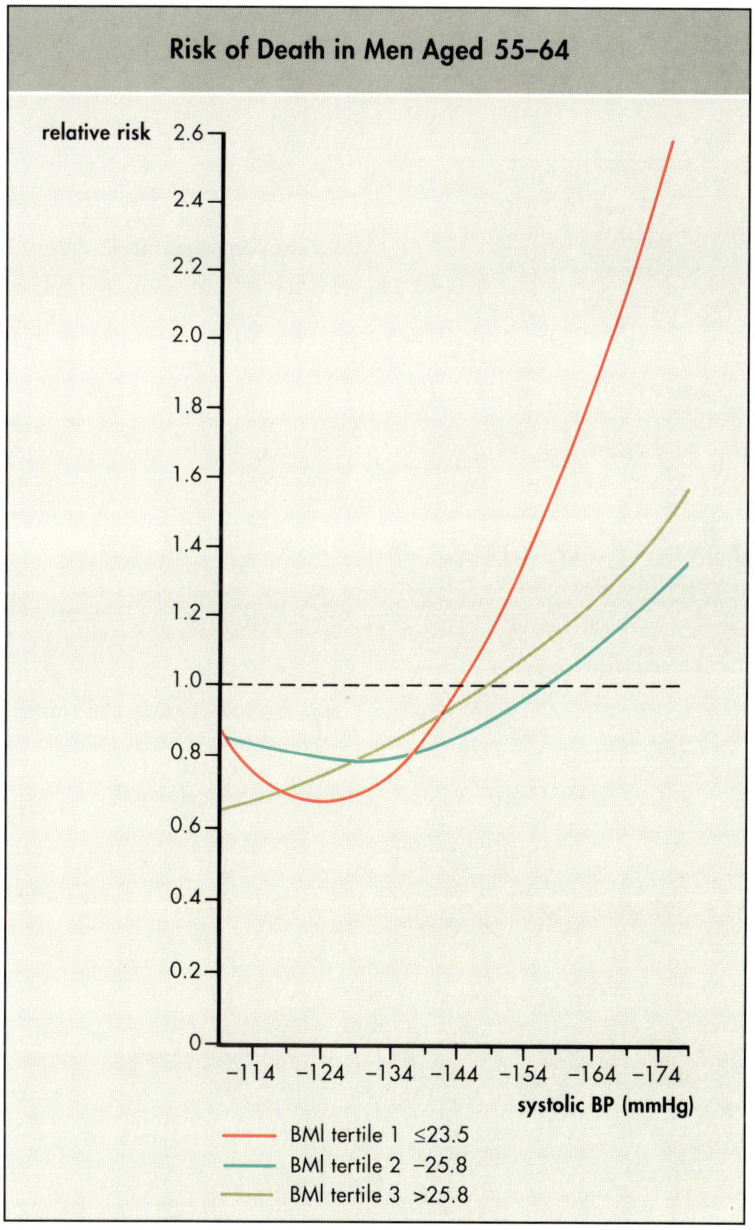

Fig. 1.61 This graph plots relative risk of death against systolic blood pressure for three body-mass tertiles. Surprisingly, the data show a higher risk for thin hypertensives. [Modified from Elliot *et al.* (1987) *J Hypertension*, **5**, s517–s519.]

weight change (Fig. 1.62). In the Framingham study the strongest predictor of an increase in systolic blood pressure was an increase in weight. In patients who became 20% above ideal weight, the risk of hypertension was eight times greater than in a group who were 10% underweight. The risk was greatest in those who gained weight during the third and fourth decades of life, after which the relationship weakened. Studies in which body weight has been reduced dietetically in obese hypertensive subjects have in the main confirmed that a significant fall in blood pressure can be produced. Hovell, in an analysis of the available literature, concluded that a weight loss of 12kg could be expected to produce a blood pressure fall of 21/13mmHg and a weight loss of 3kg a fall of 7/4mmHg (Fig. 1.63). These reductions could be observed both in drug-treated and non drug-treated patients. The mechanism which produces the fall in blood pressure is unknown. Supplementing the diet with sodium to prevent any negative sodium balance has not, in the majority of studies, prevented the fall in blood pressure. There is however evidence for a reduction in sympathetic nervous system activity, in that circulating catecholamines and pulse rate fall with dietary weight reduction. This provides an attractive, although unconfirmed, explanation for the effect.

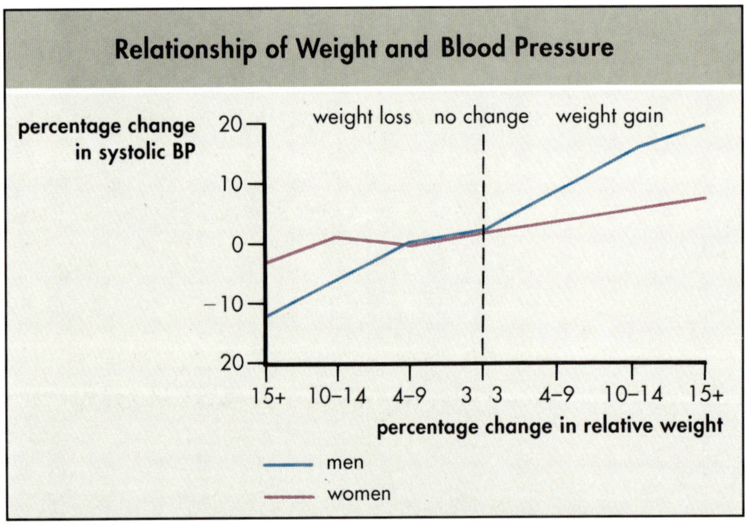

Fig. 1.62 Increase of weight in underweight individuals, or loss of weight in the obese, both tend to restore blood pressure levels to the population mean.

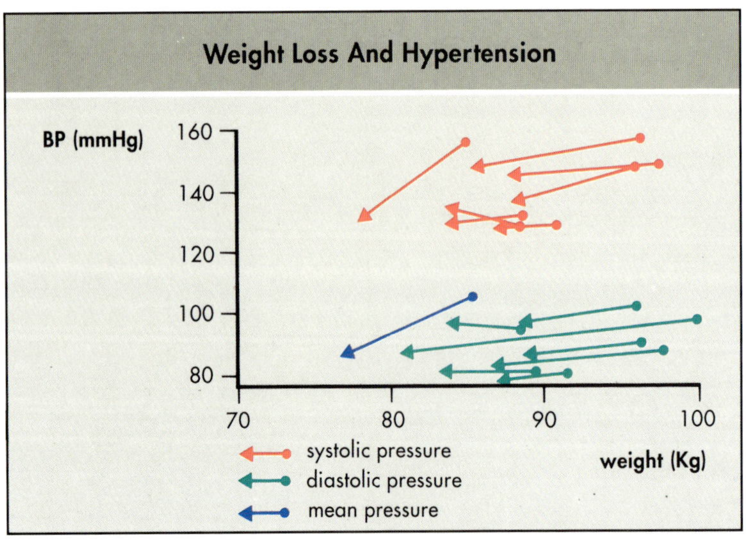

Fig. 1.63 An analysis of the major controlled trials of weight reduction in hypertension. In all but one, a significant fall is observed.

Alcohol

Despite the considerable logistical difficulties involved in assessing alcohol intake by questionnaire, almost all epidemiological studies have shown a relationship to hypertension (Fig. 1.64). Heavy drinking is associated with increased blood pressure in both sexes and in all racial groups studied. Some surveys have demonstrated a J-shaped relationship between alcohol and blood pressure with slightly lower blood pressures in moderate drinkers (those consuming 2–3 units of alcohol a day, a unit being defined as a single measure of spirits, a glass of wine or half a pint of beer). It has been argued that this result is an artefact, due to the contamination of the total abstention category by heavy drinkers who deny consuming any alcohol.

The relationship between alcohol and blood pressure has been confirmed by experiments with heavy drinking hypertensive subjects, in which alcohol has been withheld from them and then readministered. Blood pressure can be respectively lowered and raised by these manoeuvures. These studies were however of only a few days duration; the long-term effects of alcohol administration or withdrawal in man have not been systematically studied.

Diabetes

The incidence of hypertension is increased among diabetics. Conversely, insulin resistance, glucose intolerance and hyperinsulinaemia are all more common in hypertensive patients (Fig. 1.65). These abnormalities are independent of treatment with agents such as thiazide diuretics, but are observed in several situations associated with hypertension (in addition to type 2 diabetes) such as obesity, renal failure and glucocorticoid excess. The nature of the physiological link is unknown.

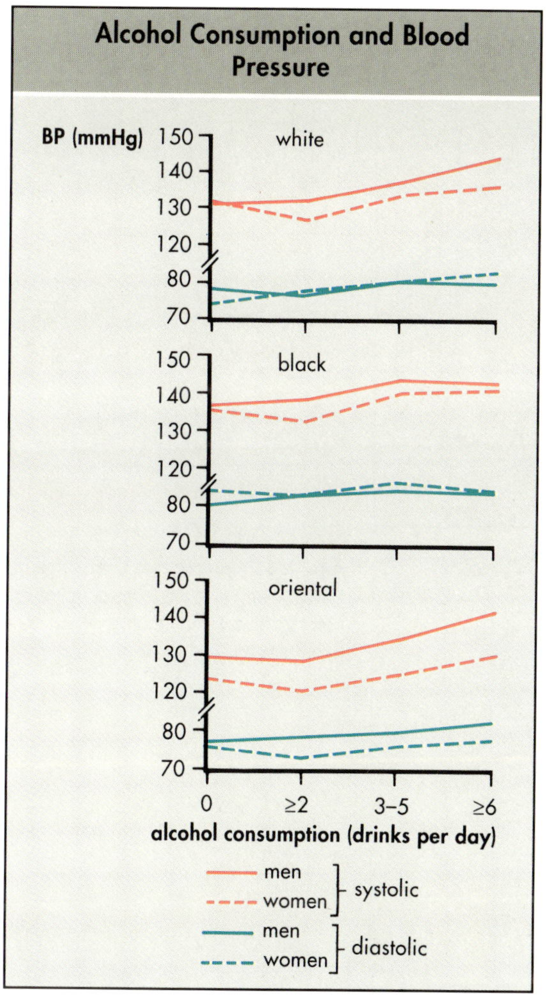

Fig. 1.64 Heavy alcohol consumption is associated with a high mean blood pressure in most populations.

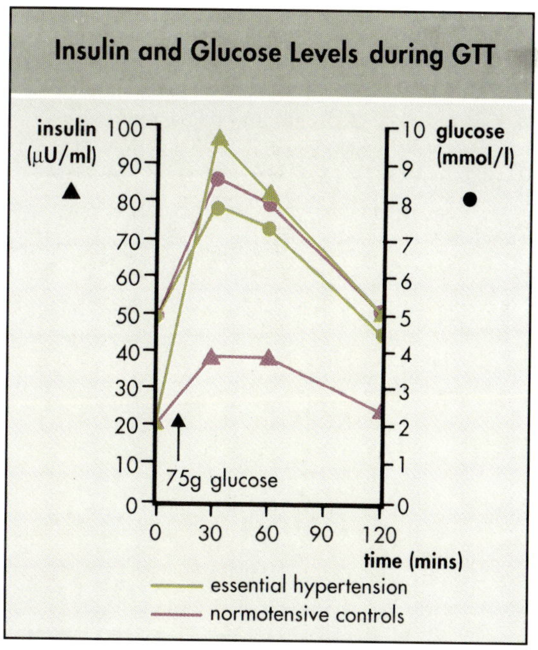

Fig. 1.65 Hypertensive patients demonstrate a marked hyperinsulinaemia, as shown by these GTT data. [Modified from Singer *et al.* (1985) *Hypertension*, **7**, 182–186.]

A further interesting association has recently been described. Parents of subjects with diabetes and proteinuria have been found to have higher blood pressures than parents of diabetic subjects without proteinuria. It has therefore been suggested that diabetic nephropathy results from an association between diabetes and a genetic predisposition to essential hypertension. Support for this has been obtained in studies of erythrocyte lithium–sodium counter transport (Fig. 1.66), which may be a genetic marker for essential hypertension (see chapter 3). This was found to be elevated only in diabetic patients who showed proteinuria.

Other Factors

Some community surveys have shown that smokers tend to have a slightly lower blood pressure than non-smokers, although the risk of complications is much higher. However, two studies, one from Birmingham and one from Glasgow, have indicated that the malignant phase of hypertension is significantly more common in subjects who smoke (Fig. 1.67). One explanation of this association is that smoking precipitates disseminated intravascular coagulation, which may play a role in the malignant phase of hypertension.

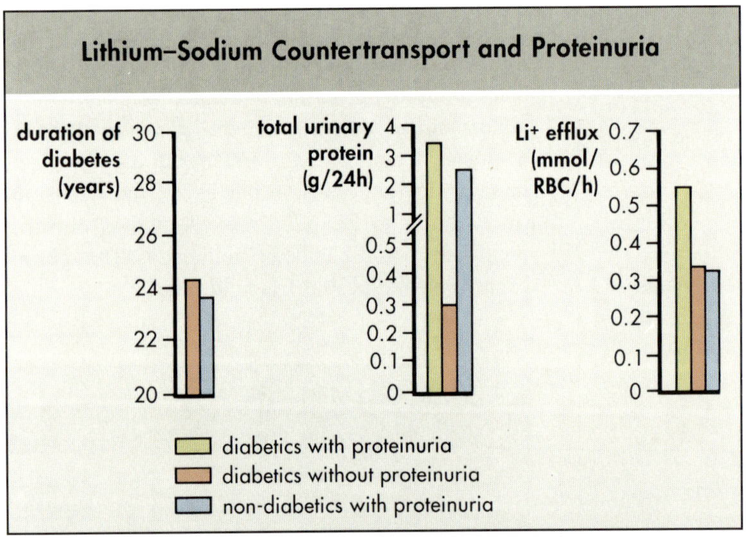

Fig. 1.66 Lithium–sodium countertransport has been found to be elevated only in proteinuric diabetics, as these results show. [Modified from Viberti in *ACE Inhibition and Renal Function*, RSM Round Table Series, **3**, 70–75.]

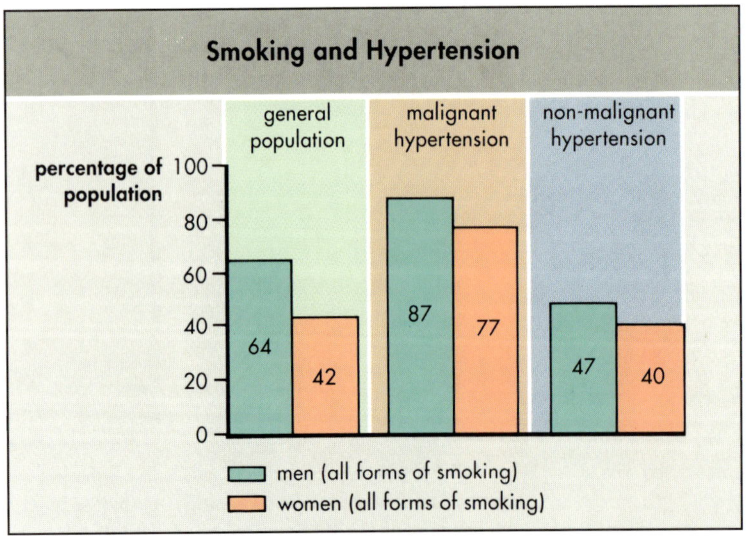

Fig. 1.67 Two studies have shown that smoking is much more common among patients with malignant hypertension.

Smoking is also significantly more frequent among subjects with renovascular hypertension (due to atheroma or fibromuscular dysplasia).

Blood pressures tend to be lower in hard water areas (Fig. 1.68). While this could be related to a higher calcium intake, a possible role for as yet unrecognized social factors has not been excluded.

Several studies have shown hypertension to be more prevalent in the lower social groups. Furthermore, the poorer health care to which these groups are subject leads to under-diagnosis of hypertension and less adequate treatment. This situation is compounded by the fact that racial minorities contribute disproportionately to the lower social classes and so genetic and environmental factors may be intermingled (see above). Identifying such relationships is particularly difficult when attempts are made to identify the effect of occupational stress on blood pressure. Amongst manual workers certain occupational groups (bus drivers for example) show a higher incidence of elevated pressure. Whilst this is not related to age, sex or social class, it would reflect (in addition to stress) exposure to factors such as different degrees of physical activity, disruption of diet and sleep and exposure to atmospheric pollution and noise.

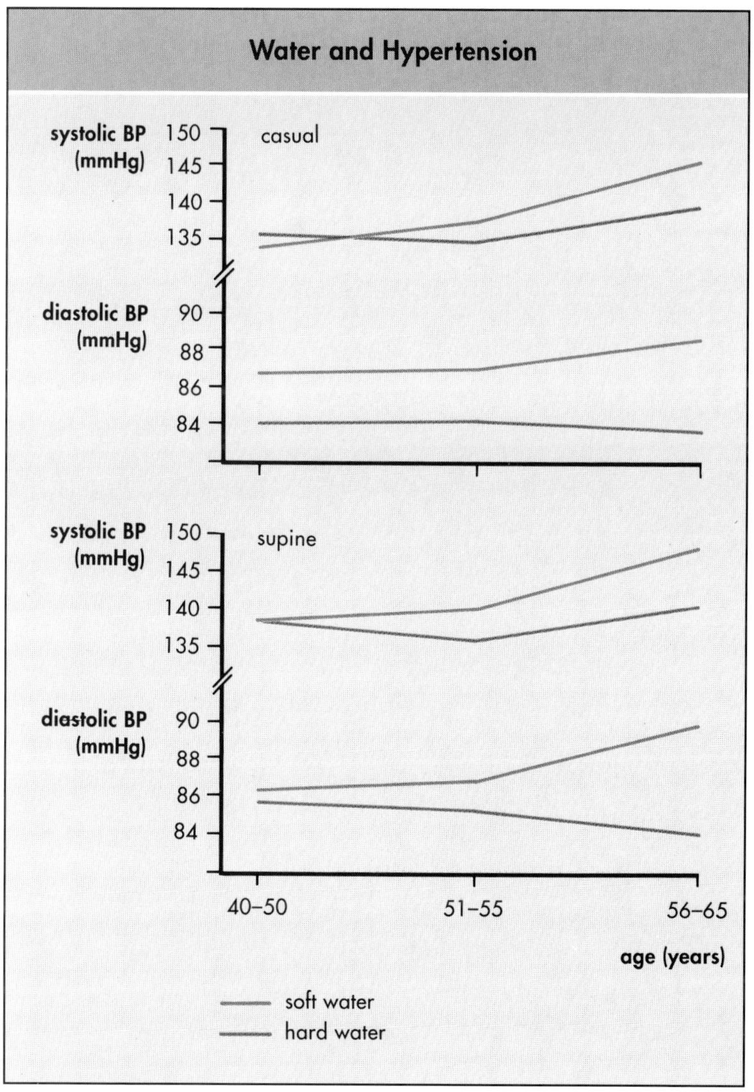

Fig. 1.68 Blood pressure tends to be lower among patients living in hard-water areas.

FURTHER READING

Acheson, R. M. (1973) Blood pressure in a national sample of US adults. Percentile distribution by age, sex and race. *Inter J Epidemiol*, **2,** 293-301.

Bursztyn, P. (1987) *Nutrition and Blood Pressure.* London: John Libby.

Dawber,T.R. (1980) *The Framingham Study.* Cambridge, Massachusetts: Harvard University Press.

Kesteloot H. & Joossens, J.V. (1980) *Epidemiology of Arterial Blood Pressure.* The Hague: Martinus Nijhoff.

Paul, O. (Ed), (1975) *Epidemiology and Control of Hypertension.* New York: Stratton.

Paul, O. (1979) Epidemiology of Hypertension. In *Arterial Hypertension.* Edited by Paul, Gross and Robertson. London: Pitman Medical.

Seedat, Y.K. (1983) Race, Environment and Blood Pressure. *J Hypertension,* **1,** 7-12.

Society of Actuaries (1959) *Build and Blood Pressure Survey.* Volumes I & II. Chicago: Society of Actuaries.

CHAPTER 2

Mechanisms of Blood Pressure Control

INTRODUCTION

The circulation is a closed system in which the fluid content (the blood) is driven by a pump (the heart). Pressure within this system is the product of two opposing forces: the output of the pump and the resistance to flow offered by the system. Although the human circulation is an extremely complex system, this generalization is still valid. Blood pressure is related to the output of blood from the heart and the resistance to flow offered by the small arteries and arterioles.

The first complication occurs because these two factors are not independent of one another. Changes in cardiac output or peripheral resistance influence each other through several mechanisms.

- Cardiac output changes in response to alterations in resistance to flow, as a result of intrinsic changes in the heart, and as a result of pressure changes monitored by the arterial baroreceptors;
- Changes in cardiac output may trigger local mechanisms which regulate peripheral resistance through alterations in tissue perfusion;
- Structural changes in the resistance vessels or in the heart may change their properties and give rise to compensatory changes elsewhere.

Although the numerous regulatory and counter-regulatory mechanisms for blood pressure do not maintain it at a constant level, it is normally kept within the physiologically acceptable range, although temporary requirements may override this control.

CARDIAC OUTPUT

The heart acts as an intermittent pump which expels blood from the left ventricle during systole. The total output of blood from the heart is therefore determined by the amount of blood expelled with each beat (stroke volume) multiplied by the number of beats per minute (heart rate). Cardiac output at rest is approximately 5–5.5l/min. (This gives a cardiac index of 3.0–3.5 l/m^2body surface.)

Cardiac output can increase 5–6-fold during strenuous exercise. The fact that blood pressure does not rise commensurately indicates that total peripheral resistance is decreased in this situation, although regional resistance in different tissue beds shows quite different changes (Fig. 2.1).

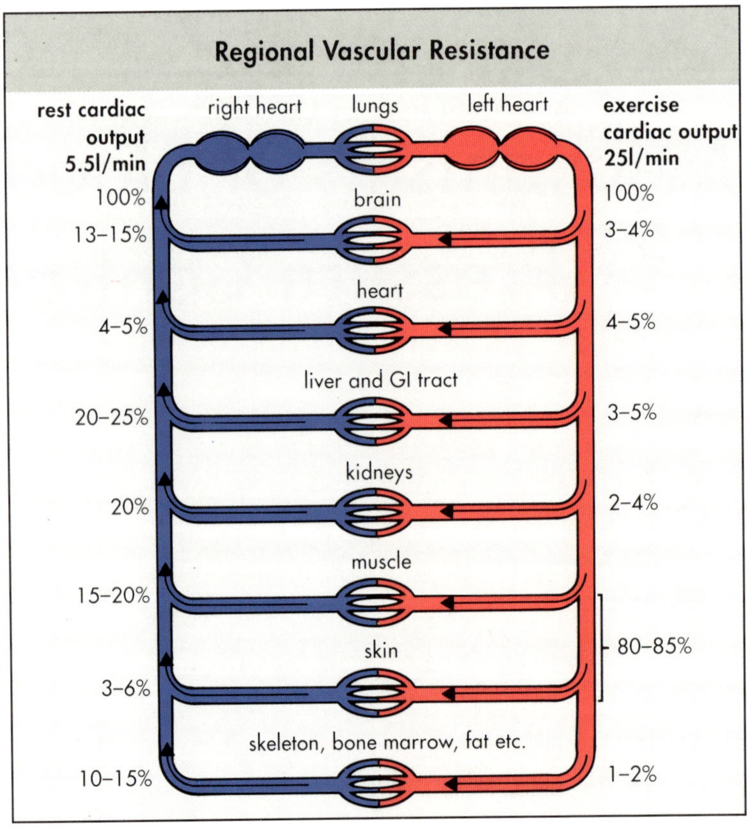

Fig.2.1 This diagram shows the flow distribution in human vascular circuits. After exercise cardiac ouput rises five-fold and regional vascular resistance alters, directing about 85% of the blood to the muscle and skin. [Modified from Folkow, B. and Neil, E. (1971) *Circulation.* Oxford: Oxford University Press.]

Cardiac output is regulated by intrinsic and extrinsic mechanisms (Fig. 2.2). The former (myocardial contractility) can be demonstrated in an isolated heart; the latter are dependent on humoral and neurogenic mechanisms (venous return and parasympathetic and sympathetic efferents).

Intrinsic Regulation of Cardiac Output

In a given period of time, the heart can only pump out the same volume of blood that it receives. However, venous return (the volume of blood entering the right atrium in unit time) varies substantially (see below). The power of adaptation that this implies is expressed by the Frank–Starling law, which states that cardiac output is proportional to filling of the heart during diastole – the cardiac muscle responds to the stretch produced by increased volumes of blood with more powerful contractions, thus increasing stroke volume. A less important contributing factor is the increase in heart rate caused by stretching of the right atrial wall. The effect of venous return on ventricular output is mediated by changes in atrial pressure. It is thus possible to express ventricular function as the relationship between output and atrial pressure. As atrial pressure is increased so either right or left ventricular output rises up to a maximum (Fig. 2.3).

The effect of changes in atrial pressure should be contrasted with the effect of altering the arterial pressure against which the cardiac pump operates (afterload). Cardiac output only falls in the face of gross arterial pressure elevation. At this point, left ventricular failure gives rise to a reduction in cardiac output.

Cardiac Hypertrophy

Thickening of the left ventricular wall occurs as a result of a sustained increased afterload. Left ventricular hypertrophy is therefore common in hypertension (see chapter 4). This has the advantage that cardiac output can be maintained against increased afterload. There are however also substantial disadvantages. For instance, the increased muscle mass may outstrip blood supply. In addition, the thickened wall is less distensible – diastolic compliance is therefore reduced. As a result, a

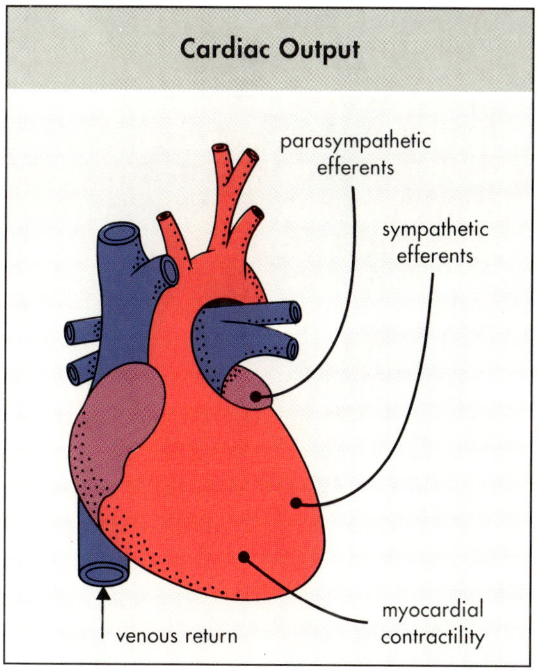

Fig. 2.2 Cardiac output depends on venous return and on cardiac factors (sympathetic and parasympathetic activity and myocardial contractility).

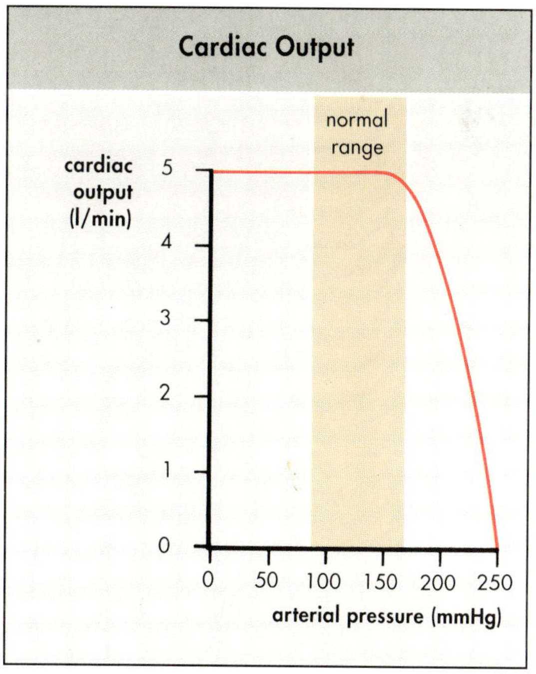

Fig. 2.3 Graph showing approximate ventricular output curves for the human heart (extrapolated from data obtained from dogs). [Modified from Guyton, A. C. (1987) The Heart. In *Textbook of Medical Physiology*. Philadelphia: W. B. Saunders.]

higher preload is required to produce a similar cardiac output in the hypertrophied compared with a normal heart. This can easily be demonstrated by perfusing isolated left ventricles from hypertensive and normotensive rats (Fig. 2.4). When afterloads observed *in vivo* are applied, the Frank–Starling curve of the hypertrophied ventricles is shifted to the right. It should be emphasized that a hypertrophied left ventricle is more effective than a non-hypertrophied ventricle against similar pressures; the hypertrophied heart under these circumstances maintains a higher cardiac output. However, the higher end diastolic pressure required to maintain cardiac output in the face of increased arterial pressure may ultimately lead to cardiac failure (see chapter 4).

Autonomic and Humoral Control of Cardiac Output

Cardiac output is regulated by sympathetic and parasympathetic (vagal) nerves (Fig. 2.5) and by circulating catecholamines.

Autonomic Control

The nervous system regulates cardiac output by changing heart rate (by adjusting the cardiac pacemaker) and stroke volume (by modifying the strength of contraction of the heart).

The sympathetic nerves, acting through β_1-receptors, maintain a tonic level of activity. A reduction or increase in this activity therefore causes a corre-

Preload and Cardiac Output

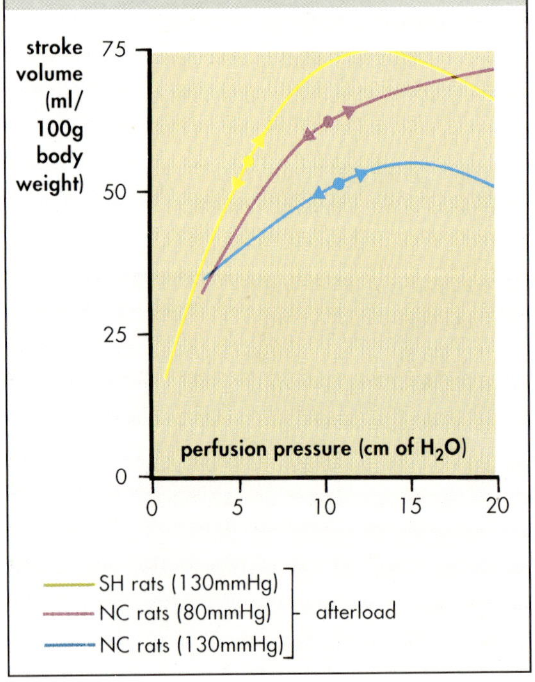

Fig. 2.4 Graph showing Frank–Starling curve for isolated perfused left ventricles of spontaneously hypertensive rats and normotensive controls, exposed to afterloads just lower than those seen *in vivo.* Left ventricular hypertrophy in the SHRs compensates for the increased afterload. However, a higher diastolic pressure is needed for a given stroke volume, due to the low compliance of the thickened wall. Also seen here is the depressed curve shown by the control rat when exposed to acute high afterload. [Modified from Noresson *et al.* (1978) *Acta Phys Scand,* **102**, 14A.]

Cardiac Nerves

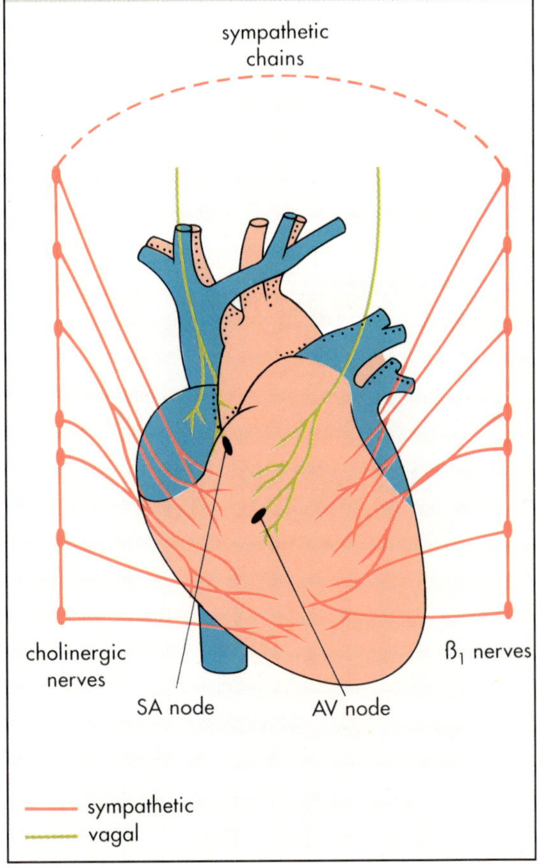

Fig. 2.5 The cardiac nerves, showing both sympathetic and parasympathetic (vagal) systems. [For source see Fig. 2.3.]

sponding reduction or increase in cardiac output and heart rate.

The vagus also maintains a level of inhibitory tone, although the activity of these fibres is much less than sympathetic efferent activity. Nevertheless, vagal inhibition does cause a significant increase both in heart rate and cardiac output.

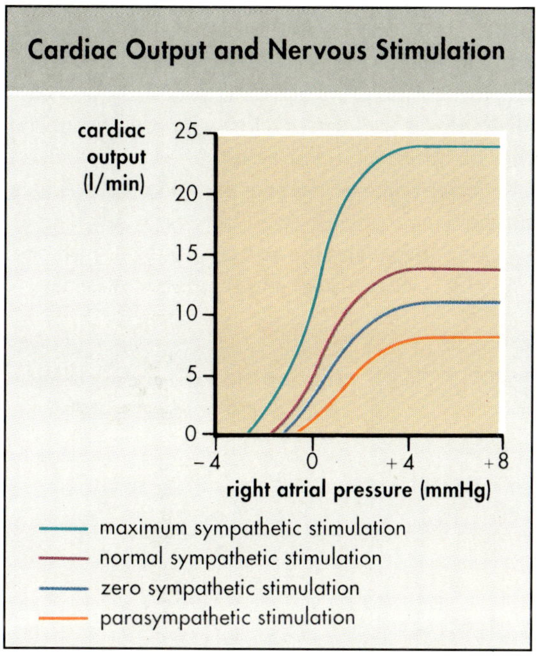

Fig. 2.6 The effect on the cardiac output curve of sympathetic and parasympathetic stimulation. [For source see Fig. 2.3.]

The overall effect of these two systems is to alter the cardiac function curve relating preload to cardiac output. Thus, for a given venous filling pressure, cardiac output is higher in the face of sympathetic stimulation or parasympathetic inhibition, and *vice versa* (Fig. 2.6).

Humoral Control

Circulating adrenaline released by the adrenal medulla also causes an increase in heart rate and stroke volume as a result of stimulation of cardiac β_1-receptors. Since adrenaline release occurs as a result of sympathetic nervous system activation, cardiac output still responds to stress or exercise even when the heart is completely denervated.

THE VENOUS CIRCULATION

The return of blood to the heart at a given moment is determined by two factors:

- the volume of blood in the venous compartment;
- the distensibility of the vessels (the venous system) in which it is contained (Fig. 2.7).

The venous system has to cope with rapid changes in the volume of contained blood in different parts of the body, when for instance an individual moves from a lying to a standing posture. Such changes in volume are produced with relatively small changes in pressure – the venous bed is very distensible when compared with the arterial bed. The change in pressure produced by a given increase in blood volume in the venous bed is

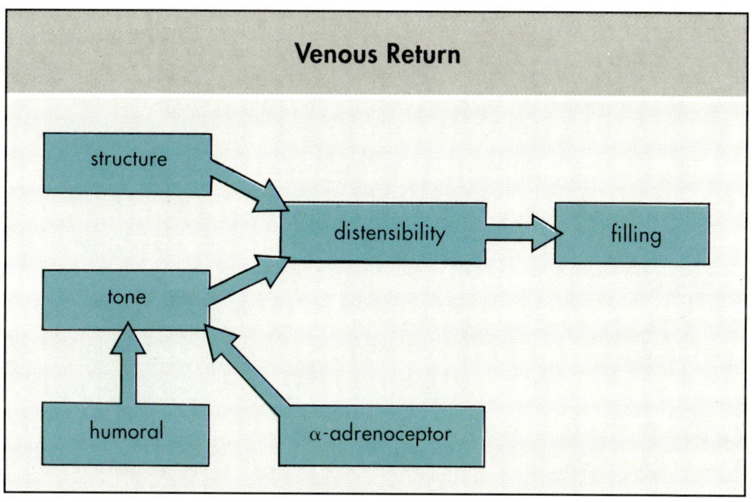

Fig. 2.7 Venous return depends upon the capacitance vessel tone and venous filling.

referred to as venous compliance. This is influenced by the distensibility of the venous wall (passive compliance) and by sympathetic nervous activity (active compliance). Humoral factors (such as the renin–angiotensin system and the kallikrein–bradykinin system) also regulate venous compliance in some situations, although the physiological role of these systems probably assumes greatest importance at physiological extremes.

Active compliance is mediated by α_1-adrenoceptors situated on the large veins which cause contraction of smooth muscle within the venous walls. Stimulation or inhibition of the sympathetic nervous system results in a shift of the capacitance vessel volume/pressure relationship to the left or the right respectively.

Compliance of the capacitance vessels is not solely due to changes in elastic recoil of the walls and vascular smooth muscle activity. The most important component is the change in geometry of the large veins. At low pressures the cross-sectional shape of vessels in the venous bed is an ellipse. As the pressure increases the vein distends and the geometry changes to that of a circle (Fig. 2.8); this increases the cross-sectional area and, therefore, the volume of the venous bed. These changes become important when the upright position is assumed. Pressure in veins below the heart increases and they assume a circular diameter increasing their volume perhaps by 500mls or more. The reduction in right atrial filling pressure and cardiac output results in a transient fall in blood pressure. This activates baroreceptor-mediated reflexes and causes reflex venoconstriction, so that the effect of venous pooling is partly offset. The importance of changes in active compliance can be seen in subjects who have been given an α-blocking drug. The normal postural fall in blood pressure is exaggerated and fainting may occur.

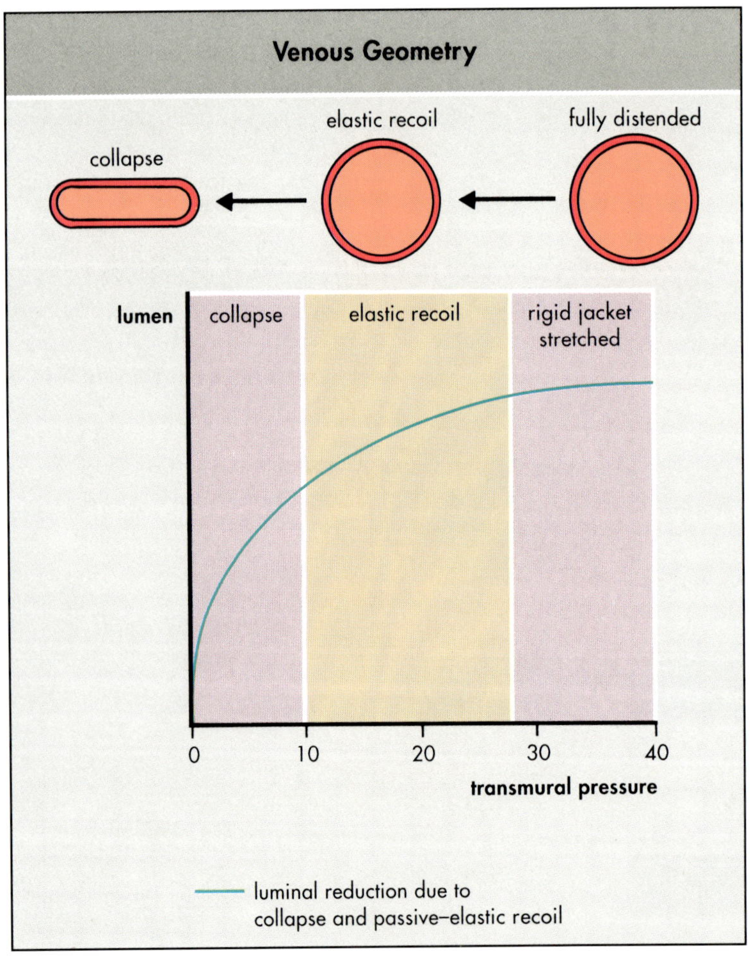

Fig. 2.8 Pressure has direct effects on the geometry and cross-sectional area of the veins.

Mean Circulatory Filling Pressure

The pressure gradient which results in venous return to the right atrium is determined by the mean circulatory filling pressure. This is the pressure in the circulation produced when the pumping action of the heart has been temporarily arrested. For obvious reasons, it is only possible to measure mean circulatory filling pressure in experimental animals, but it probably is about 7mmHg in man. The critical variables determining the mean circulatory pressure are the volume and distribution of blood within the venous bed and the degree of sympathetic efferent activity at the venous adrenoceptors. The contribution of the three major components of the systemic venous system (splanchnic venous bed, muscle and cutaneous veins) to circulatory filling pressure is regulated in slightly different ways (Fig. 2.9). Venous pressure in the splanchnic bed is controlled by cardiovascular reflexes together with extramural pressure exerted by the abdominal vessels. The cutaneous veins are regulated in response to emotional stimuli, changes in respiration and external temperature, predominantly by hypothalamic centres. The skeletal muscle veins, which have few adrenoceptors, are emptied passively by the pumping action of skeletal muscles. The other determinant of mean circulatory filling pressure, the volume of blood within the venous system, is dependent upon the overall blood volume. This can alter as a result of haemorrhage, dehydration, changes in renal excretion or by the entry of blood through the capillary system, which is regulated by the degree of contraction of the precapillary resistance vessels. Thus, dilatation of these vessels, caused by warmth or by vasodilator drugs, increases blood flow to the venous system. This responds by venodilation, increasing capacity and so restoring circulatory filling pressure to normal.

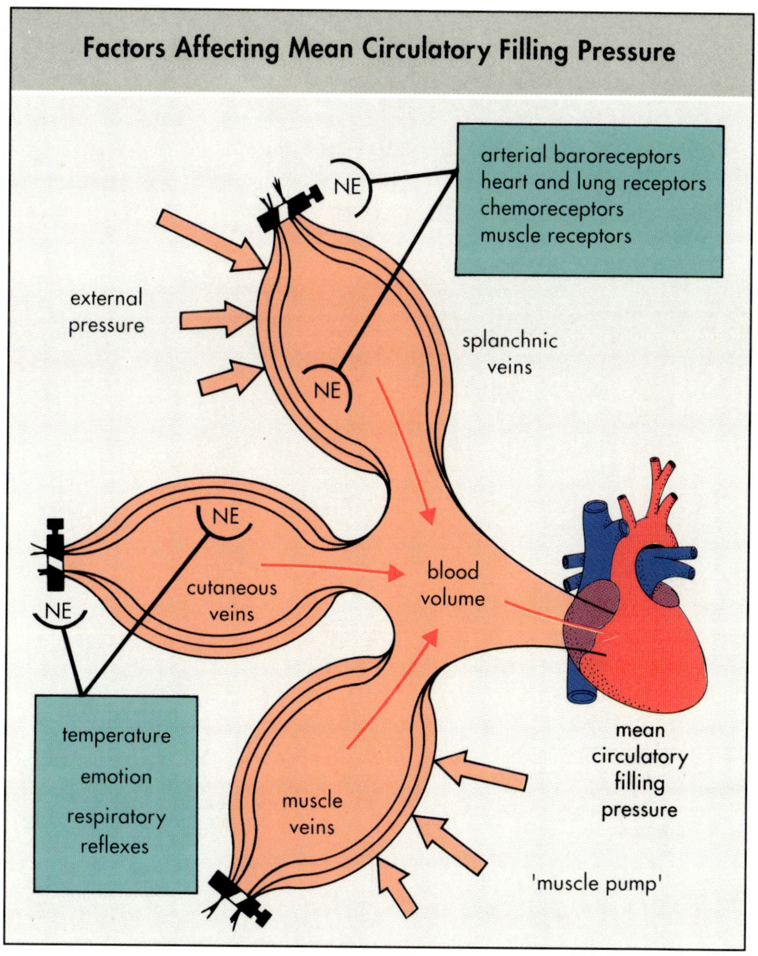

Fig. 2.9 The active expulsion of blood from the splanchnic venous bed is controlled primarily by the cardiovascular reflexes. Expulsion from the veins is governed mainly by local and central temperature changes and by emotion. [Modified from Shepherd & Vanhoutte (1974) *The Human Cardiovascular System: Facts and concepts*. New York: Raven Press.]

PERIPHERAL RESISTANCE

The mean aortic pressure of about 100mmHg in a healthy individual falls to a pressure of 10mmHg at the venous end of the capillary bed. The aorta and large arteries (Windkessel vessels) offer little resistance to flow but form a distensible reservoir bed which damps the left ventricular pressure wave. Pressure falls rapidly along the course of the smaller arteries and arterioles, which are therefore referred to as the precapillary resistance vessels (Fig. 2.10). It is important to bear in mind that overall peripheral resistance represents the sum of resistances in the various tissue beds of the body and that marked variation in the contribution of different tissue beds at different times may occur (see Fig. 2.1). In addition, the contribution of different vessels along the tree to resistance may alter with the degree of vasodilatation (see below).

The flow of fluid through a tube can be expressed by Poiseuille's formula:

$$Q = \frac{\pi r^4 (P_1 - P_2)}{8 l \eta}$$

where r is the radius of the vessel, $(P_1 - P_2)$ is the pressure gradient across its end, l the length of the vessel and η the viscosity of the fluid. Resistance, defined as the pressure gradient divided by the flow, can therefore be expressed by the following equation:

$$r = \frac{8 l \eta}{\pi r^4}$$

The important factor in this equation if r^4. Blood viscosity makes a contribution to vascular resistance in smaller vessels (10–100μm radius), but neither resistance vessel length nor blood viscosity vary sufficiently between individuals to suggest a significant contribution to blood pressure.

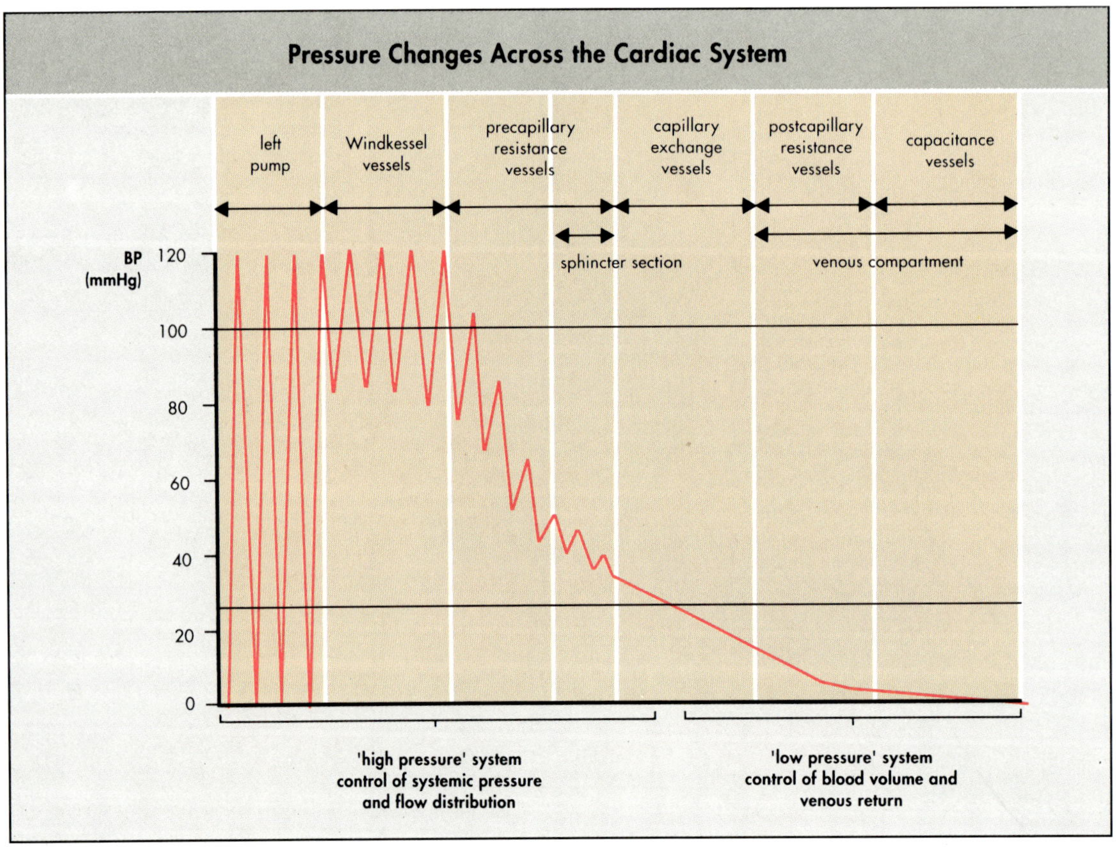

Fig. 2.10 Diagram showing the pressure across the various sections of the cardiovascular system. [For source see Figure 2.6].

The geometry of the resistance vessel is determined by contraction of vascular smooth muscle and by the intrinsic structure of the vessel. Both of these factors come into play in chronic hypertension, where the wall of the resistance vessel is thickened and the lumen reduced (see Fig. 4.2). Reduction in the radius of the resistance vessel bed can be demonstrated by inducing maximal vasodilatation pharmacologically and by warmth. Under these circumstances, vascular resistance is higher in hypertensives, despite the fact that vascular tone is making no contribution to resistance (Fig. 2.11). An increased wall-to-lumen ratio also leads to a greater degree of resistance for a given shortening of vascular smooth muscle (see Fig. 4.4). The reason for this is that vascular contractions originate from the outermost layer of the vascular smooth muscle, a result of the predominantly peripheral distribution of innervation. When smooth muscle contracts the increased wall mass is pushed into the reduced lumen. The reduction in resistance vessel radius is therefore greater than would occur in a normal vessel; the effect on resistance is amplified to the fourth power in accordance with Poiseuille's law. The role of vascular hypertrophy in hypertension is discussed further in chapter 3.

Vasoconstrictor Tone

The resistance vessels are normally under a degree of vasoconstrictor tone. This determines to some extent which vessels make the largest contribution to peripheral resistance. Thus, when arterioles are maximally dilated, slightly larger arteries become more important in determining resistance. The degree of vasoconstriction of the resistance vessels influences pressure distally as well as proximally. Vasodilatation causes an increase in capillary hydrostatic pressure and vasoconstriction reduces it, so long as the calibre of the post-capillary resistance vessels remains unchanged (Fig. 2.12). The consequent alteration in the equilibrium of Starling forces may cause changes in the partition of fluid between the vascular and extra-vascular compartments. This is an important factor in the

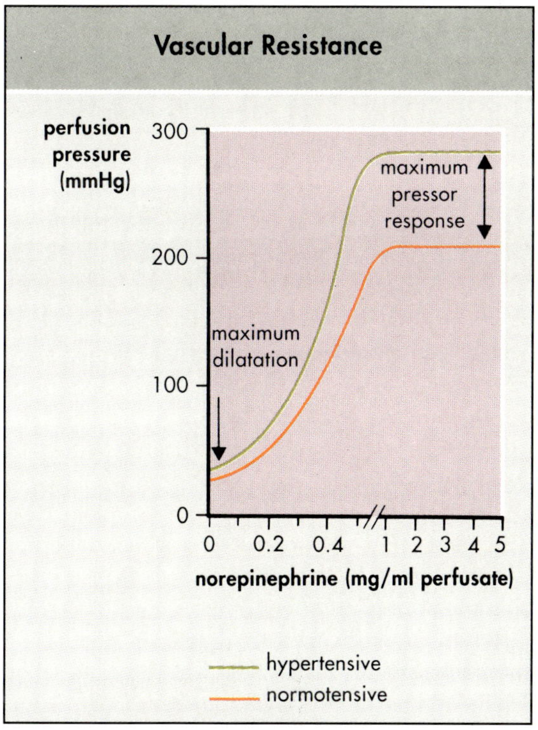

Fig. 2.11 Changes in resistance produced by vasoconstrictor agonist norepinephrine in rat hindquarters showing the effect of increased wall-to-lumen ratio produced by hypertension. [Modified from Folkow, B. (1978) *Clin Sci*, **55**, 3s–22s.]

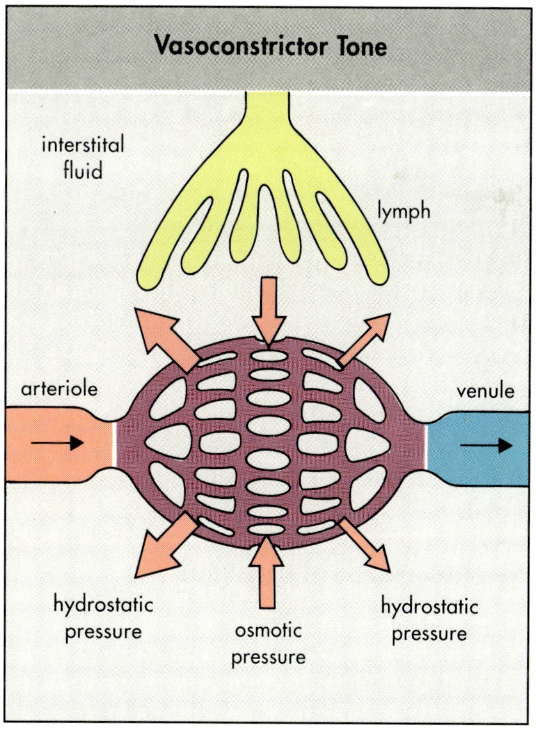

Fig. 2.12 The capillary bed is limited at each end by pre- and post-capillary resistance vessels. Fluid is retained in the capillary bed by a balance of oncotic and hydrostatic pressure.

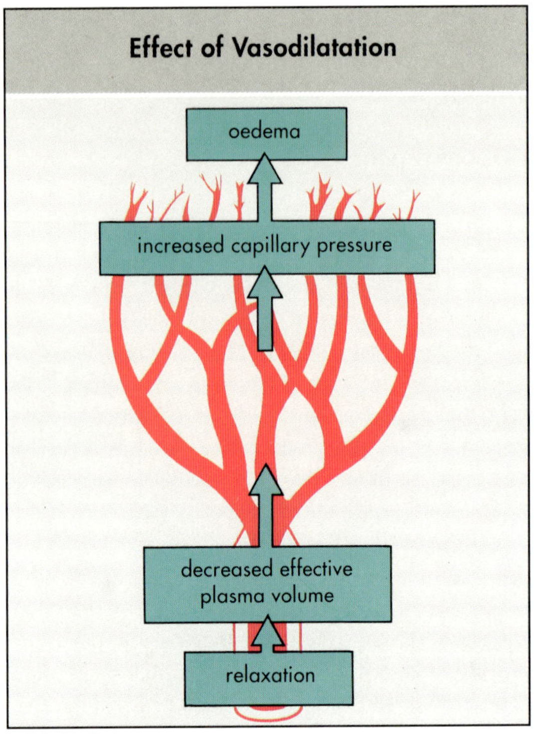

Fig. 2.13 Effect of dilatation of precapillary resistancevessels by diazoxide or warmth. This leads to transudation of fluid (shown as arrows through the capillary bed).

Factors Controlling Resistance Vessel Diameter

autonomic nervous system	catecholamines
circulating	renin–angiotensin ANF kinins vasopressin epinephrine
local humoral	metabolites histamine serotonin renin–angiotensin kallikrein–bradykinin prostaglandins EDRF endothelin
intrinsic	tone autoregulation

Fig. 2.14 Factors controlling resistance vessel diameter.

type of oedema associated with sympathetic denervation of the limb, following minoxidil therapy or prolonged exposure to a high ambient temperature (Fig. 2.13).

Vasoconstrictor tone is under the influence of local factors, circulating factors and neurogenic control. Non-neurogenic factors account for the greater part of vasoconstrictor tone. Thus, sympathetic blockade to (human) limb vessels reduces local resistance by about 50% while maximal vasodilatation is associated with a fall in resistance to 5–10% of baseline values.

Local Regulation of Resistance

The degree of smooth muscle contraction is influenced by the supply and removal of metabolites and by local humoral factors (Fig. 2.14). Vasoconstrictor tone is influenced by the oxygen supply, although the role of oxygen demand as a determinant of resistance under normal physiological circumstances is still debated. Supply of glucose and some B-group vitamins (thiamine and nicotinic acid) may also become rate-limiting under some circumstances. In addition to this, in the face of diminished blood flow the following vasodilator metabolites accumulate:

- carbon dioxide;
- lactic acid;
- adenosine and adenosine phosphates;
- histamine;
- potassium and hydrogen ions.

Autoregulation

The capacity to autoregulate is a fundamental property of vascular smooth muscle. If the perfusion pressure of an artery or arteriole is raised by increasing flow, the smooth muscle will contract to normalize the blood flow even at the expense of maintaining a high proximal pressure (Fig. 2.15). This is probably simply a consequence of the removal of vasodilator metabolites. Conversely, when perfusion pressure is lowered resistance vessels dilate. The result is preservation of blood flow within quite narrow limits over a wide range of

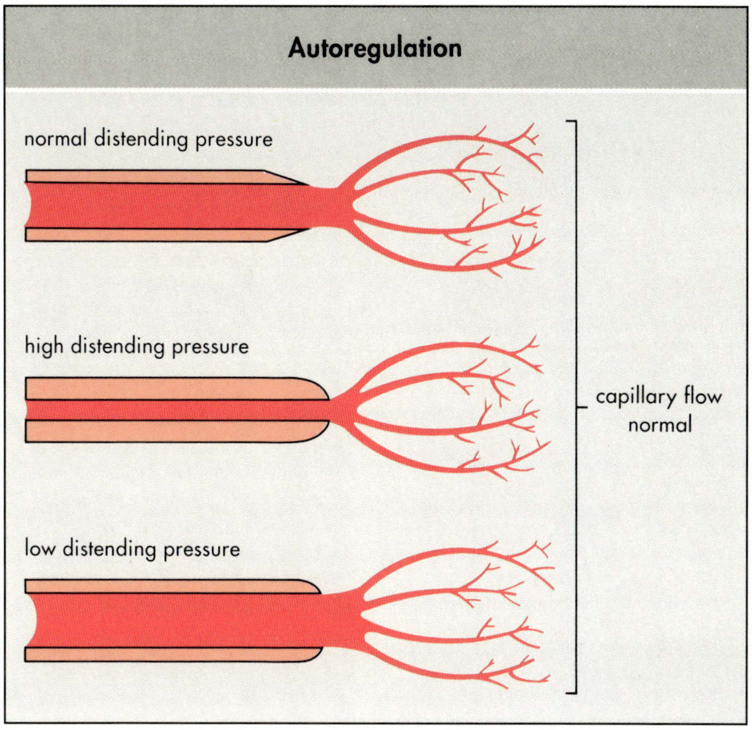

Fig. 2.15 The concept of autoregulation. Increased perfusion pressure causes vascular constriction. Reduced pressure causes vasodilation. In all cases, capillary flow is constant.

pressures (Fig. 2.16). This process, known as autoregulation, has an important homeostatic function in protecting tissues from over- or under-perfusion. The autoregulatory pressure range does, of course, have limits. Perfusion pressures outside the autoregulatory range cause blood flow to increase or decrease in proportion to pressure.

Not all tissues can autoregulate. For instance, renomedullary blood flow is closely related to pressure over the physiological range of renal perfusion pressures. After a stroke or head injury the cerebral vasculature loses its capacity to autoregulate. As a result, therapeutic blood pressure lowering after a stroke may cause a reduction in cerebral blood flow and cerebral infarction (see chapter 10).

The autoregulatory range is altered by resistance vessel hypertrophy. Thus, the upper limit of the autoregulatory range is elevated in chronic hypertension (see Fig. 2.16). The cerebral vasculature is thus protected against increased cerebral blood flow, local oedema and hypertensive encephalopathy. The trade-off, however, is a similar elevation of the lower limit of the autoregulatory range. A reduction in blood pressure to levels which a

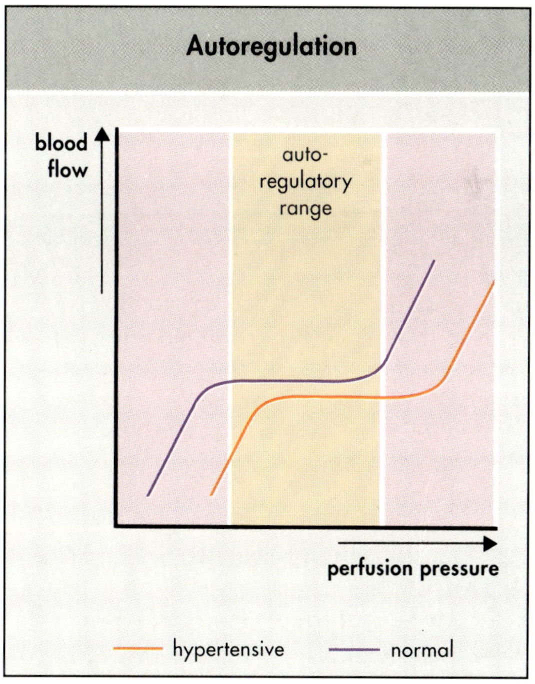

Fig. 2.16 Autoregulatory curve of the renal cortex and cerebral vessels, showing that if pressure is raised or lowered, flow remains constant over a certain range; beyond this range, flow and pressure are proportional to each other. In hypertension, the autoregulatory range is raised.

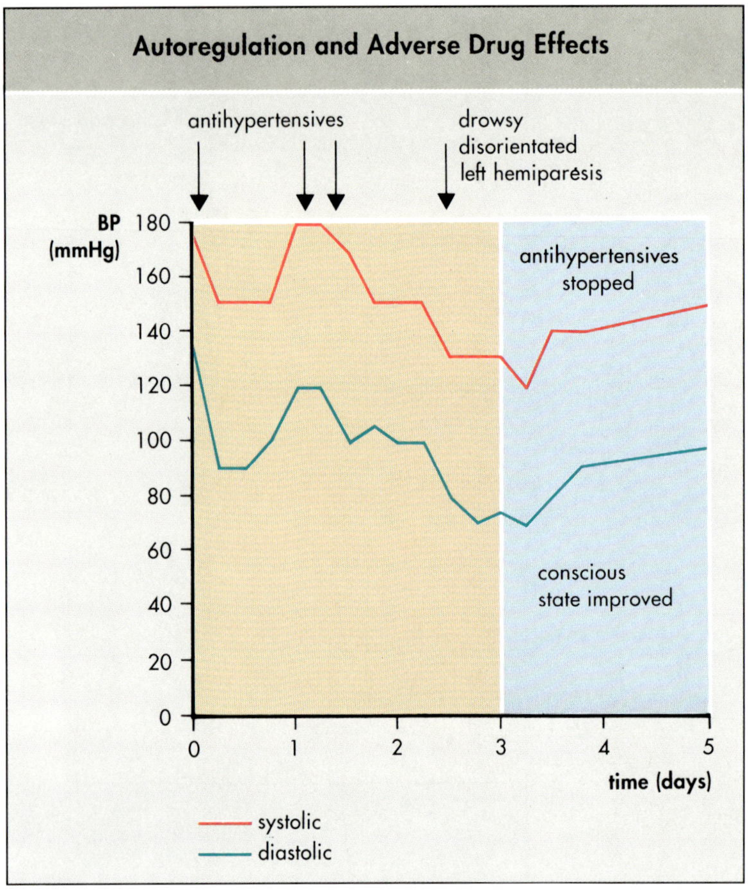

Fig. 2.17 The consequences of excessive lowering of blood pressure. A severely hypertensive patient was treated with antihypertensive drugs. After two days blood pressure control was imperfect and further, different drugs were prescribed. Over the next 24 hours blood pressure fell gradually; at the same time the patient became drowsy and disorientated and developed weakness on the left side of the face. A brain scan was normal. With the blood pressure at 130/75mmHg, therapy was stopped. Over the next two days blood pressure rose steadily and the patient became more alert. However, signs of parietal lobe dysfunction became more obvious; the patient was dysphasic and dyspraxic. [Modified from Ledingham, J. & Rajagopalan, B. (1979) *Q J Med*, **48**, 25–41.]

healthy individual would tolerate therefore produces a fall in cerebral blood flow in hypertensive patients. There are many case reports of patients who have developed cerebral infarction as a result of rapid pharmocological lowering of blood pressure to levels generally regarded as quite acceptable (mean blood pressure of 90–100mmHg in patients whose normal mean pressure was 160–180mmHg) (Fig. 2.17).

LOCAL HUMORAL REGULATION OF BLOOD FLOW

A number of vasoactive substances are produced locally by resistance vessels. They probably play an important role in the local regulation of blood flow in response to specific local stimuli such as tissue injury. Their role in the sustained increase in peripheral resistance observed in hypertension is more controversial.

Vasodilator Factors

Kallikrein–Kinin System

Kallikrein is an enzyme synthesized by several organs, including the kidneys, salivary glands and pancreas (Fig. 2.18). Renal kallikreins release the decapeptide lysyl bradykinin (Kallidin) from kininogens while glandular kallikrein forms bradykinin from these precursors. Both bradykinin and kallidin are potent vasodilators. Locally released kinins also increase capillary permeability – high local concentrations produce oedema. Kinins also cause vasodilatation indirectly by activating prostaglandin synthesis with the consequent production of prostacyclin and PGE_2. There is evidence to support a local role for the generation of kinin in mediation of vasodilatation associated with inflammation. Local kinins may be involved in renal blood flow control, but their role in other tissue beds is uncertain.

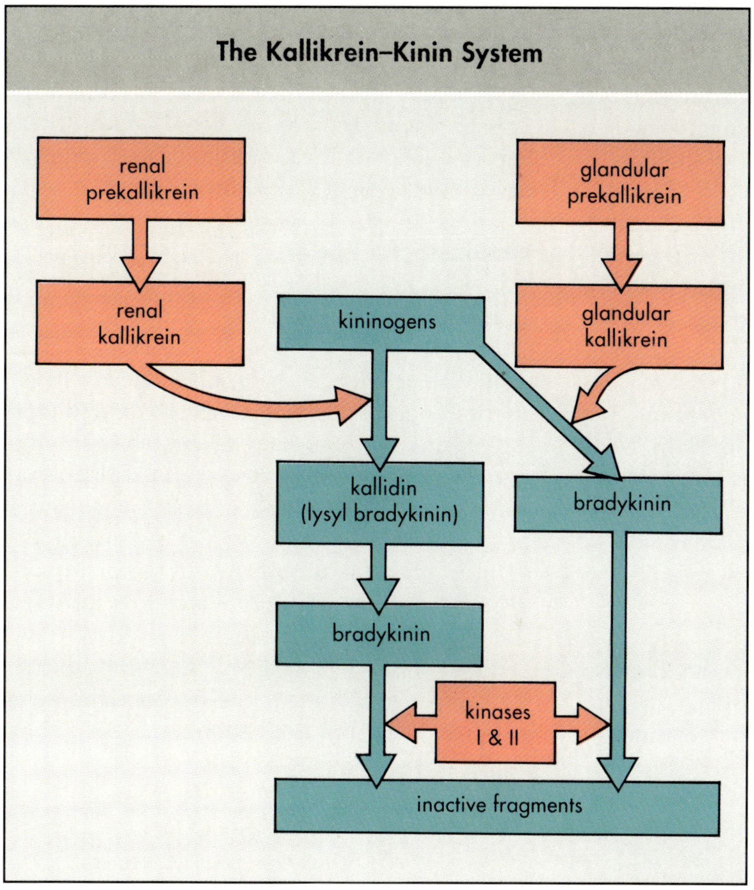

Fig. 2.18 The kallikrein–kinin system.

Histamine

Histamine causes both vasodilatation and increased permeability. There is no evidence that it has a role in the overall regulation of peripheral resistance.

Endothelial-derived Relaxant Factor

Acetylcholine normally causes relexation of the rabbit aorta. If the endothelium is removed by rubbing this action is lost (Fig. 2.19). The endothelium must therefore release locally a factor which relaxes smooth muscle in response to stimuli such as acetylcholine. A similar endothelial mechanism mediates the vasodilator response to histamine, bradykinin and substance P. Local release of EDRF can be demonstrated by perfusing two arteries in sequence. Active material which relaxes the second vessel is then demonstrable on stimulating the first. Studies such as this have shown that the material has a half-life of only a few seconds.

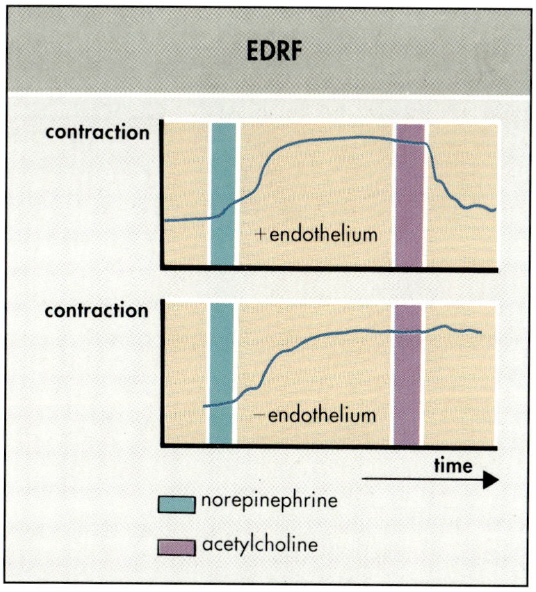

Fig. 2.19 Endothelial derived relaxant factor. Rabbit aorta is contracted with norepinephrine. It can normally be relaxed wiith acetylcholine, but this response is not seen when the endothelium is removed.

Recently EDRF has been identified as nitric oxide, a metabolite which is also responsible for the relaxation of vessels produced by nitrates and sodium nitroprusside and which acts through the cyclic GMP second messenger system. Whether other relaxant factors are involved in addition to nitric oxide is unknown.

There are marked regional differences and species differences in the EDRF response. However, it has now been demonstrated not only in the aorta but also in muscular arteries and pre-capillary resistance vessels. Its role in the overall regulation of resistance is unknown but it may be of importance when endothelial damage has occurred (for instance in association with atheroma). Depression of EDRF has been demonstrated in both large vessels and resistance vessels of some experimental models of hypertension.

Prostacyclin

This prostanoid is derived from endothelial membrane phospholipids (Fig. 2.20). Prostacyclin synthesis is stimulated by bradykinin, thrombin, platelet derived growth factor (PDGF) and adenine nucleotides. Prostacyclin has a short half-life in the blood stream (1–2 minutes) but may play an important role in the local regulation of resistance. Some studies have shown a reduction in urinary prostacyclin metabolites in subjects with essential hypertension, although whether this is a primary or secondary change is unknown.

Vasconstrictor Factors

Renin–Angiotensin System

Renin-like activity can be demonstrated in larger arteries. Some of this activity may be derived from the plasma by the uptake of circulating renin; some may be due to proteases other than renin that are, nevertheless, able to release angiotensin from renin substrate. However, recent studies using molecular biological techniques have demonstrated renin mRNA in aortae. In addition, some vascular beds release angiotensin II when perfused with synthetic media, suggesting that all the components of the renin–angiotensin system are present within the beds themselves. Such locally derived angiotensin II could act as a local

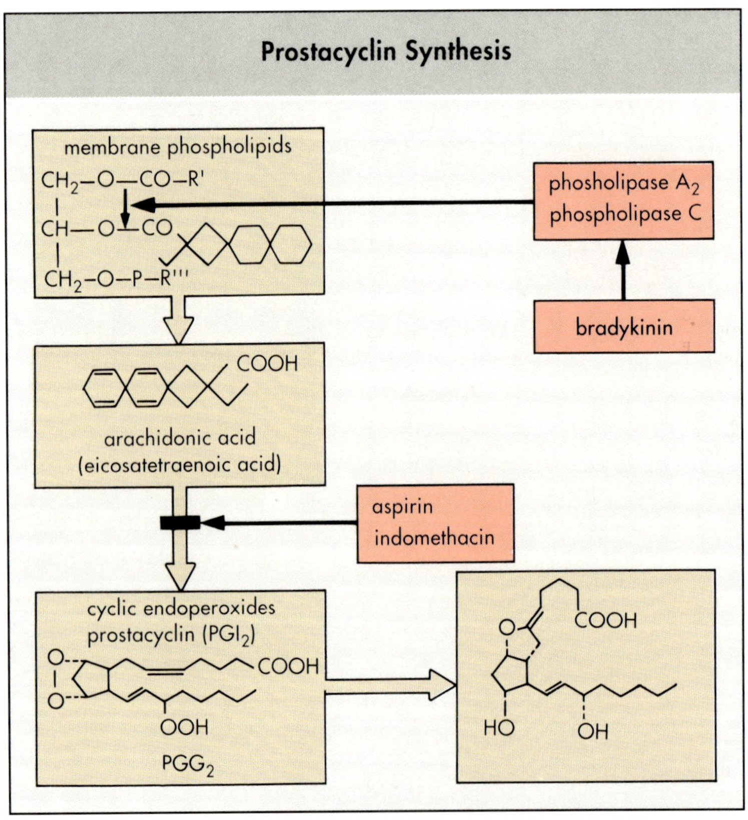

Fig. 2.20 Prostacyclin is derived from endothelial membrane phospholipids.

vasoconstrictor system and also – through interaction with presynaptic α_2-receptors – potentiate sympathetically induced vasoconstrictor tone (Fig. 2.21). Thus, vasoconstriction in isolated mesenteric blood vessels produced by electrical stimulation is potentiated by renin substrate and inhibited by blockade of the renin–angiotensin system.

Endothelin

Endothelin is a 21 amino acid polypeptide produced by cultured pig aortic endothelial cells (Fig. 2.22). It is the most potent vasoconstrictor agent known. In contrast to EDRF it has a prolonged action (40–60 minutes) in isolated arteries, which

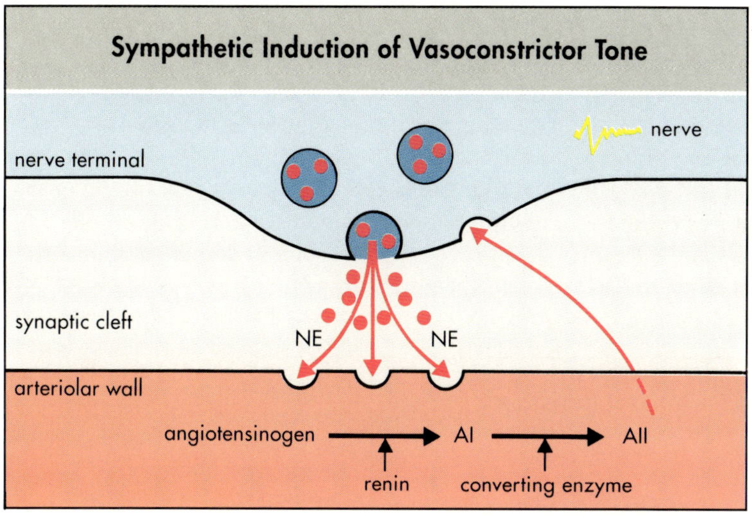

Fig. 2.21 Angiotensin II generated within the arteriolar wall potentiates the constrictor response to nerve stimulation by acting on presynaptic receptors in the nerve terminal.

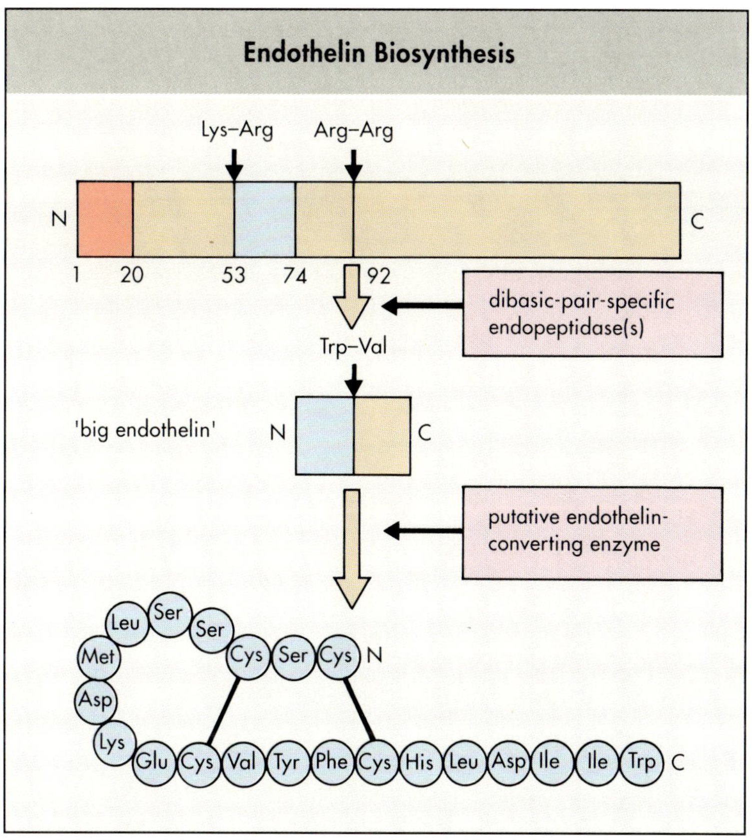

Fig. 2.22 Possible pathway of endothelin biosynthesis. The putative secretory signal sequence and the endothelin sequence are shown by the red and blue boxes respectively.

is mediated by voltage dependent calcium channels. Endothelin's long duration of action probably precludes any involvement in acute regulation of blood pressure, although it may be of importance in regulating local blood flow in response, for instance, to injury.

Serotonin

This powerful vasoconstrictor (5-hydroxytriptamine) is released locally from platelets. It is synthesized in a number of tissues, including the enterochromaffin cells of the gastrointestinal mucosa, the brain and peripheral nervous system (particularly in the gastrointestinal tract). Platelet stores are formed by uptake and not by synthesis. Although serotonin may be important in the regulation of blood pressure, this is through its role as a neurotransmitter. There is no evidence that locally derived serotonin is important in the overall regulation of resistance.

Circulating Factors

Some of the systems which play a local role may also be important systemically. This is most obvious in the case of the renin–angiotensin system which is discussed below. Some workers have postulated a systemic role for the kallikrein–kinin system. Thus, a competitive antagonist of bradykinin has been reported to raise blood pressure when injected in high concentrations into rats. It has further been argued that some of the blood pressure lowering action of converting enzyme inhibitors is due to decreased kinin clearance although this explanation is still debated (see

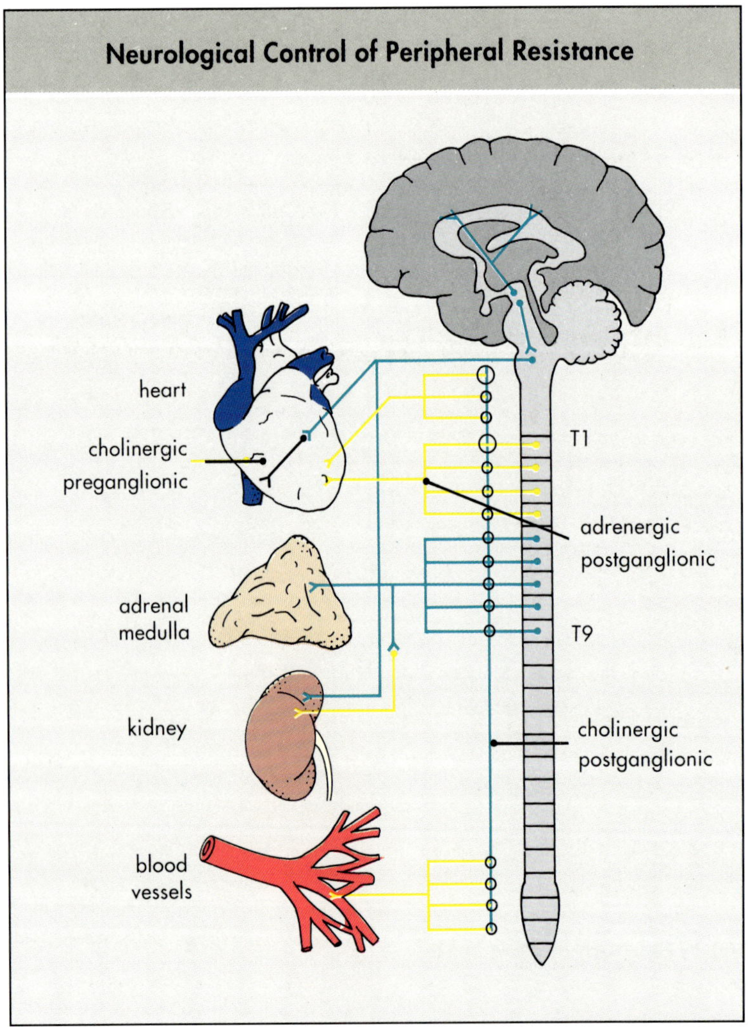

Fig. 2.23 Efferent pathways of the autonomic nervous system involved in blood pressure control. The neurohumoral transmitter of all preganglionic fibres and all postganglionic parasympathetic fibres is acetylcholine. Of the latter the most important is the vagal parasympathetic supply to the heart, activation of which causes slowing of the cardiac rate. Most postganglionic sympathetic fibres are adrenergic (the transmitter is norepinephrine). These fibres are important in vasomotor control and also in some renal functions influencing blood pressure (renin secretion, fluid and electrolyte secretion. The adrenal medulla is functionally analogous to a sympathetic ganglion, although the principal catecholamine released is epinephrine rather than norepinephrine.

chapter 9). While vasopressin has a vasoconstrictor action, the plasma levels necessary to produce an effect on blood pressure are higher than the levels needed to produce an antidiuretic action. Under normal physiological conditions plasma levels of vasopressin are probably not important in blood pressure regulation.

Circulating norephinephrine for the main part represents an overflow of neurotransmitter from the sympathetic neuronal junction: very little is secreted by the adrenal medulla. The pressor action of norepinephrine is the result of an action upon vascular α-receptors causing vasoconstriction. Epinephrine secreted by the adrenal medulla has a mixed action upon both α-vasoconstrictor and ß-vasodilator adrenoceptors – it causes an increase in blood flow to cardiac muscle, skeletal muscle and liver and a decrease in blood flow to kidneys, skin and gastrointestinal tract (the fight or flight reaction).

Neurological Control of Peripheral Resistance

Sympathetic nerves contain vasoconstrictor and, to a more limited degree, vasodilator fibres (Fig. 2.23). The vasoconstrictor fibres release norepinephrine into the neuroeffector cleft in the outer part of the vascular media. Noradrenaline binds to α-receptors to initiate contraction.

There are also vasodilator sympathetic nerve fibres to skeletal muscle resistance vessels; they use acetylcholine as a neurotransmitter, binding to post-synaptic cholinergic receptors. These mediate increased skeletal muscle blood flow at the initiation of exercise.

In addition to the above, salivary glands, some gastrointestinal glands and the external genitalia are all supplied by parasympathetic vasodilator nerves. These are, however, not of importance in the regulation of overall resistance.

Efferent sympathetic innervation of blood vessels is therefore responsible for α-mediated vasocontriction, while ß-adrenoceptors responding to circulating epinephrine induce vasodilatation and a decrease in peripheral resistance.

The classification of adrenoceptors into α and ß types has been taken further, giving distinct subclasses which have different properties and different responses to specific drugs (Fig. 2.24). $ß_1$-mediated effects include tachycardia and increased myocardial contractility, associated with a decreased refractory period. Activation of $ß_2$-receptors produces skeletal and coronary vessel

Adrenoceptor Responses

effector organs		adrenergic impulses	
		receptor type	responses
kidney		$ß_2$	renin secretion
heart	S-A node	$ß_1$	increase in heart rate ++
	atria	$ß_1$	increase in contractility and conduction velocity ++
	A-V node	$ß_1$	increase in automaticity and conduction velocity ++
	His-Purkinje system	$ß_1$	
	ventricles	$ß_1$	increase in contractility, automaticity, conduction velocity and rate of idioventricular pacemakers +++
veins (systemic)		$\alpha_1 ß_2$	constriction +; dilatation ++
arterioles	coronary	$\alpha_1 ß_2$	constriction +; dilatation +
	skin and mucosa	α	constriction +++
	skeletal muscle	$\alpha_1 ß_2$	constriction ++; dilatation ++
	cerebral	α	constriction (slight)
	pulmonary	$\alpha_1 ß_2$	constriction +; dilatation +
		α	constriction +++
	abdominal		constriction +++
	viscera; renal		dilatation +

Fig 2.24 Table showing responses of α,ß, and $ß_2$ adrenoceptors.

dilatation, bronchial and uterine muscle relaxation, hyperglycaemia, lactic acidaemia and an increase in free fatty acids. There are also ß-receptors situated on the pre-synaptic membrane of the neuronal cleft which are activated by low concentrations of norepinephrine (acting as a positive feedback mechanism). By contrast, presynaptic α-receptors turn off norepinephrine secretion (a negative feedback mechanism). There are important pharmacological differences between peripheral, pre- and post-synaptic α-receptors. They have therefore been reclassified as α_2 and α_1 receptors. Some α_2-receptors (for instance those within the CNS) are located on the post-synaptic membrane (Fig. 2.25). The terms pre- and post-synaptic α-receptors are therefore misleading and should be discarded.

The autonomic nervous system may also have an indirect effect on blood pressure, influencing renin secretion and sodium excretion by the kidney.

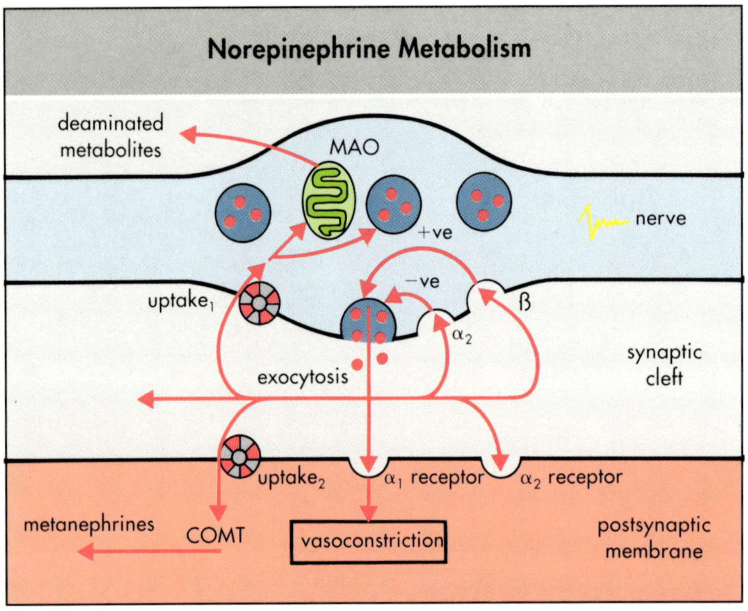

Fig. 2.25 Metabolic pathways in the storage, release and clearance of norepinephrine from a nerve ending. NE = norepinephrine. MAO = monoamine oxidase. COMT = catechol-O-methyltransferase.

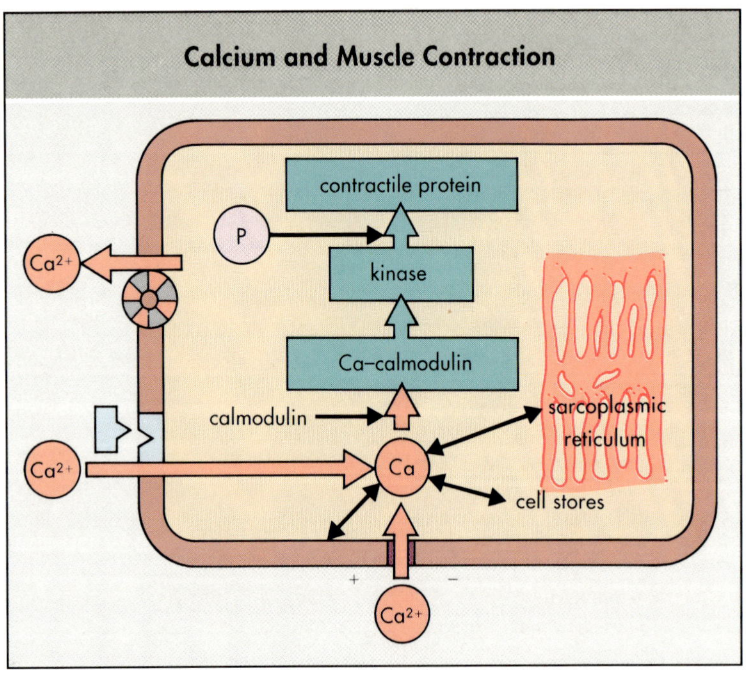

Fig. 2.26 Calcium-mediated pathways for contraction of vascular smooth muscle.

SECOND MESSENGER SYSTEMS

Contraction of vascular smooth muscle is initiated by phosphorylation of the myosin light chain of the contractile protein actomyosin. The chain of events leading to phosphorylation is triggered by the binding of a hormone or neurotransmitter to a receptor on the cell's surface. The linkage between the process occurring on the outer surface of the cell membrane and contraction is termed 'chemo-mechanical coupling' and is achieved by second messenger systems (Fig. 2.26).

The immediate stimulus to myosin light chain kinase activation is a rise in free intracellular calcium which binds calmodulin, a receptor protein. The resulting calcium–calmodulin complex activates myosin light chain kinase. Three systems mediate the increase in cytosolic calcium and therefore vascular smooth muscle contraction. These are:

- a voltage operated calcium channel which responds to depolarization of smooth muscle cell membrane.
- a receptor-regulated calcium channel responding, for instance, to noradrenaline;
- an increase in water soluble phosphoinostides, of which inositol trisphosphate is probably the most important (Fig. 2.27).

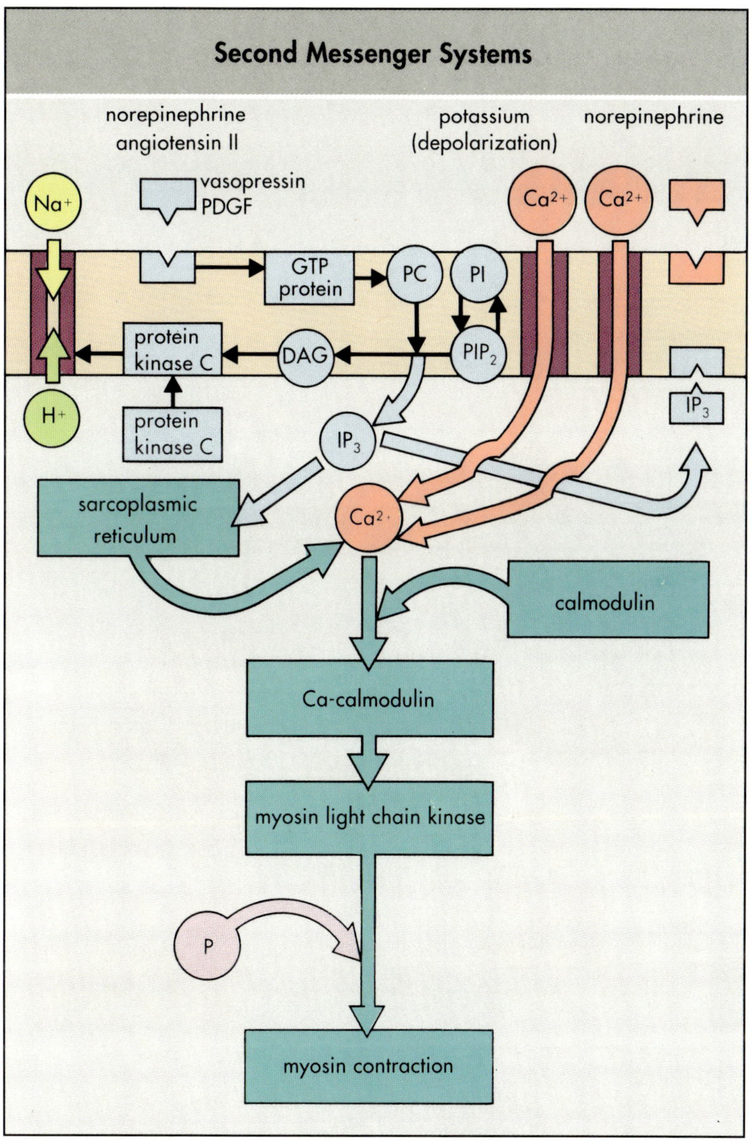

Fig. 2.27 The phosphoinositide second messenger system and other transmembrane pathways mediating vascular smooth muscle contraction.

The Water Soluble Phosphoinositides

These compounds are chemical second messengers which stimulate the release of calcium from intracellular stores. They are produced by hydrolysis of phosphatidyl inositol bisphosphate (PIP_2) as a result of activation of the enzyme phospholipase C. PIP_2 is the result of phosphorylation of membrane phosphatidyl inositol. All of these phospholipids are normal components of the cell membrane. The phosphoinositol second messenger system therefore provides a system with transmits information from the lipid environment of the cell membrane to the aqueous intracellular enviroment. The hydrolysis of PIP_2 also releases diacyl glycerol. This remains within the cell membrane and is an activator of protein kinase C. This enzyme is a regulator of the sodium–proton exchange and therefore of intracellular pH which is concerned with cell growth and differentiation. (It is now clear that the phosphoinositide–diacylglycerol system may regulate growth and differentiation independendently of cell alkalinization.) As a result, the same messenger system which is intimately concerned with contraction may also be involved with structural changes (Fig. 2.28). This may explain why substances such as angiotensin II, which exert their effect through the phosphoinositide system, also have a trophic action in vascular smooth muscle cultures. The link between agonist binding to a receptor and activation of phospholipase C may involve the GTP binding protein, a special membrane signal protein which is also involved in the regulation of second messenger systems that mediate relaxation (see below).

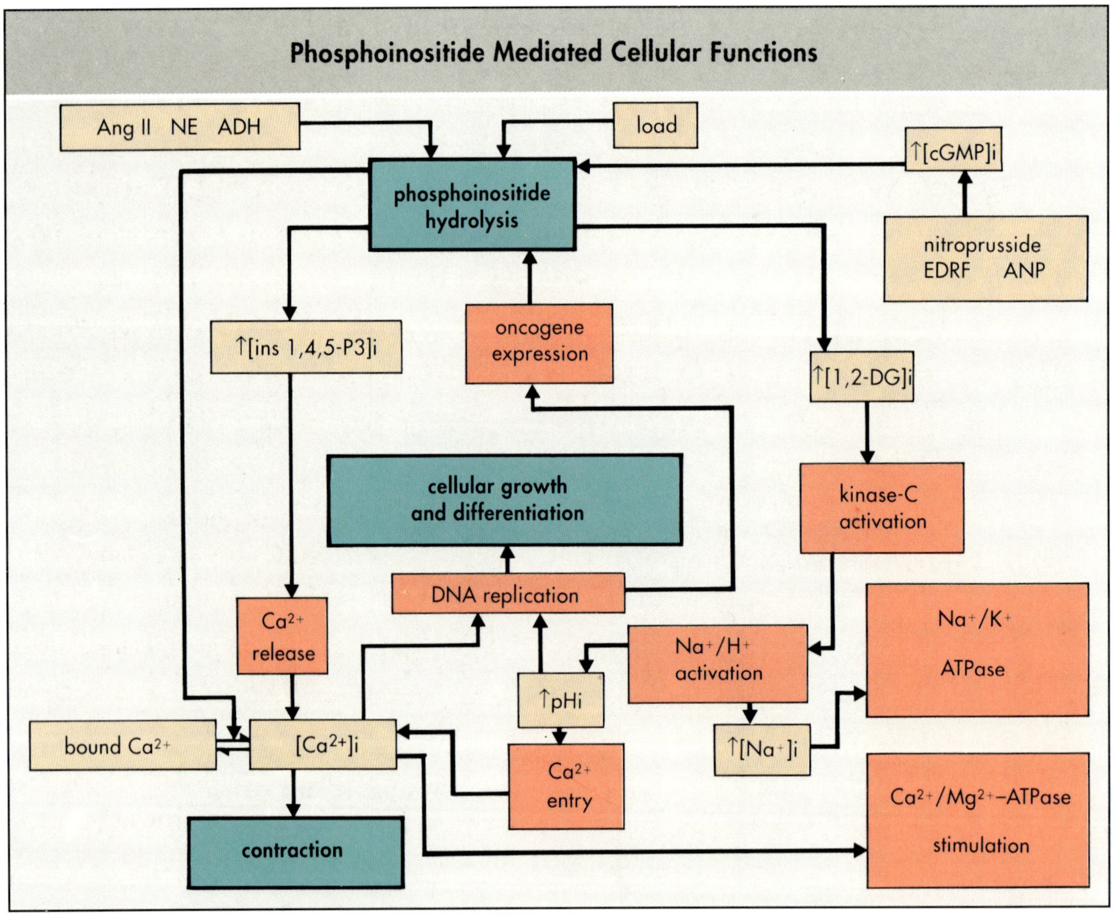

Fig. 2.28 Cellular functions mediated or influenced by phosphoinositide lipids in smooth muscle.
EDRF = endothelial-derived relaxing factor; ANP = atrial natriuretic peptide. [Modified from Heagerty, A. M. & Ollerenshaw, J. D. (1987) *J Hypertension*, **5**, 515–524.]

Intracellular Messengers

Two intracellular chemical messengers mediate relaxation of vascular smooth muscle, namely cyclic AMP (cAMP) and cyclic GMP (cGMP).

cAMP is formed when a ß-agonist combines with its receptor. The receptor stimulation causes a change in the configuration of the GTP binding protein. This activates adenylate cyclase and cAMP is generated (Fig. 2.29). cAMP decreases smooth muscle tone in two ways:

- by increasing the incorporation of free calcium into the intracellular stores;
- by decreasing the calcium sensitivity of the contractile protein.

cGMP is generated by guanylate cyclase. This enzyme occurs in two quite distinct forms, one soluble and the other membrane-bound. The soluble form is activated by drugs such as nitrate, sodium nitroprusside and arachidonic acid and its immediate metabolite. Atrial natriuretic factor and EDRF are believed to activate membrane-bound (particulate) guanylate cyclase. Cyclic GMP relaxes vascular smooth muscle by reducing free (second messenger) calcium levels.

Smooth Muscle Contraction

Phosphorylation of the myosin light chain induces the formation of cross bridges between filaments of the contractile protein. The formation of these cross bridges causes the movement of filaments which gives rise to contraction (Fig. 2.30). This occurs at relatively high free cytosolic calcium levels. As calcium falls after stimulation of the smooth muscle cell, the cross bridges are converted into non-phosphorylated latch bridges which require a much lower energy expenditure to maintain tonic vasoconstriction. It has been estimated that skeletal muscle would require 300 times as much ATP to maintain a similar vascular resistance, Relaxation occurs when cytosolic calcium falls to a low level and all cross bridges are inactivated.

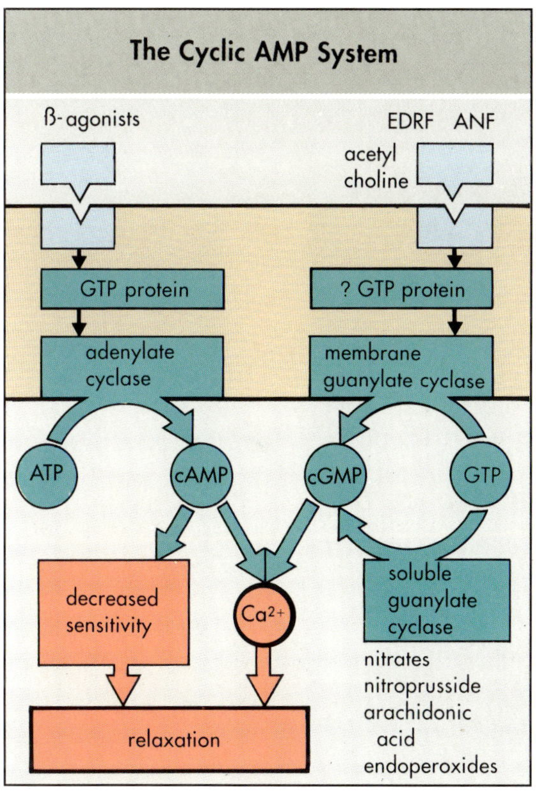

Fig. 2.29 The cyclic AMP system for mediation of smooth muscle relaxation.

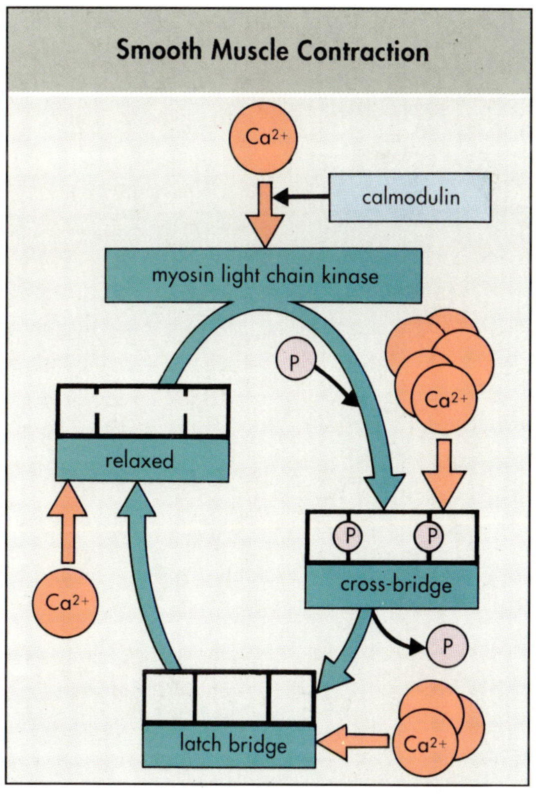

Fig. 2.30 The molecular mechanism of smooth muscle contraction.

CENTRAL REGULATION OF BLOOD PRESSURE

Both cardiac output and peripheral resistance are regulated by the brain stem vasomotor centre, which integrates information received from the higher nervous centres and from the circulatory baroreceptors through afferent fibres. This centre is situated in the reticular substance of the lower third of the pons and the upper two-thirds of the medulla. Thus, when the brain stem is transected above the lower third of the pons, blood pressure is maintained. However when the brainstem is transected just below this level, blood pressure falls substantially. Transection experiments of this sort have indicated that the upper and lateral parts of the vasomotor centre are excitatory while the medial and lower parts are inhibitory. Stimulation of the latter areas therefore causes a fall in blood pressure. Direct inhibitory and excitatory fibres descend the spinal cord where they form synapses with efferent fibres to the heart and blood vessels (Fig. 2.31). The vasomotor centre is also closely associated with the dorsal motor nucleus of the vagus through which cholinergic (parasympathetic) vagal fibres are conveyed to the heart. These fibres are inhibitory and maintain a constant inhibitory tone to the heart. Fibres from the vasomotor centre maintain sympathetic tone to the blood vessels.

The level of tonic activity exerted by the vasomotor centre on the heart and blood vessels is modified by impulses from other parts of the brain. Impulses from baroreceptor afferents are conveyed through the nucleus of the tractus solitarius. Lesions to this structure therefore block inhibitory impulses from the arterial baroreceptors and cause increased activity in the excitatory part of the

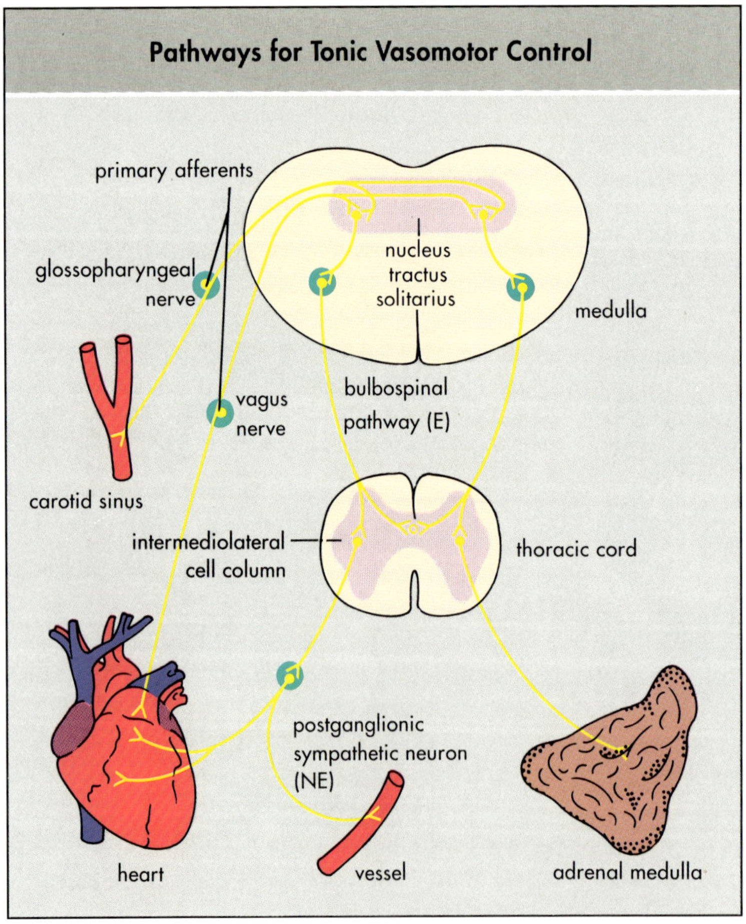

Fig. 2.31 Pathways for tonic vasomotor control and baroreceptor reflex pathway.

vasomotor centre, a massive increase in sympathetic efferent activity and severe hypertension. The vasomotor centre is also influenced by the activity of higher areas of the brain. These include the mid-brain, hypothalamus and cerebral cortex (Fig. 2.32). Separate centres of the hypothalamus have excitatory or inhibitory actions on the vasomotor centre. Thus, nuclei situated in the anterior part of the hypothalamus cause a mild pressor or depressor effect while nuclei in the posterior lateral part of the hypothalamus cause mainly pressor reactions when stimulated. There is particular interest in the anteroventral third ventricular (AV3V) region. The excitatory activity of this part of the hypothalamus seems to be essential for development of experimental renovascular and DOC–salt hypertension.

An important function of the vasomotor centre is to provide an integrated circulatory response to stimuli from the outside environment and from within the circulation. Thus, in response to acute stress, increased sympathetic efferent activity regulated by the vasomotor centre causes widespread peripheral vasoconstriction and increased tone in the capacitance vessels. This raises mean circulatory filling pressure and increases cardiac output; decreased vagal tone and increased sympathetic drive serves to increase cardiac output still further. When cerebral perfusion pressure falls below the autoregulatory range, reduced blood flow to the vasomotor centre causes ischaemia with accumulation of local metabolites. The vasomotor centre responds by causing a massive increase in sympathetic outflow with vasoconstriction, increased cardiac output and hypertension. The same response is observed when intracranial pressure is raised, compressing the arteries to the brain stem (the Cushing reaction – see Fig. 2.33).

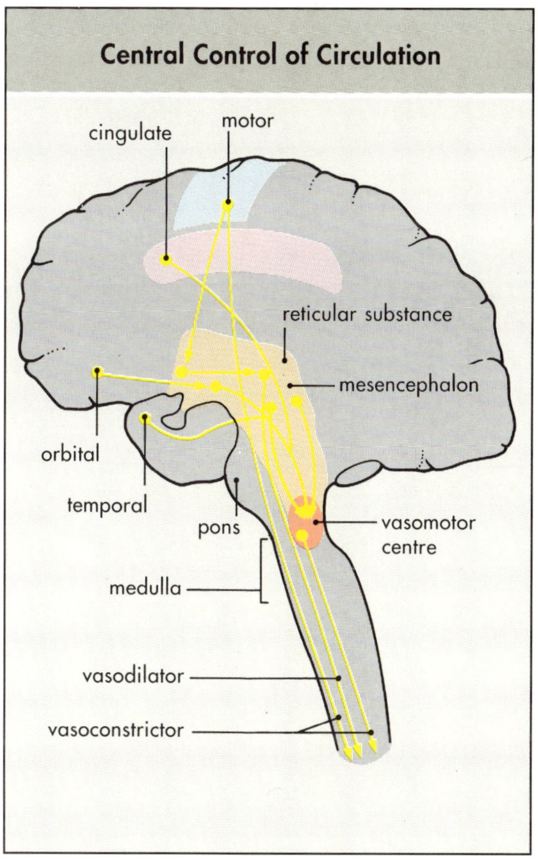

Fig. 2.32 A number of areas in the brain play important roles in the circulatory regulation.

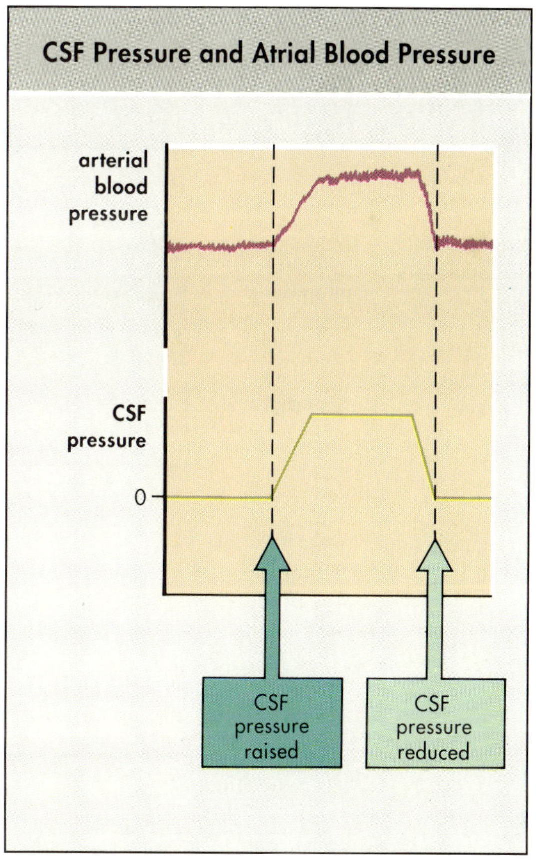

Fig. 2.33 The effect of CSF pressure on atrial blood pressure.

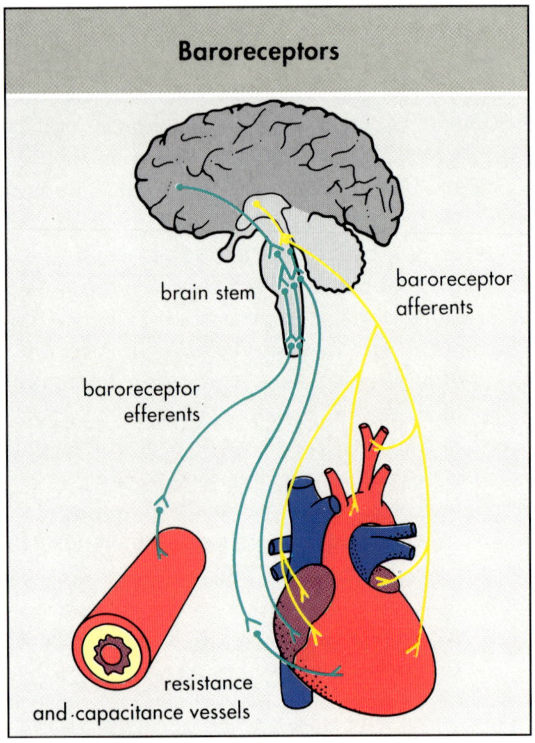

Fig. 2.34 Diagram showing the baroreceptors and their links to the central nervous system.

The Arterial Baroreceptors

The baroreceptors are stretch receptors situated in the wall of a blood vessel or in the heart. The most important baroreceptors in blood pressure regulation are situated in the carotid sinus, lying on the internal carotid artery just above the bifurcation and supplied by the 9th cranial (glossopharyngeal) nerve through Hering's nerve. The aortic baroreceptors lie on the walls of the aortic arch and are supplied by the vagi and sympathetic afferents to the spinal cord (Fig. 2.34).

The carotid and aortic baroreceptors respond to increased perfusion pressure by an increase in discharge rate (Fig. 2.35). When blood pressure is stable the impulses in afferent fibres from the baroreceptors are phasic, showing a burst with systole and no activity during diastole. Baroreceptors respond to a stable elevation in blood pressure by an initial increase, until discharge is almost continuous, followed by a steady reduction (resetting, see below).

Arterial baroreceptor reflexes influence heart rate, atrioventricular conduction and peripheral resistance. The overall activity of these reflexes in

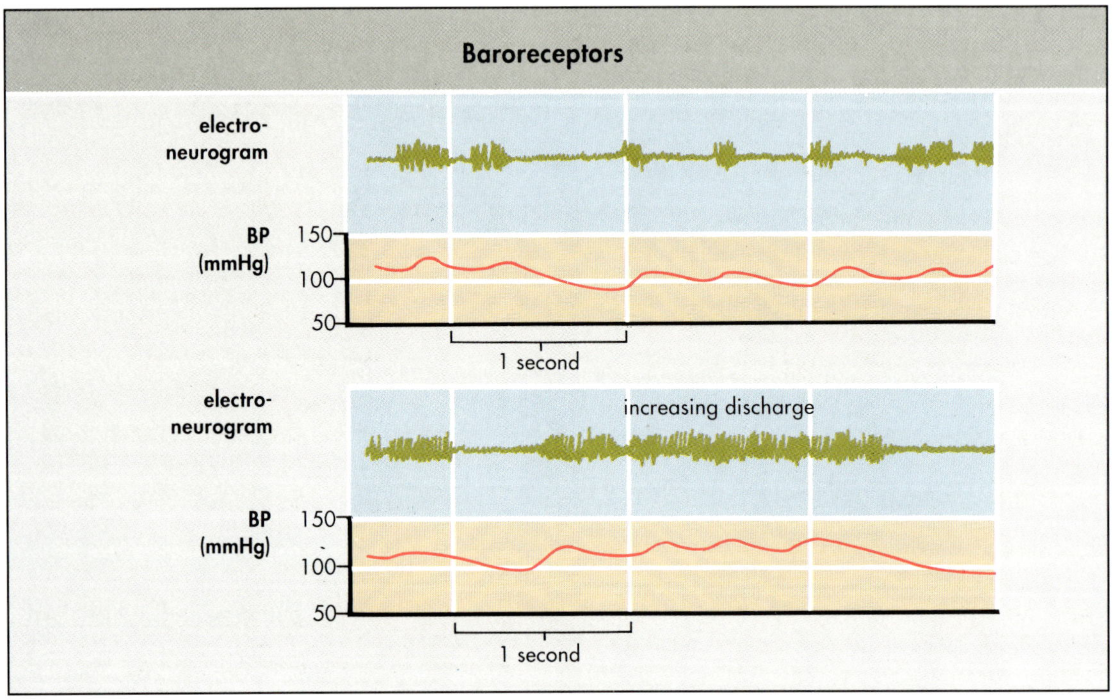

Fig. 2.35 Record of action potentials from baroreceptors showing that elevation of systemic blood pressure is associated with a reduction in frequency of impulses, while a fall in blood pressure is associated with increased frequency.

the regulation of heart rate can be assessed by injecting a drug which raises blood pressure without having any direct effect on the heart – the degree of slowing of heart rate is a measure of baroreceptor activity. The most frequently used drug is phenylephrine, an α-agonist without direct action on the heart. Blood pressure can be raised 20–30mmHg acutely using a bolus injection (Fig. 2.36); sustained elevation can be produced by a steady infusion (the ramp method). Since the sympathetic effects of baroreceptor stimulation develop more slowly than vagal effects, the ramp method is superior for assessing both components. The sympathetic component of the baroreceptor reflex can be assessed by blocking cardiac ß-receptors with propranolol, while vagal inhibition of heart rate can be blocked by the anti-cholinergic drug atropine. Using these agents it has been possible to show that the reduction in heart rate produced by increased arterial pressure is mediated through an increase in vagal tone to the heart. The increased heart rate produced by a blood pressure reduction also appears initially to be largely mediated by the vagus, but after a few seconds sympathetic activation also plays a part. Complementary changes can be demonstrated in peripheral resistance. Thus, elevation of perfusion pressure to the arterial baroreceptors inhibits vasomotor tone and *vice versa*. Atropine does not influence the baroreceptor mediated changes in peripheral resistance, indicating that cholinergic sympathetic fibres do not have a role in its production.

The two major groups of arterial baroreceptors probably play rather different roles. Thus in dogs the aortic baroreflex plays little part in the response to lowered blood pressure, while the carotid arteries appear to be important in protecting the circulation from the effects of both high and low blood pressures (Fig. 2.37). Activation of the carotid baroreceptors produces effects on both peripheral resistance and cardiac output, while aortic baroreceptor activity predominantly influences peripheral resistance. Because the aortic baroreceptor is inaccessible in man it has not been possible to assess its contribution adequately. However, direct stimulation of the vagus nerve at operation has produced little in the way of circulatory effects suggesting that, in these circumstances at least, the aortic baroreceptor is not of great importance.

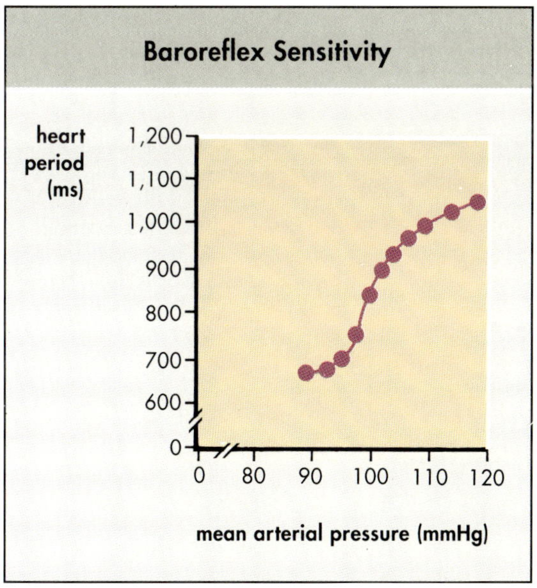

Fig. 2.36 Baroreflex sensitivity measured by changes in heart period (R–R interval on the ECG) after an injection of phenylephrine.

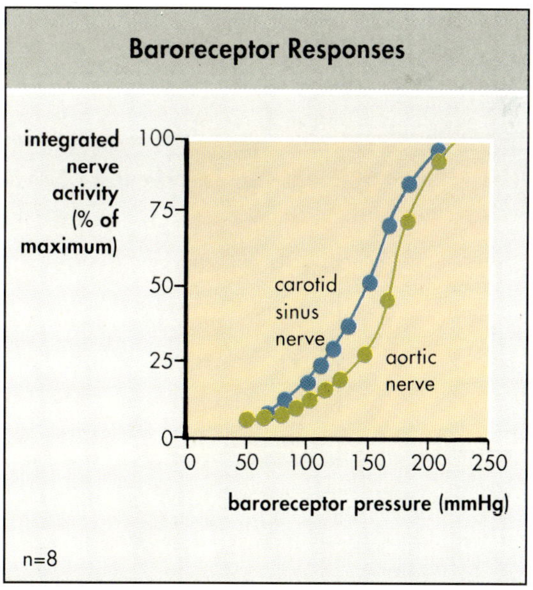

Fig. 2.37 Responses of afferent nerves from carotid and aortic baroreceptors to changes in pressure. Note that the aortic receptors are less sensitive to lower pressures. [Modified from Shepherd, J. T. (1982). In *Blood pressure Measurement and Systemic Hypertension*. Edited by Arntzenius, A. C. *et al.* Breda: Medical World Press. pp. 321–337.]

Other Baroreceptors

Low pressure baroreceptors are situated in the pulmonary vasculature and in both atria. They are innervated by vagal and spinal afferent fibres. Atrial receptors are activated by changes in atrial volume induced, for instance, by respiration. The cardiopulmonary receptors have an important influence upon the vasomotor centre. Thus, changes in intrathoracic blood volume sufficient to influence central venous pressure, but insufficient to alter arterial pressure produce reflex dilatation or constriction of the forearm resistance vessels. When intrathoracic blood volume is reduced further, constriction of splanchnic resistance vessels and tachycardia are produced as a result of activation of the arterial baroreceptors.

Other high pressure receptors are contained in the ventricles (mainly the left ventricle). They are regularly activated during ventricular systole: discharge rate increases with an increase in end diastolic pressure.

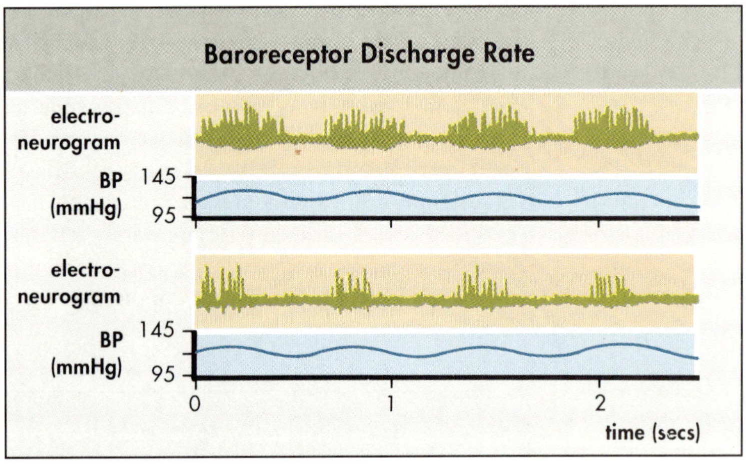

Fig. 2.38 Electroneurograms of carotid sinus nerve in the dog during sinusoidally varying pressures. Top: Normotensive. Bottom: Hypertensive. Note the resetting of the response in the hypertensive animal.

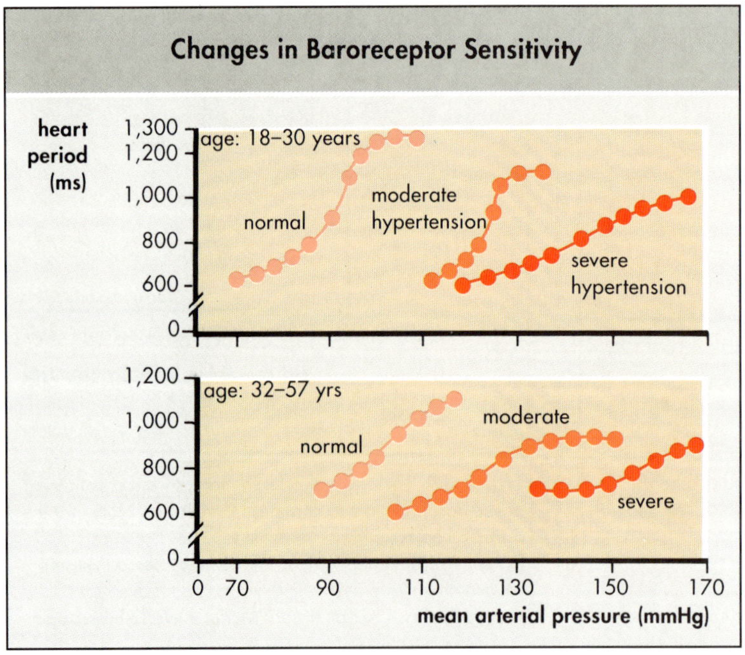

Fig. 2.39 A phenylephrine test reveals the changes in baroreceptor sensitivity caused by hypertension and by ageing. Note the change in sensitivity and the resetting in the hypertensives. [Modified from Korner *et al.* (1974) *Clin Exp Pharmacol Physiol,* **1**, 65–76.)

Changes in Baroreceptor Responsiveness

Responsiveness of baroreceptors can be altered in two ways:

- The set point is altered when the threshold blood pressure at which discharges occur is shifted – there is no alteration in the increase in discharge rate produced by a given increment in blood pressure;
- The sensitivity is altered when the change in discharge rate induced by a given change in blood pressure is either increased or decreased.

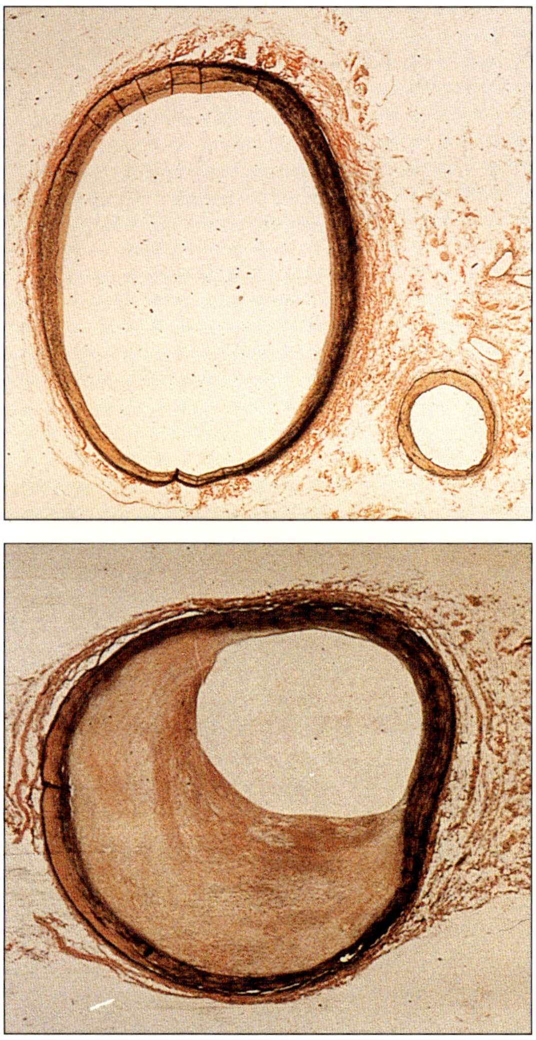

Fig. 2.40 Top: Histology of normal carotid in the region of the carotid sinus. Bottom: Similar histology in aged individual showing thickening of carotid arterial wall with extensive subendothelial fibrosis.

Resetting can be demonstrated by setting up sustained hypertension. An acute rise in blood pressure induces a rapid increase in carotid baroreceptor impulse discharge (Fig. 2.38). Discharge rate falls rapidly over the next few seconds and then more slowly over the next day or two until it has returned to normal levels despite the elevation of blood pressure. Thus, the baroreceptors perform a short-term buffering function but soon adapt to higher (or lower) blood pressure levels. Resetting shifts the curve relating pulse interval and pressure but does not alter its shape.

Changes in sensitivity of the baroreceptor responses can be assessed by the phenylephrine test (Fig. 2.39). Diminished sensitivity (a lesser degree of bradycardia for a given blood pressure elevation) occurs with ageing and in hypertension. It produces a reduction in the slope of the curve which relates pulse interval to blood pressure. The reason for diminished sensitivity is probably thickening and rigidity of the arterial wall in the region of the baroreceptors (Fig. 2.40). Thus, an artificial increase in rigidity produced by medial calcification (induced by hypercalcaemia) causes a similar reduction in baroreflex sensitivity (Fig. 2.41). Decreased sensitivity can also be demonstrated after blockade of the α-mediated efferent limb of the reflex. It is also seen in patients with autonomic dysfunction (multisystem atrophy or Shy–Drager syndrome), where degenerative changes are found in the spinal and peripheral sympathetic efferent pathways.

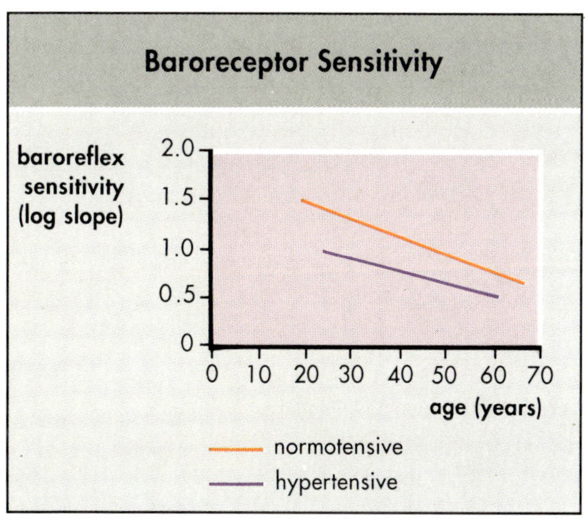

Fig. 2.41 Baroreceptor sensitivity, measured by pulse interval, changes on raising the blood pressure. Sensitivity declines with age.

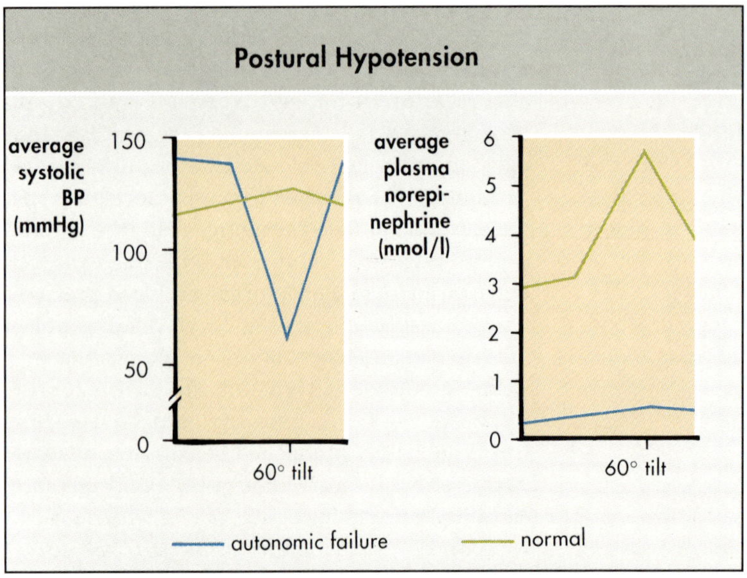

Fig. 2.42 Effect of a 60° tilt on the blood pressure in normal and blocked subjects. The results show the importance of the sympathetic nervous system in the control of capacitance vessel time, and therefore venous return, to the heart.

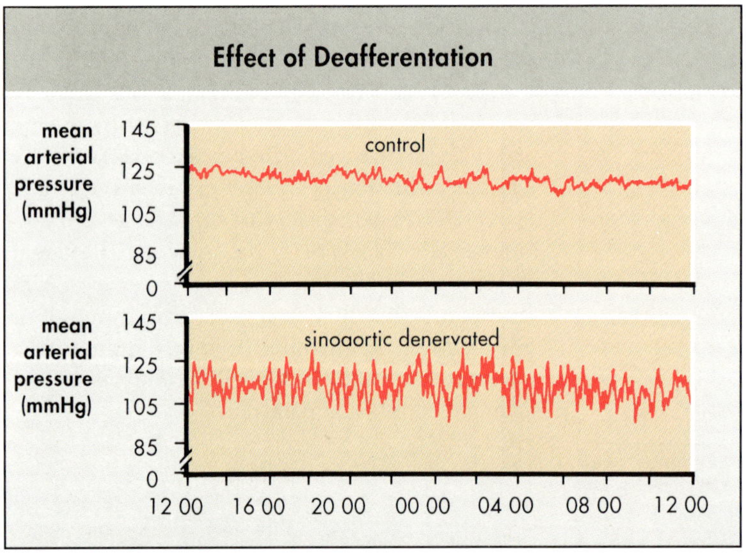

Fig. 2.43 These data demonstrate the role of the baroreceptors. Blood pressure was measured for 24 hours after the baroreceptor denervation. Blood pressure variability is greatly increased, but mean blood pressure, at least acutely, does not change.

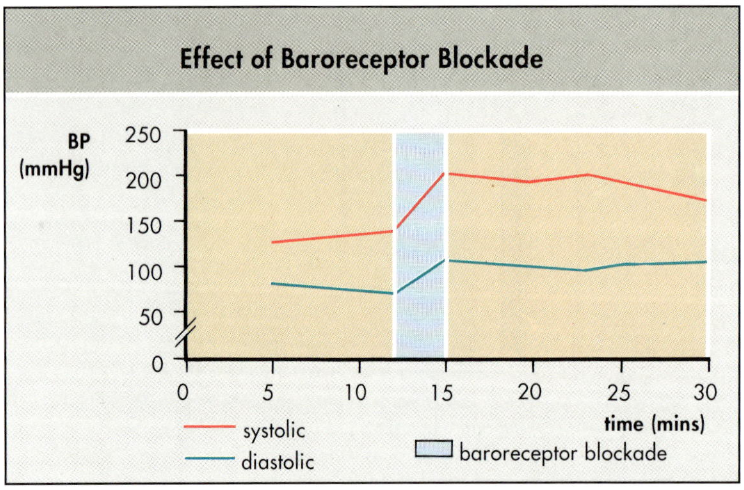

Fig. 2.44 Arterial pressure is increased almost immediately following local anaesthetic of the 9th and 10th cranial nerves in a normal subject pretreated with atropine.

Profound postural hypotension occurs as a result of diminished or absent sympathetic efferent nerve activity; this can be inferred from measurements of plasma norepinephrine, which are reduced in these patients (Fig. 2.42).

Although baroreceptor reflexes are of great importance in the minute-by-minute control of blood pressure, there is little support for the view that they are involved in the pathogenesis of hypertension. When the reflexes are abolished by deafferentation, the variability of blood pressure is increased but the mean blood pressure over a 24 hour period is not influenced (Fig. 2.43). This observation has been disputed – some reports have shown deafferentation has apparently producing sustained hypertension in animals. There is less evidence for this effect in humans. One normotensive subject is reported to have developed labile hypertension, followed several years later by established hypertension, after bilateral denervation of the carotid sinus. In other case reports, however, hypertension following surgical denervation of carotid sinuses has subsided within hours or days. While the diminution in baroreflex sensitivity observed in the elderly probably does not play a role in hypertension, it assumes great clinical importance when blood pressure is lowered pharmacologically (Fig. 2.44). Under these circumstances the elderly are particularly predisposed to postural hypotension (see chapter 6).

THE RENIN–ANGIOTENSIN SYSTEM

Renin is a proteolytic enzyme which hydrolyses an α-globulin substrate to form the decapeptide angiotensin I (Fig. 2.45). The C-terminal dipeptide fragment of angiotensin I is then split off by a converting enzyme to form the octapeptide angiotensin II, which is the main effector hormone of the system. Angiotensin II is then rapidly degraded by plasma and tissue aminopeptidases and endopeptidases to smaller peptide fragments.

Renin

Renin is a highly specific aspartyl proteases. It belongs to a family of enzymes which includes pepsin, chymosin and cathepsin D. They all have two aspartyl residues in the catalytic site and are all inhibited by pepstatin.

Renin-like enzymes can be demonstrated in a wide variety of tissues other than the kidney, including the uterus, chorion, salivary glands, arterial walls, adrenal glands, brain and liver. Some of this apparent activity is probably not due to renin, but is caused by other aspartyl proteases. However, molecular biological techniques have now demonstrated renin-specific mRNA in these tissues indicating that local synthesis of Preprorenin (for which it codes) is occurring. Other evidence suggests that, at least in vascular tissue,

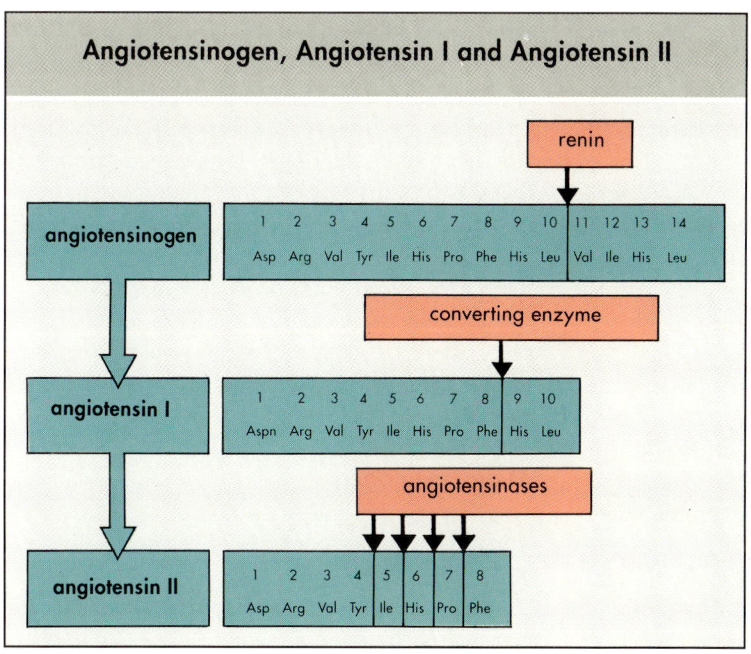

Fig. 2.45 Biochemical structures of N-terminal end of the human angiotensinogen, angiotensin I and angiotensin II molecules. Cleavage points for renin and converting enzyme are shown.

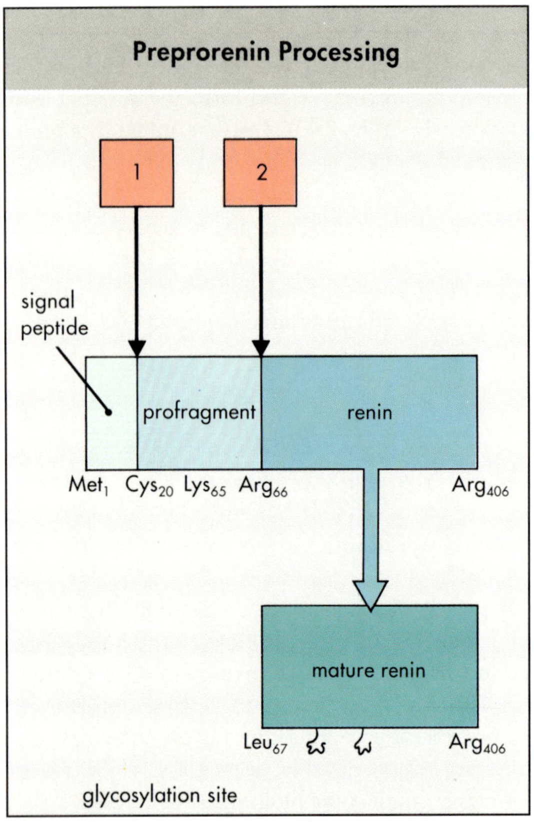

Fig. 2.46 Processing of pre-prorenin into renin by cleavage of the signal peptide and then the pro fragment.

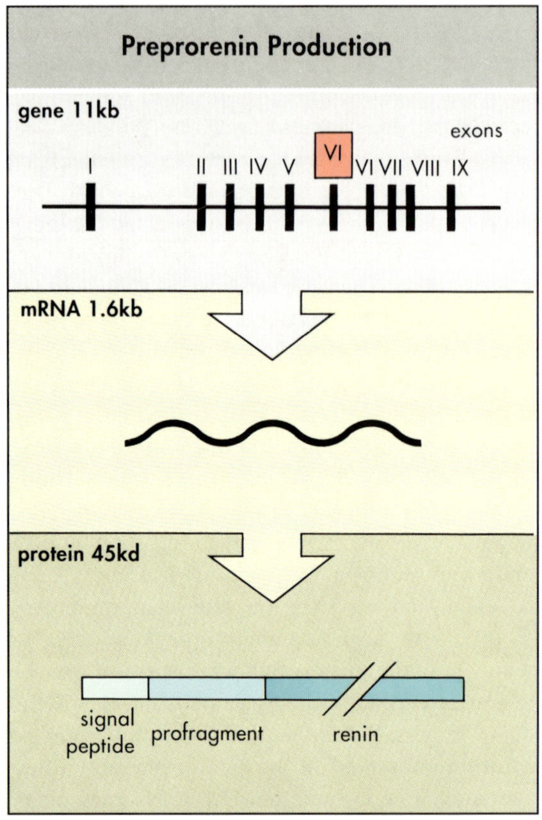

Fig. 2.47 The renin gene contains 9 coding regions (exons) with intervening non-coding regions (introns). Note that the gene product is probably pre-prorenin which is processed to renin within the cell.

this is activated to renin (see above). The role of extrarenal renin remains hypothetical, although vascular renin synthesis has been implicated in pathogenesis of increased peripheral resistance in hypertension.

The amino acid sequence of renin has been determined. Human renal renin is a glycoprotein (mol. wt 38,000). The three dimensional structure of renin has not been fully elucidated but the active site probably consists of a cleft between two lobes containing the two aspartic acid residues.

Renin synthesis and secretion has been studied both in the submaxilllary gland and the kidney. The primary transcription product is a larger molecule called Pre-prorenin which is cleaved to form a short signal peptide and prorenin (Figs 2.46 & 2.47). The signal peptide directs the Pre-prorenin into the secretory pathway (endoplasmic reticulum and Golgi apparatus). Prorenin is rapidly converted in the Golgi apparatus to active renin which is simultaneously incorporated into storage granules. Most of the active renin stored in the juxtaglomerular apparatus is released as such. Other tissues however (particularly the chorion) release prorenin (Fig, 2.48). It now seems probable that this precursor prorenin is identical with inactive renin which has been recognised in plasma and kidney extracts for many years. Thus, the renin activity of blood or kidney extracts can be substantially increased by exposure to çold, acid or proteolytic enzymes such as kallikrein or trypsin. How far activation of inactive renin forms a physiological regulator *in vivo* is unknown.

Angiotensinogen

Angiotensinogen consists of a group of compounds with molecular weights 61,400–65,400. The proportion of higher molecular weight forms is increased by the oral contraceptive pill and by

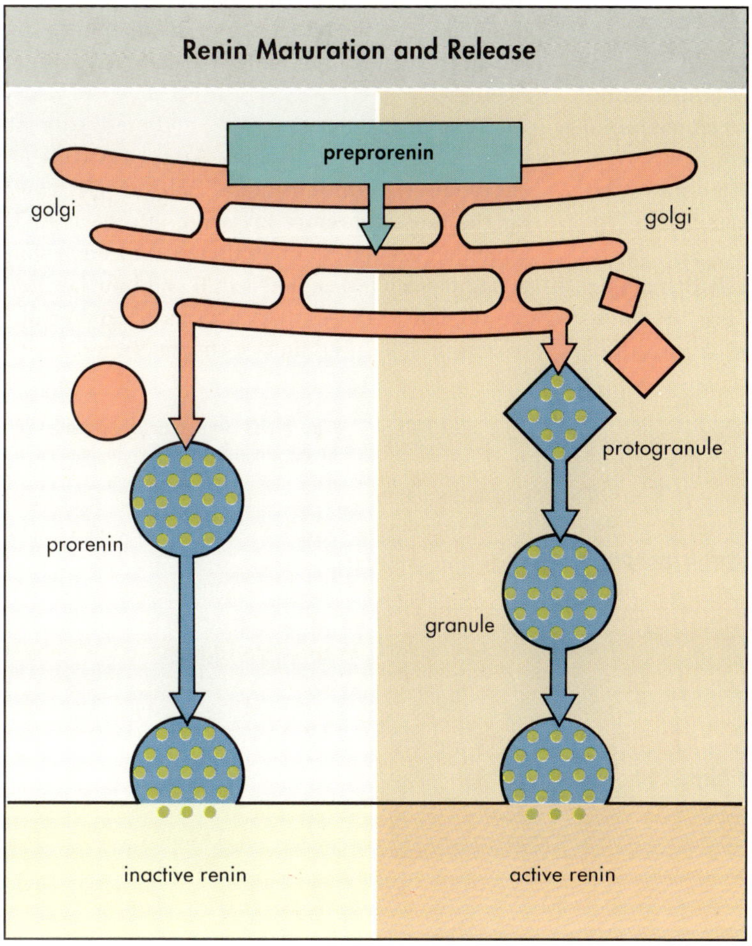

Fig. 2.48 Proposed model for the maturation and release of human renin. Pathway 1 would be predominent in the juxtaglomerular apparatus whereas pathway 2, which involves no processing of inactive renin into active renin, would be predominent in the Chorionic tissue. [Modified from Galen *et al.* (1986) Unpublished data.]

pregnancy. The complete amino acid sequence has now been defined. The first ten amino acids at the amino terminal end of the molecular comprise the sequence for angiotensin I. Splitting of the angiotensinogen molecule between amino acids 10 and 11 (leucine and valine) releases angiotensin I.

Angiotensinogen concentrations in plasma are approximately 1–2μg/ml. As this is approximately 10,000 times the normal molar concentration of circulating angiotensin I and II, angiotensinogen concentration is not usually a rate-limiting factor. Hepatic synthesis and secretion of angiotensinogen are increased by oestrogens, glucocorticoids, thyroid hormones and angiotensin II. Synthesis and secretion also rise following bilateral nephrectomy and are slightly elevated in hypertension. Angiotensinogen concentration is reduced after administration of converting enzyme inhibitors, in chronic liver disease, nephrotic syndrome and adrenal insufficiency (Fig. 2.49).

Clinical Conditions
increase
oestrogen therapy, oral contraceptives
pregnancy
glucocorticoid therapy
Cushing's disease, adrenocortial tumours
malignant hypertension
essential hypertension
decrease
adrenal insufficiency
converting enzyme inhibition
cirrhosis of the liver
nephrotic syndrome

Fig. 2.49 A number of clinical conditions are associated with change in plasma angiotensinogen levels.

Angiotensin I Converting Enzyme

Angiotensin converting enzyme (ACE) is a dipeptidyl-carboxypeptidase which removes the terminal dipeptide (histidyl leucine) from the C-terminal of angiotensin I to form the active octapeptide angiotensin II. It can also remove the C-terminal dipeptide of des-Asp[1]-angiotensin I to producing angiotensin III.

ACE is identical with kininase II, the major enzyme responsible for inactivating bradykinin. It is bound to the cell membranes of vascular endothelial cells and renal endothelial cells. It is also present on the brush border of gut epithelium and in the testes. It is widely distributed within the brain.

Besides cleaving angiotensin I and bradykinin, it has been reported that ACE hydrolyses encaphalins, neurotensin and Substance P. How far the blood pressure lowering effects of ACE inhibition are due to inhibition of the conversion of angiotensin I to angiotensin II and how far they are related to these other actions of converting enzyme is still uncertain (see chapter 9).

Primary Structures of the Angiotensins

	amino acid position 1	2	3	4	5	6	7	8	9	10
angiotensin I	Asp	Arg	Val	Tyr	Val Ile (ox)	His	Pro	Phe	His	Leu
angiotensin II	Asp	Arg	Val	Tyr	Val Ile (ox)	His	Pro	Phe		
angiotensin III		Arg	Val	Tyr	Ile	His	Pro	Phe		

Fig. 2.50 Amino acid sequences of the angiotensins.

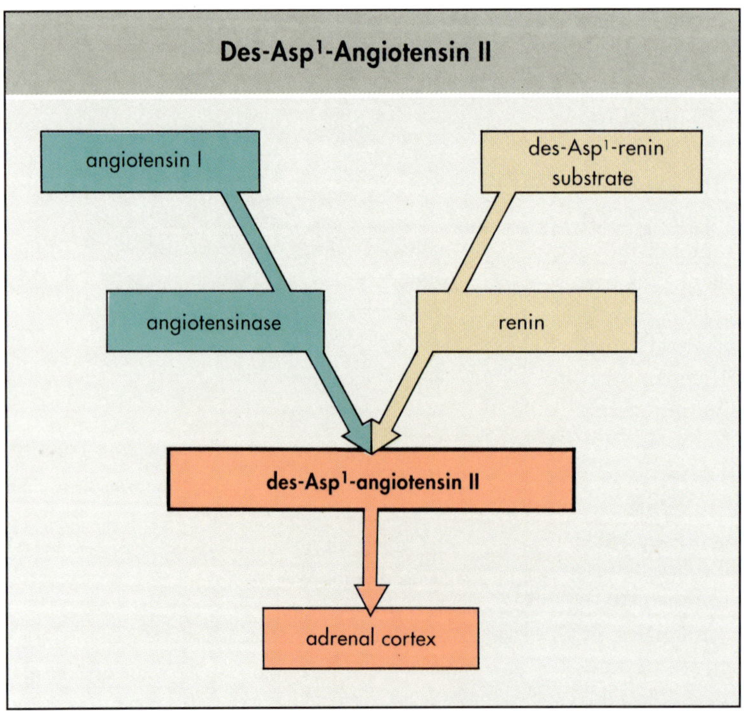

Fig. 2.51 The heptapeptide des-Asp[1]-angiotensin II can be formed from either angiotensin I or partially degraded renin substrate.

The Angiotensins

Angiotensin II is formed from angiotensin I both in the tissue bed and in circulation (the relative importance of these two sites is uncertain). Angiotensin II is quickly inactivated by aminopeptidases after a half life of 15–30 seconds. The heptapeptide des-Asp[1]-angiotensin II or angiotensin III has some biological activity. It is formed by cleavage of the N-terminal aspartate residue from angiotensin II (Fig. 2.50). However, it can also be formed by the action of converting enzyme on the nonapeptide des-Asp[1] angiotensin II (Fig. 2.51). The physiological role of this compound is still uncertain although it has been postulated that it forms an alternative pathway for the synthesis of biologically active angiotensin.

Secretion of Renin

Most circulating renin is derived from the kidney, where it is secreted by the cells of the juxtaglomerular apparatus (Figs 2.52 & 2.53). This is essentially a modified segment of the afferent arte-

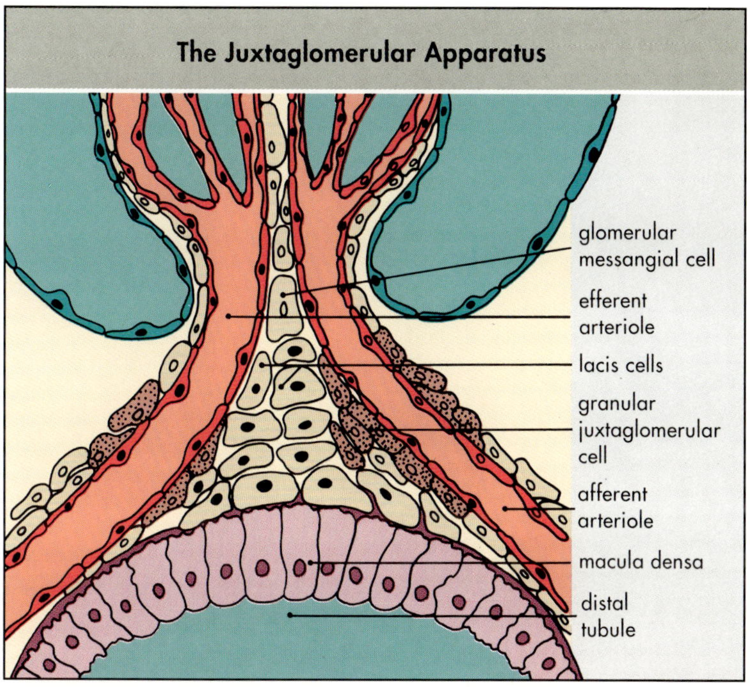

Fig. 2.52 Diagram of the components of the juxtaglomerular apparatus.

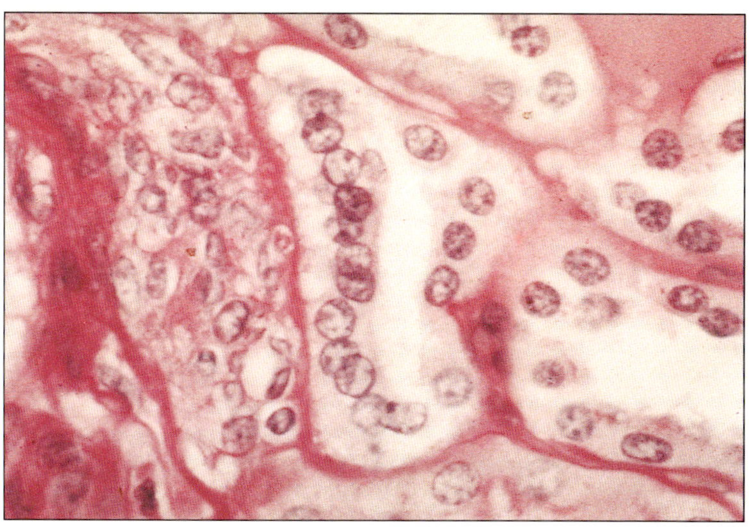

Fig. 2.53 Histology of the normal juxtaglomerular apparatus.

riole and serves both as a baroreceptor and a source of renin, which is stored within histologically visible granules (Fig. 2.54). An important component of the juxtaglomerular apparatus is the macula densa, a specialized part of the distal tubule. This acts as a chemoreceptor responding to changes in the sodium or chloride load imposed by the tubular fluid reaching the distal tubule. Increased renin secretion occurs in response to three groups of stimuli:

- a fall in renal perfusion pressure, monitored by the arterial baroreceptors – renin secretion is therefore influenced by activation of systemic baroreceptor reflexes;
- extracellular fluid volume depletion, probably recognised by its effects upon blood pressure and tubular fluid composition;
- ß-adrenoceptor stimulation in the JGA (Fig. 2.55).

These stimuli are of course often closely related; the secretion of renin can be regarded as a homeostatic attempt to maintain blood pressure in the face of threats from haemorrhage or shock.

At least two second messenger systems regulate renin secretion. cAMP stimulates renin secretion (mediating the response, for instance, to ß-agonists) while intracellular calcium inhibits renin secretion, mediating the response to increased circulating angiotensin II (Fig. 2.56).

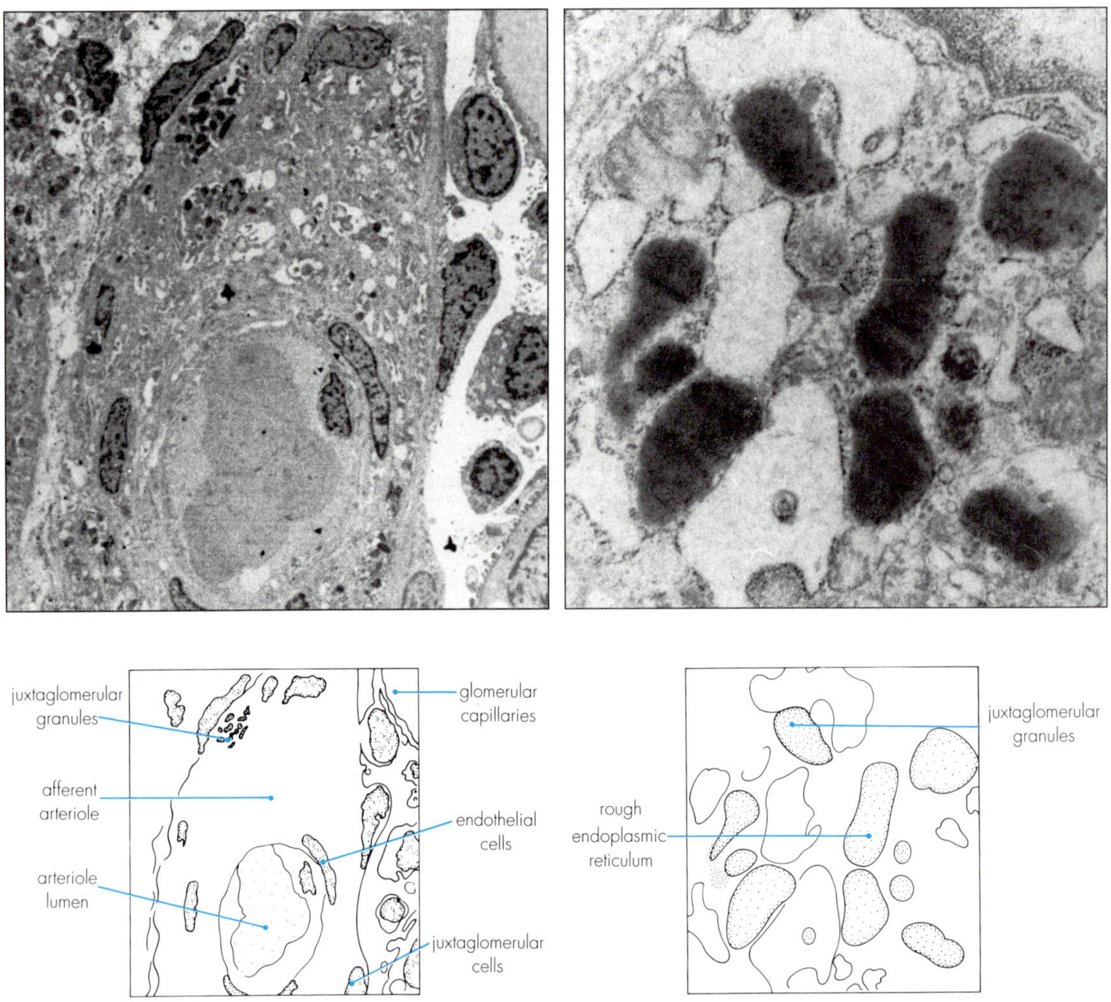

Fig. 2.54 Afferent arteriole of renal glomerulus adjacent to capillary vascular tuft. Left: The modified smooth muscle cells of the arteriole wall contain JG granules. Right: Details of modified smooth muscle cell in arteriole wall can be seen. These electron micrographs come from a patient with Bartter's syndrome in which marked hyperplasia of the JG apparatus can be observed.

Renin Secretion
renin secretion controlled by
ß-receptor stimulation
α-receptor inhibition
decreased extracellular fluid
decreased perfusion pressure plasma sodium, plasma potassium and plasma ADH

Fig. 2.55 Factors controlling renin secretion.

Regulation of Renin Release

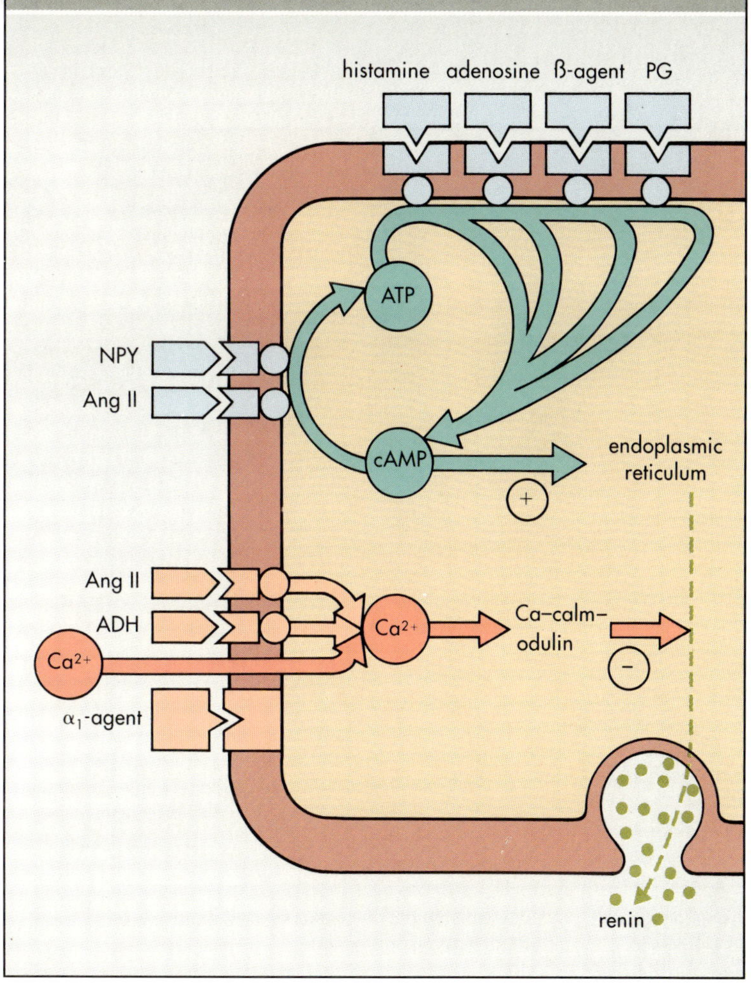

Fig 2.56 Signal transduction coupling in the regulationof renin release from the juxtaglomerular cell.

Circulatory Actions of the Renin–Angiotensin System

The renin-angiotensin system may maintain or elevate blood pressure in several ways (Fig. 2.57). These are:

- a direct vasoconstrictor effect upon vascular smooth muscle mediated through the phosphoinositide second messenger system;
- an indirect action upon the area prostrema of the medulla oblongata and sub-fornical region of the third ventricle, causing an increase in sympathetic efferent nerve activity through the vasomotor centre;
- facilitation of sympathetic nervous activity by enhancing the release of norephinephrine into the synaptic cleft when the sympathetic nerves are stimulated;
- stimulation of the zona glomerulosa causing aldosterone secretion and sodium retention;
- a direct action (in low doses) causing sodium retention – higher pressor doses of renin produce natriuresis and diuresis.
- increased drinking through an action on hypothalamic drinking centres;
- an action of angiotensin II on cell growth may

The complexity of the renin–angiotensin system's action is well illustrated by the slow pressor effect of angiotensin II. When angiotensin II is infused chronically in doses too low to have acute pressor action, pressure rises slowly several days. The cause of this phenomenon is unknown although sodium retention, sympathetic activation and vascular structural changes have been suggested.

Antihypertensive drugs have important actions upon renin secretion (Fig. 2.58). In general a fall in

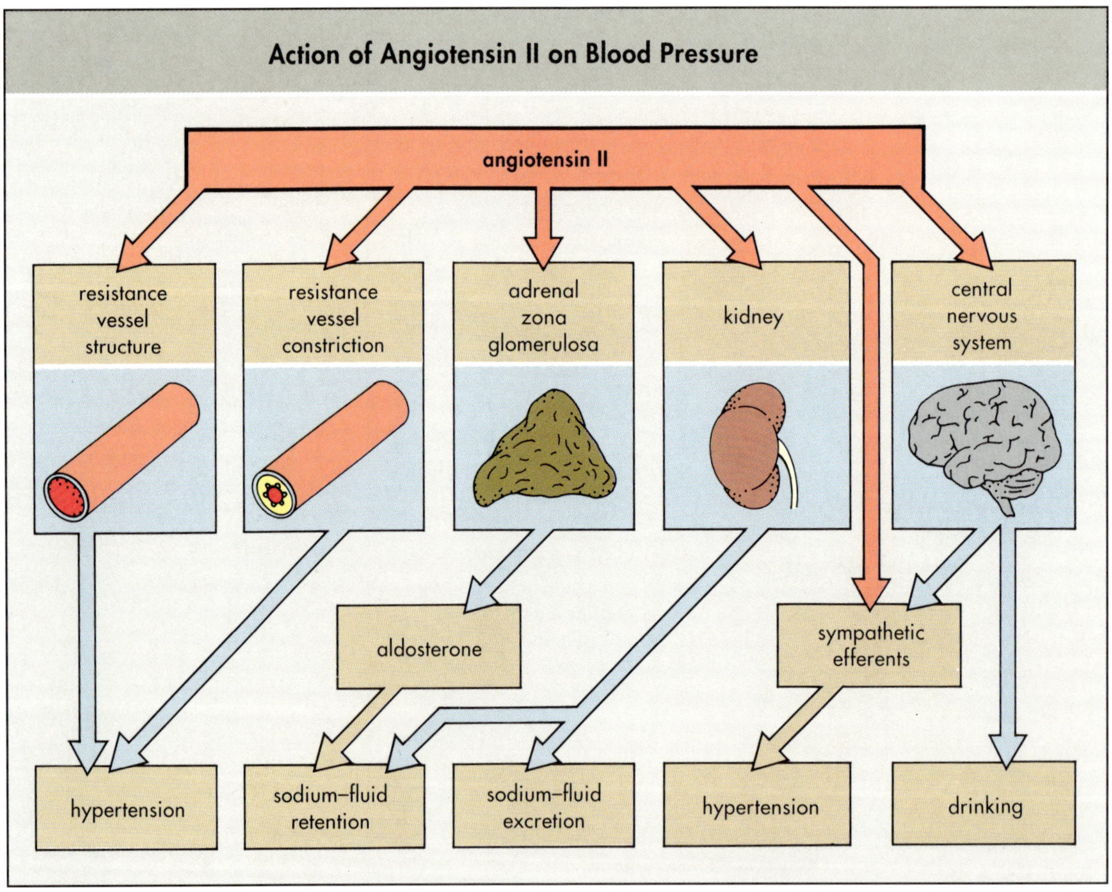

Fig. 2.57 Diagram of action of angiotensin II on blood pressure showing effect of angiotensin upon peripheral resistance vessels, autonomic effects of angiotensin II, action of angiotensin II on zona glomerulosa and direct effect of angiotensin II on the kidney.

Renin Secretion
renin secretion decreased by
sympathetic inhibition ß-adrenoceptor blockade
renin secretion increased by
sympathetic nerve stimulation vasodilatation reduced perfusion pressure inhibtion of sodium and chloride transport

Fig. 2.58 The effect of antihypertensive drugs and dietary salt changes upon renin secretion.

renin perfusion induced by antihypertensive therapy increases renin secretion: hyperreninaemia is seen particularly after vasodilator and diuretic therapy. However, antihypertensive drugs which reduce adrenergic stimulation (methyldopa, clonidine or ß-blockers) will reduce renin secretion despite the fall in blood pressure.

MINERALOCORTICOID HORMONES

Certain adrenal cortical hormones, of which aldosterone is the most important, are synthesized by the zona glomerulosa of the adrenal cortex and stimulate transepithelial sodium tranport (Figs 2.59 & 2.60). This causes a reduction in sodium

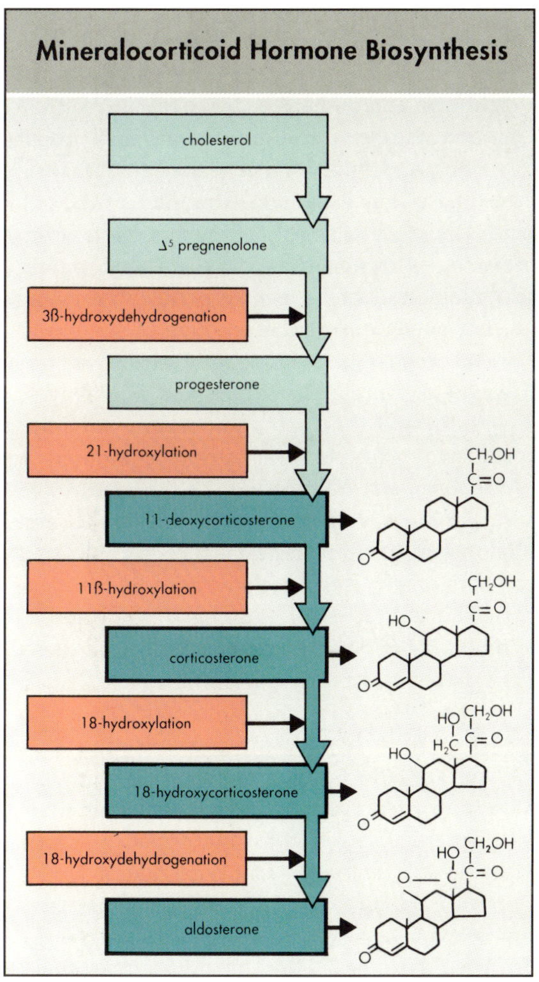

Fig. 2.59 Synthetic pathways of mineralocorticoid hormones.

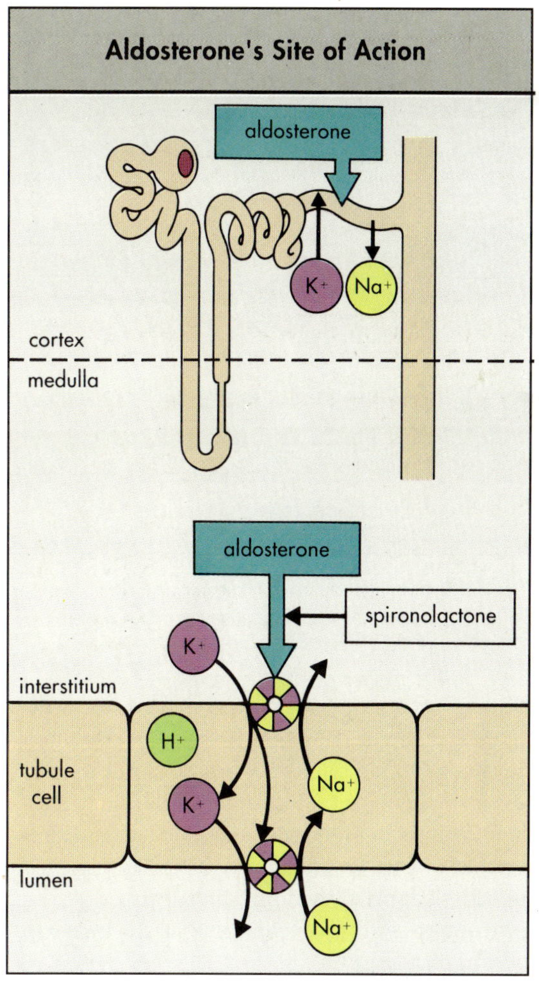

Fig. 2.60 Diagram showing aldosterone's site of action on the renal tubule and its effect on sodium, potassium and proton exchange.

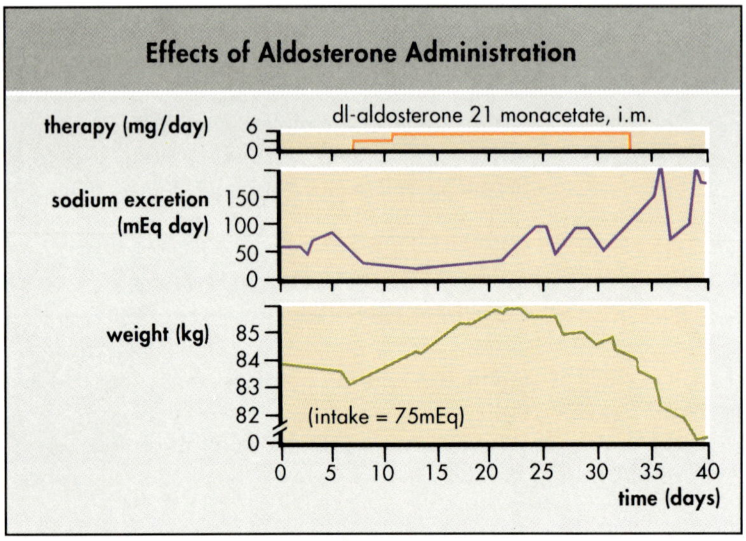

Fig. 2.61 The effect of aldosterone on sodium balance showing initial sodium retention and then escape, emphasizing that oedema does not usually occur when aldosterone is administered.

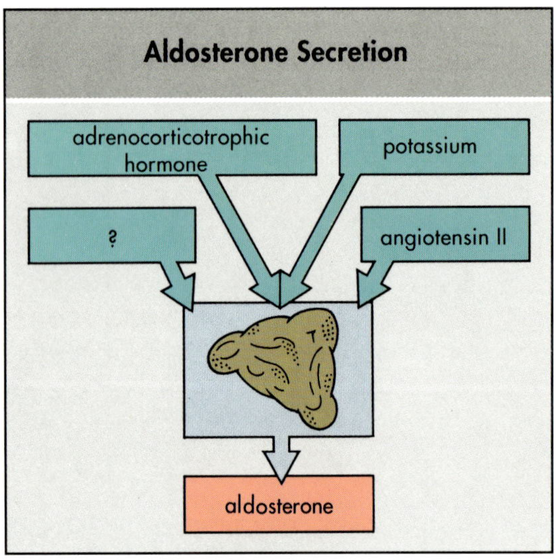

Fig. 2.62 Control of aldosterone secretion showing renin, ACTH, and potassium ion acting upon the adrenal zona glomerulosa.

and an increase in potassium content of both the faeces and the urine. In the absence of diarrhoea the change in faecal electrolytes does not usually have any significant effect upon sodium or potassium balance, but the renal effects of mineralocorticoid hormones are more important. They act at a specific segment of the distal tubule (the sodium–potassium exchange site) to increase sodium reabsorption and potassium secretion so that urinary sodium falls and potassium excretion rises. The result therefore is an expansion in the extracellular fluid volume with decrease in plasma potassium. Sodium and fluid retention does not proceed indefinitely (Fig. 2.61). After a few days of weight gain and perhaps oedema, urinary sodium excretion rises until sodium output equals input so sodium and fluid balance reach equilibrium at the expense of an expanded extracellular fluid volume. The mechanism of escape is uncertain but there is evidence that it is at least partly attributable to increased renal perfusion pressure causing enhanced tubular rejection of sodium. It has also been suggested that atrial natriuretic peptide may play a role, since levels rise progressively as sodium and fluid retention occurs. An additional factor is the putative 'natriuretic hormone'.

Aldosterone secretion (Fig. 2.62) is controlled mainly by the renin–angiotensin system. Angiotensin II stimulates mineralocorticoid secretion both *in vivo* and in isolated zona glomerulosa cells. The second major stimulus for aldosterone secretion is the potassium ion, which has a direct effect on isolated zona glomerulosa cells. Adrenocorticotrophic hormone (ACTH) and a reduction in serum sodium concentration have less marked effects upon aldosterone secretion. Atrial natriuretic peptide inhibits the stimulation of aldosterone secretion by angiotensin II. Other workers have suggested that dopamine may also exert an inhibitory effect upon aldosterone secretion in man. Less well characterized factors have also been described. Thus, an aldosterone stimulating protein has been isolated from the urine which may represent the excretory product of a pituitary hormone.

ATRIAL NATRIURETIC PEPTIDE

Mammalian atria contain granules that, when injected into the circulation, lower blood pressure and induce natriuresis and diuresis. The active principles were shown to be a family of peptides derived from a stored 126 amino acid precursor (Fig. 2.63). While this precursor has little or no biological activity, removal of the 28 C-terminal amino acids yields the major active circulating peptide which, in humans, is designated hANP 99–126. The stimulus for this compounds release is provided by an increase in atrial pressure induced, for instance, by volume expansion or cardiac failure. Elevated levels are also observed in hypertension. Atrial natriuretic peptide causes natriuresis, diuresis and reduced aldosterone, renin and vasopressin secretion. The cardiovascular effects are more complex. Relaxation of the capacitance vessels occurs with a fall in cardiac output. Concentrations required to lower peripheral resistance acutely in man are high, although sustained elevations within the physiological range may have an important physiological effect. In some experimental models, such as the 2-kidney 1-clip Goldblatt hypertensive rat and the spontaneously hypertensive rat (see chapter 3), vessels appear to be more sensitive to the vasodilator actions of ANP. Most isolated resistance vessels do not respond to physiological quantities of ANP, although rat renal arcuate artery does show a dilator response.

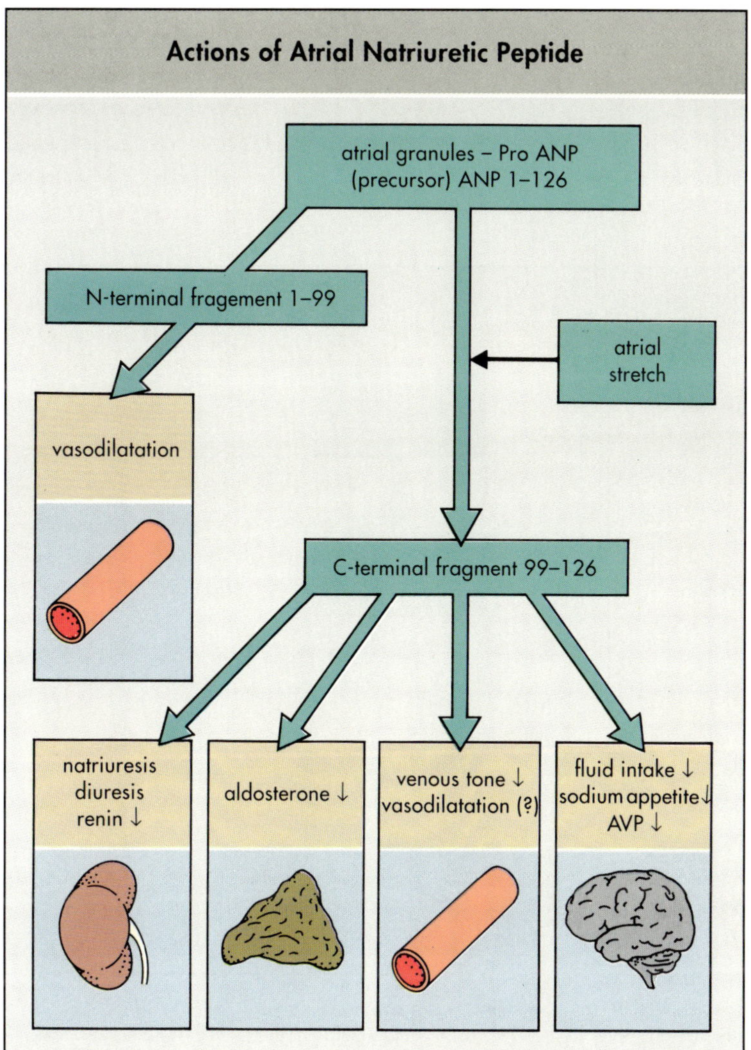

Fig. 2.63 Actions of atrial natriuretic peptide on blood pressure, sodium and fluid balance.

RENAL EXCRETION OF SODIUM AND WATER

Retention of sodium and water in bilaterally nephrectomized patients causes elevated blood pressure (see chapter 3). The regulation of sodium and water excretion by the kidney is therefore an important mechanism for blood pressure control. An increase in systemic pressure increases renal tubular rejection of sodium and water, probably through changes in the peritubular hydrostatic fluid pressure (Fig. 2.64). Guyton has emphasized the importance of this process in blood pressure regulation. As blood pressure increases the resultant negative sodium and water balance tends to return blood pressure to normal. Guyton described this as a system of infinite gain – blood pressure is restored to baseline levels rather than being only partly restored, as is the case with the baroreceptor reflexes. The role of changes in the natriuresis–diuresis blood pressure relationship will be discussed further in chapter 3. However, it should be noted here that processes which inhibit diuresis will, by blocking this compensatory response, tend to elevate blood pressure. In addition to increased activity of the renin–angiotensin system, which has already been discussed, other factors which may be of importance in this context are increased sympathetic drive to the kidney and reduction in renal mass.

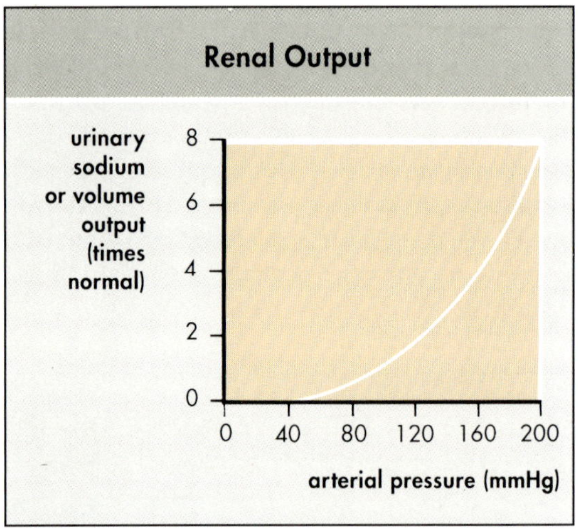

Fig. 2.64 A typical renal output curve, showing pressure diuresis and natriuresis.

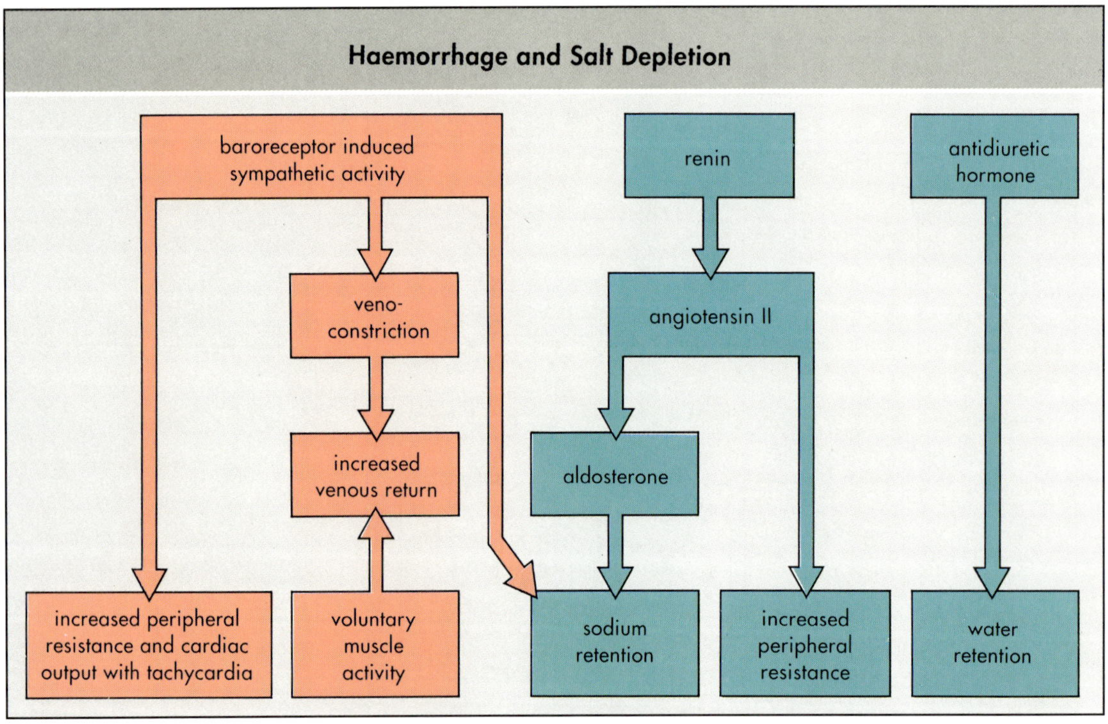

Fig. 2.65 Summary of the various mechanisms which maintain blood pressure in the face of haemorrhage or salt depletion, i.e. rapid mechanisms (sympathetic nervous system), slow mechanisms (renin–angiotensin) and then aldosterone with retention of fluid.

OVERALL CONTROL OF BLOOD PRESSURE

The maintenance of blood pressure is clearly of critical importance to the preservation of well-being. There are many mechanisms by which blood pressure can be controlled (Fig. 2.65). The interaction between these mechanisms normally serves to keep blood pressure within well-defined limits (Fig. 2.66). Acute blood pressure variability is controlled by sympathetic efferent activity under the influence of baroreceptor afferents and higher centres within the central nervous system. Hormonal systems (the renin–angiotensin system is the most important of these) have a less immediate effect on blood pressure. Slower adjustment processes include the resetting of the discharge activity of baroreceptors and changes in body fluid, determined by alterations in the excretion of sodium and water by the kidney. In addition there may be changes in the partition of fluid between the plasma and interstitial fluid spaces due to alterations in the balance of pre- and post-capillary resistance. Other changes which may be of equal importance are slower, since they consist of structural alterations in the resistance vessels due to increased load and, possibly, humoral and neurogenic stimulation. These systems interact with each other in a complex fashion – if one system is inactivated for some reason, the others may increase their activity to compensate. Essential hypertension is a multifactorial disorder – for this reason the unravelling of its pathogenesis remains an extremely daunting task.

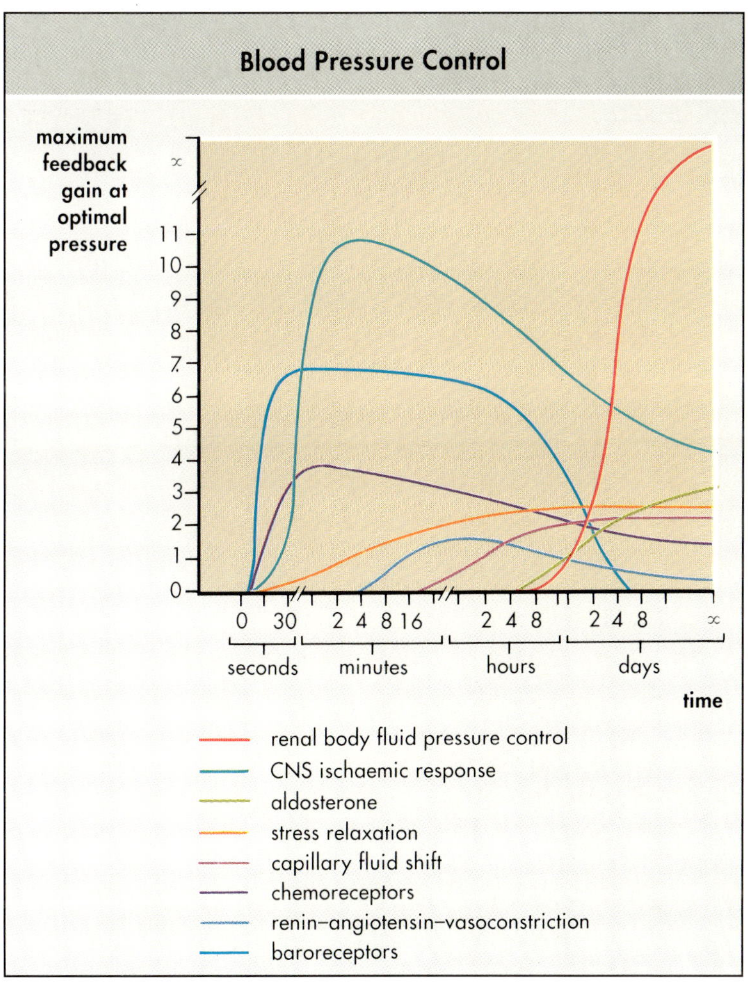

Fig. 2.66 Time-course of changes on arterial control systems after an initial disturbance in arterial pressure.

FURTHER READING

Folkow, B. & Neil, E. (1971) *Circulation* Oxford: Oxford University Press.

Guyton, A. C. (1987) *Textbook of Medical Physiology*. Philadelphia: W. B. Saunders.

Hackenthal, E. & Taugner, R. (1986) Hormonal signals and intracellular messengers for renin secretion. *Molecular and Cellular Cardiology*, **47**, 1–12.

Horman, F. (1985) The molecular basis of second messenger systems for regulation of smooth muscle contractility. *Journal of Hypertension*, **3** (Suppl 3), S3-S8.

Lang, R. E., Unger, R. & Ganten D. (1987) Atrial natriuretic peptide: a new factor in blood pressure control. *Journal of Hypertension* , **5**, 255–272.

Mancia, G. & Mark, A. L. (1984) Arterial baroreflexes in humans. In *Handbook of Physiology: The Cardiovascular System III*. USA: American Physiological Society.

Murphy, R. A. & Mros, S. (1983) Control of tone in vascular smooth muscle. *Arch Intern Med*, **143**, 1001–1005.

Proceedings of a Symposium on the Renin–Angiotensin System. Biochemistry (1983) Pharmacology and Clinical Aspects. *Clinical Exp Hypertension*, **A5** (7 & 8).

CHAPTER 3

Pathogenesis and Experimental Models

INTRODUCTION

In all clinical and experimental forms of chronic hypertension, blood pressure is maintained by an elevated peripheral vascular resistance. The physiological systems that are involved in controlling blood pressure are:

- the renin–angiotensin system;
- the control of sodium and water balance;
- the autonomic nervous system;
- the humoral systems (other than the renin–angiotensin system);
- structural changes in the resistance vessels.

Each of the above has been implicated in the pathogenesis of hypertension (Fig. 3.1). Important information has been provided not only by studies in man, but through the development of experimental models of hypertension.

EXPERIMENTAL MODELS OF HYPERTENSION

Hypertension has been induced in laboratory animals by a range of interventions (Fig. 3.2) and by selective inbreeding.

Goldblatt originally showed that the constriction of both renal arteries in a dog produced a slow, progressive rise in blood pressure. Hypertension in other animals can be created by constricting a single renal artery, leaving the opposite kidney *in situ* (Goldblatt 2-kidney 1-clip hypertension). The severity of this form of hypertension can be increased by removing the unclipped kidney (Goldblatt 1-kidney, 1-clip hypertension).

The physiological changes in the two Goldblatt models are quite distinct. The combination of unilateral nephrectomy and renal artery clipping in

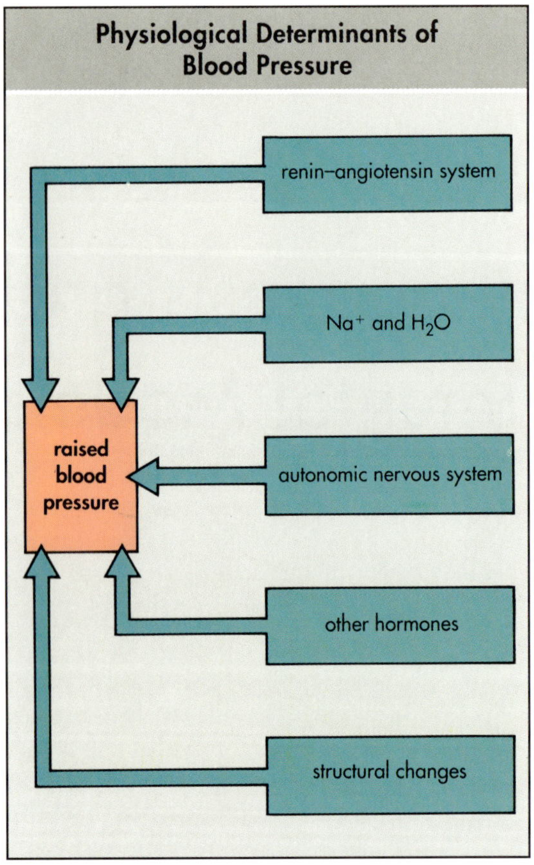

Fig. 3.1 A number of physiological systems are important in the control of blood pressure.

Experimental Models

name	procedure	effect: renin	effect: sodium balance
Goldblatt 2-kidney 1-clip	clip 1 renal artery	↑ then normal	↓ or normal
Goldblatt 1-kidney 1-clip	clip 1 renal artery contralateral nephrectomy	↓ or normal	↑
DOC–salt	regular deoxycorticosterone injections, saline to drink and contralateral nephrectomy	↓	↑
cellophane wrap	cellophane-induced perinephritis, either bilateral or unilateral with contralateral nephrectomy	↓ or normal	↑
coarctation	constriction of aorta between renal arteries	↑ then normal	?
adrenal regeneration	adrenal enucleation, unilateral nephrectomy, unilateral adrenalectomy, saline to drink	normal	normal

Fig. 3.2 The various experimental models of hypertension. Each have a specific effect upon sodium and renin levels.

the Goldblatt 1-kidney 1-clip model causes sodium retention while renin levels remain stable. However, in the Goldblatt 2-kidney model renin is elevated in the early stages. In DOC salt hypertension, one kidney is removed, deoxycorticosterone acetate (a potent mineralocorticoid) is injected and 1% saline supplied as drinking water. The net result of these manoeuvres is to impair the animals capacity to excrete a sodium load. It seems likely that the deoxycorticosterone also has a peripheral effect upon the resistance vessels.

Cellophane wrap hypertension probably causes cortical ischaemia as a result of perinephritis.

Constriction of the aorta between the two renal arteries produces a non-excretory distal kidney which releases large quantities of renin into the circulation.

Adrenal regeneration hypertension is a curious form which has not been extensively investigated. Enucleation of one adrenal gland is combined with contralateral nephrectomy and adrenalectomy and animals are given 1% saline to drink. Hypertension develops in association with hyperplasia of the adrenal remnant. This hypertension is not explicable by sodium retention, and it seems possible that adrenal regeneration is associated with increased secretion of certain hypothalamic peptides (γ-MSH peptides). This model seems to have no obvious counterpart in man.

Several groups have developed genetic strains of hypertensive rat (Fig. 3.3).

- The spontaneously hypertensive rat (SHR) is the most commonly used animal. Further inbreeding of this strain gave rise to a stroke-prone group of SHRs. SHR strains show increased sympathetic activity in the early phase of hypertension.
- The Milan strain shows transient sodium retention during the early phase of hypertension.
- The Otago genetically hypertensive rat shows increased vascular sensitivity to noradrenaline.
- The Sabra strain is particularly susceptible to DOC–salt hypertension.
- The Dahl salt-sensitive strain develops hypertension only on exposure to high salt intake.

Genetic Hypertension

strain	control	characteristics
Dahl–sensitive	Dahl–resistant	hypertensive on exposure to high salt diet
genetically hypertensive	Wistar–Otago	increased pressor responsiveness
Lyon hypertensive	Sprague–Dawley	moderate hypertension
Milan hypertensive	Wistar	moderate hypertension
Sabra hypertensive	Sabra	DOC–salt sensitive hypertension
spontaneously hypertensive (SHR)	Wistar–Kyoto	early increased sympathetic activity
spontaneously hypertensive stroke-prone (SHR–SP)	spontaneously hypertensive	prone to cardiovascular disease

Fig. 3.3 A large number of genetic strains of hypertensive rat have been developed.

PHYSIOLOGICAL MECHANISMS OF BLOOD PRESSURE CONTROL

The Renin–Angiotensin System

Renin-Dependent Hypertension

The renin–angiotensin system plays a major role in hypertension in a few, fairly unusual clinical situations (Fig. 3.4). For instance, there is little doubt that the renin–angiotensin system is responsible for hypertension in patients with renin-secreting tumours, although other factors are clearly also involved (Fig. 3.5). Blood pressure, for example, is higher than would be expected from circulating levels of renin and angiotensin II. It seems probable that resistance vessel hypertrophy (induced by elevated blood pressure) amplifies the effect of humoral agents in such cases (see below).

The blood pressure of patients with terminal renal disease on haemodialysis sometimes fails to respond to the removal of sodium until a bilateral nephrectomy has been carried out (Fig. 3.6). In situations such as this, renin secretion secondary to renal damage is probably also responsible for blood pressure elevation. These patients have very high renin, angiotensin II and aldosterone levels and their blood pressures respond to infusion of the angiotensin II blocker saralasin. It seems likely that the normal mechanisms that control renin secretion are disturbed in such patients, resulting in renin hypersecretion and hypertension.

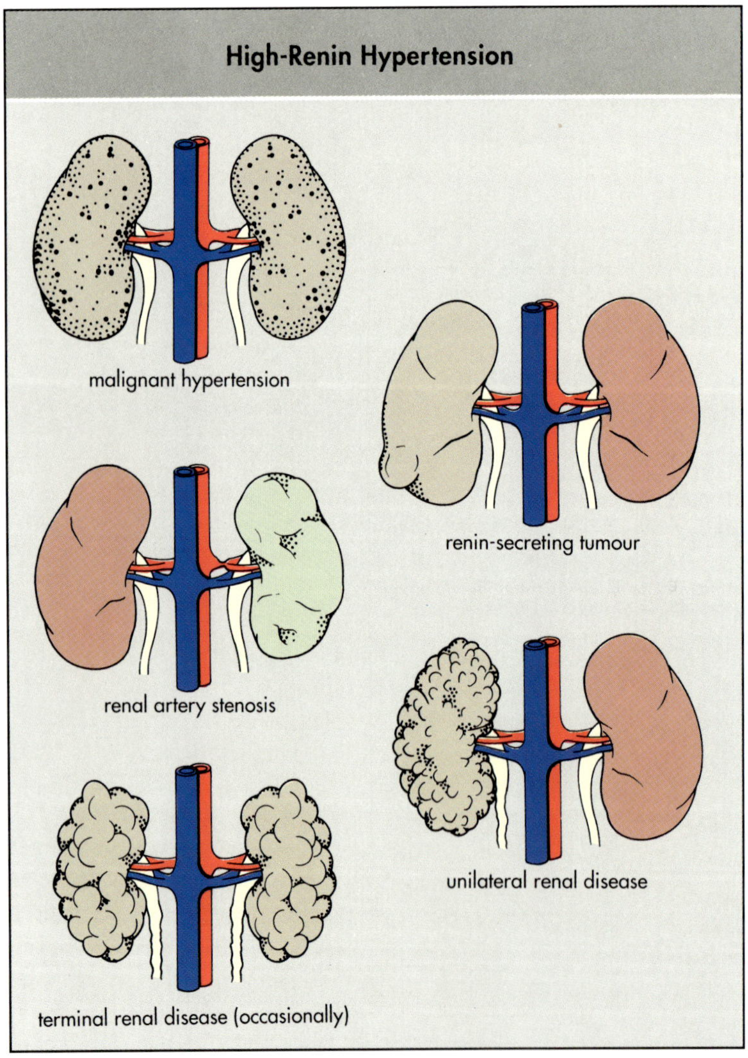

Fig. 3.4 Clinical states in which the renin–angiotensin system may be involved.

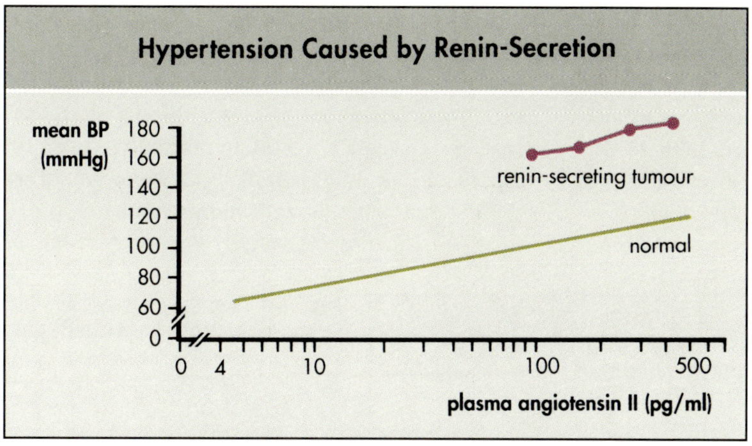

Fig. 3.5 Hypertension caused by a renin- secreting tumour. [Modified from Brown, J. J. *et al.* (1979) *Hypertension,* **1**, 159–168.]

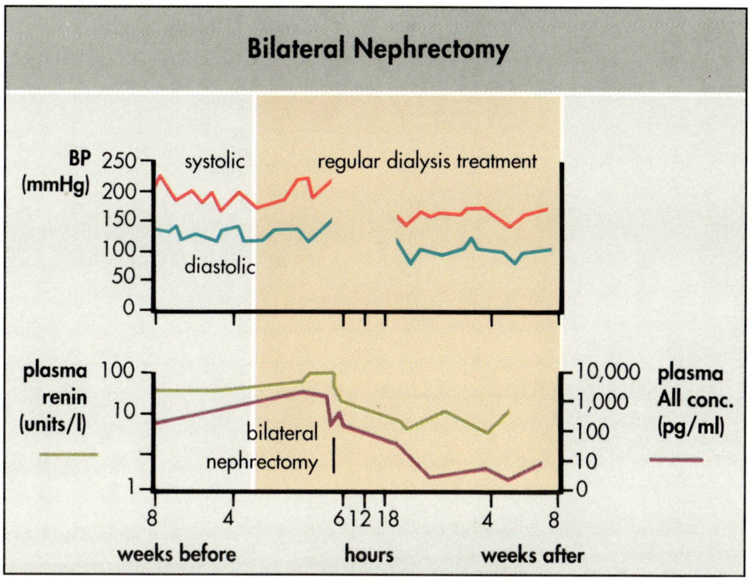

Fig. 3.6 A patient on dialysis with high renin levels and very high blood pressure whose blood pressure was controlled by bilateral nephrectomy. Bilateral nephrectomy was associated with a fall in plasma renin.

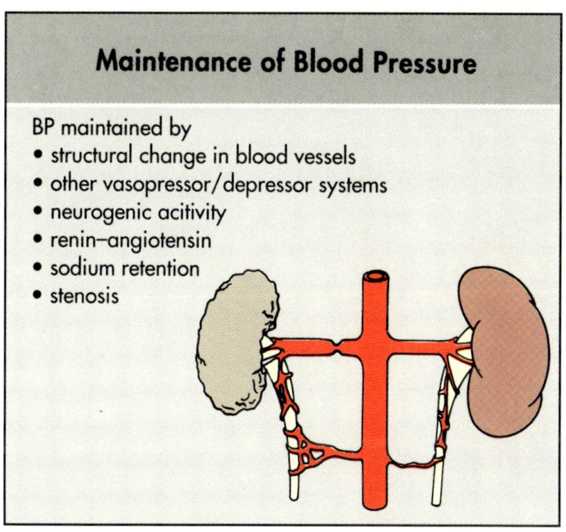

Fig. 3.7 Possible factors involved in maintaining blood pressure in patients with hypertension due to unilateral renal artery stenosis.

Renin in Other Forms of Hypertension

The role of the renin–angiotensin system in hypertension associated with unilateral renal disease is much more controversial. Thus several factors contribute to blood pressure maintenance in this model (Fig. 3.7). There are two major difficulties in studying the role of renin in human renovascular hypertension. Firstly, atheromatous renal artery stenosis is frequently found at necropsy in patients who are normotensive; since essential hypertension is a common disorder, association between the two must often be coincidental. Secondly, it is rarely possible to follow the natural history of the disease from the very outset. Thus, if renin were important in the early phase of hypertension, it might not be apparent if only patients with established renovascular hypertension were studied. One approach is to study the blood pressure response when a renal artery stenosis is corrected surgically. In some patients, surgery corrects both high plasma renin and high blood pressure. In others, corrective renal artery surgery restores blood pressure to normal even when preoperative plasma renin is not elevated. Furthermore, surgery sometimes corrects an elevated preoperative plasma renin activity, but has little effect upon the level of hypertension (Fig. 3.8). In the latter case it seems that other factors (such as resistance vessel hypertrophy) may be responsible for maintaining blood pressure (Fig. 3.9). In some patients with high renin levels however, the renin–angiotensin system is important, as

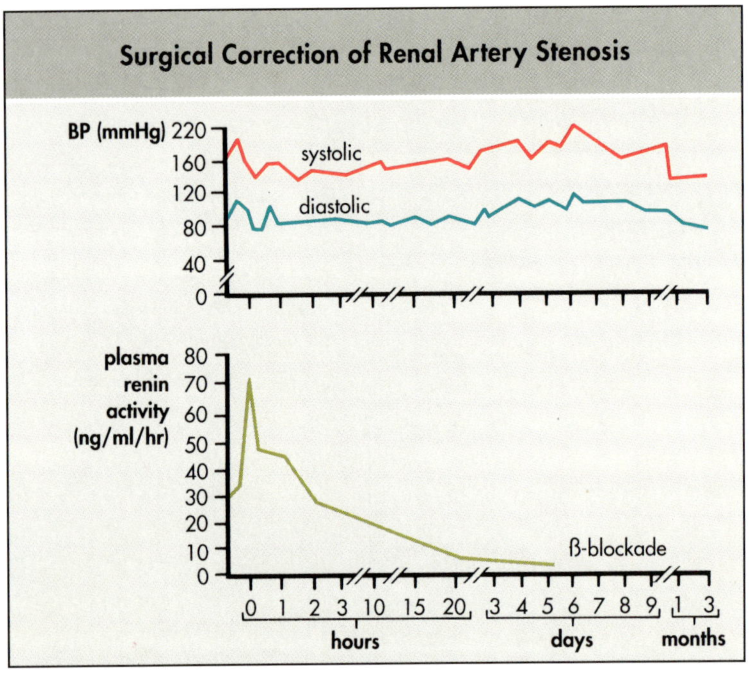

Fig. 3.8 Surgical correction of renal artery stenosis (in humans) can have the effect of reducing renin levels to normal while blood pressure remains elevated.

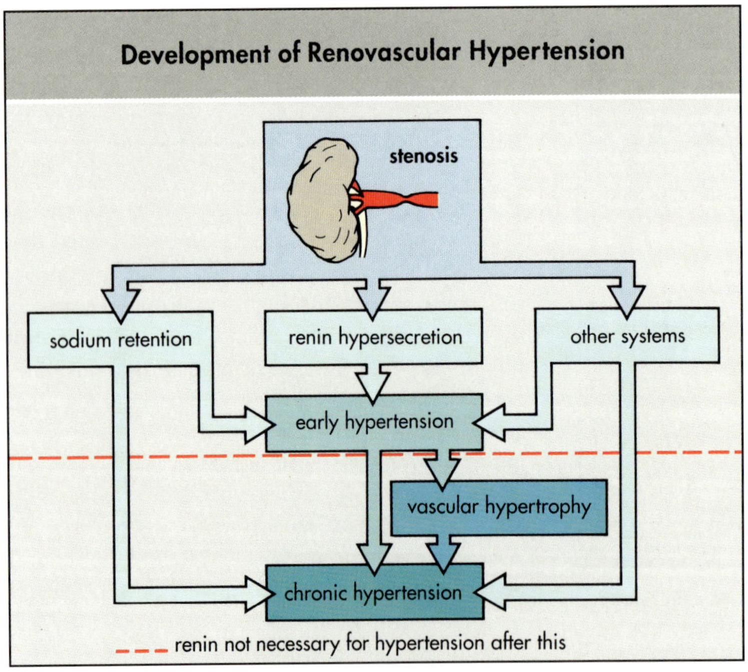

Fig. 3.9 A possible sequence of events in the development of renovascular hypertension.

demonstrated by the drop in blood pressure which follows inhibition of the renin–angiotensin system (Fig. 3.10).

The changes in the renin–angiotensin system can most easily be followed in Goldblatt 2-kidney 1-clip hypertension (Fig. 3.11). Immediately after a constricting clip is placed on the renal artery there is a transient rise in plasma renin; this is probably due to the acute fall in renal perfusion pressure and to the handling of the kidney itself. This is often associated with a rise in blood pressure which lasts a few hours and then returns to normal. A variable latent period then follows, after which pressure gradually rises over days or weeks. This early phase of hypertension is almost always associated with an elevated plasma renin.

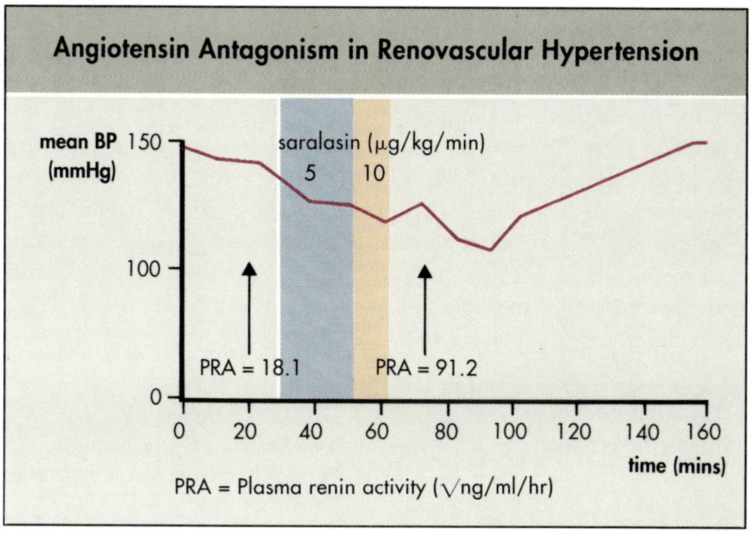

Fig. 3.10 The effect of saralasin on a patient with hypertension due to renal artery stenosis. Blood pressure falls, but does not return to normal.

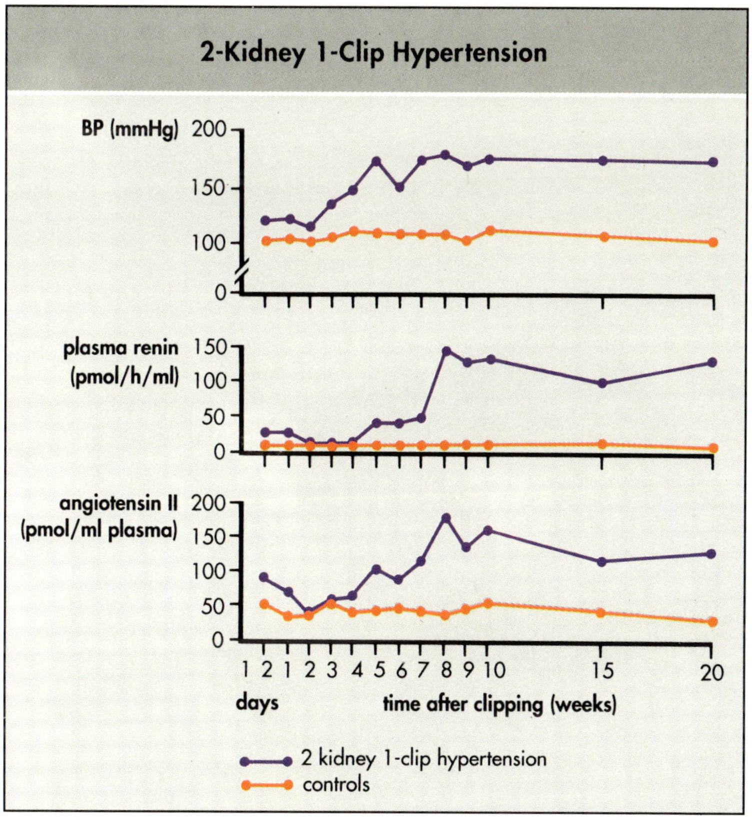

Fig. 3.11 Use of Goldblatt 2-kidney 1-clip hypertension allows the sequence of changes in the renin–angiotensin system to be followed. [Modified from Morton, J. & Wallace, E. (1983) *Clin Sci*, **64**, 359–370.]

There is a direct correlation between plasma renin and blood pressure. In addition, blockade of the renin–angiotensin system, with the competititve antagonist saralasin for instance, substantially reduces blood pressure. When blood pressure has been elevated for some time, the renin–angiotensin system seems to become less important. Plasma renin and angiotensin II levels fall and the blood pressure response to saralasin is not observed (Fig. 3.12). Despite this, when the constricting clip is removed from the renal artery, blood pressure falls within a few hours (Fig. 3.13), suggesting that other renal mechanisms are important in blood pressure maintenance. The rapid fall in blood pressure does not exclude a role for hypertrophy of the resistance vessel bed. An increase in the wall-to-lumen ratio of the resistance vessels can be demonstrated and, as one might expect, gives rise to generalized hyperreactivity (see chapter 2). The swiftness of the fall does suggest, however, that the relaxation of renal ischaemia produces an acute reduction in the vasomotor tone of the resistance vessels. The renomedullary lipid vasodepressor system could be involved here; after the renal artery is deconstricted, vasodepressor lipids can be detected in the renal venous effluent and the medullary interstitial cells degranulate.

These changes in plasma renin are dependent upon the presence of an intact contralateral kidney. This kidney prevents sodium and water retention and actually undergoes a perfusion pressure natriuresis and diuresis as blood pressure rises, so that in more severe hypertension sodium balance is negative. When that intact kidney is removed, clipping a single kidney (Goldblatt 1-kidney 1-clip hypertension) produces sodium retention and normal or low plasma renin throughout the course of the hypertension (Figs 3.14 & 3.15).

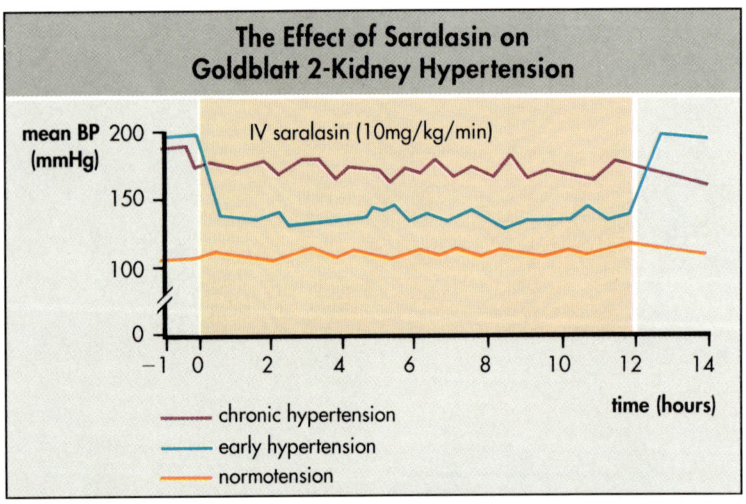

Fig. 3.12 The effect of saralasin infusion on Goldblatt 2-kidney hypertension. Only a small fall in blood pressure is produced in chronic hypertension and blood pressure remains higher than normal. A much larger response is seen in early hypertension when renin levels are high. [Modified from Bing, R. F. *et al.* (1981) *J Lab Clin Med*, **98**, 302–310.]

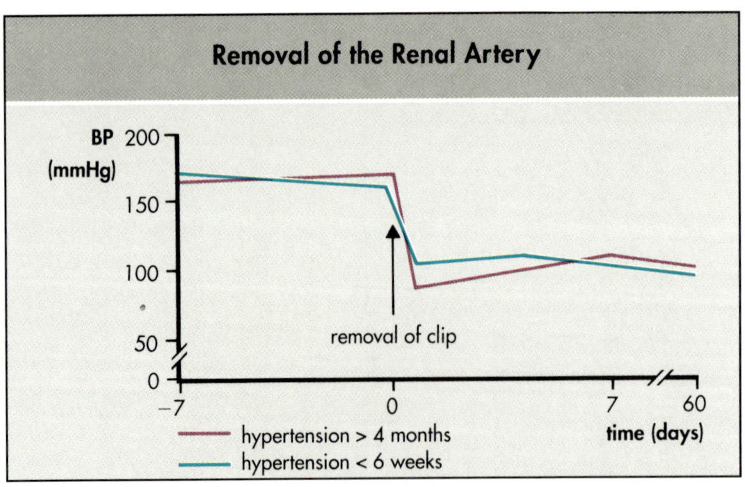

Fig. 3.13 When the renal artery clip is removed, blood pressure shows an immediate fall. This holds true for both long-standing and chronic hypertension. [Modified from Thurston, H. *et al.* (1980) *Hypertension*, **2**, 256–265.]

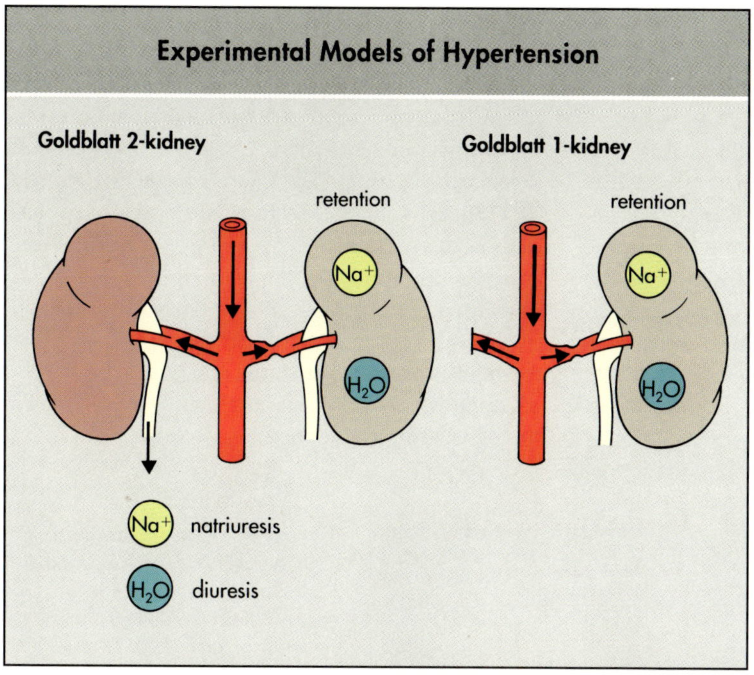

Fig. 3.14 Models of Goldblatt 2-kidney and 1-kidney hypertension.

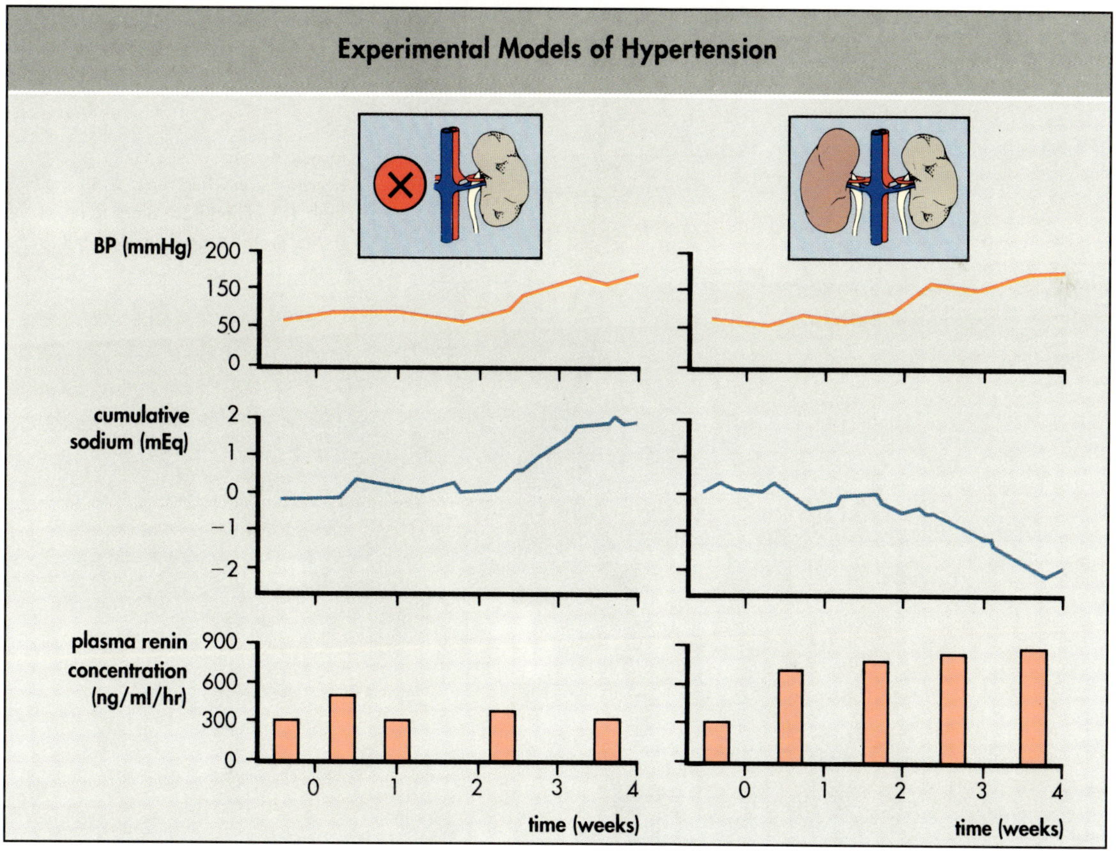

Fig. 3.15 Experimental Hypertension. Left: Goldblatt 1-kidney model. Renal ischaemia on one side with the kidney removed on the other side. The ischaemic kidney gives rise to sodium retention – renin levels are normal or low. Right: Goldblatt 2-kidney model. The untouched kidney undergoes high perfusion pressure natriuresis due to systemic hypertension. Renin levels are elevated.

The Slow Pressor Action of Angiotensin II

When angiotensin II is infused into normal human subjects or into animals in doses too low to cause an acute rise in blood pressure, blood pressure rises gradually over a period of days (Fig. 3.16). This hypertension is not attributable to stimulation of aldosterone secretion, since it is not prevented by adrenalectomy and cannot be mimicked by chronic aldosterone infusion. This slow pressor effect is clearly important as a possible mechanism whereby the renin–angiotensin system could maintain blood pressure even when plasma levels are normal or only marginally raised. Its mechanism is still controversial, but one explanation which has been put forward is that it is the direct effects of angiotensin II on the kidney which cause sodium retention. This has arisen from the observation (in some studies) that blood pressure has been lowered by sodium depletion and restored by sodium loading. The interaction of angiotensin II with sympathetic nervous system activity has also been suggested as a possible explanation (see chapter 2) although there is no evidence for increased sympathetic nervous system activity when the slow pressor effect of angiotensin II is operative. More recently, the effects of angiotensin II upon smooth muscle proliferation have been invoked as an explanation.

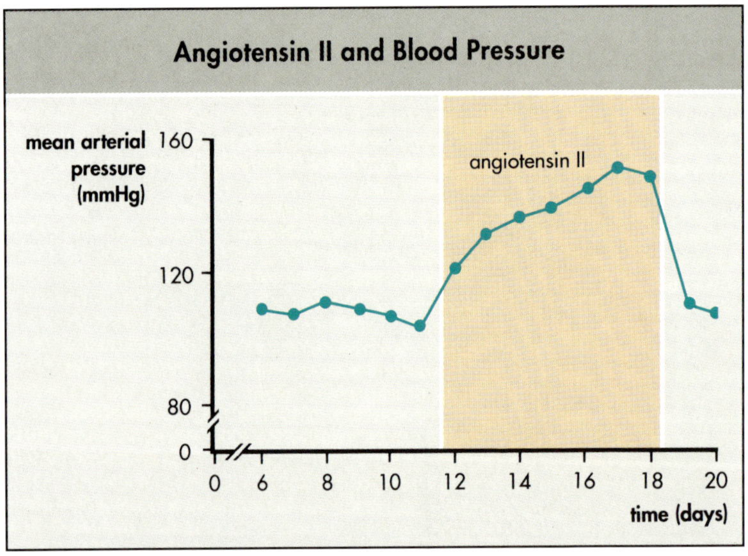

Fig. 3.16 When angiotensin II is administered to rats over a period of 7 days, blood pressure shows a steady increase. [Modified from Brown, A. J. *et al.* (1981) *Amer J Physiol*, **241**, H381–H386.]

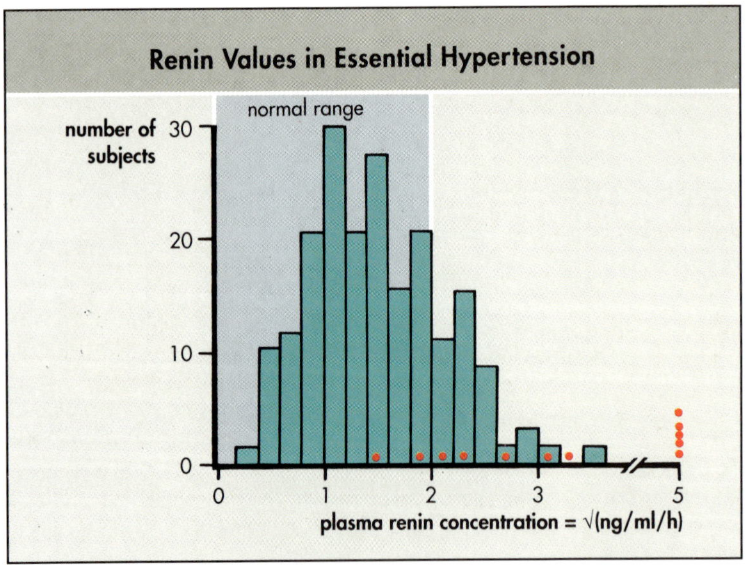

Fig. 3.17 The distribution of renin values in essential hypertension. A small group have elevated renin levels, but in most patients renin levels are normal or low. Red dots show values for patients with malignant hypertension.

The Renin–Rngiotensin System in Essential Hypertension

There is no persuasive evidence to implicate the renin–angiotensin system in human essential hypertension. Plasma renin levels fall within the normal range in the majority of patients with essential hypertension, although a minority (approximately 15%) have slightly elevated values (Fig. 3.17). This category (high-renin hypertension) includes some patients with malignant hypertension and some young patients showing evidence of activation of the sympathetic nervous system (which is a stimulus to renin release).

About one-third of patients with essential hypertension have plasma renin levels which lie at the lower end of the normal range. They show a subnormal response to stimuli such as sodium depletion, diuretics (Fig. 3.18) or diazoxide and a low renin level when plasma renin is standardized to sodium intake or excretion (Fig. 3.19). This is known as low-renin hypertension. Patients with low-renin hypertension tend to be older than those with normal- or high-renin hypertension. However, although renin levels fall with age and in spite of the fact that this effect is more marked in hypertensive individuals, ageing alone does not explain the nature of low-renin hypertension.

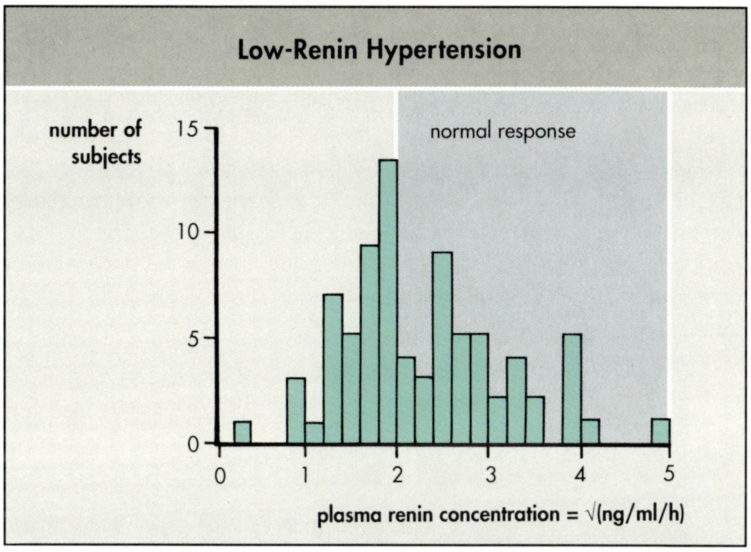

Fig. 3.18 Plasma renin levels in a group of subjects with essential hypertension who had been receiving bendrofluazide for seven days. Patients with low-renin hypertension have an impaired renin response compared with normal subjects.

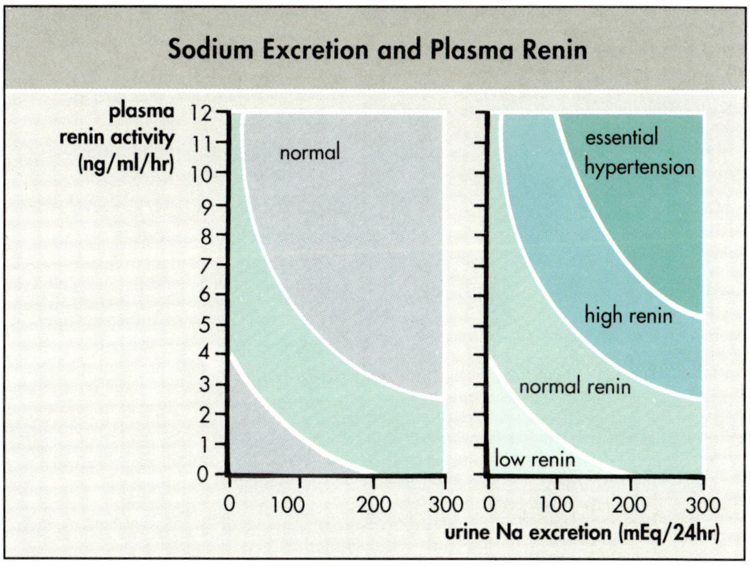

Fig. 3.19 Nomogram relating twenty-four hour sodium excretion and plasma renin activity in normotensive and hypertensive subjects. Urinary sodium excretion is used as an index of sodium intake; thus lower sodium intakes are associated with higher values of plasma renin. Note that with normal dietary sodium intake (100–200mmol/day), changes in dietary salt contribute little to changes in plasma renin. In hypertensive subjects the relationship is lost, a result of the presence of groups of patients with disproportionately high or low plasma renin activities.

When low-renin hypertension was first described it was suggested that it represented a discrete form of essential hypertension, with a distinct aetiology analagous to mineralocorticoid hypertension. It was thus concluded that sodium retention, perhaps related to an unknown mineralocorticoid, caused hypertension and renin suppression. This hypothesis has not stood the test of time. There is no evidence that patients with low renin hypertension form a discrete subgroup when plasma renin is measured in an unselected group of essential hypertensives (under these circumstances the classification of low renin hypertension is arbitrary). Furthermore, different stimuli (see above) do not give concordant results, and the proportion of low renin hypertensive patients in a hypertensive population varies according to the method of stimulation used. Prolonged antihypertensive treatment can influence renin responsiveness (Fig. 3.20). Several months' treatment with diuretics can normalize the plasma renin response, an effect which can last for at least several weeks. Although early studies suggested that extracellular fluid volume was expanded in patients with low renin hypertension, this result has not been confirmed in more recent studies. When properly matched groups are compared, there is no difference between the body fluid volume and sodium content in low renin hypertension and that found in other forms of essential hypertension (Fig. 3.21).

It has been shown, however, that patients with low renin hypertension show a particularly good blood pressure response to diuretics and salt restriction. This is probably because the renin–angiotensin system normally helps to maintain blood pressure in the face of sodium and fluid losses. Where the renin response is impaired, therefore, a disproportionate blood pressure reduction is produced. A similarly enhanced response to sodium depletion can be observed after pharmacological blockade of the renin–angiotensin system with, for instance, converting-enzyme inhibitors (see chapter 9).

It seems likely therefore that the reduction in renin responsiveness is not secondary to volume expansion. From one point of view, low renin levels in hypertension could be seen as a normal physiological response of the juxtaglomerular apparatus to an increase in perfusion pressure. However, histological changes in the afferent arteriole of the glomerulus may also play a role. Hyaline nephrosclerosis (Fig. 3.22) is commonly

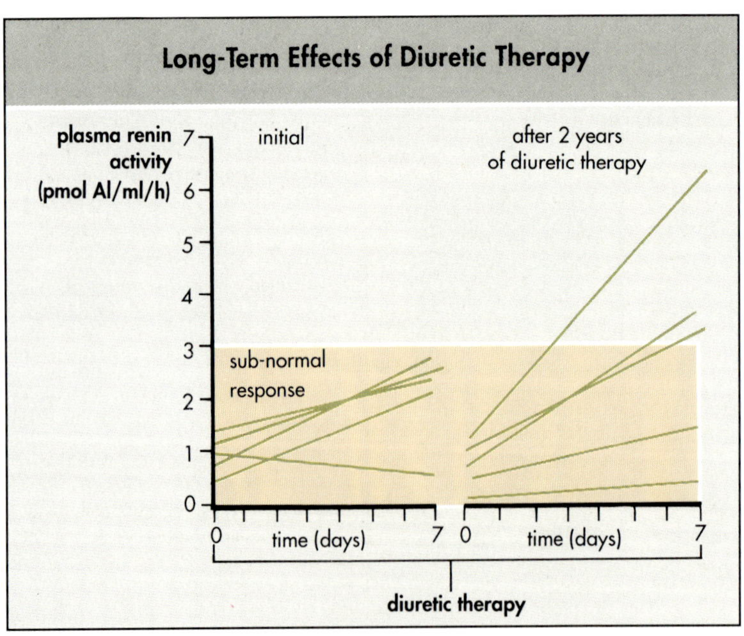

Fig. 3.20 The response of plasma renin to seven days of diuretic therapy in five patients with low-renin hypertension. Plasma renin would normally rise to values above 3.0pmol AI/ml/hr. After two years of treatment with diuretics, medication was stopped for a month and plasma renin did not differ significantly from initial untreated levels. However, the responsiveness to diuretics was substantially increased in three patients who then no longer met the criteria for low-renin hypertension, indicating that treatment can substantially modify the classification of patients. [Modified from Swart, S. S. *et al.* (1982) *Clin Sci*, **63**, 121–125.]

observed with both aging and hypertension, and both factors affect the incidence of such changes additively. Hyaline nephrosclerosis affects the elasticity of the arteriole and may, therefore, influence juxtaglomerular responsiveness to alterations in perfusion pressure, just as changes in the carotid arterial wall may affect the carotid baroreceptor mediated reflexes. Hyporeninaemic hypoaldosteronism may occur in association with diabetes in elderly subjects with vascular disease, perhaps for the same reason. It has also been suggested that patients with low renin hypertension

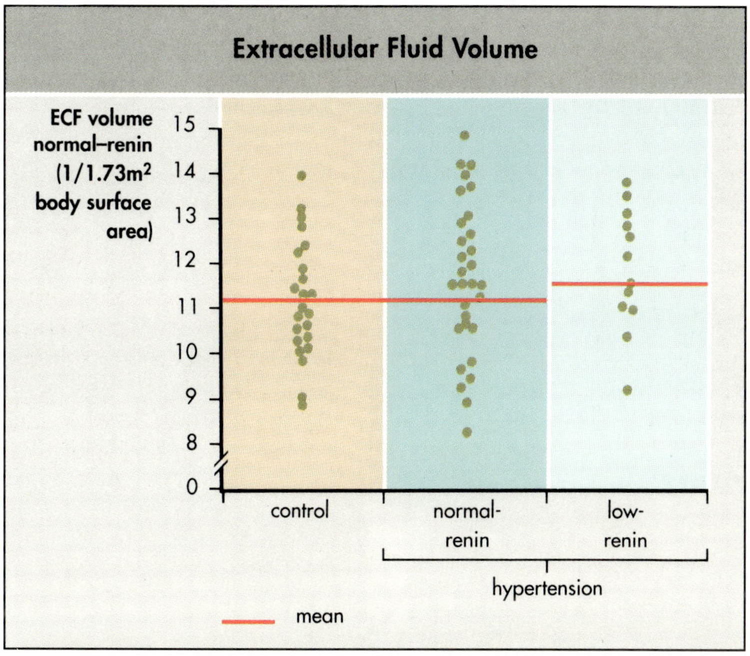

Fig. 3.21 Extracellular fluid volume in normal individuals and patients with either low-renin or normal-renin essential hypertension.

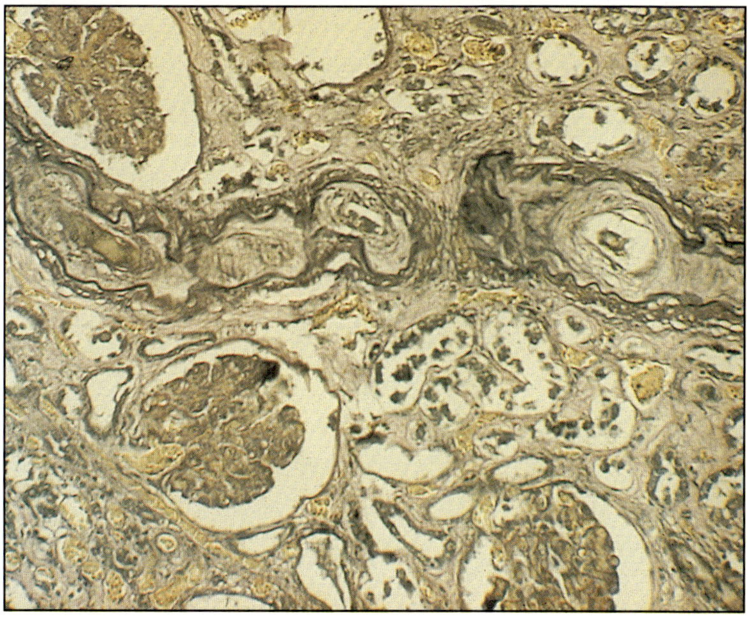

Fig. 3.22 Histology of a glomerulus from a patient with essential hypertension, showing benign nephrosclerosis with hyaline changes. This is particularly marked in the afferent arteriole (stained yellow).

have a lower level of sympathetic neuronal activity, which may in turn influence renin secretion. It therefore seems probable that low renin hypertension is not a homogeneous pathogenetic entity; according to this explanation, several factors influence juxtaglomerular responsiveness (Fig. 3.23). This explanation would be consistent with the observation that renin levels and renin responsiveness in hypertension form a continuum, with no evidence of discrete subgroups.

Sodium and Fluid

Observations noting the effect of salt upon the circulation have been found in very early Chinese writings, although the connection between salt and blood pressure has been recognised in the West only since the beginning of this century.

Sodium-Dependent Hypertension

In some clinical situations, elevated blood pressure can be directly attributed to increased body sodium (Fig. 3.24). For instance, in patients maintained on dialysis after bilateral nephrectomy, there is a close correlation between sodium balance, exchangeable sodium and blood pressure (Fig. 3.25). As patients retain sodium between each dialysis, blood pressure rises – as sodium is removed at dialysis, blood pressure falls again. When diseased kidneys are *in situ* the relationship between sodium and blood pressure is often less clear-cut. Indeed, in some cases hypertension is worsened by dialytic removal of sodium and fluid in association with very high renin levels. When an animal with normal kidneys or with Goldblatt 2-kidney 1-clip hypertension has its sodium and

Factors Influencing Juxtaglomerular Responsiveness

process	consequences	renin secretion
raised renal perfusion pressure	increased pressure in JGA baroreceptor	–
raised renal perfusion pressure	pressure natriuresis causing sodium depletion	+
change in renal tubular sodium reabsorption (?)	inhibition of natriuresis	–
increased sympathetic activity (some patients)	stimulation of JGA ß-receptors	+
decreased sympathetic activity (? some patients)	inhibition of JGA ß-receptors	–
benign nephrosclerotic change or age or hypertension	increased rigidity of JGA wall	–
malignant hypertension	fibrinoid necrosis of JGA wall	?
treatment	stimulation/inhibition of JGA by a variety of mechanisms	±

Fig. 3.23 Influences upon renin which are probably responsible for the observed abnormalities in hypertension. (JGA=juxtaglomerular apparatus.)

fluid balance altered by dialysis, the relationship between sodium and blood pressure is not seen unless sodium removal is sufficient to cause circulatory collapse. The kidneys therefore appear to possess buffering mechanisms which protect blood pressure against the pressor and depressor effects of salt loading and depletion. One of these systems is undoubtedly the renin–angiotensin system; the reno-medullary antihypertensive system of Muirhead may also be important in this respect, although its physiological role is less well defined (see below).

Hypertensive States Attributable to Sodium

- mineralocorticoid excess
- bilateral nephrectomy
- terminal renal disease
- iatrogenic
- dialysis

Fig. 3.24 Clinical hypertensive states in which sodium excess appears to play a role.

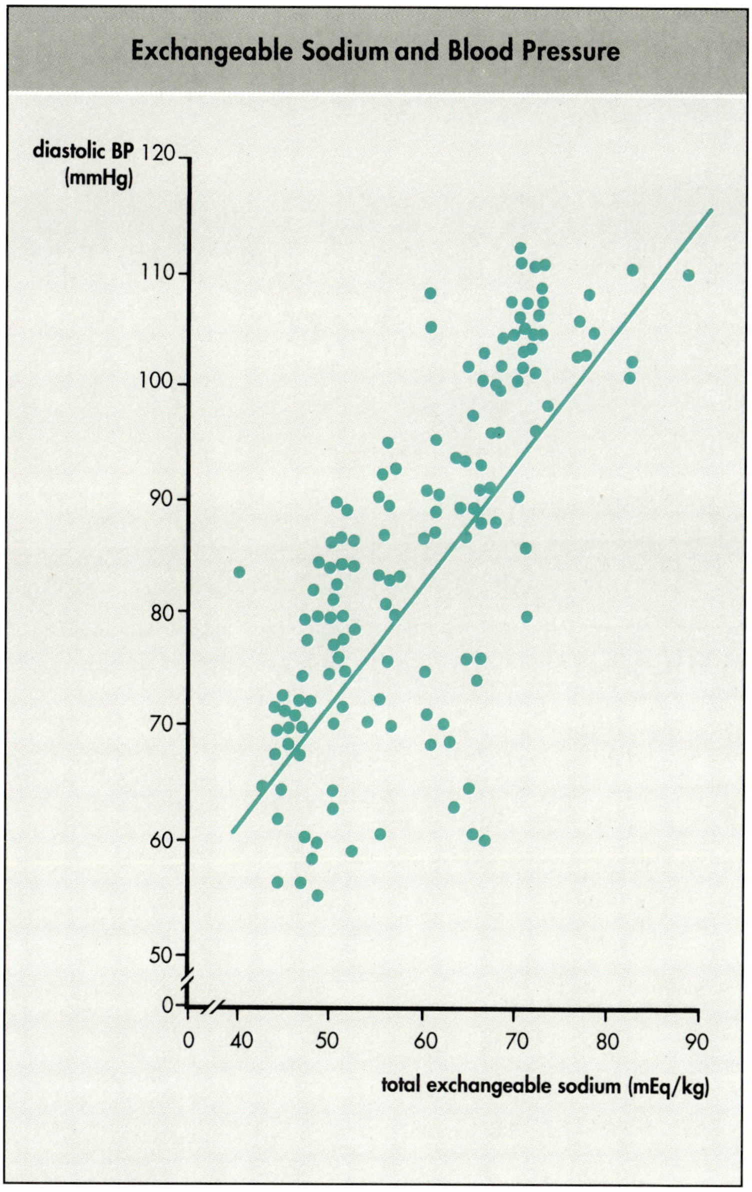

Fig. 3.25 The relationship between exchangeable sodium and blood pressure in patients with terminal renal failure showing that high blood pressure is usually associated with sodium retention.

The Autoregulatory Hypothesis

How does sodium elevate blood pressure (Fig. 3.26) when the confounding effect of the kidney is removed? It is important to bear in mind that the pressor effect of sodium is observed when sodium loading is isotonic, that is when there is no change in serum sodium. Sodium is therefore acting through extracellular or plasma volume expansion. Guyton and his co-workers have put forward a hypothesis which is a development of that of Borst and Ledingham and based upon the sequence of events which was observed when partially nephrectomized dogs were loaded with salt (Fig. 3.27). An early rise in blood pressure was associated with an elevation of cardiac output, which returned to normal levels as peripheral resistance increased. It was suggested that volume expansion produced an increase in venous return to the heart, thereby elevating stroke volume and cardiac output (see chapter 2). This, it was argued, produced tissue overperfusion, which in turn resulted in a protective autoregulatory vasoconstriction, reducing peripheral flow to normal

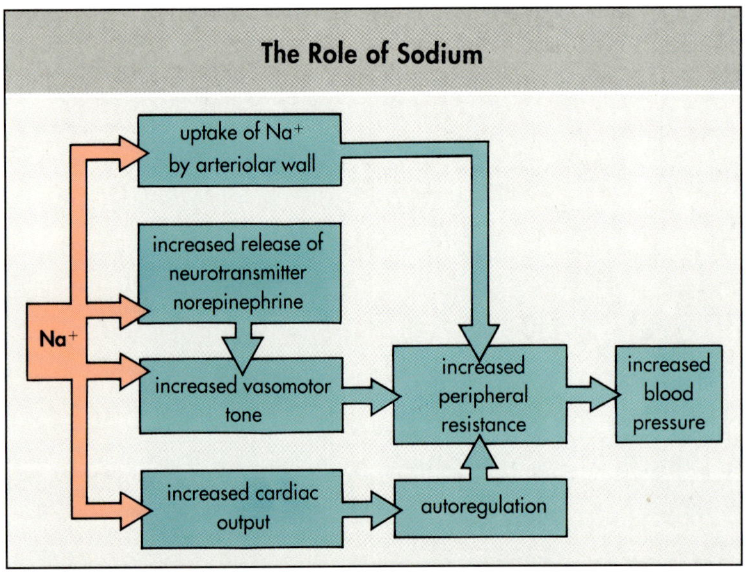

Fig. 3.26 Postulated effects of sodium in producing high blood pressure.

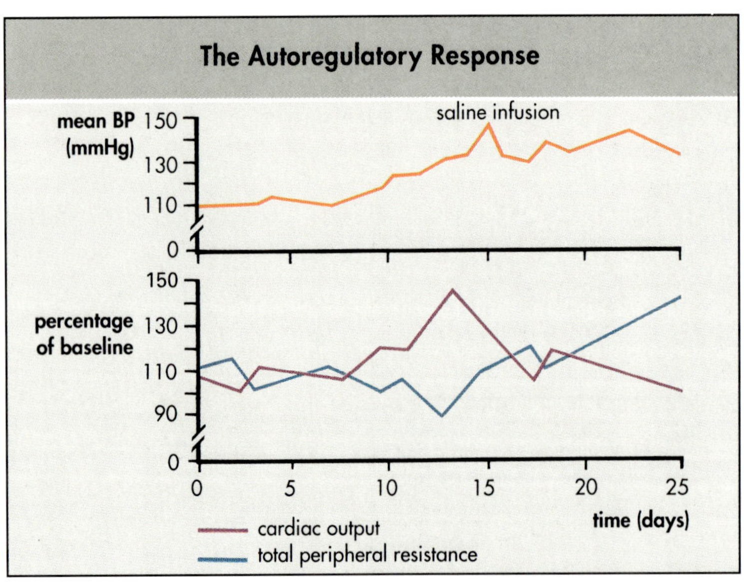

Fig. 3.27 Guyton's experiment on partially nephrectomized dogs – when sodium-loaded, the rise in pressure is initially associated with a rise in pressure is initially associated with a rise in cardiac output and a subsequent rise in peripheral resistance.

levels at the expense of an elevated blood pressure. The second part of Guyton's theory puts forward an explanation for volume expansion. Normally, any rise in blood pressure produces a perfusion pressure natriuresis and diuresis which restores blood pressure to normal. Unlike the blood pressure reduction produced by baroreceptors, for example, pressure natriuresis and diuresis proceed until blood pressure is restored to normal (Fig. 3.28), unless prevented by other systems. Hypertension can only therefore occur, Guyton argues, if the normal pressor diuresis and natriuresis is inhibited so that the response curve relating pressure to natriuresis and diuresis is shifted to the right (Fig. 3.29). This could occur as the result of a genetic abnormality in kidney function or as a result of the action of aldosterone, angiotensin II, or increased sympathetic nervous system activity. Thus, the renal control of sodium balance is critical even in models such as the Goldblatt 2-kidney 1-clip, where high angiotensin II levels help to restrict the natriuresis and diuresis which would otherwise limit blood pressure elevation.

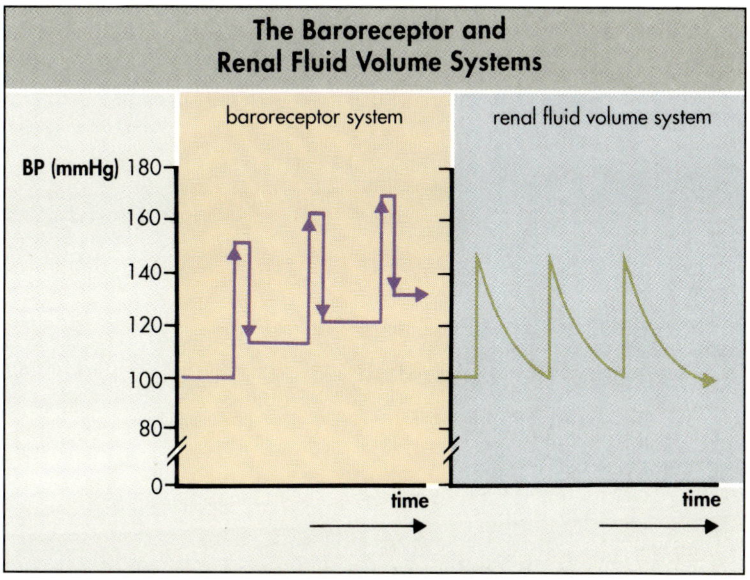

Fig. 3.28 The action of the baroreceptor and renal fluid volume systems in returning arterial pressure to within normal limits after blood pressure has been raised by external influence. Note that the baroreceptors do not return blood pressure completely to normal, whereas the renal fluid volume system does. Guyton describes the latter as 'a system of infinite gain'.

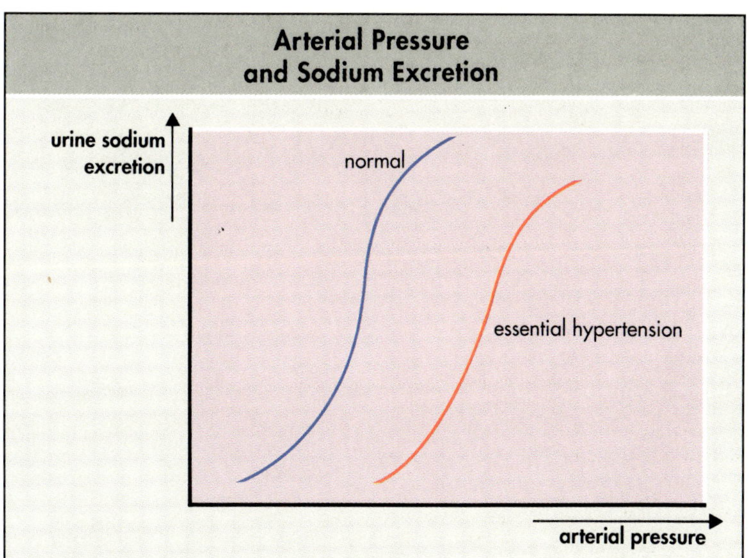

Fig. 3.29 The relationship between increased arterial pressure and urinary sodium excretion. For any given pressure, urinary sodium excretion is lower in hypertensive subjects.

Many physiologists still accept Guyton's hypothesis. However, it has been criticized in the light of subsequent experimental work. The extent to which the whole body autoregulatory mechanism occurs in the intact animal remains uncertain: it frequently appears to be overridden *in vivo*, although it can be demonstrated in some (but by no means all) tissue beds. When hypertension is induced, either by infusing saline into patients on dialysis or by discontinuing mineralocorticoid antagonists in patients with primary aldosteronism, the haemodynamic sequence of events described by Guyton is frequently either not seen or seen to occur over widely differing periods of time. In some complex clinical situations, other factors may substantially modify the haemodynamic pattern. Anaemia in patients with renal failure is associated with an increase in cardiac output and a decrease in peripheral resistance. Correction of anaemia by transfusion restores the haemodynamic pattern to normal. In other forms of hypertension the first event associated with elevation of blood pressure may be an increase in peripheral resistance without any initial increase in cardiac output. Thus a primary increase in peripheral resistance has frequently been described in experimental models of hypertension (Fig. 3.30). Even where the initial rise in cardiac output occurs at the point of induction of experimental hypertension, it may not be a *sine qua non* for hypertension, but could simply be a manifestation of postoperative sodium and fluid retention or venoconstriction.

The failure to observe a chronic perfusion pressure natriuresis and diuresis in either experimental or clinical hypertension is accepted. However, it should be borne in mind that any initial negative sodium and water balance produced by an increase in renal perfusion pressure will inevitably set up potent renal conservation of sodium and water. This will cause a secondary shift in the perfusion pressure natriuresis/diuresis curve. Distinguishing between such a primary change in renal function and a secondary effect is difficult.

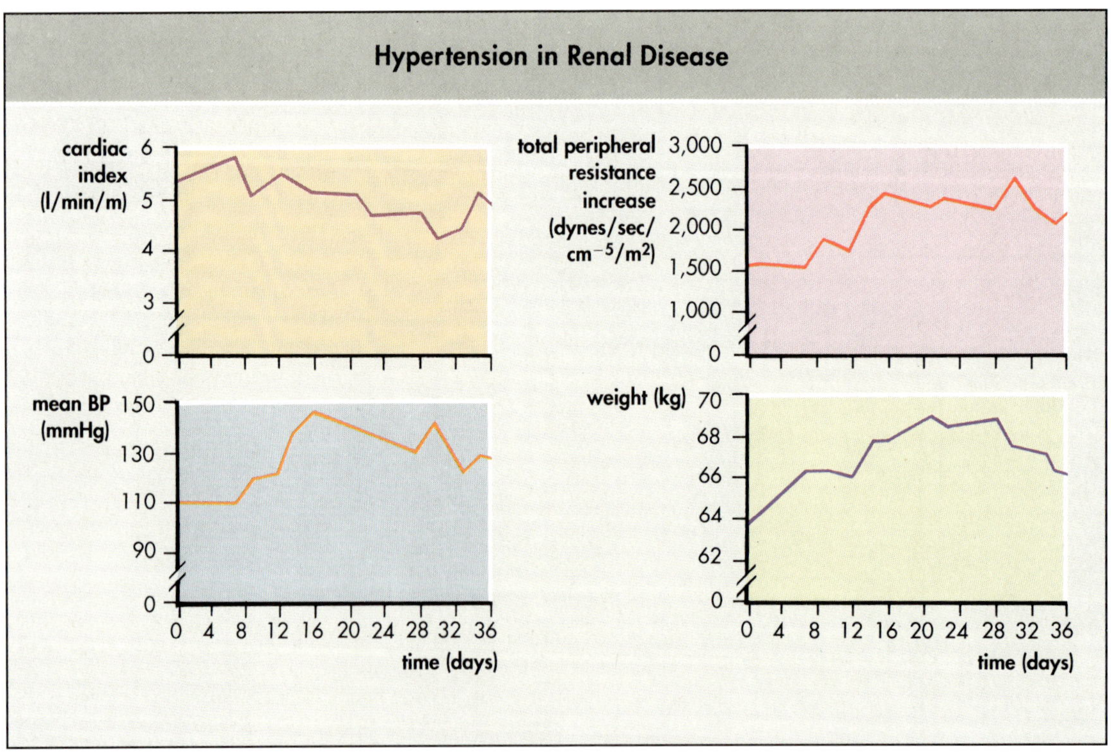

Fig. 3.30 Patients with renal disease often develop hypertension associated with sodium retention, a result of increased peripheral resistance without early elevation of cardiac output.

The Cell Sodium Hypothesis

It is not surprising that more interest has been focussed upon the direct or indirect action of sodium upon peripheral blood vessels. The earlier hypothesis, put forward by Tobian's group, suggested that sodium and fluid retention by the arteriolar wall increased wall thickness. This would impinge upon the lumen of resistance vessels and so cause an elevation in peripheral resistance (Fig. 3.31). The quantity of sodium in the arterial wall was shown to be elevated in several forms of experimental hypertension, although it was uncertain whether the extra sodium lay in the extracellular fluid compartment (perhaps bound osmotically) or within cells. However, it now seems likely that this change in vessel electrolyte content was a product of the structural changes produced by hypertension, rather than a cause of hypertension in its own right. It is possible that an expansion of extracellular space in the arterial wall occurred, with increased non-osmotic binding of sodium by the extra collagen which is associated with hypertensive structural change. It should also be recalled that one of the primary characteristics of hypertensive resistance vessels is increased maximal contraction (see chapter 3). It is difficult to explain this in terms of waterlogging of the vessel wall which would, if anything, cause weakening of contractile ability.

Blaustein has postulated a more indirect link between sodium retention and blood pressure. In some tissues (most notably the heart) there is a sodium–calcium exchanger. This is a transporter which moves calcium ions out of the cell. It is powered by the passage of sodium ions down the concentration gradient from extracellular to intracellular fluid. Elevation of intracellular sodium will therefore reduce this gradient and reduce the extrusion of calcium. Any process which increases intracellular sodium will thus also increase intracellular calcium through inhibition of this

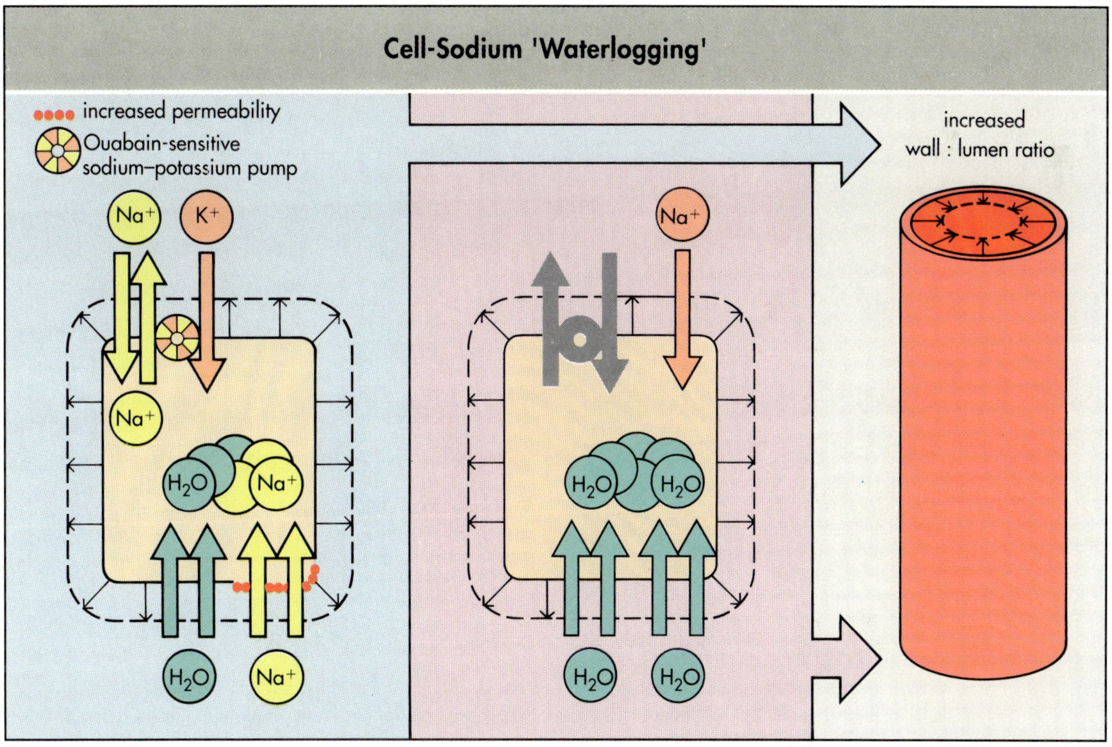

Fig. 3.31 Tobian's group proposed that sodium and fluid retention give rise to hypertension by increasing the wall-to-lumen ratio in arteriolar walls, thereby elevating peripheral resistance. A net influx of sodium into the cell could occur as a result of increased membrane permeability, or through inhibition of the ouabain-sensitive sodium–potassium pump.

exchanger (Fig. 3.32). Since calcium is an important second messenger for vasoconstriction, increases in intracellular sodium will elevate blood pressure through generalized vasoconstriction. Why should intracellular sodium be elevated? It has been suggested that a positive sodium balance stimulates the secretion of a natriuretic hormone which reduces renal tubular reabsorption of sodium. This hormone has ouabain-like properties which inhibit the sodium pump – its source is probably the hypothalamus. This inhibitory property, so important in mediating natriuresis, also has the undesirable effect of reducing sodium extrusion by vascular smooth muscle and therefore (via the sodium–calcium exchanger) promoting vasoconstriction (Fig. 3.33).

This imaginative hypothesis has attracted widespread interest and many studies have been directed at testing it. One of the major difficulties is that the ouabain-like natriuretic hormone has not yet been characterized. It is, therefore, only possible to measure it by indirect assay. Sodium pump activity is inhibited by a wide range of biological compounds, including fatty acids and several steroids, and it has been very difficult to exclude such confounding factors in experimental studies. There is no consensus on whether volume expansion inhibits sodium pump activity in tissues other than the renal tubule. Although vascular smooth muscle probably does contain a

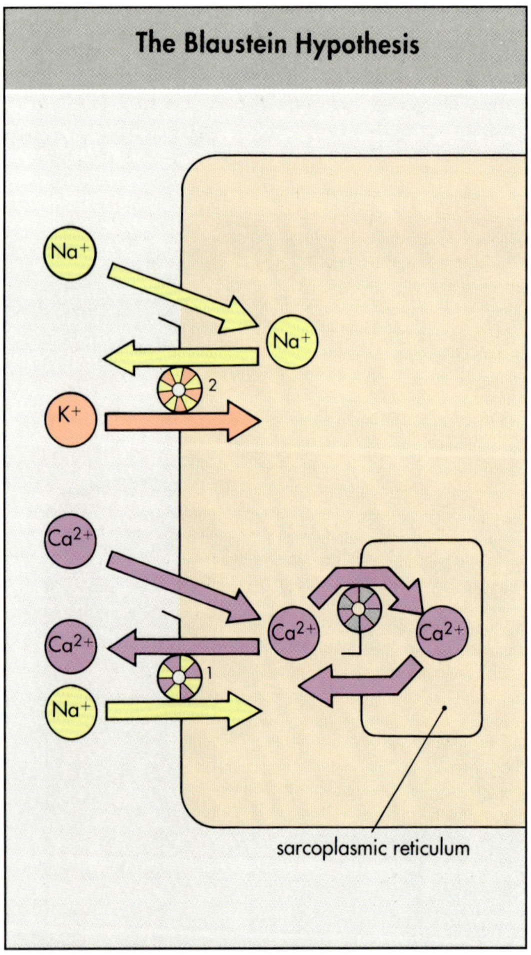

Fig. 3.32 Smooth muscle contractility may be increased by a rise in intracellular calcium caused by inhibition or failure of a postulated exchanger (1) in muscle cell walls which is responsible for an exchange of sodium for calcium (Blaustein). This pump is separate from the sodium–potassium pump (2) inhibited by ouabain.

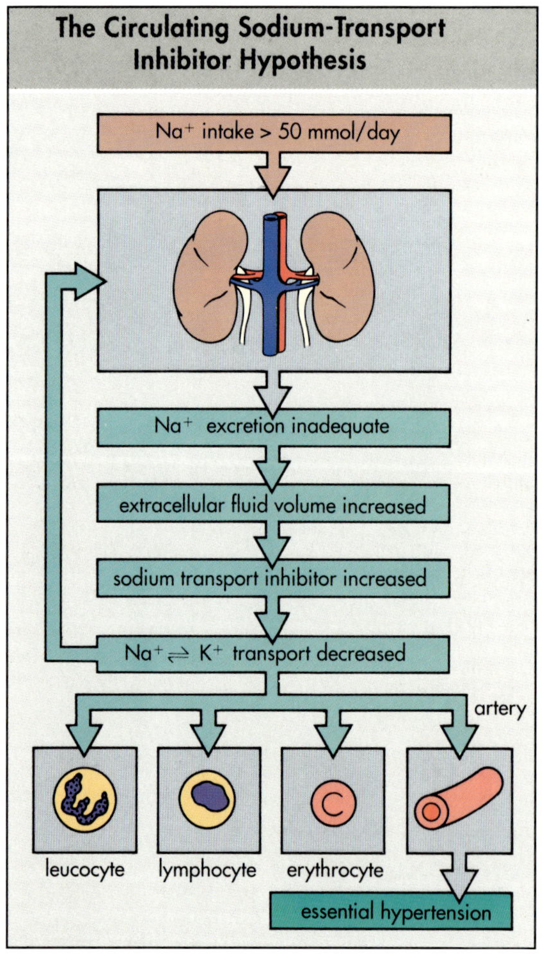

Fig. 3.33 The circulating sodium transport inhibitor hypothesis. Sodium retention stimulates the secretion of a natriuretic hormone which has additional effects on vascular smooth muscle and blood cells, inhibiting sodium–potassium transport and thereby indirectly increasing intracellular calcium (cf. Fig. 3.32).

sodium–calcium exchanger, it may not operate within the normal physiological range. Ouabain causes vasoconstriction in isolated resistance vessels, but this is transient and may well be related to inhibition of the sodium pump in pre-synaptic neurones, where calcium also acts as a second messenger regulating neurotransmitter release.

Sodium Interaction with the Nervous System

High sodium intake has an important effect upon the sympathetic nervous system – the amount of neurotransmitter released per impulse is increased (Fig. 3.34). Whether similar changes occur in the vasomotor centre and the higher centres which regulate it is unknown; if they do, this would provide an important mechanism for linking changes in sodium balance and blood pressure.

Sodium in Other Forms of Hypertension

Several unusual clinical forms of hypertension are associated with extracellular fluid volume expansion. It is, for instance, observed in primary aldosteronism and in its experimental analogue, DOC–salt hypertension. In Conn's syndrome there is a correlation between exchangeable sodium and blood pressure (Fig. 3.35). Blood pressure lowering by potassium-retaining diuretics or by removal of the adenoma returns exchangeable sodium to

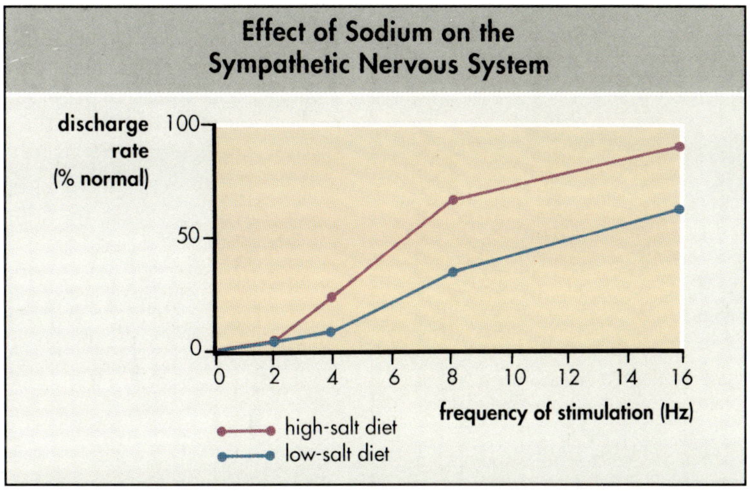

Fig. 3.34 The relationship between sympathetic fibre discharge rate and neurogenic response was examined in two groups of rats. One group had been kept on a high-salt diet, the other on a low-salt diet. The former showed a markedly higher response across the greater part of the frequency-range. [Modified from Folkow and Ely (1987) *J Hypertension*, **5**, 389.]

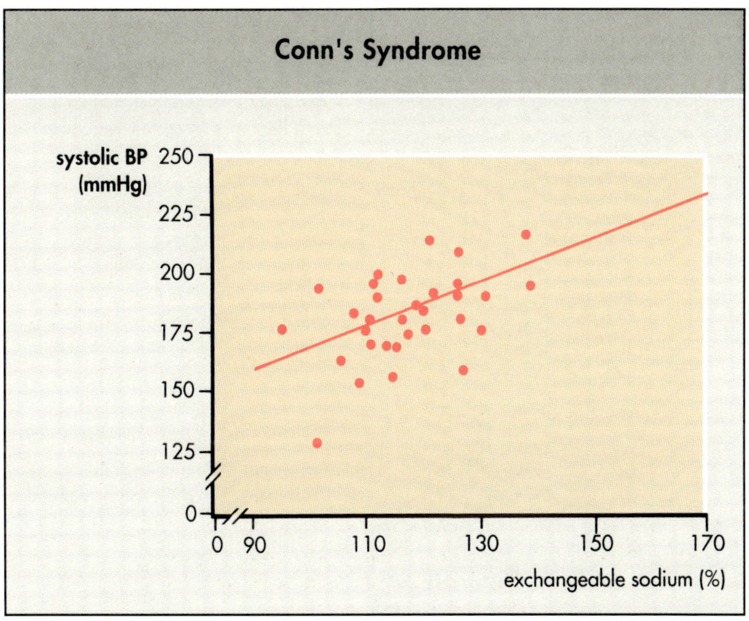

Fig. 3.35 The correlation between exchangeable sodium and blood pressure demonstated in patients with Conn's syndrome suggests that volume expansion is related to hypertension. [Modified from Beretta-Piccoli *et al.* (1983) *J Hypertension*, **1**, 197–205.]

normal (Fig. 3.36). It therefore seems likely that volume expansion does contribute to hypertension. However, mineralocorticoid hormones such as deoxycorticosterone also have a cellular effect on vascular smooth muscle increasing its permeability to sodium and enhancing sodium turnover. This direct effect may contribute to the elevation in peripheral resistance.

Secondary changes in the resistance vessels assume importance in maintaining blood pressure in the chronic state. In DOC–salt hypertension, when DOC is stopped blood pressure usually remains elevated despite the fact that exchangeable sodium is normal.

Mineralocorticoid-like syndromes are seen in patients who ingest liquorice or carbenoxolone. These agents appear to have an action upon the renal metabolism of cortisol which results in metabolites with mineralocorticoid-like activity being formed. Non-steroidal anti-inflammatory drugs interfere with sodium and water excretion by inhibiting the synthesis of renal prostanoids, which have a diuretic and natriuretic action.

The Dahl rat has been used extensively as a model of sodium-dependent hypertension. Dahl was able, by a process of selective inbreeding, to develop a strain of rat which became hypertensive when given high salt loads (Fig. 3.37). Blood pres-

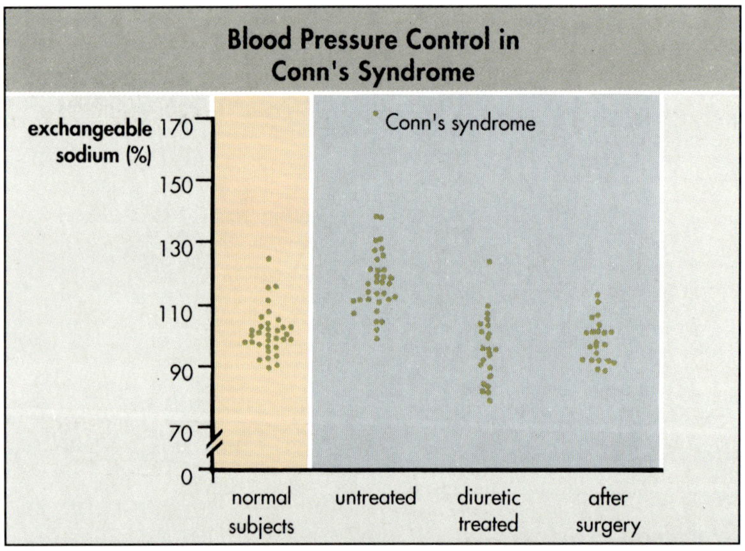

Fig. 3.36 Exchangeable sodium in patients with Conn's syndrome, showing untreated patients, patients on diuretics and patients after removal of the adenoma. (For source see Fig. 3.35.)

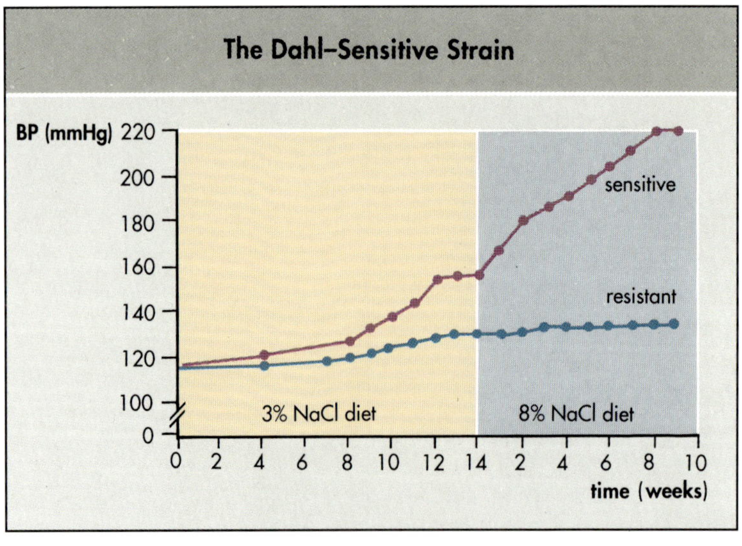

Fig. 3.37 The Dahl salt-sensitive strain becomes hypertensive when extremely high salt-loads are administered. It is compared here with a salt-resistant strain.

sure remained elevated even when a normal salt diet was resumed. Cross-circulation studies suggested that a circulating factor was responsible for hypertension in the Dahl salt-sensitive strain; salt resistant strains could have salt-sensitivity induced by linking circulations with salt sensitive rats. Salt sensitivity could also be transmitted by transplanting a kidney from a salt sensitive to a salt resistant strain (Fig. 3.38). The Milan strain of rat shows a similar phenomenon. There are however difficulties in extrapolating from these models to man. Firstly, the amount of salt required by the Dahl rat is extremely high, even allowing for the its higher metabolic rate. Further, as Dahl Pointed out, hypertension is also produced by other noxious stimuli. Although the ouabain-like natriuretic hormone is a possible candidate as the agent which produces hypertension in the Dahl rat, it has not been possible to show inhibition of the sodium pump in the vascular smooth muscle in this strain. Indeed, although turnover of sodium seems to be increased, studies show body sodium to be unchanged. The Milan strain of rat, on the other hand, does show a transient increase in body sodium during the development of hypertension. Data on the most commonly used genetic model of hypertension (the SHR) are contradictory in this respect, with some groups demonstrating an early, minor increase in plasma volume. In the established phase of hypertension, however, there is no evidence of sodium retention. A major increase in sodium in the diet exacerbates hypertension in this model. In other models of hypertension, for instance the Goldblatt 2-kidney 1-clip model, blood pressure can be increased by severe sodium restriction and the same phenomenon has been demonstrated in non-hypertensive laboratory strains of rat (Fig. 3.39). Whether or not this is a non-specific stress response remains unclear.

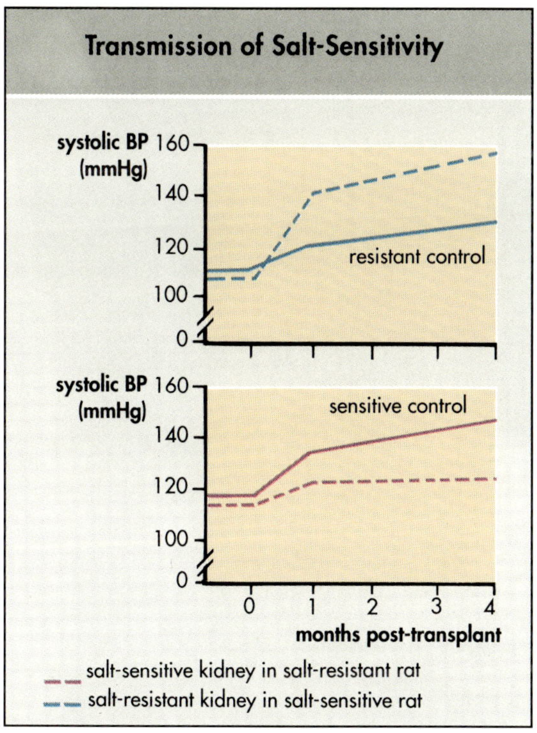

Fig. 3.38 The effect of a kidney transplant between salt-sensitive and salt-resistant strains of rat is to produce hypertension in the salt-resistant strain.

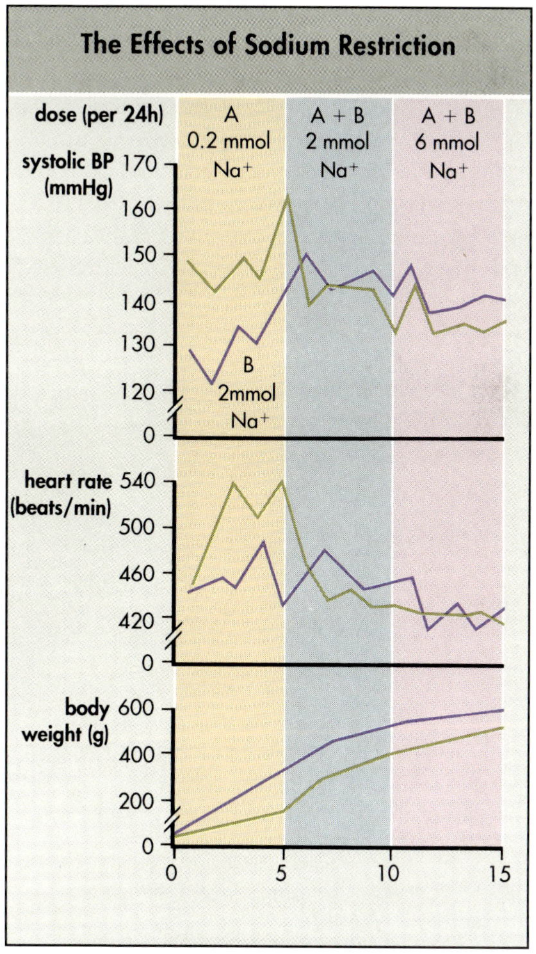

Fig. 3.39 Changes in blood pressure, heart rate and body-weight in normal rats placed alternately on low and normal salt intakes. [Modified from Webb *et al.* (1987) *J Hypertension,* **5**, 525–532.]

Sodium in Essential Hypertension

Dahl suggested a relationship between salt intake and blood pressure. Certain cultures, he pointed out, which were free of essential hypertension and which failed to show any increase in blood pressure with age, appeared also to have a low salt (sodium) intake (Fig. 3.40). These cultures tended to be technologically unadvanced, obtaining their salt from vegetable ash, which is high in potassium and low in sodium. A First World diet, by contrast, is relatively high in sodium and low in potassium content. Furthermore, salt ingestion in the early months of life is often high, because of the relatively high salt content of artificial baby foods and cows milk. Although the correlation between salt intake and blood pressure that Dahl reported was a close one, cross-cultural information is extremely difficult to come by. However, the Intersalt Study has examined this relationship by studying 24-hour urinary sodium in over 10,000 individuals from 52 different cultures. This showed a weak relationship between urinary sodium and systolic blood pressure, although there was no significant relationship with diastolic blood pressure when confounding factors, such as body weight and alcohol intake, were eliminated.

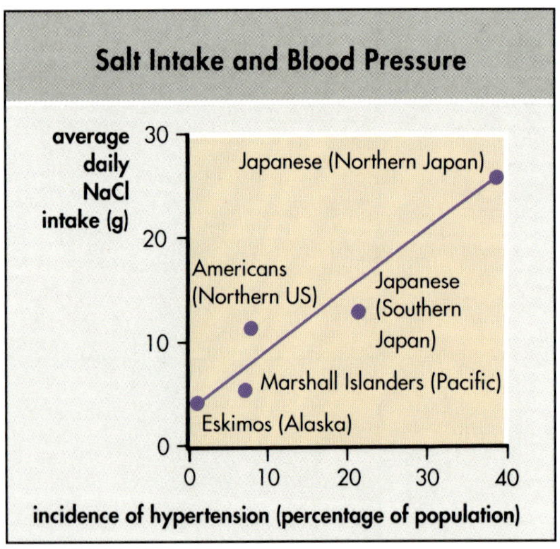

Fig. 3.40 Having studied a number of races, Dahl reported a correlation between estimated salt intake and the incidence of hypertension.

There is difficulty, however, in interpreting the results, since four cultures with very low sodium intakes and low blood pressures weighted the relationship. The correlation actually did not exist over the range of sodium intakes found in Western society (Fig. 3.41). There were, however, stronger relationships between sodium intake and the rise in blood pressure with age (Fig. 3.42). Other studies have shown a rise in blood pressure in rural populations as they as they become urbanized, and these changes are also associated with an

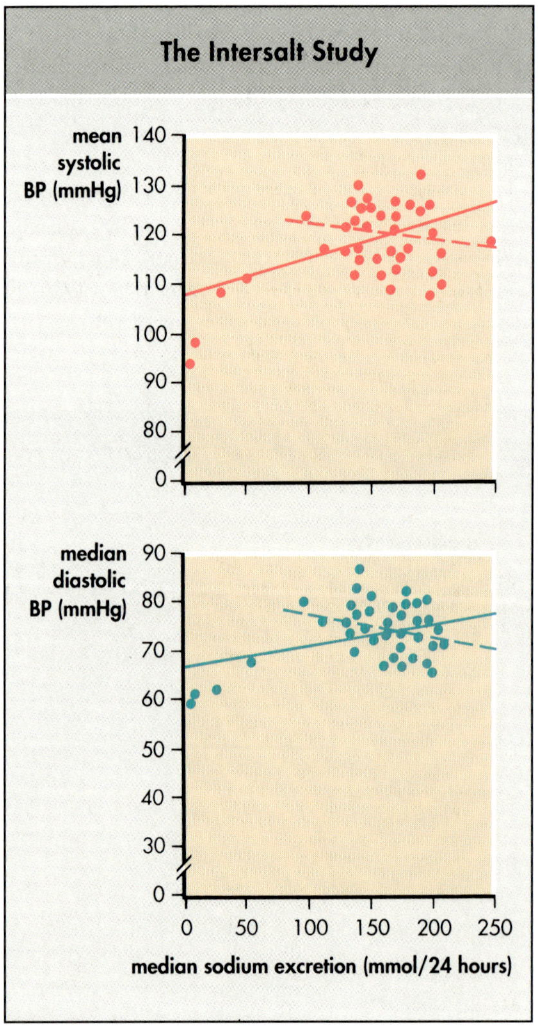

Fig. 3.41 The relationship between sodium excretion and blood pressure in the Intersalt Study. The continuous line shows the relationship in all 52 centres studied. The dotted line shows the relationship excluding 4 centres in which the sodium intake was very low. Note how these four centres, where sodium intake is well below levels found in Western societies, weight the relationship. [Modified from Intersalt Study (1988) *Brit Med J*, **297**, 319–328.]

increase in sodium and a decrease in dietary potassium. These changes in blood pressure may occur within months so the effect should be easy to reproduce by dietary change in humans. Studies of blood pressure and sodium intake in single societies have in general failed to demonstrate a relationship. The largest of these, the Scottish Heart Health Study (7,354 subjects), showed a small correlation disappearing when the data were corrected for bodymass index and alcohol and potassium intake. Exactly how much such epidemiological associations owe to causal relationships is, at present, unknown.

An alternative and widely held view is that salt intake acts as a marker of the 'civilizing process' or, in other words, urban stress. For example, a recent study showed that women entering a closed religious order showed no rise in blood pressure with age – a control group of women showed the typical 'Western' rise in blood pressure with age. This difference was not related to diet (see Fig. 3.68). If the salt hypothesis is correct, dietary salt in most Western populations is excessively high. The fact that only a minority of people develop frank hypertension might therefore be related to genetic susceptibility. There may be an analogy with the Dahl strain of rat. If only genetically sensitive individuals develop hypertension in the face of a high salt intake, a close correlation between salt intake and blood pressure would not be anticipated and the relevance of salt may be underestimated. On these grounds it has been suggested that the blood pressure response to salt loading and salt restriction identifies a group of 'salt sensitive' hypertensives. Although some subjects undoubtedly respond to salt restriction by a significant reduction in blood pressure (Fig. 3.43), there

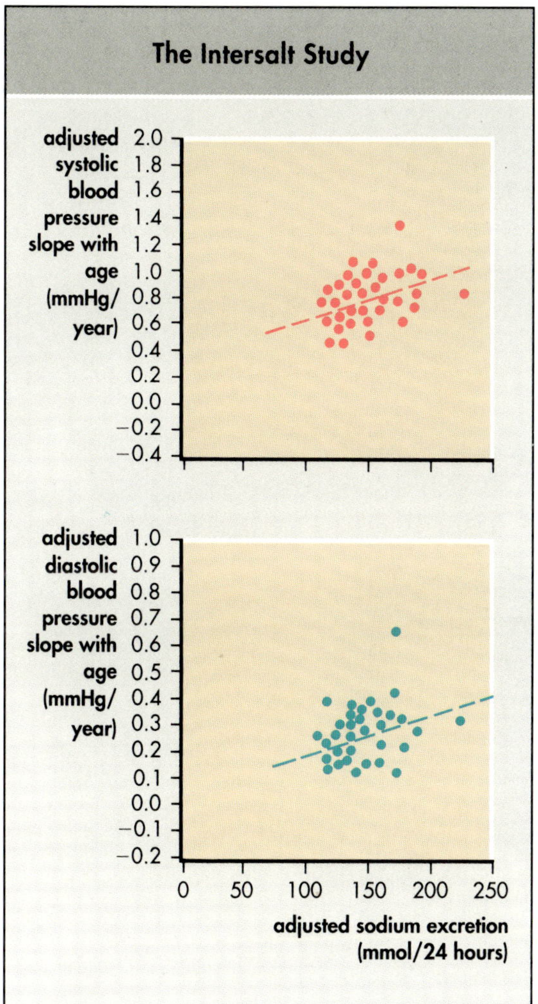

Fig. 3.42 Relationship between increase of blood pressure with age and sodium excretion in the Intersalt Study, after values have been adjusted for differences in alcohol intake and body mass index. (For source see Fig. 3.41.)

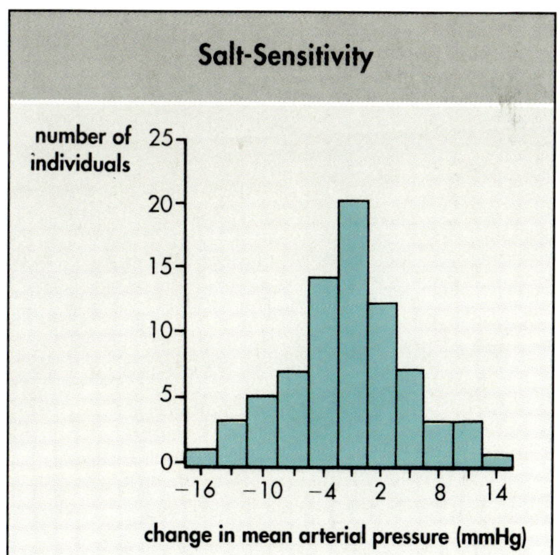

Fig. 3.43 Distribution of blood pressure responses recorded when normotensive adults were subject to a reduction of dietary sodium to less than 65mEq per day for four weeks. Note that, although some significant reductions occurred, mean arterial blood pressure in some individuals actually increased over the period of salt restriction. [Modified from Luft, F. C. (1988) *Hosp Pract*, **October 13th Edn,** 73–80)

is no evidence at present that such individuals form a discrete, genetically defined, 'salt sensitive' group. The phenomenon of 'salt sensitivity' may at least partly reflect impaired responsiveness of the renin–angiotensin system to sodium depletion since this systen normally helps to maintain blood pressure (see chapter 2).

The Central Nervous System

Central nervous system mechanisms which control efferent sympathetic activity may occasionally be involved by disease, leading to hypertension. Lesions of the nucleus tractus solitarius, for instance, produce severe hypertension, tachycardia, high circulating catecholamine levels and evidence of sympathetic nervous system activation (Fig. 3.44). This combination may result in confusion with phaeochromocytoma. The aetiology of the hypertension is probably through interference with the afferent limb of cardiovascular reflexes within the brain stem. Higher lesions, such as those involving the anteromedial nucleus of the hypothalamus, are thought to cause hypertension by destruction of sympathetic inhibitory areas. In man hypertension is occasionally seen in brain stem encephalitis, poliomyelitis, tumours of the fourth ventricle and cerebellum, as well as in

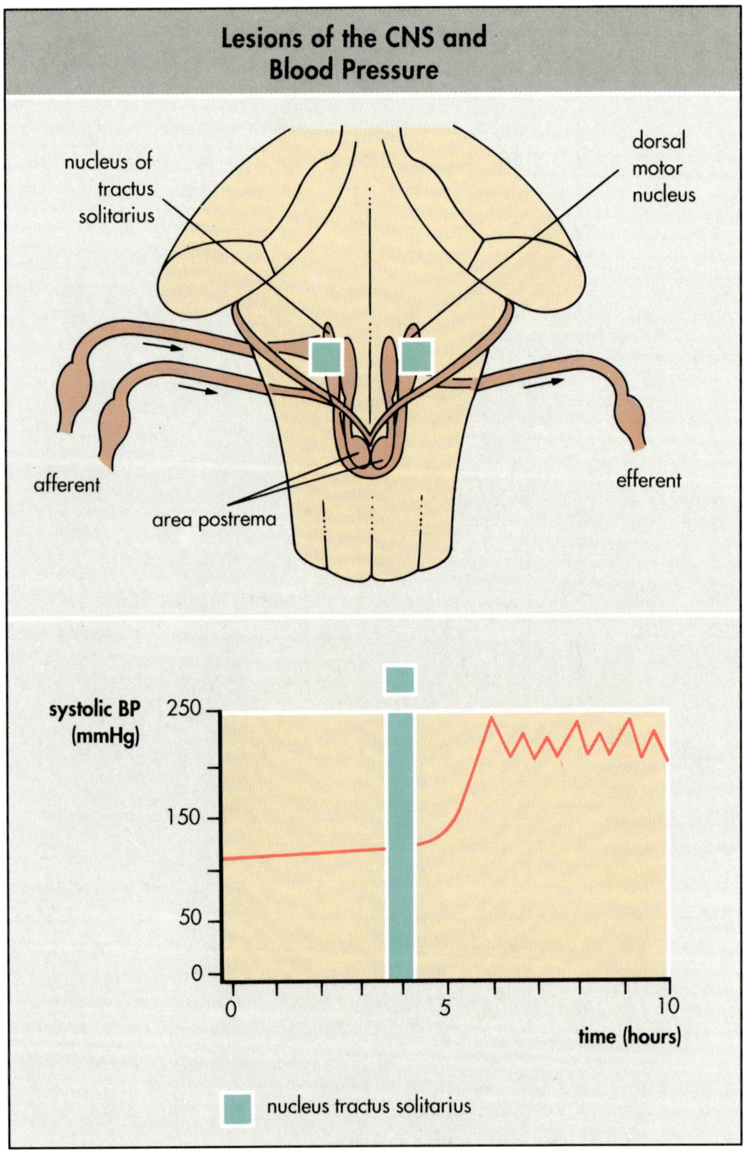

Fig. 3.44 Lesions of the nucleus tractus solitarius produce severe paroxysmal hypertension in rats.

association with acute elevation of intracranial pressure (the Cushing response; see chapter 2). Acute brain stem ischaemia may also cause hypertension on occasions. Transection of the spinal cord above the second thoracic segment releases autonomic reflexes from higher inhibition and causes acute, frequently severe paroxysmal hypertension in response to bladder or rectal stimulation. A full bladder of which the subject is unaware is a major stimulus.

In some genetic models of hypertension, such as the SHR, there is evidence that the sympathetic nervous system is overactive during the earliest phases of hypertension (Fig. 3.45). Thus, the SHR shows a greater increase in pulse rate and cardiac output in response to stress than do matched controls (Fig. 3.46). This hyperreactivity seems to precede hypertension and originate from the limbic hypothalamic system. In addition, it has been observed that peripheral noradrenergic nerves in SHRs release slightly more transmitter per nerve impulse than those in normotensive controls. Folkow has suggested that this enhanced alerting response is important in causing structural changes in essential hypertension and in the SHR (see below). When hypertension is fully established in the SHR there is no evidence of increased sympathetic nervous system activity.

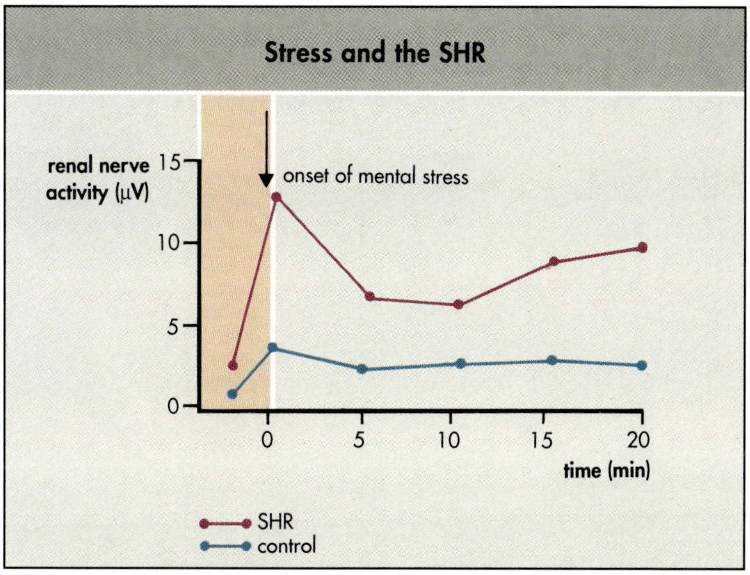

Fig. 3.45 Renal nerve activity in the SHR increases in response to stress.

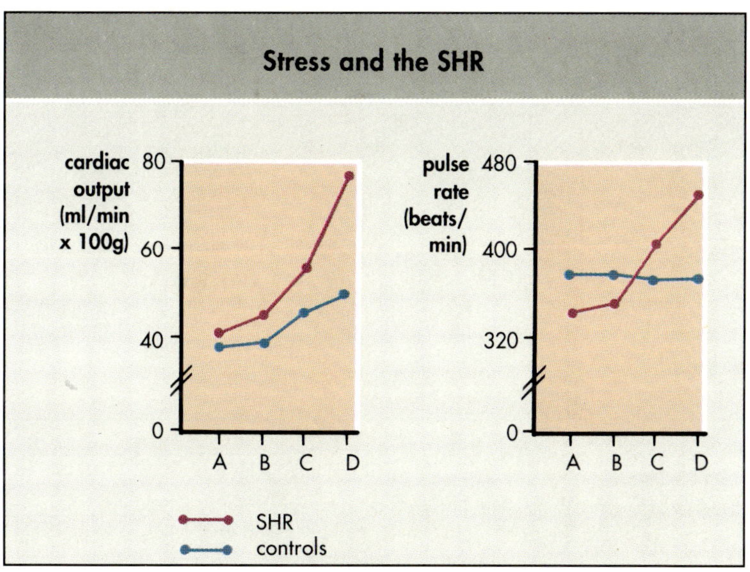

Fig. 3.46 When subjected to stress, spontaneously hypertensive rats (SHRs) showed a much greater increase in cardiac output and pulse rate compared with normotensive controls.

A similar situation may exist in human essential hypertension. It is of course much more difficult to identify a pre-hypertensive phase. However, subjects with a family history of hypertension are at risk of hypertension later in life (although of course this by no means applies to all such individuals). In several studies these have shown increased pulse rate and blood pressure response when exposed to mental stress or cold (Fig. 3.47). In another study, patients with borderline elevation of blood pressure were monitored for twenty years. In many subjects the earliest phases of hypertension were associated with an increase in cardiac output, which slowly returned to normal as peripheral resistance rose. The increased cardiac output and heart rate observed in the early stages of hypertension in these subjects therefore resembled the defence reaction observed in SHRs and was suggestive of enhanced sympathetic nervous system activity. When autonomic influences upon the heart are blocked by cholinergic and ß-blockade, the high cardiac output of subjects with mild hypertension is normalized (Fig. 3.48), indicating that it is due to the autonomic nervous system. Many epidemiological studies have shown a correlation between pulse rate and blood pressure.

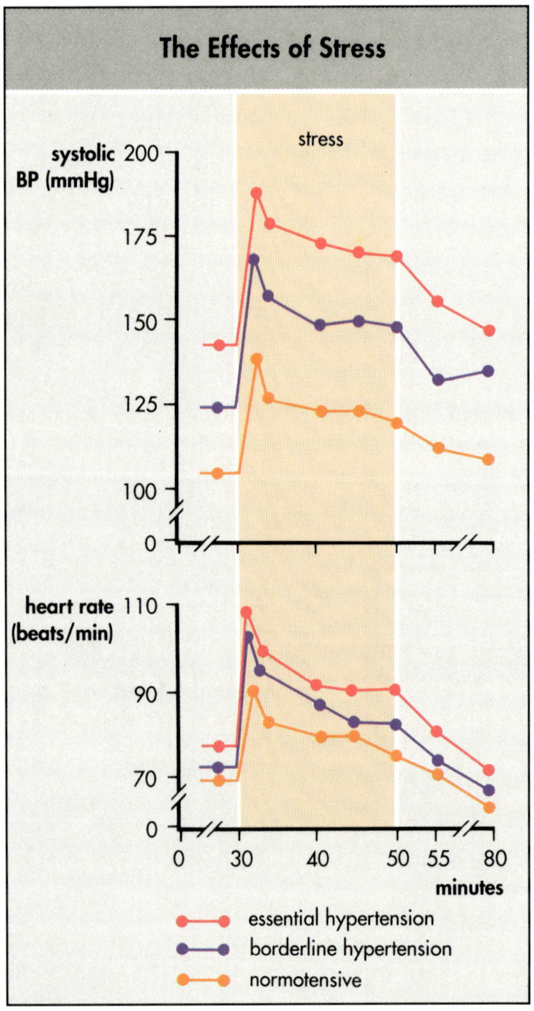

Fig. 3.47 Normotensive and hypertensive humans respond in characteristic ways. [Modified from Eliasson, K. *et al.* (1983) *J Hypertension,* **1**, 134.]

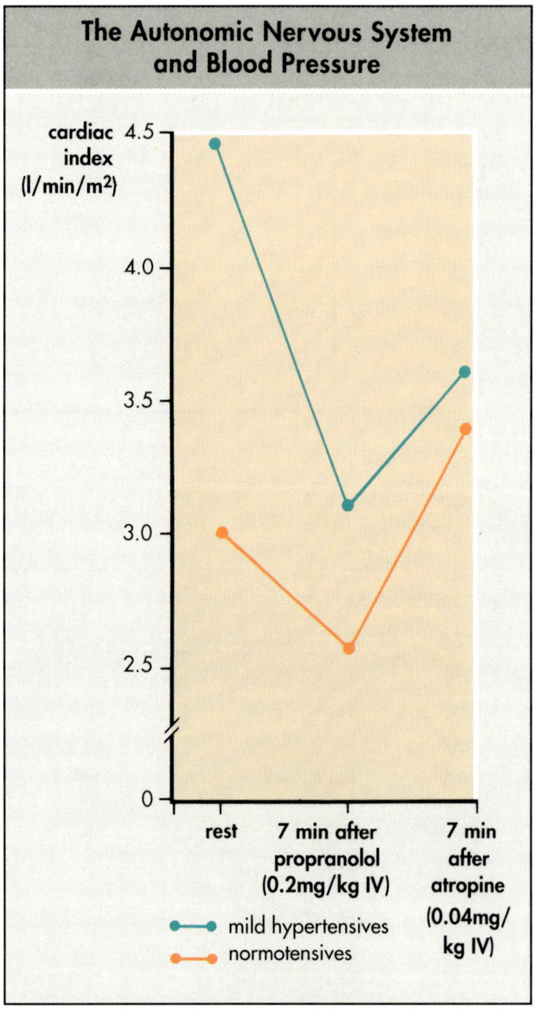

Fig. 3.48 When normotensives and mild hypertensives are subjected to a blockade of the autonomic nervous system, the cardiac output of the latter is brought into line with that of the former. [Modified from Julius, S. *et al.* (1988) *J Cardiovasc Pharmacol*, **12**, s121–s129.]

The determination of sympathetic nervous activity in man is extremely difficult. Although the newer physiological and biochemical techniques provide more insight, they are by no means foolproof. Plasma norepinephrine is derived mainly from peripheral sympathetic nerve endings, with little or no contribution from the central nervous system or adrenal glands (Fig. 3.49). It has been suggested that plasma norepinephrine is a fair determinant of sympathetic activity, and indeed in some circumstances it can be shown to correlate with activity of sympathetic muscle fibres (Fig. 3.50). However, other tissues do contribute substantially to the total plasma norepinephrine, so that the value of this measurement as an assessment of sympathetic nervous activity is limited. Furthermore, the circulating levels of this neurotransmitter are determined by many factors including neuronal and extra-neuronal uptake, metabolism and clearance by a number of organs. Consequently, the interpretation of differences in levels between individuals and between groups must be approached with caution. Early claims that plasma norephinephrine was elevated in hypertensive subjects have not been substantiated by later studies, in which subjects were more

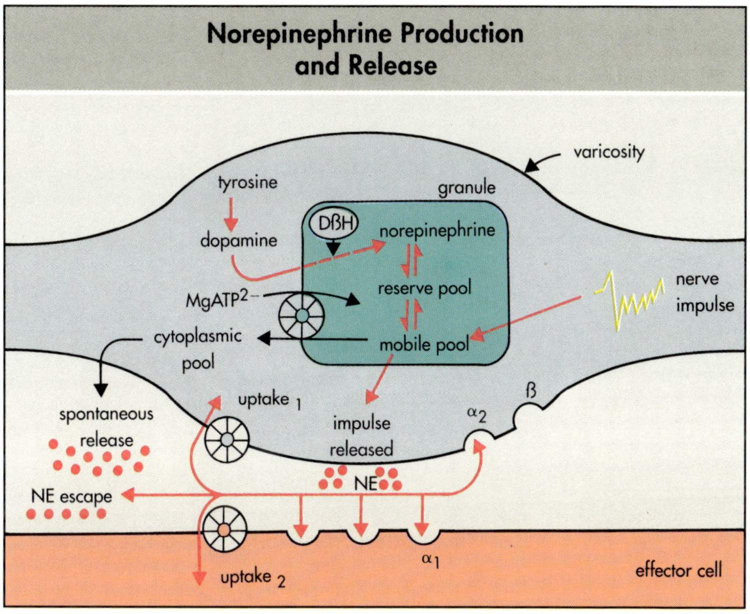

Fig. 3.49 The production and release of norepinephrine from sympathetic nerve endings. (DßH = dopamine ß-hydroxylase; NE = norepinephrine.)

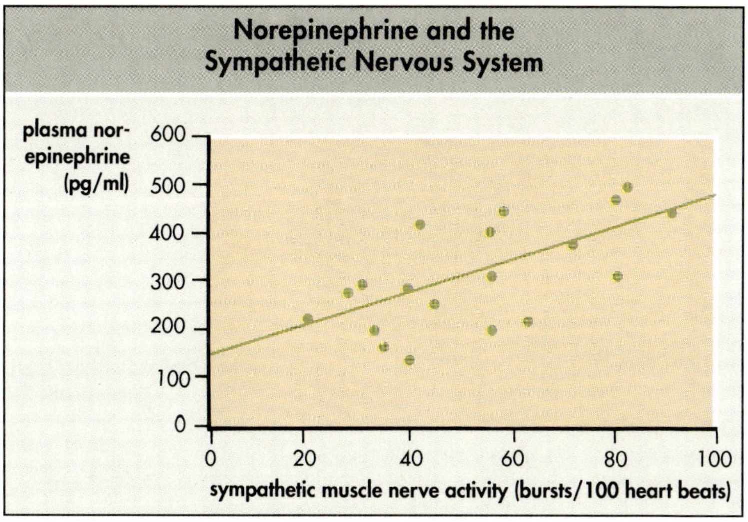

Fig. 3.50 The relationship between sympathetic muscle nerve activity (measured in bursts of activity per one hundred hearbeats) and plasma norepinephrine in a group of normal subjects.

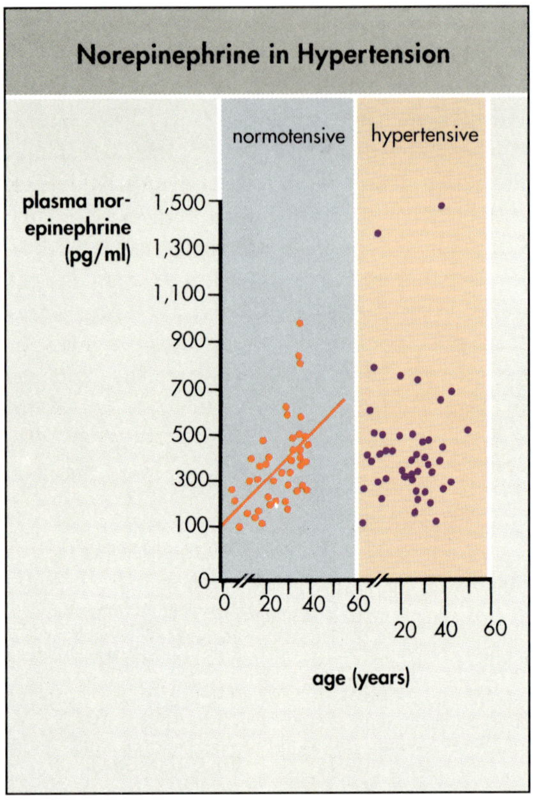

Fig. 3.51 The relationship between plasma norepinephrine and age in a control normotensive population and in subjects with essential hypertension. The loss of a relationship in hypertensives is due to younger hypertensives having a higher plasma norepinephrine.

closely matched for age, sex, race and familiarity with the environment in which plasma samples were obtained. There is, however, considerable evidence that younger hypertensives have levels significantly higher than age-matched controls (Fig. 3.51). This is in contrast to older subjects, in whom no differences are found and in whom there is no relationship between norepinephrine and absolute blood pressure (Fig. 3.52).

It is possible that the reactivity of blood vessels to sympathetic activity is increased. Distler and his co-workers demonstrated that in hypertensive subjects the normal inverse correlation between plasma norephinephrine and the pressor response to norepinephrine infusions was altered. In hypertensive patients with high plasma norephinephrine levels the pressor response to norepinephrine was not reduced appropriately – in patients with normal or low norephinephrine the reactivity to exogenous norepinephrine was disproportionately increased (Fig. 3.53). It was concluded from these studies that both sympathetic nervous activity and vascular reactivity to norepinephrine were important determinants of arterial pressure in hypertensive subjects. In conclusion, the central nervous system is of major importance in blood pressure control through the autonomic nervous system. It has not been possible, however, to detect evidence of increased activity consistently in sustained hypertension. Even

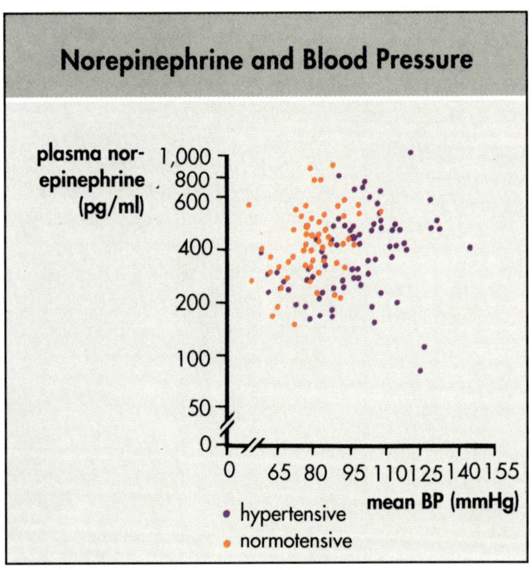

Fig. 3.52 There is no clear relationship between norepinephrine and blood pressure in normotensive and hypertensive patients.

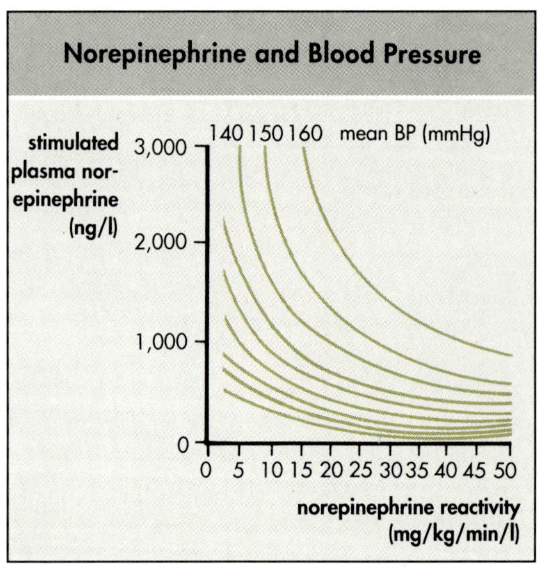

Fig. 3.53 The response of blood pressure to norepinephrine is dependent not only on sympathetic nerve activation but also vascular responsiveness.

where there is such evidence, the role of such abnormalities is uncertain.

Measurement of the activity of the second messenger systems which mediate vasoconstriction is still in its infancy. However, it is known that generation of phospho-inositides is increased in the aorta, both basally and after stimulation with noradrenaline in spontaneously hypertensive rats (Fig. 3.54). This enhanced activity is seen only in young animals, in the early stages of hypertension. It is not seen in established hypertension. It has not so far been possible to measure intracellular calcium in vascular smooth muscle. Platelets have been used as a debatable analogue; several groups have reported an increase in platelet calcium both in SHRs and in human essential hypertensives.

It is extremely difficult to study genuine hypersensitivity of the resistance vessels in man and distinguish it from hyperreactivity due to an increased wall-to-lumen ratio (see chapter 2). Recently, however, it has been possible to isolate subcutaneous resistance vessels from hypertensive subjects and from subjects genetically predisposed to hypertension. In these studies no hypersensitivity to any agonist could be detected (Fig. 3.55) suggesting that both in the early and established phase of essential hypertension secondary messenger systems are not overactive. The major change demonstrable in essential hypertension was a substantial increase in the wall-to-lumen ratio of the resis-

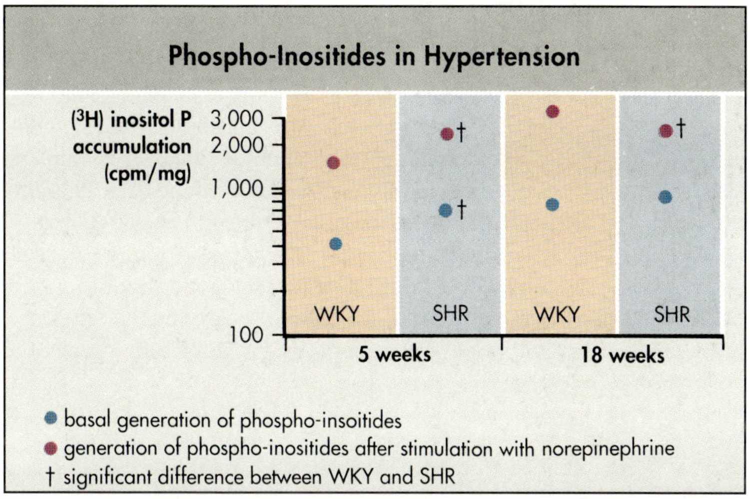

Fig. 3.54 Generation of second messenger phospho-inositides by aortae of spontaneously hypertensive rats (SHR) and their controls (WKY). Note the increased generation in young animals which is lost in mature hypertensives. [Modified from Heagarty *et al.* (1986) *Brit J Pharmacol*, **89**, 803–807.]

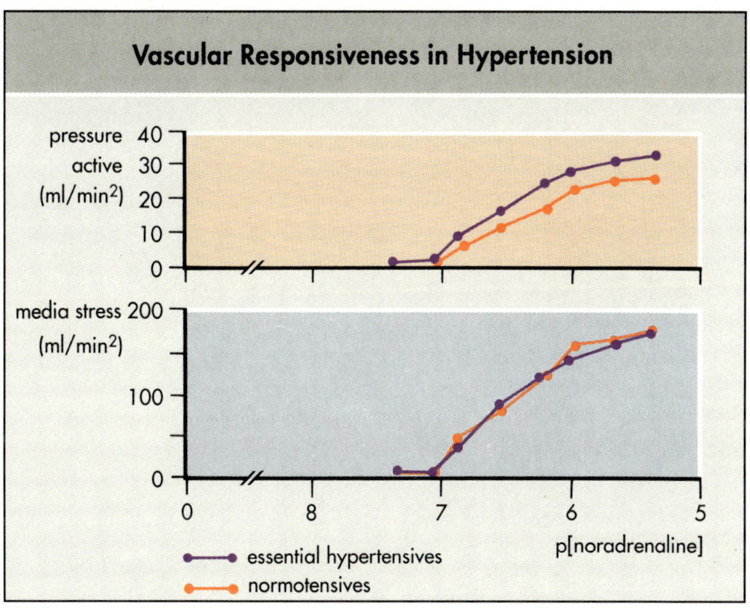

Fig. 3.55 The dose-response curves of isolated subcutaneous resistance vessels to noradrenaline. The responses, expressed as active pressure and media stress, show no real difference in sensitivity between hypertensives and normotensives. [Modified from Aalkjaer *et al.* (1987) *Circ Res*, **61**, 181–186.]

tance vessel (Fig. 3.56), which was great enough to account for the rise in blood pressure if similar changes were observed throughout the resistance vessel bed.

Resistance Vessels in Hypertension

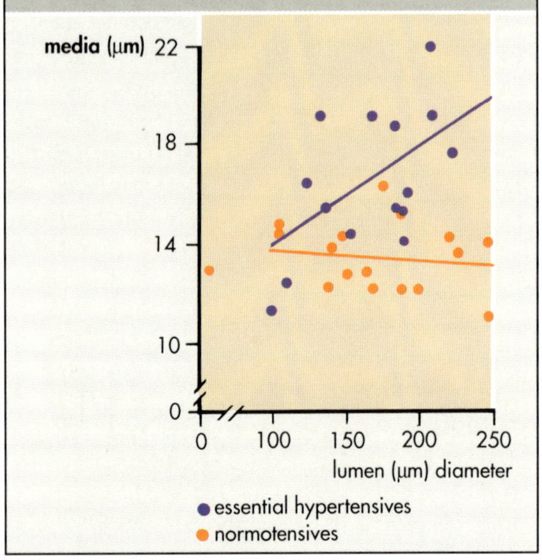

Fig. 3.56 This study noted a substantial increase in wall-to-lumen ratio of subcutaneous resistance vessels in subjects with essential hypertension. (For source see *Fig. 3.55*).

Other Humoral Systems

There is no reason to believe that there is either overactivity of the other pressor systems (described in chapter 2) or underactivity of depressor systems. However, a renomedullary vasodepressor system may participate in some models of renovascular hypertension (Fig. 3.57). Thus, subcutaneous or intraperitoneal transplants of renal medullary interstitial cells prevent or reverse some forms of experimental hypertension (Fig. 3.58). When the constricting clip is removed from the renal artery in Goldblatt hypertension, blood pressure falls rapidly within a few hours. This fall is not necessarily related to changes in the renin–angiotensin system or in sodium excretion. It can however be partially blocked by chemical destruction of the renal medulla (Fig. 3.59). Muirhead and his co-workers have shown that as blood pressure falls during reversal of renovascular hypertension, an antihypertensive, non-prostanoid, neutral renomedullary lipid can be detected in the renal venous effluent. At the same time, the renomedullary interstitial cells degranulate. In other studies, the clipped kidney has been removed from rats with Goldblatt 2-kidney 1-clip hypertension and perfused with blood from normal, conscious rats in a closed circulation

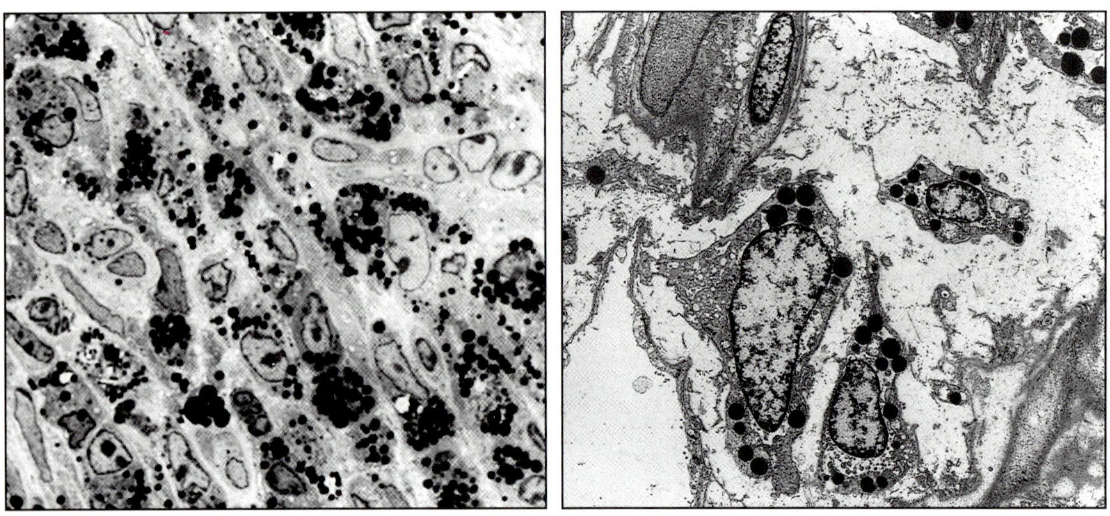

Fig. 3.57 Renal papillae in the rat. (Left) Section of fragmented rat renal papilla transplant. Secretion from this transplant lowered the blood pressure of a hypertensive recipient. Note the lipid granules which have been stained with toluidine blue. (Right) Electron micrograph from the papilla of a normal rat. Round dark granules are seen stained with osmiom. The clear surroundings are due to glycosaminoglycans which are secreted by the interstitial cells. Courtesy of Prof. E. E. Muirhead.

system. Removal of the constricting clip from the isolated kidney gave rise to a profound fall in blood pressure in the recipient animal (Fig. 3.60). It was postulated that the humoral agent released from the kidney had a direct inhibitory effect on sympathetic activity as shown directly by splanchnic nerve electrodes. The chemical nature of the renomedullary neutral lipid is still unknown.

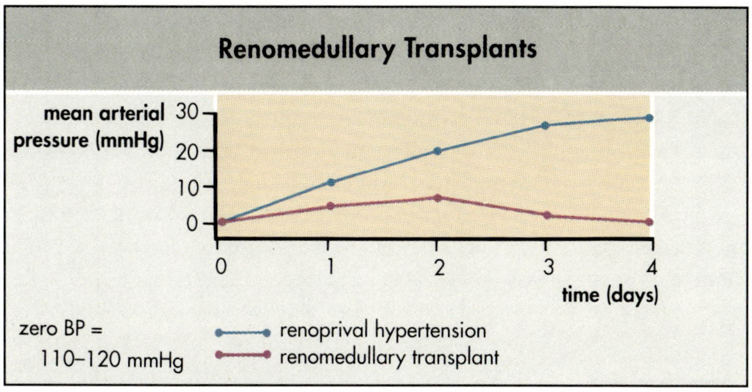

Fig. 3.58 Renomedullary transplants improved renoprival hypertension of the dog in this study. [Modified from Tobian & Azar (1971) *Trans Assoc Am Physicians*, **84**, 281–288.]

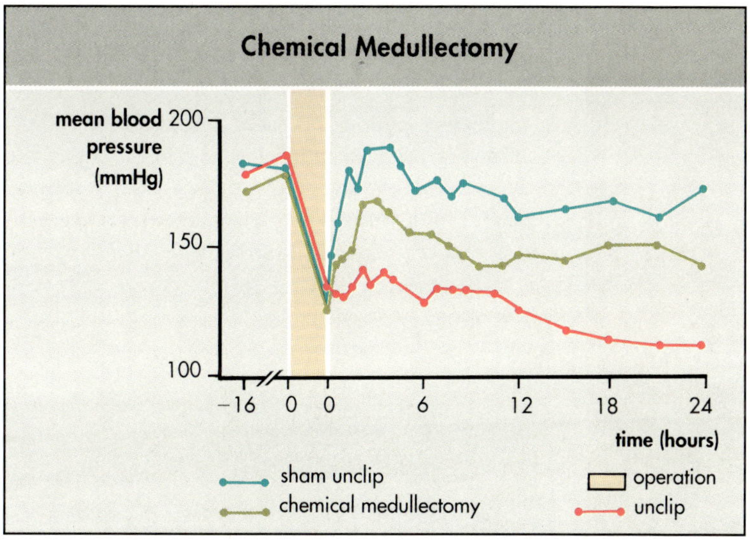

Fig. 3.59 In this study a number of rats were given Goldblatt 2-kidney 1-clip hypertension. Some days later, all these rats were operated on. Some had the clip removed others were simply opened and then closed again (sham unclip). A number of the unclipped rats were chemically medullectomized. The mean blood pressures for all these rats were followed for 24 hours. [Modified from Bing *et al.* (1981) *Clin Sci*, **61**, 335s–338s.]

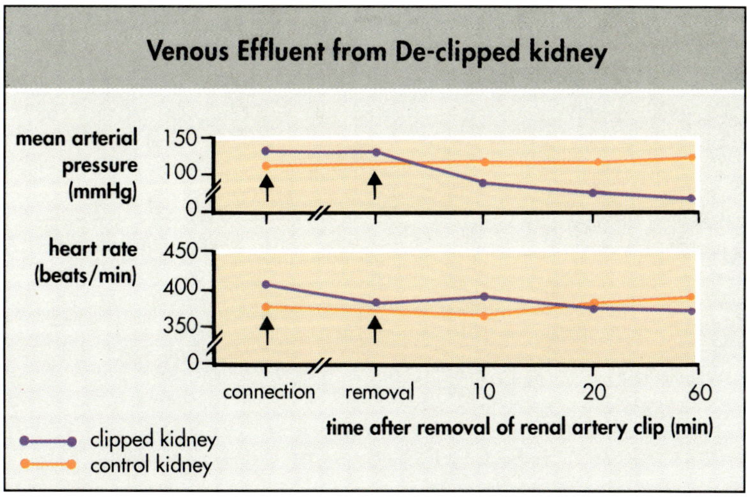

Fig. 3.60 Effect of perfusate from an isolated kidney on a recipient rat. When a previously ischaemic kidney was unclipped, the venous effluent lowered blood pressure in the recipient without influencing heart rate. [Modified from Gothberg G. *et al.* (1981) *Hypertension*, **4**, II-101–II-110.]

Structural Changes and Blood Pressure Maintenance

Chronic hypertension, whatever the cause, is associated with an increase in the wall to lumen ratio of the resistance vessels. This can be demonstrated on routine histology (Fig. 3.61) and on morphometry of the living blood vessel maintained *in vivo*. There is also functional evidence for these structural changes. When isolated tissue beds or isolated resistance vessels are exposed to vasoconstrictor or vasodilator stimuli, there is a resistance increase at maximal vasodilatation, an increase in maximal contraction and an alteration in the slope of the dose response curve (see chapter 2). These changes are seen with any constrictor or dilator stimulus. All these features are characteristic of increased wall-to-lumen ratio in the resistance vessel. Structural change in resistance vessels therefore amplifies the effect of any other factors which maintain vasoconstrictor tone – increased sympathetic nerve activity or raised levels of circulating angiotensin II, for example. Such changes could therefore be of great theoretical importance both in the maintenance of high levels of blood pressure and in the high peaks of blood pressure which hypertensive patients show on exposure to stress. Structural changes are slow to reverse, and there is still controversy over the extent to which they can be reversed in humans. In the rat, functional evidence of increased resistance vessel wall-to-lumen ratio persists for several weeks after renovascular hypertension is corrected surgically. Treatment of genetically hypertensive rats with antihypertensive medication has yielded variable results – some agents failed to have any detectable effect upon hypertrophy. However, drug induced regression of structural changes, if carried out for a sufficient period and early enough in the course of hypertension, may have an important impact on the natural history of the disease. For example, when blood pressure of spontaneously hypertensive rats is prevented from rising with antihypertensive drugs, it remains below that of untreated animals even after the drugs have been discontinued (Fig. 3.62). It should be noted, however, that

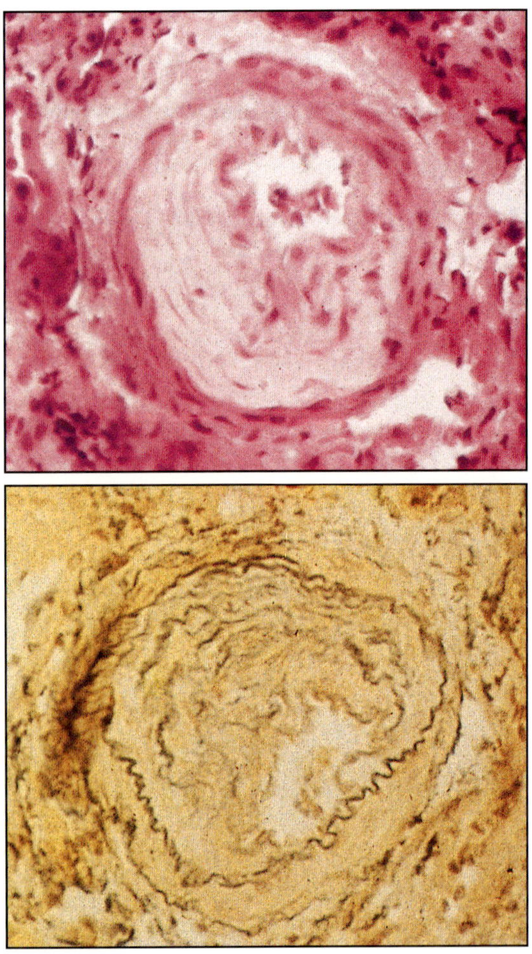

Fig. 3.61 Small artery from hypertensive patient. (Top) Intimal hyperplasia and hypertrophy. (Bottom) Duplication of the internal elastic lamina.

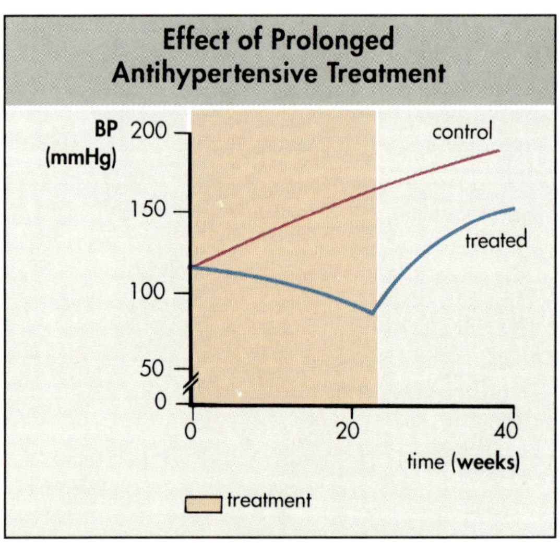

Fig. 3.62 Effect of prolonged treatment with antihypertensive drugs in evolution of blood pressure in the spontaneously hypertensive rat. Even after treatment was discontinued blood pressure remained lower in previously treated animals.

blood pressure does rise progressively after drugs are withdrawn. A similar phenomenon can be observed in man. In the MRC Trial, when either bendrofluazide or propranolol were withdrawn from mildly hypertensive patients after several years therapy, blood pressure climbed only slowly over the next few months (see Fig. 1.14). It should be emphasized that blood pressure did ultimately return to the pretreatment values. Furthermore, even a period of several months is much shorter than the period required for hypertension to develop initially, suggesting that the processes responsible for blood pressure elevation (which may include structural changes) were proceeding at an accelerated rate.

The major factor causing the increased wall-to-lumen ratio of the resistance vessels is unquestionably exposure to increased pressure. Thus, when resistance vessel beds are 'protected' by a constricting clip (Fig. 3.63), vascular hypertrophy is not seen to the same extent. In some studies of coarctation-induced hypertension distal structural changes could be observed, suggesting that either humoral or neurogenic factors were responsible.

Since hypertrophy has such important functional consequences, any predisposition to develop it could be of great significance. Both norepinephrine, angiotensin II and other vasoconstrictors cause vascular smooth muscle cells in tissue culture to proliferate (Fig. 3.64). In addition, smooth muscle cell division in tissue culture is much more rapid in cells from SHRs than in controls. On these grounds it has been suggested that an inherited predisposition to vascular hypertrophy, or an acquired predisposition as a result of high sympathetic nerve activity or high local concentrations of angiotensin II, could be important in the pathogenesis of hypertension. Such evidence should be reviewed with caution. There are many phenotypic differences between the SHR and its control strain, most of which are unrelated to blood pressure differences.

Folkow has postulated that recurrent transient hypertension, a result of repeated episodes of environmental stress, sets up structural changes which are then responsible for maintaining blood

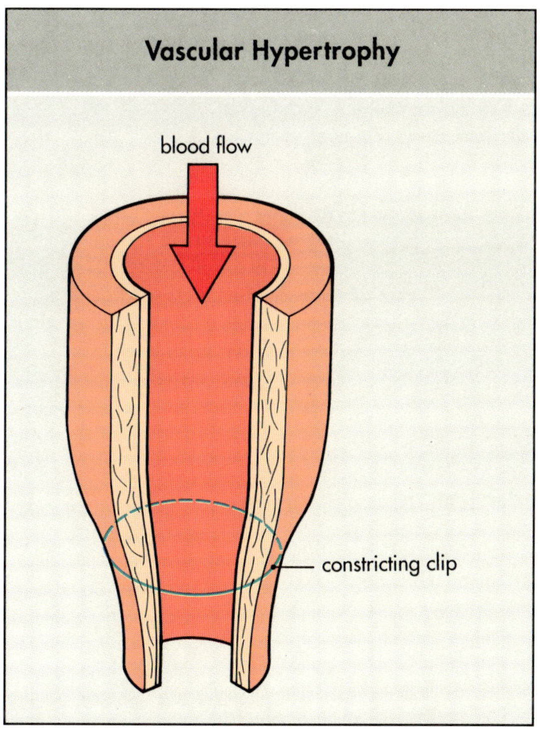

Fig. 3.63 When the aorta is constricted, wall thickness is greatly increased in the proximal part. Some thickening has also been reported in some studies in vessels originating in the distal aorta, indicating a possible role for circulating or neurogenic factors.

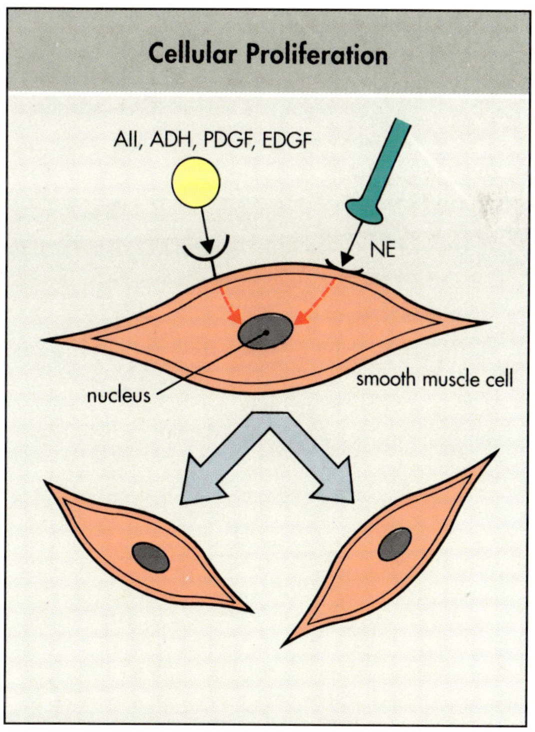

Fig. 3.64 Some factors which cause vasoconstriction may also in some circumstances cause growth and proliferation.

pressure. Thus, the rise in blood pressure which is observed in spontaneously hypertensive rats is moderated by isolation from environmental stimulation, although such isolation does not reduce blood pressure to normotensive levels (Fig.3.65). Henry has carried out the complementary experiment of exposing mice to increased stress in a social conflict cage (Fig. 3.66). Mice placed in these

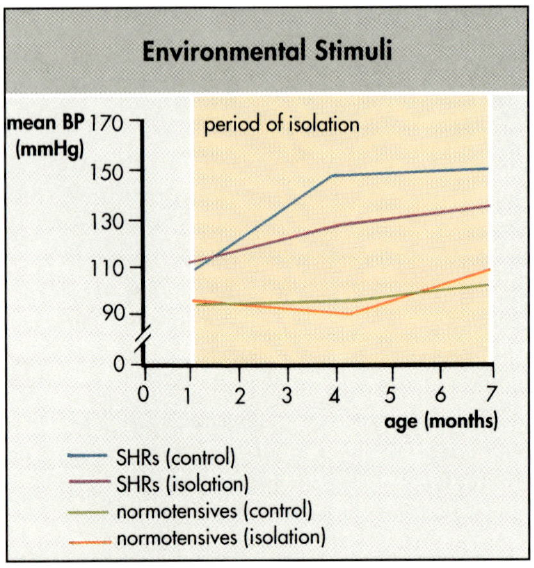

Fig. 3.65 Effect of isolating spontaneously hypertensive rats and a normotensive control strain from extraneous stimuli. The spontaneously hypertensive strain shows a significantly lower blood pressure indicating the importance of environmental stimuli acting upon a genetic predisposition.

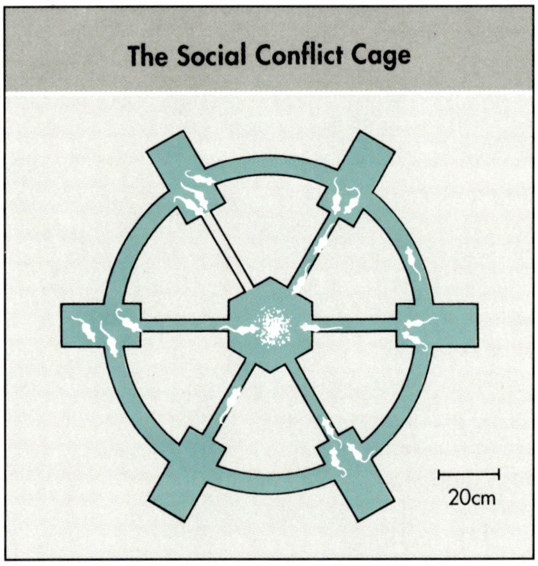

Fig. 3.66 Henry's social conflict cage. Mice have to complete with each other to gain access to food. [Modified from Henry, J. P. & Stephens, P. M. (1977) *Stress, Health and the Environment: A Sociobiologic Approach to Medicine*. Berlin: Springer Verlag.]

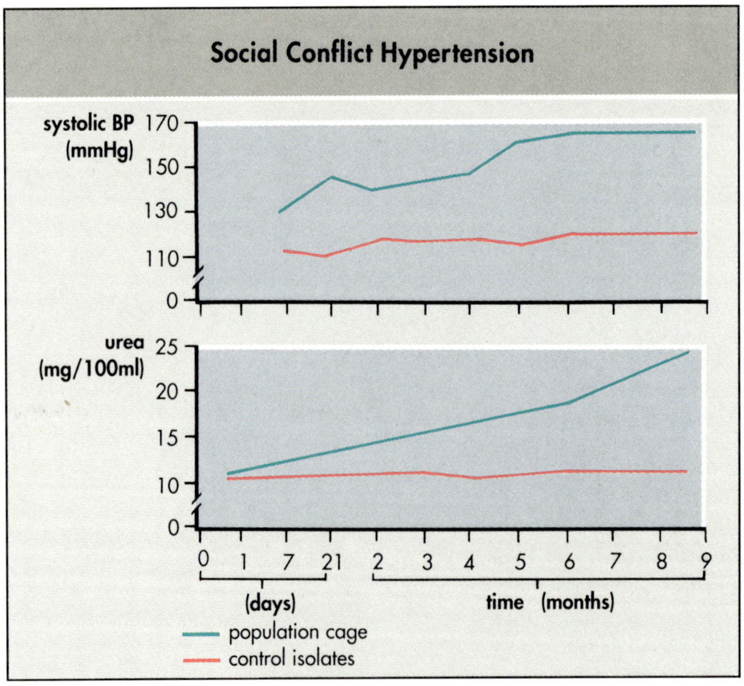

Fig. 3.67 As hypertension becomes more severe in animals exposed to social conflict, there is evidence of progressive target organ damage, shown here by deteriorating renal function. Renal function in control animals stayed within normal limits.

cages are exposed to competitive stress in their attempts to obtain food, territory and mates. Under these circumstances blood pressure rises progressively with, ultimately, renal and vascular damage (Fig. 3.67). It is more difficult to distinguish a role for stress in man. However, a 20 year follow-up study of nuns in a closed order showed no rise in blood pressure with age, compared with women of the same background who remained in the community (Fig. 3.68).

Genetic predisposition to hypertension could therefore elevate blood pressure via structural changes in two ways. Increased transient pressor responses to stress as a result of sympathetic overactivity could cause hypertrophy through exposure of resistance vessels to increased pressure. In addition, vessels could be genetically susceptible to pressure load. This theory is extremely attractive; it explains how environmental factors such as stress and diet, which may cause relatively small changes in blood pressure, sympathetic nerve activity or humoral responses, may interact with genetic predisposition to produce sustained hypertension. Furthermore, this theory may indicate important lines of research into drug-specific effects upon structure, since if either sympathetic activation or angiotensin II are involved, there should be important differences between various antihypertensive agents.

CELLULAR CHANGES IN HYPERTENSION

Several membrane functions are subtly altered in a number of different tissues in hypertension (Fig. 3.69). Early studies suggested that the sodium content of red cells was increased. However, patients and controls were not always well matched in these studies; although important ethnic differences have been observed in red cell sodium, these

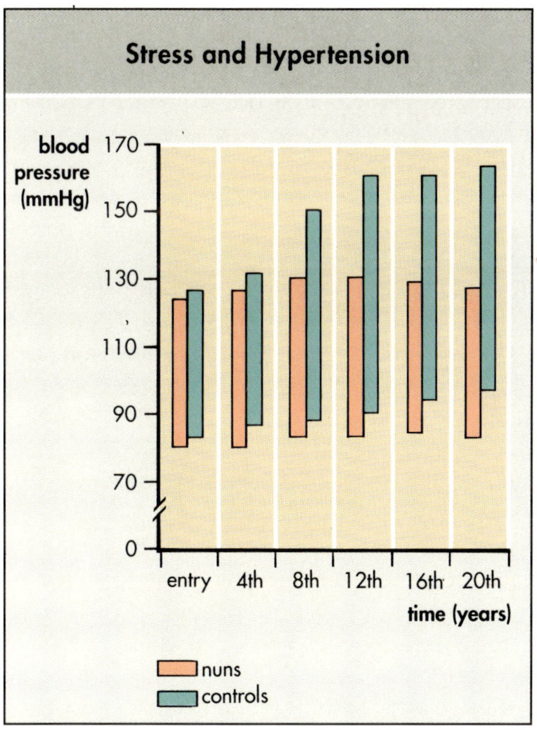

Fig. 3.68 A twenty year follow-up study of women from the same community who either entered a convent or remained as lay people. This showed a progressive rise of blood pressure in the latter, but not in the former. This difference could not be related to diet. [Modified from Timio, M. *et al.* (1988) *Hypertension*, **12**, 457–461.]

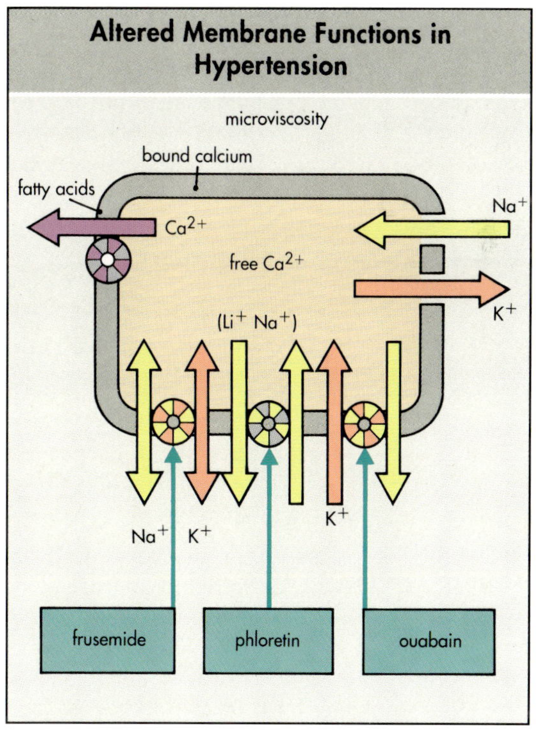

Fig. 3.69 Summary of systems which have been reported as abnormal in erythrocytes, leucocytes, and platelets in essential hypertension.

findings have not been universal in hypertensives. Nevertheless, these observations have stimulated research into abnormalities in membrane ionic fluxes. A number of systems have been studied.

The Ouabain-Sensitive Sodium Pump

The sodium pump extrudes three sodium ions in exchange for two potassium ions and is the major regulator of intracellular sodium and potassium. No consistent difference has been found in the sodium pump in red cells, but a reduction in its activity (rate constant for ouabain sensitive sodium transport) has been observed in the leucocytes of patients with essential hypertension.

Sodium–Potassium Cotransport

This system, which is sensitive to loop diuretics, moves pairs of sodium and potassium ions in both directions across the cell membrane. Whilst it may, under extreme physiological conditions, contribute to net changes in sodium and potassium, normally the effects in each direction are equal. Earlier reports suggested inhibition of this system in erythrocytes with essential hypertensives, but in other populations this phenomenon could not be confirmed (activity of the system was actually increased in one or two populations). Again, ethnic factors appeared to be of considerable importance.

Lithium–Sodium Countertransport

This system exchanges one lithium ion for one sodium ion and is inhibited by phloretin. Lithium is probably acting as a marker for sodium, so that the system exchanges internal and external sodium ions. It does not therefore contribute to any net changes in sodium. Considerable interest has however attached to this system since, in another mode, it may act as a sodium–proton exchanger and therefore regulate intracellular pH, an important regulator of cell differentiation and proliferation (see below). In a number of studies, erythrocyte sodium–lithium countertransport has been shown to be elevated both in hypertensives and in normotensives with a strong family history of hypertension. However, large epidemiological studies have shown a closer relationship with serum lipids than with blood pressure. It seems likely that modulation of this system is dependent upon alteration in membrane lipids.

Calcium ATPase

This system, which is important in the extrusion of calcium, shows reduced activity in both spontaneously hypertensive rats and in patients with essential hypertension.

Bound Calcium

Calcium binding to the inner surface of the erythrocyte cell membrane is reduced in patients with essential hypertension and in their relatives. The cells in which these observations have been made do not of course participate in blood pressure elevation. There have been few studies of vascular tissue in man because of its limited accessibility. However, it has been possible to show correlations between leucocyte sodium transport and sodium transport in the resistance vessel. How far other changes in erythrocyte membrane function are reflected in vascular smooth muscle in man is unknown. In experimental models of hypertension, such as the DOC–salt model and the SHR, sodium turnover is increased and smooth muscle cells are slightly depolarized. If also true of resistance vessels this would result in increased vasoconstrictor tone through the opening of calcium channels.

The explanation of the multiple disturbances in membrane function is still controversial. On the strength of the demonstration of sodium pump inhibition in the leucocyte, it has been suggested that circulating natriuretic hormone is both acting as a sodium pump inhibitor and causing hypertension (see above). However, it has not been possible to show sodium pump inhibition in vascular smooth muscle in most experimental models, or consistently in the human erythrocyte. This hypothesis also does not explain the other disturbances, both in transport pathways and calcium binding. It seems more likely that these disturbances represent alterations in the physicochemical properties of cell membranes. Erythrocyte membrane fluidity has been shown to be decreased in essential hypertension, and the sodium pump, sodium–lithium counter-transport and sodium–potassium co-transport can all be modified by changing the lipid composition of the membrane in which they are operative.

If this is the case, it is possible that the altered lipid environment also modifies the activity of second messenger systems (in particular the phosphoinositide system) which regulate vasoconstrictor tone as well as cell growth and differentiation. Minor changes in the activity of these systems could, over a period of time, have important effects on both vasoconstriction and on the structural increase in vascular resistance. There is little direct evidence in favour of this explanation at the moment. However, the observation that the phosphoinositide system is overactive in the early stage of development of hypertension in the SHR and the demonstration of vascular smooth muscle alkalinization in this model, both point to possible participation of second messenger systems.

CONCLUSIONS

Only in one or two rare instances is it possible to point to a single cause of hypertension. It is perhaps unsurprising that in human essential hypertension, which is a multifactorial condition, a number of possible processes are at work. The evidence we have points to a modest degree of overactivity of the sympathetic nervous system in the early stages of essential hypertension. This overactivity may be causal, but there may be an additional element of overactive vascular second messenger systems (Fig. 3.70). Structural changes in the peripheral vasculature maintain blood pressure at a later stage in the evolution of hypertension, although these can be overridden by manoeuvres or drugs which reduce vascular tone. Structural changes may be the result of pressure surges caused by autonomic overactivity. Resetting of baroreceptors and alterations in baroreceptor sensitivity appear to be secondary to blood pressure elevation. It seems possible that genetic predisposition, neurogenic drive and perhaps some humoral systems are all important in

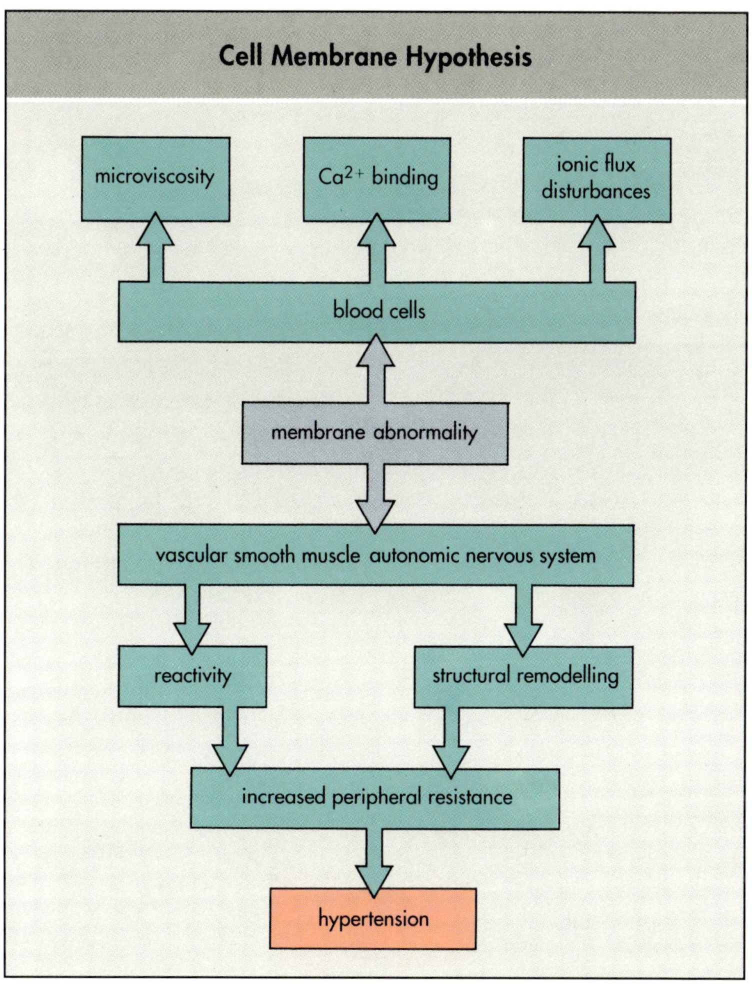

Fig. 3.70 Proposed sequence of events in the pathogenesis of hypertension according to the cell membrane hypothesis.

predisposing to these structural changes in certain individuals (Fig. 3.71). Genetic and environmental influences interact with these processes at several levels to create sustained elevated blood pressure.

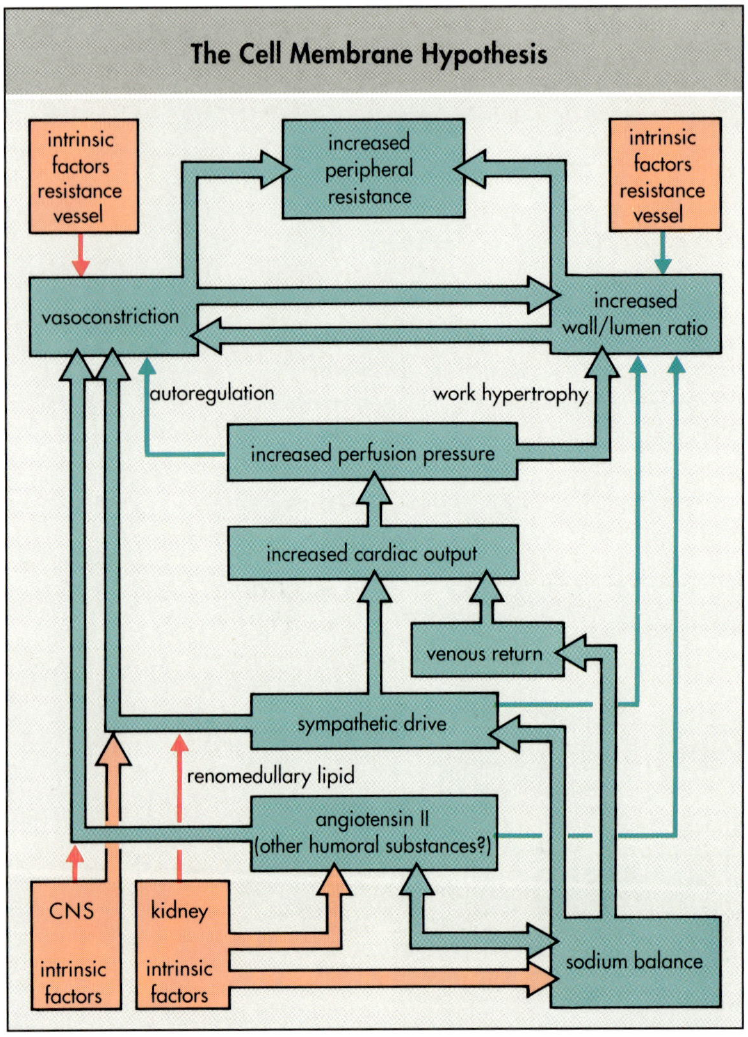

Fig. 3.71 Interrelationships between the various blood pressure regulatory systems in hypertension. Intrinsic changes in activity of the vascular, central nervous or renal regulatory systems may have multiple effects on mutually interacting systems. Established processes are shown by broad arrows, postulated processes by thin arrows.

CHAPTER 4

Pathological Consequences of Hypertension

INTRODUCTION

There are a number of interacting systems that can initiate a rise in blood pressure. However, hypertension in its chronic phase is maintained by additional factors, including structural changes in peripheral blood vessels. This pathological process is self-perpetuating.

While both experimental and epidemiological data indicate that increased peripheral resistance is a consequence of raised blood pressure, it is important to bear in mind that an increase in peripheral resistance itself causes a rise in arterial pressure. Increased perfusion pressure can result in a variety of distinct changes in the blood vessels, such as wall hypertrophy, intimal hyperplasia, fibrinoid necrosis, Charcot–Bouchard aneurysms and atheroma (Fig. 4.1). This is not to imply that hypertension itself is the only factor involved, since genetic predisposition and environmental factors also have considerable effects (see chapter 1).

VASCULAR EFFECTS OF HYPERTENSION

Vascular Hypertrophy

Hypertension leads directly to harmful effects on blood vessel walls, promoting a compensatory response which eventually causes wall hypertrophy. The increased load imposed by systemic hypertension produces hypertrophy of the media. This is associated with duplication of the internal elastic lamina and fibrous thickening of the intima (Figs 4.2 & 4.3). Interestingly, similar changes are occasionally seen in patients with chronic diarrhoea and Bartter's syndrome. Both of these conditions are associated with low blood pressure and high plasma renin – it is possible, therefore, that factors other than hypertension *per se* contribute to the hypertrophic process.

In experimental studies a number of vasoconstrictor substances (noradrenaline, angiotensin II, vasopressin and endothelin, an endothelial-derived peptide) have been identified as smooth

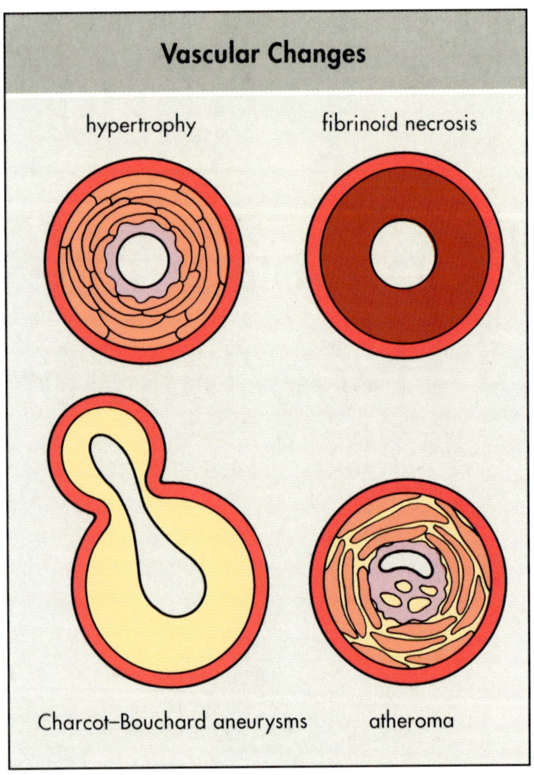

Fig. 4.1 Hypertension produces several types of structural change in the blood vessel wall. Some, such as hypertrophy, are adaptive while others are the result of structural damage.

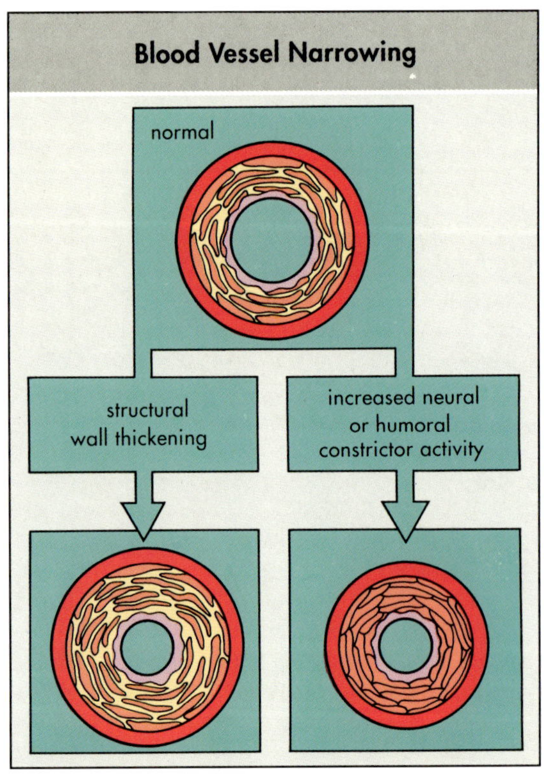

Fig. 4.2 Blood vessel walls in hypertension may be narrowed in two ways: structural hypertrophy increases the wall-to-lumen ratio or there may be increased smooth muscle contraction producing vasoconstriction.

muscle mitogens. Arterial smooth muscle hypertrophy induced by angiotensin II is associated with the accumulation of both proto-oncogene and growth factor mRNA. Several studies are currently underway to determine the pattern of oncogene message accumulation induced by a variety of mitogens in hypertrophy and hyperplasia. The role of these agents and of other growth factors (insulin, insulin-like growth factor, ß-transforming growth factor, growth hormone and platelet-derived growth factor) in the pathogenesis of smooth muscle hyperplasia is yet to be clarified, as does the role of hypertrophy in hypertension.

The most clearly understood consequences of wall hypertrophy are the alterations in peripheral resistance. Resistance to blood flow is increased even when the vessels are fully dilated. This increased resistance is secondary to functional factors such as altered sympathetic tone.

Any increase in wall-to-lumen ratio has additional haemodynamic consequences because, for any given degree of vascular smooth muscle contraction, vascular resistance will increase more in a hypertrophied vessel (see chapter 3 & Fig. 4.4). This results in hyperresponsiveness even to normal vasoconstrictor stimuli. Such hyperresponsiveness is a consequence, rather than a cause of hypertension. However, once developed it could provide a mechanism by which hypertension becomes self-perpetuating.

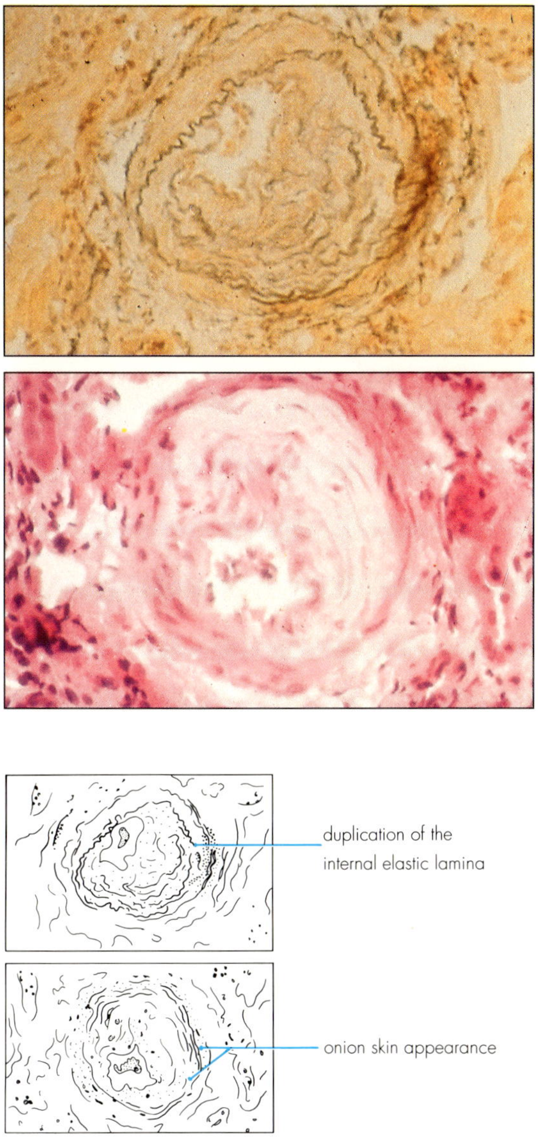

Fig. 4.3 Tranverse section of a small artery from a hypertensive patient. There is duplication of the internal elastic lamina (top) and intimal hyperplasia and hypertrophy (bottom).

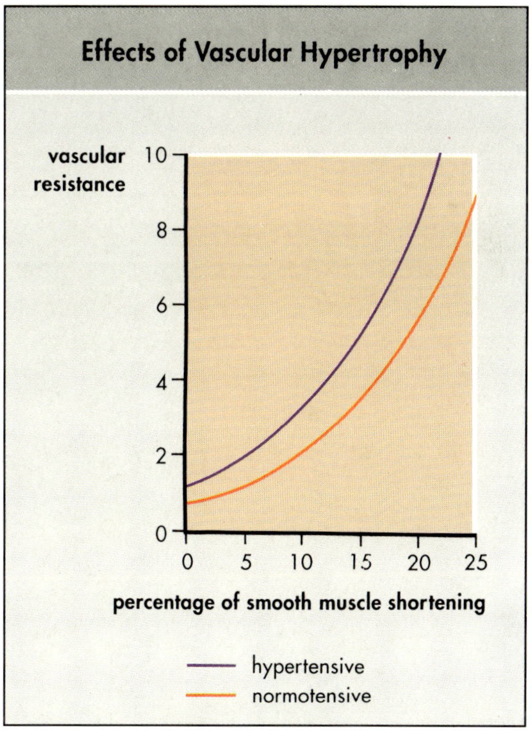

Fig. 4.4 Response of normal and hypertrophied vessels to vasoconstrictor stimuli. The hypertrophied vessel with an increased wall-to-lumen ration shows increased resistance to flow at maximal vasodilatation and a greater increase in resistance for a given degree of smooth muscle contraction.

As hypertension enters the accelerated or malignant phase, intimal hyperplasia or 'onion skinning' becomes more extensive. This results in progressive narrowing of the lumina. In the kidney, involvement of interlobular arteries leads to ischaemic atrophy of nephrons distal to vascular lesions. These changes probably play a major role in initiating and maintaining the vicious circle of malignant hypertension.

Fibrinoid Necrosis

Like vascular hypertrophy, fibrinoid necrosis is a hallmark of malignant hypertension (Fig. 4.5), although it is sometimes seen when the blood vessels are affected by other processes such as scleroderma or irradiation. It is a serious disorder, involving disruption of the vascular endothelial wall and an increase in permeability to plasma

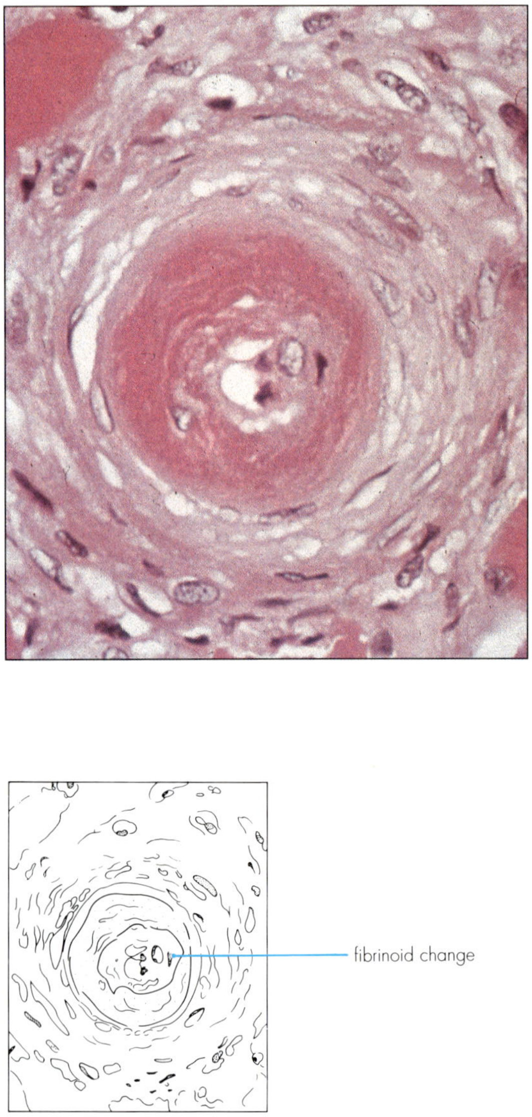

Fig. 4.5 Small artery from patient with malignant hypertension showing fibrinoid necrosis of the blood vessel wall.

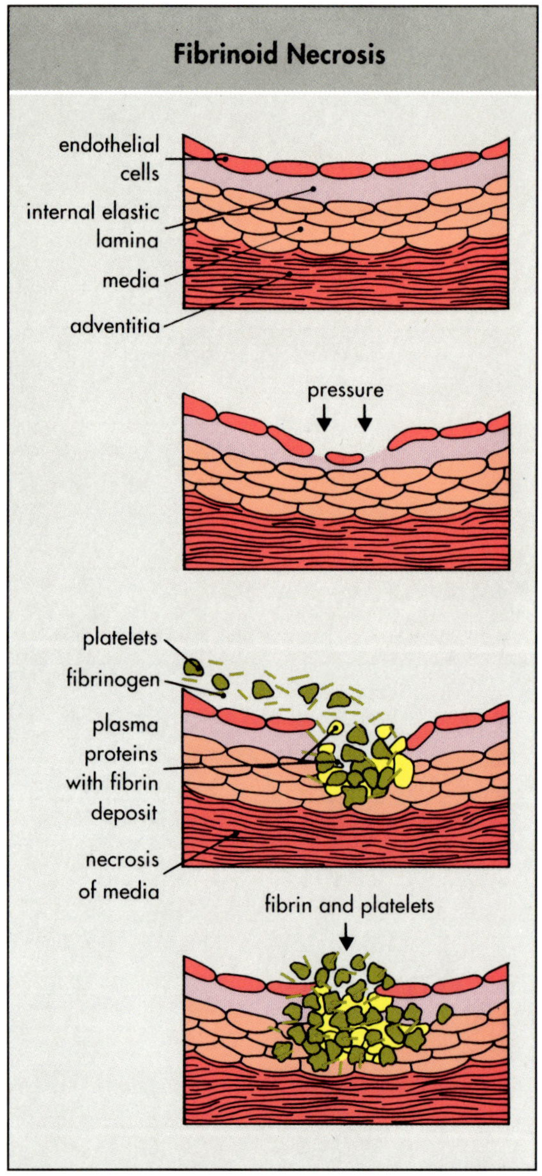

Fig. 4.6 Development of fibrinoid necrosis in malignant hypertension. There is insudation of plasma proteins into the media of the blood vessel wall with fibrin and platelet deposition on the endothelial surface.

proteins, which exude into the media and cause local tissue destruction. The wall structure is destroyed and replaced by a fibrin-like material that includes fibrinogen, γ-globulin, albumin and complement (Fig. 4.6). Fibrinoid necrosis is a sign of severe blood vessel damage. Clinically it is associated with florid fundal changes, including papilloedema (Figs 4.7 & 4.8). The level of blood pressure elevation at which fibrinoid necrosis occurs depends largely on the duration of hypertension and the rate at which the blood pressure has risen. Long-standing hypertension appears to afford some degree of protection – fibrinoid necrosis in such patients tends to occur only when blood pressure levels are very high. Conversely, in short-duration hypertension (in pregnancy, in glomerulonephritis or in children) fibrinoid necrosis occurs at lower blood pressure levels.

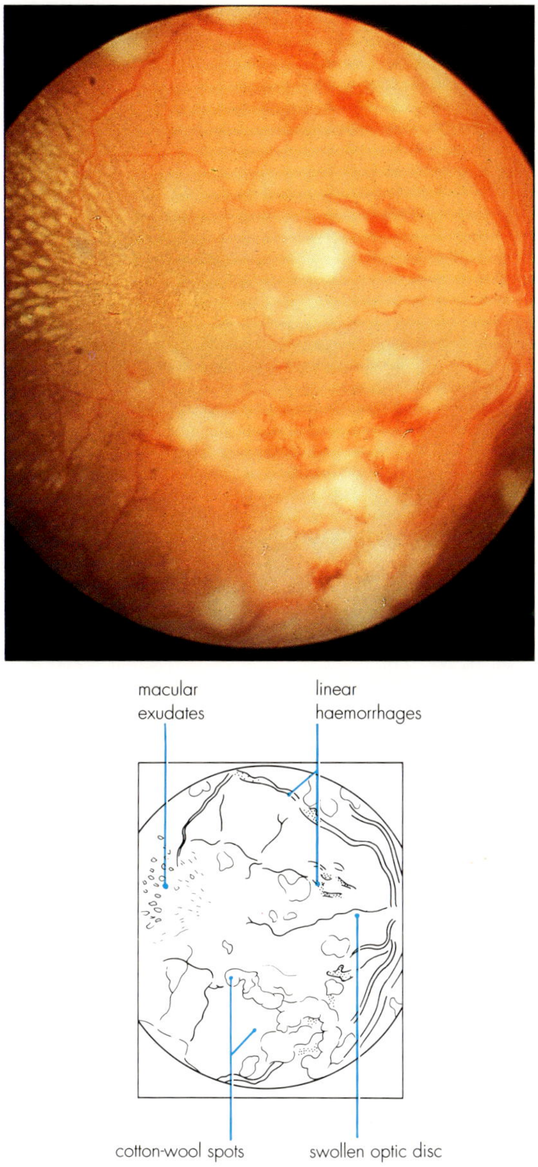

Fig. 4.7 Fundal photograph of a patient with severe renal hypertension showing a macula star with extensive exudates, haemorrhages and papilloedema. Courtesy of Prof. A. Garner.

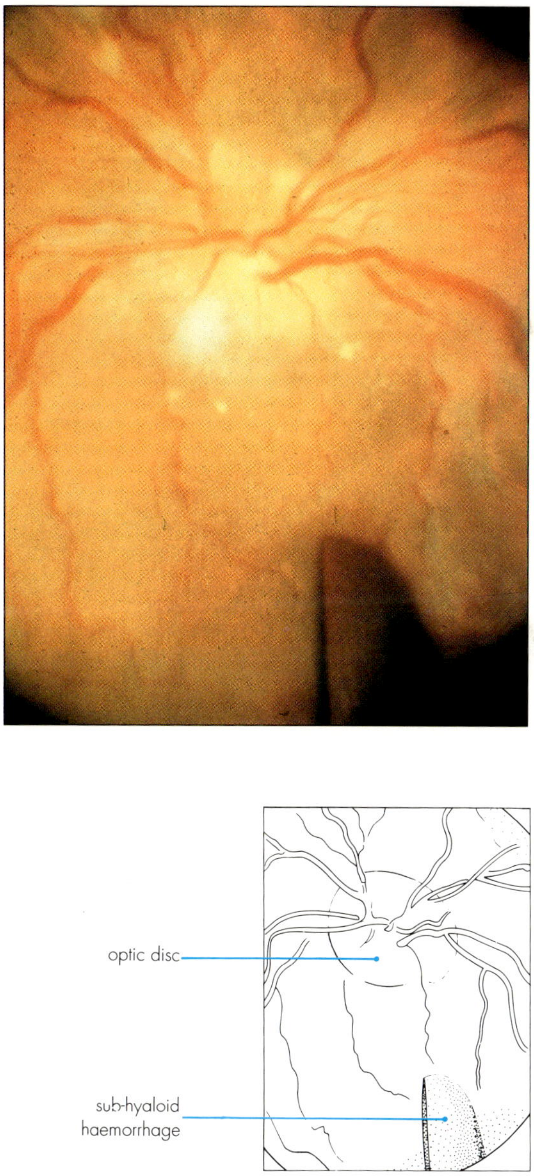

Fig. 4.8 Fundus from a patient with malignant hypertension showing papilloedema and a sub-hyaloid haemorrhage.

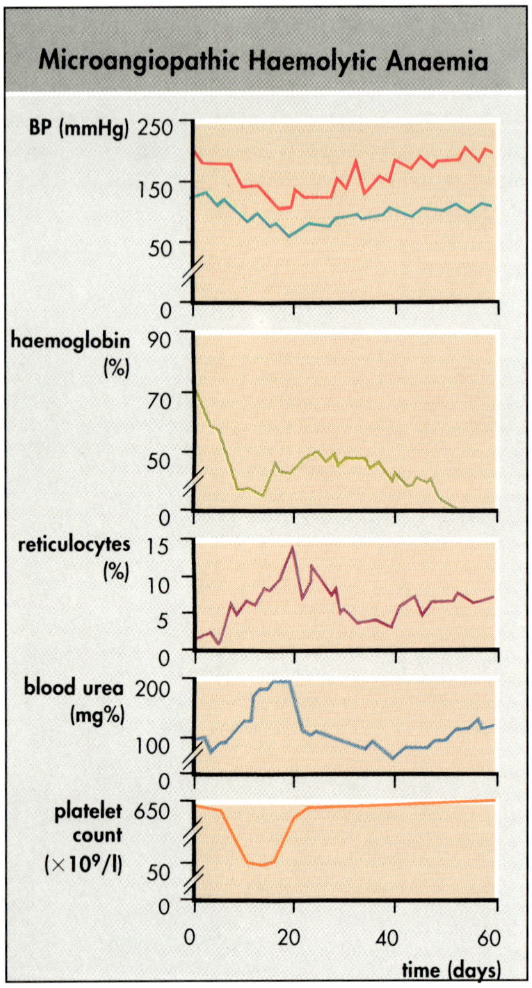

Fig. 4.9 Microangiopathic haemolytic anaemia occurring in a patient with malignant hypertension. The haemolytic anaemia was associated with reticulocytosis and renal failure.

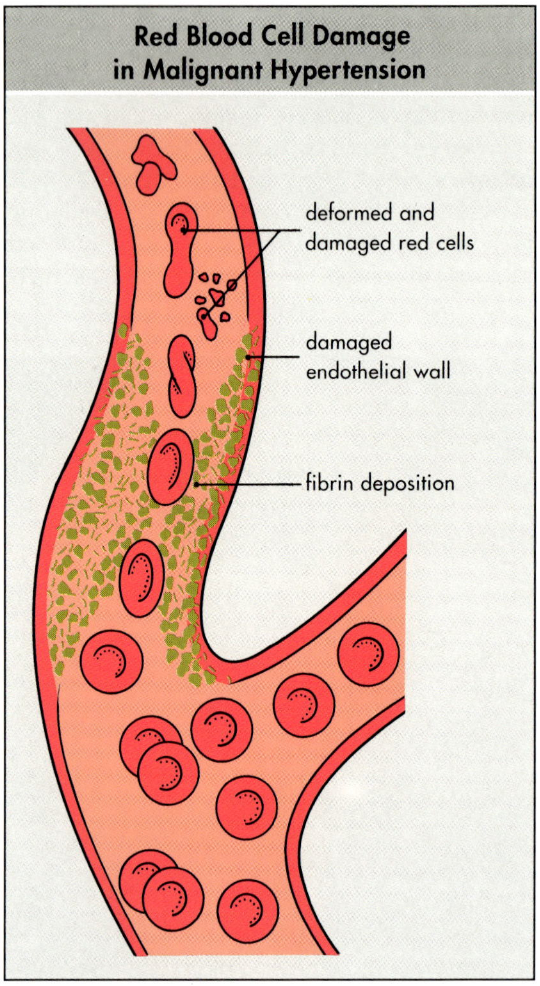

Fig. 4.10 Deformity and damage to red cells occurs as a result of their passage through a fibrin meshwork in the peripheral vessels.

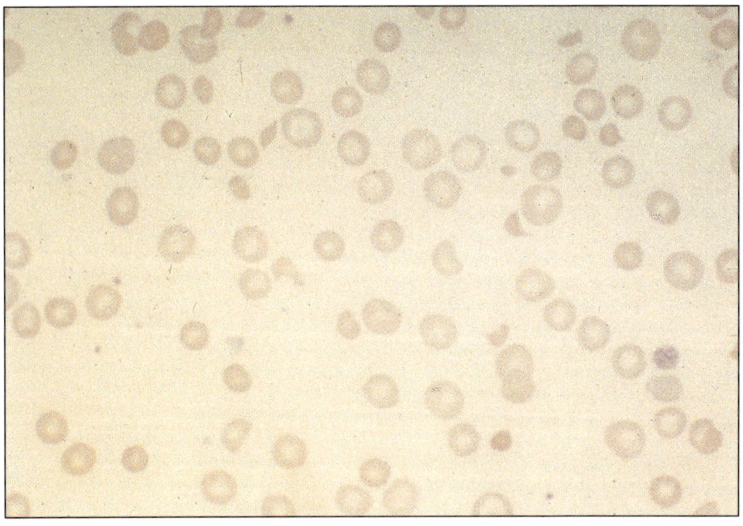

Fig. 4.11 Blood film from a patient with intravascular coagulation showing deformed and fragmented red cells (burr cells). Courtesy of Prof. S. N. Wickramsinghe.

Microangiopathic Haemolytic Anaemia

The fibrin and platelet deposition and arteriolar wall thrombosis caused by malignant hypertension leads to the development of microangiopathic haemolytic anaemia (Fig. 4.9). Red cells are damaged as they pass through the fibrin mesh so that the peripheral blood film shows deformed red cells (burr or helmet cells) and a diminished platelet count (Figs. 4.10 and 4.11). There is also an increased titre of fibrin degradation products in the plasma and urine with accelerated fibrinogen catabolism. In severe cases, microangiopathic haemolytic anaemia may give rise to acute renal failure (Fig. 4.12). Although fibrinoid necrosis and microangiopathic haemolytic anaemia can be life-threatening, both can be reversed by effective anti-hypertensive treatment.

Arteriosclerosis

'Hardening of the arteries' is common in elderly patients and is associated with calcification of the media of the larger vessels (Mönckeberg's sclerosis). This is a consequence of ageing rather of than of hypertension.

Atheroma

Atheroma formation is accelerated in the hypertensive subject. It principally involves medium-sized arteries in the coronary and cerebral circulations together with the aorta and lower limb vessels (Fig. 4.13). lesions are characterized morphologically by lipid deposition, smooth muscle proliferation and fibrosis (Fig. 4.14). Early lesions, described as fatty streaks, are raised

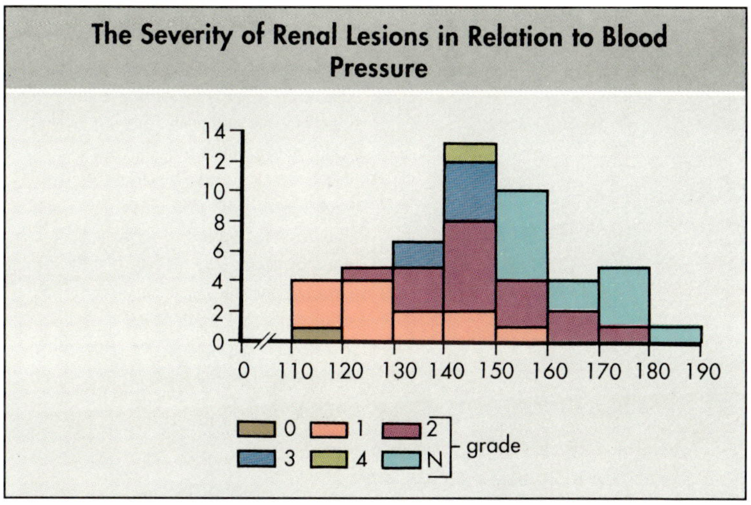

Fig. 4.12 The histological severity of the renal lesion in hypertensive patients (progressing from grade 0 to 4 and fibrinoid necrosis, N), is related to the diastolic blood pressure level.

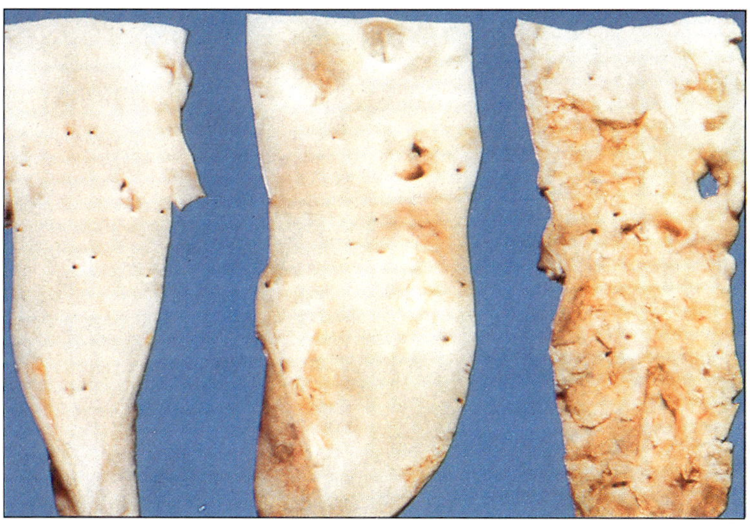

Fig. 4.13 Aortae from a young normotensive (left), a middle-aged normotensive (centre) and an elderly hypertensive patient (right). Artheroma was most severe in the elderly hypertensive patient, shown on the right; the young normotensive individual on the left was relatively free from atheroma.

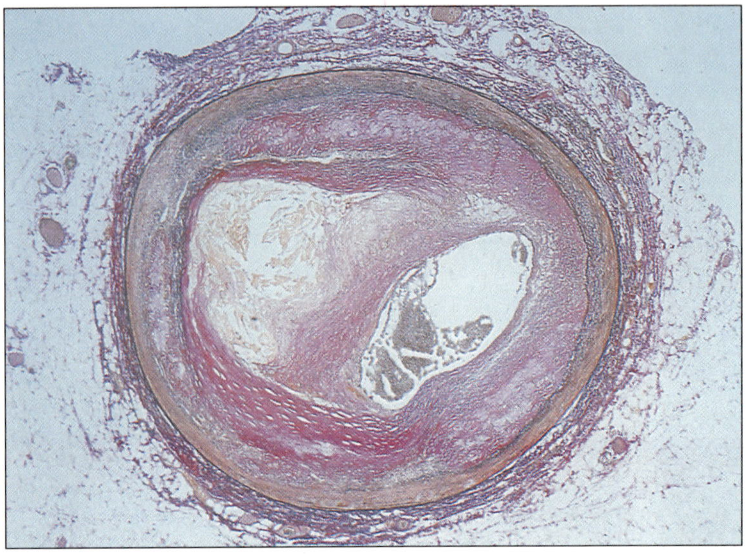

Fig. 4.14 Histological section of coronary artery showing classical atherosclerotic lesion. Fatty debris is the major plaque constituent. Courtesy of Prof. A. E. Becker and Prof. R. H. Anderson.

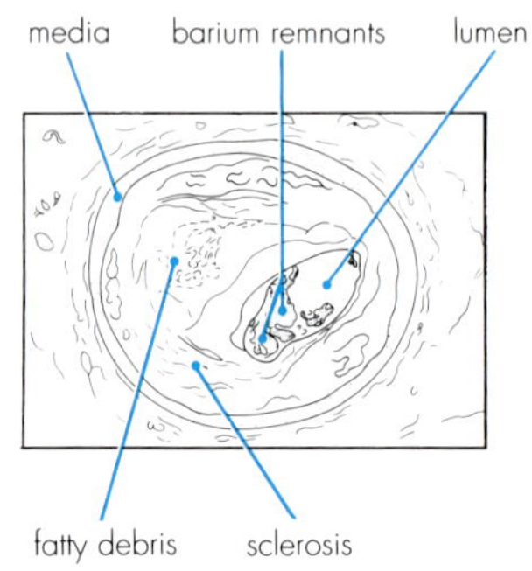

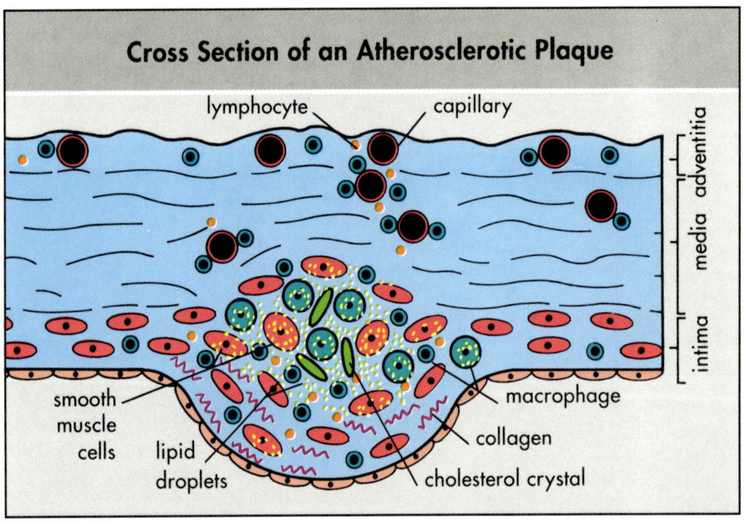

Fig. 4.15 Schematic representation of a cross-section through an atherosclerotic plaque. The medial smooth muscle cells are not drawn in. Overlying endothelium is intact in this example. There is a 'cap' with smooth muscle cells and collagenous bands. Underneath is the core region with abundant extracellular lipid and foam cells. Macrophages are widely distributed and lymphocytes can be seen in the cap and to the sides of the core. Adventitial capillaries are gravitating toward the intimal lesion. [For source see Figure 4.17.]

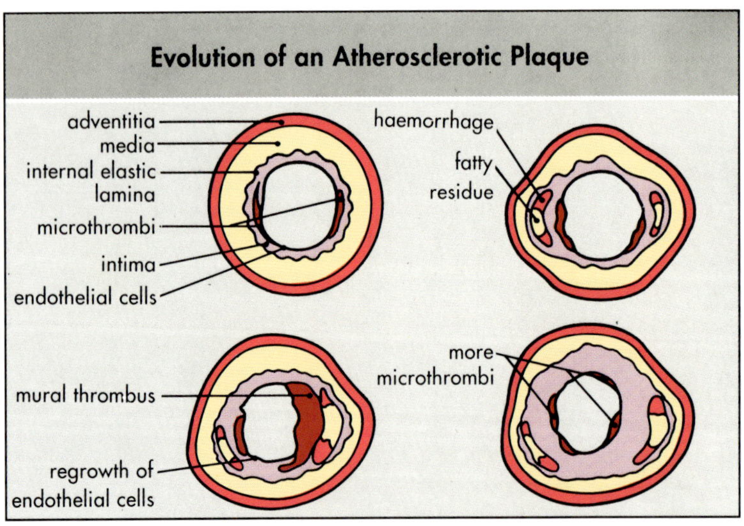

Fig. 4.16 Evolution of an atheromatous plaque. According to the thrombosis theory, the deposition of mural thrombi on an ulcerated area is followed by re-endothelialization, leaving a haemorrhagic fatty residue in the subendothelial region. The atheromatous plaque may then be the site of further mural thrombi.

yellow deposits consisting of subendothelial aggregations of foam cells. These cells, derived largely from macrophages and to a lesser degree from smooth muscle cells, contain lipid droplets. It is probable that fatty streaks develop into fibrofatty plaques (Fig. 4.15), which have the following structure:

- a fibrous cap of smooth muscle cells, collagenous bands and a few leucocytes;
- a cellular component of macrophages, smooth muscle cells and T lymphocytes;
- a deep necrotic cone of cell debris, foam cells, lipid droplets, cholesterol and calcium.

Proliferation of small blood vessels around the edges of atheromatous lesions is occasionally seen.

Thrombosis commonly arises during the development of atheromatous plaques (Fig. 4.16). Mural thrombi form on ulcerated plaques, which re-endothelialize in some cases. Haemorrhage into ulcerated plaques may initiate the thrombotic process, leading to total occlusion of the lumen with, for example, consequent myocardial or cerebral infarction.

One of the more plausible hypotheses explaining atherogenesis is that the process follows damage to or dysfunction of the vascular endothelium, resulting in adhesion of platelets and monocytes. Monocytes then penetrate between the endothelial cells and contribute to the cellular component of plaques in the form of monocyte-derived macrophage foam cells. Platelet adherence to the endothelium causes the release of platelet-derived growth factor, which in turn leads to smooth muscle cell migration and proliferation (Fig. 4.17).

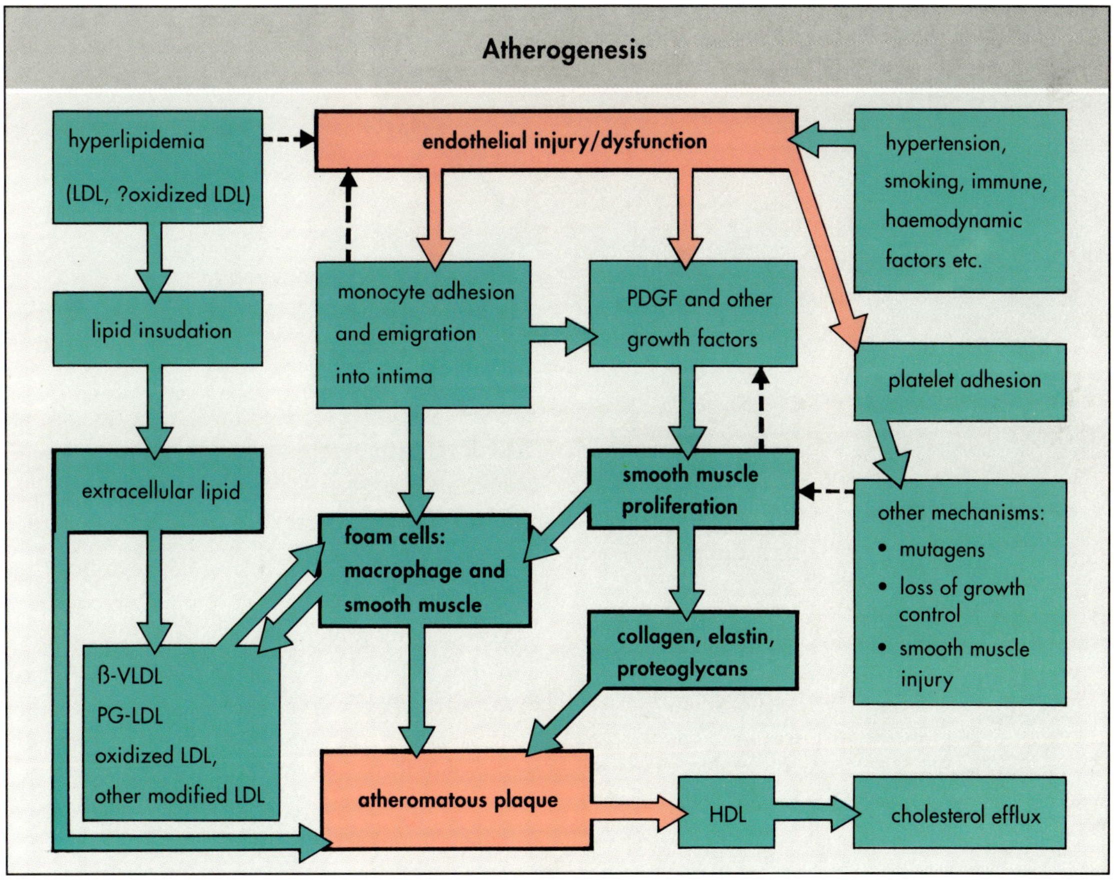

Fig. 4.17 Schematic diagram of a hypothetical sequence of events and cellular interaction in atherogenesis. PG-LDL = proteoglycan–low density lipoprotein; HDL = high density lipoprotein. [Modified from Cotran R.S., and Munro J. M. Pathogenesis of atherosclerosis: recent concepts. In Grundy S. M. and Bearn A. G. (eds). The role of cholesterol in atherosclerosis: New therapeutic opportunities, philadelphia, Hanley and Belfus, 1988, p.5.]

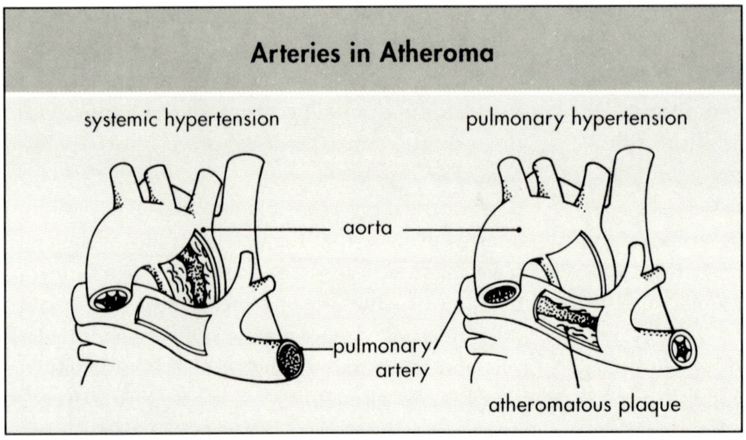

Fig. 4.18 Atheroma is usually more marked in the aorta, which is exposed to a higher transmural pressure than the pulmonary artery. In the presence of pulmonary hypertension, however, atheroma develops in the pulmonary artery.

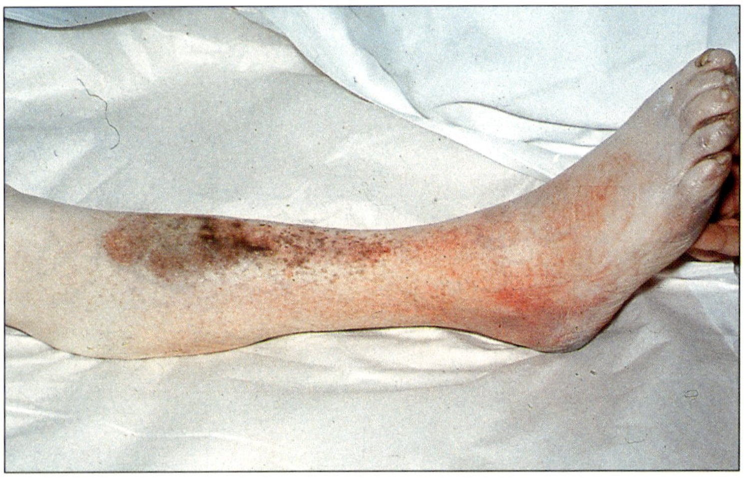

Fig. 4.19 Gangrene of the leg secondary to peripheral vascular disease.

A number of factors are putatively involved in increased monocyte adhesion and migration into the intima. The process may be enhanced in hyperlipidaemic states. The lipid content of the foam cells is mainly cholesterol ester, probably derived from a modified form of low density lipoprotein (LDL) taken up by monocytes. The scavenger receptors which bind modified LDL are distinct from classical LDL receptors, which are regulated by the cholesterol requirements of the cell and are probably responsible for the main bulk of LDL accumulation. Extracellular lipid deposits also accumulate within the atheromatous plaques and are derived from insudation from the lumen and from degenerating foam cells.

The enhanced atherogenesis associated with high blood pressure levels is incompletely understood. The pulmonary artery, for example, which is not usually exposed to high perfusion pressures, is usually free of atheroma. However, atheroma does develop in the presence of pulmonary hypertension (Fig. 4.18). Atheromatous lesions occur in both clinical and experimental coarctation, particularly in vessels exposed to a high perfusion pressure. Hypertension may act synergistically with other factors. Thus, in monkeys subjected to experimental coarctation and fed a high cholesterol diet, atheroma developed in the vessels proximal to the coarctation. When a low cholesterol diet was given, only vascular hypertrophy could be demonstrated in these vessels. In general, essential hypertensives are more likely to show an atherogenic plasma lipoprotein profile – this could partly explain the increased atheroma when compared to normotensives. Nevertheless, it is likely that either blood pressure itself, or some other factor(s) involved in the pathogenesis of high blood pressure, may accelerate atheroma formation. For example, endothelial abnormalities have been described in experimental models of hyper-

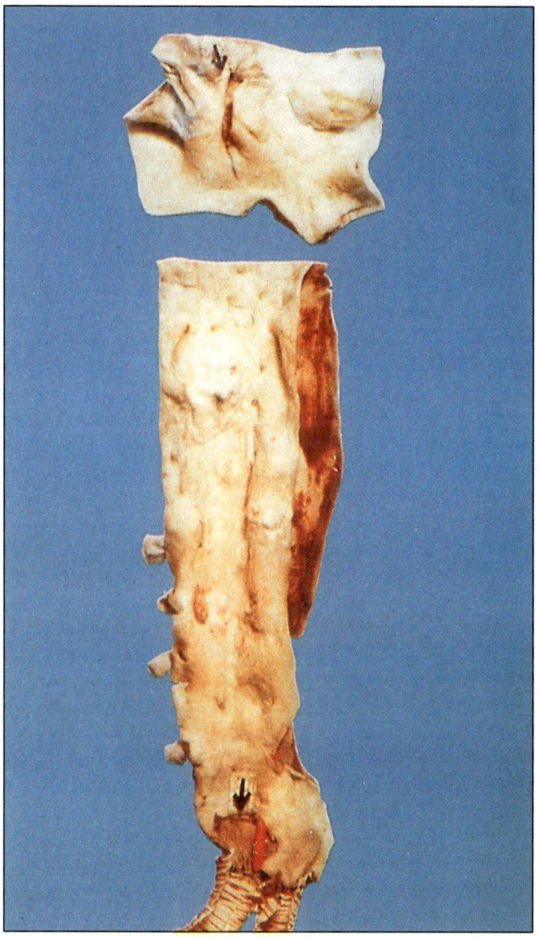

Fig. 4.20 Dissection of the aorta. The site of the re-entry of blood is marked by an arrow.

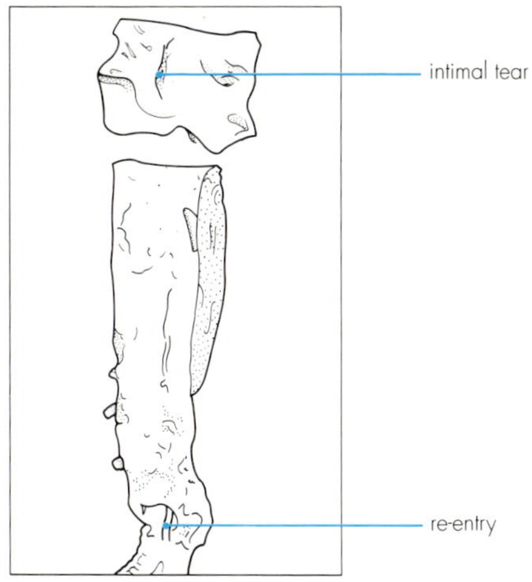

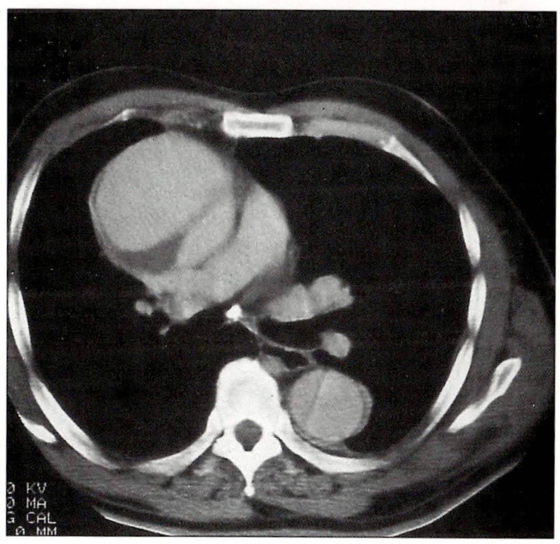

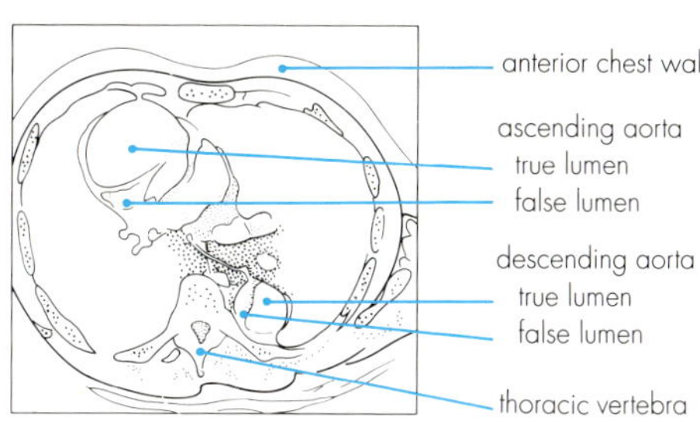

Fig. 4.21 CT scan of dissecting aneurysm of the aorta showing dissection of the media by extravasated blood. Dissection commonly begins in the ascending aorta.

tension and could play a role in atherogenesis if present in human hypertension. The haemodynamic effects of raised blood pressure or of turbulence at certain points, for example at the aortic bifurcation, could alter the properties of the endothelium and facilitate cell adhesion and migration. The similarity of smooth muscle proliferation in both atheroma and hypertension implies some common pathogenetic stimulus.

Atheroma is clinically important in the development of cerebrovascular, cardiovascular and peripheral vascular disease (Fig. 4.19). Although not sequelae of atheroma, dissecting aneurysms of the aorta (Figs 4.20 & 4.21) are usually associated with atheroma and are more common in hypertensive individuals. The immediate predisposing cause is a systemic degeneration of the aortic media with rupture of the vasa vasorum in the degenerated area and intramural haemorrhage.

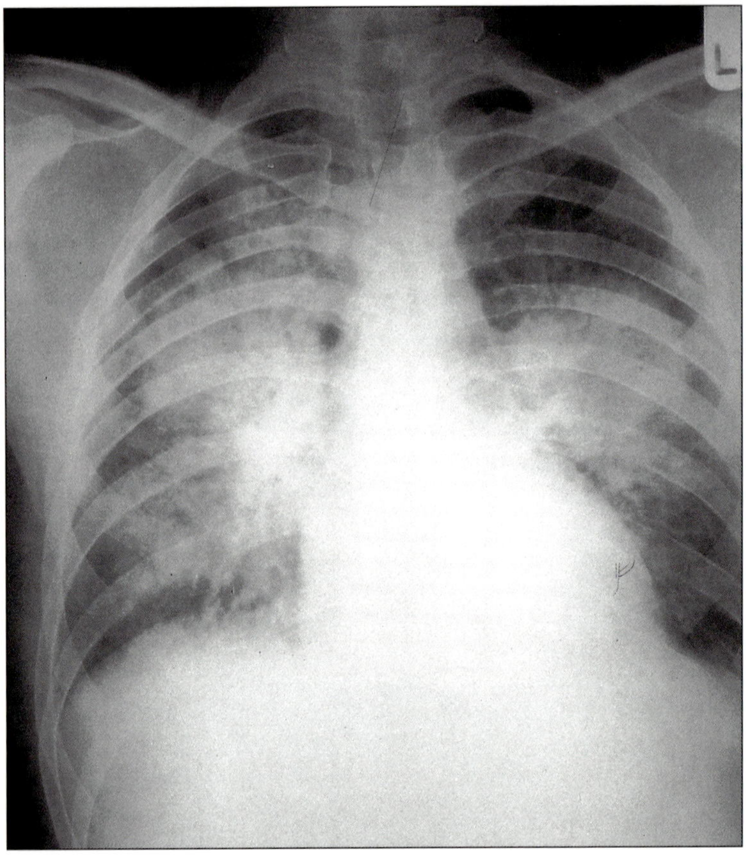

Fig. 4.22 X-ray showing left ventricular failure in a hypertensive patient with typical bat's wing appearance at the hila.

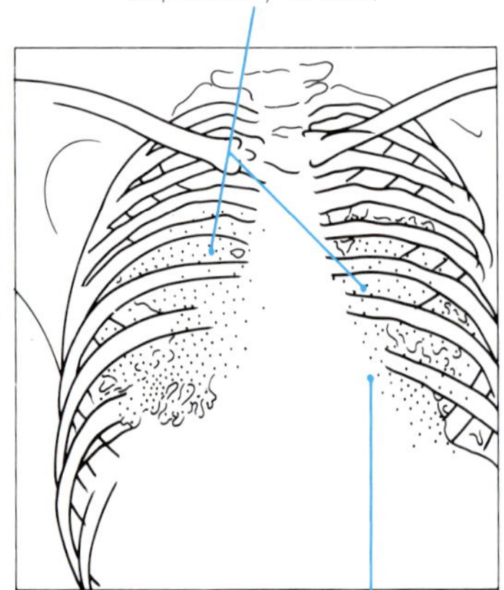

CARDIAC EFFECTS OF HYPERTENSION

Systemic arterial hypertension causes an increase in both cardiac work and left ventricular hypertrophy. However, this hypertrophy is probably not solely the result of arterial hypertension. There is evidence that neurohumoral influences, particularly cardioadrenergic drive, may play a modulating role in the development of hypertrophy, with noradrenaline acting as a potential mitogen on the cardiac myocyte in much the same way as it has been implicated (along with other growth factors) in vascular smooth muscle hypertrophy. Thus, although they lower blood pressure to similar degrees, different drugs have quite distinct effects on left ventricular hypertrophy. Diuretics, vasodilators such as hydralazine or minoxidil and peripheral α-antagonists such as prazosin or urapidil produce little or no regression. On the other hand, centrally acting antihypertensives such as methyldopa, calcium antagonists and ACE inhibitors all reduce left ventricular mass.

Another consequence of ventricular hypertrophy in the hypertensive subject is an increase in arrhythmias. The reason for this is unclear.

Ventricular hypertrophy is not necessarily a beneficial compensatory change, because a reduction in left ventricular compliance may impair the ability of the heart to increase its stroke volume in response to increased demand. Thus, stroke volume in hypertensive subjects tends to be lower than in normotensive subjects.

The slight decrease in cardiac performance produced by left ventricular hypertrophy is not usually associated with definable clinical symptoms. The development of left ventricular failure can be a gradual process, with shortness of breath on exertion progressing slowly to full-blown cardiac decompensation. Left ventricular failure may also present as a medical emergency, with paroxysmal nocturnal dyspnoea or pulmonary oedema (Fig. 4.22). In left ventricular failure cardiac output cannot be sustained in the face of the systemic arterial pressure. Pulmonary venous pressure

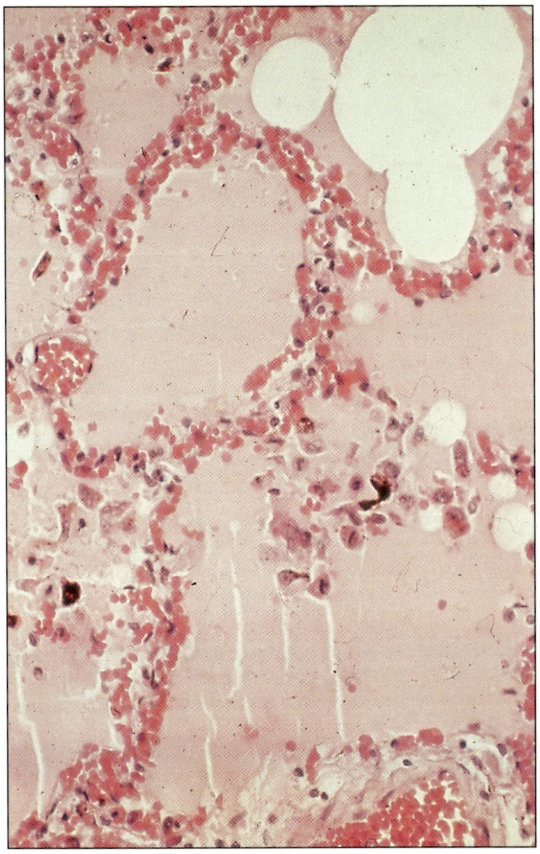

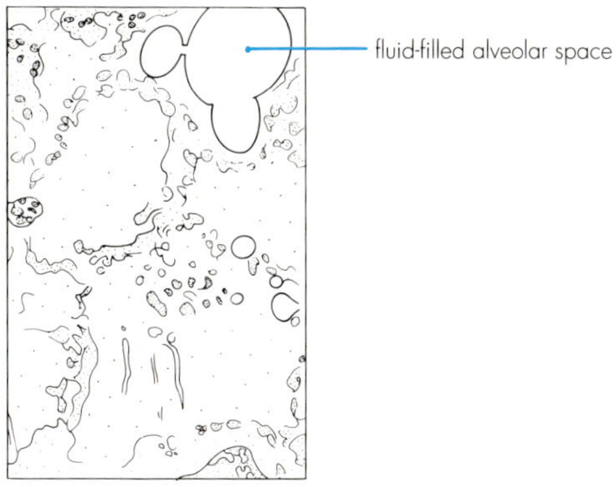

Fig. 4.23 Histology of the lung in pulmonary oedema with dilatation of the blood vessels and widening of the alveolar septa.

therefore rises, causing an increase in the hydrostatic pressure gradient across the pulmonary capillary endothelium. The resulting disturbance in the Starling equilibrium causes transudation of fluid when the critical threshold is passed, and pulmonary oedema occurs (Fig. 4.23).

The capacity of the left ventricle to cope with the load imposed by hypertension may be influenced by several factors. These include the following:

- the degree of blood pressure elevation;
- the biochemical composition of the myocardium;
- the effects on myocardial function of progressive hypertrophy;
- the combined effects of age and genetic factors;
- coronary atheroma (Fig. 4.24), closely associated with hypertension, which can compromise blood flow to the enlarged heart;
- drug treatment – administration of sympatholytic drugs may remove or impair the effect of the sympathetic drive which would otherwise have assumed increasing importance in maintaining cardiac output in this critical situation.

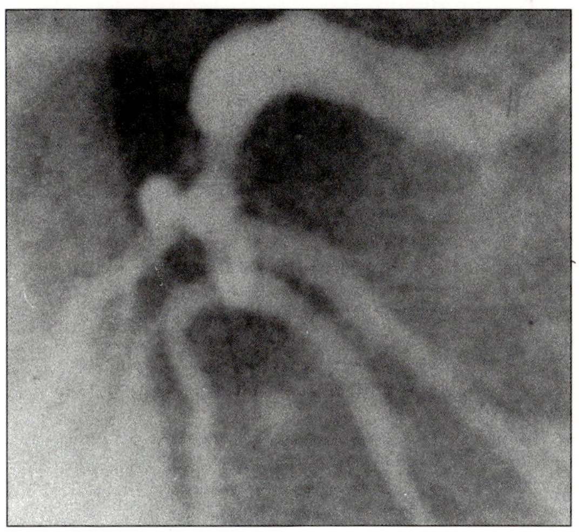

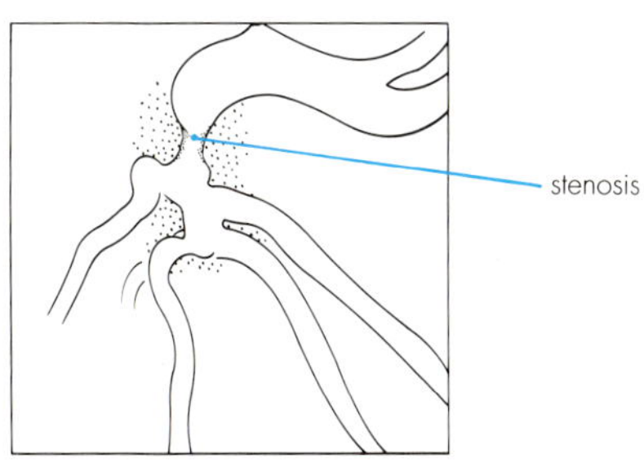

Fig. 4.24 Coronary angiogram from a young hypertensive patient showing critical narrowing of the right coronary artery.

PATHOLOGICAL CHANGES IN THE CENTRAL NERVOUS SYSTEM

Hypertension is the most important risk factor in cerebrovascular disease. Atheroma has a major role in cerebral thrombosis, one of the most common cerebrovascular diseases. Other harmful effects of hypertension include encephalopathy, cerebral haemorrhage, lacunar stroke, embolization of cerebral vessels, transient ischaemic attacks and multi-infarct syndrome (Fig. 4.25).

Hypertensive Encephalopathy

Hypertensive encephalopathy is the result of a marked elevation in blood pressure above the autoregulatory range (the range at which protective constriction of the cerebral resistance vessels prevents an increase in cerebral blood flow). The breakdown of autoregulation is associated with increased cerebral perfusion. This does not occur evenly throughout the cerebral arterial tree. There are therefore focal areas of vasodilatation associated with intervening areas of vasoconstriction, giving a 'string of sausages' effect (Fig. 4.26). The vasodilatation occurs only in the abnormal sections of the arterial tree. Originally it was thought that the vasoconstricted segments of the arterial tree were responsible for the pathogenesis of encephalopathy. It is now believed that autoregulation has broken down in the dilated segments, which have therefore become unprotected and abnormally permeable. This increased permeability can be demonstrated with carbon particles, which readily pass through the blood vessel wall from the plasma (Fig. 4.27). In practice, this results in cerebral oedema. Clinically it is associated with both focal neurological signs and generalized clinical manifestations (Fig. 4.28).

The blood pressure at which encephalopathy occurs varies between patients, just as the autoregulatory range of blood pressure varies (Fig. 4.29). In long-standing hypertension the autoregulatory range is probably elevated as a result of sustained hypertension. Thus the upper threshold for encephalopathy is also raised. However, in hypertension of short duration, for example hypertension of pregnancy and of phaeochromocytoma,

Cerebral Complications
encephalopathy
cerebral haemorrhage
cerebral thrombosis
lacunar stroke
embolism
transient ischaemic attacks
multi-infarct dementia

Fig. 4.25 Cerebral complications of hypertension.

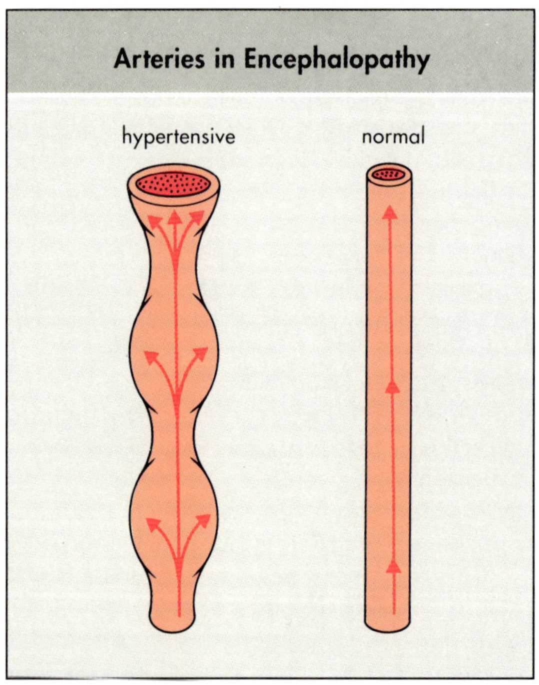

Fig. 4.26 Appearance of cerebral arteries in hypertensive encephalopathy. the 'string of sausages' effect is due to focal dilatation of the artery.

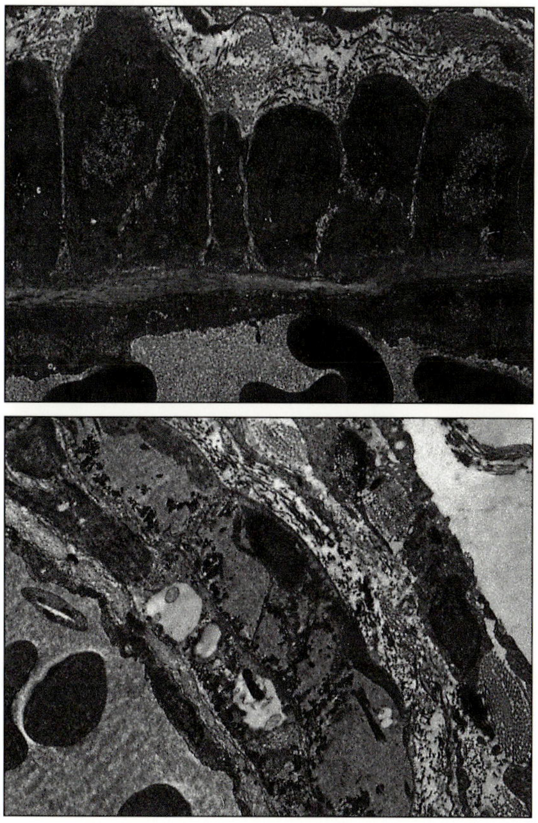

Fig. 4.27 Electron micrographs of a normal rat arteriole (top) and an arteriole showing hypertensive damage (bottom). Increased permeability to carbon particles can be demonstrated experimentally in the dilated segments. Courtesy of Dr F. S. Goldby.

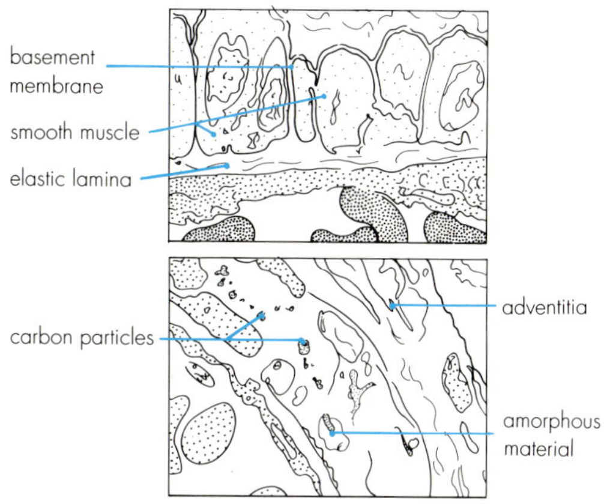

Clinical Features of Encephalopathy

- confusion
- headache
- seizure
- coma
- visual disturbance
- dysarthria
- hemianaesthesia
- dysplasia
- hemiparesis

Fig. 4.28 Clinical features of encephalopathy.

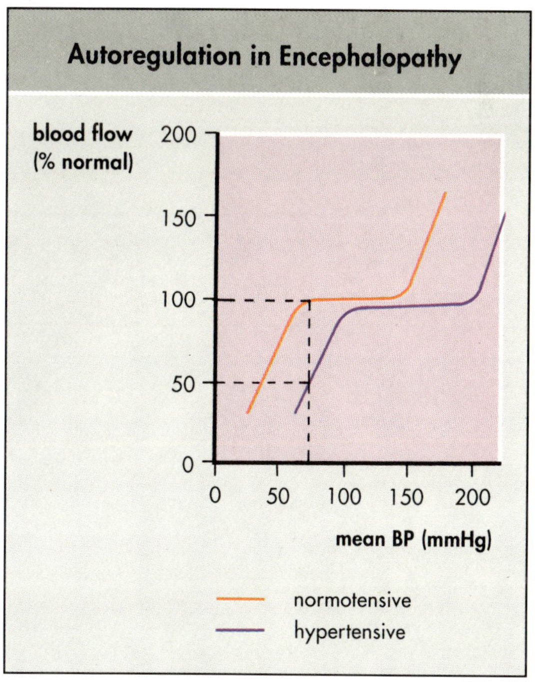

Fig. 4.29 Autoregulatory curves of cerebral blood vessels in hypertensive and normotensive patients. The curve of the hypertensive patients is displaced to the right.

there is a greater chance of encephalopathy occurring at lower pressures (Figs 4.30 & 4.31).

Although patients with hypertension of long duration are relatively protected from encephalopathy by this elevation of their autoregulatory range, they may become more liable to cerebral insufficiency because of a rise in the lower limit. Cerebral infarction (Fig. 4.32) could therefore be produced by overenthusiastic and rapid antihypertensive therapy in patients with long-standing hypertension, despite the fact that blood pressure had been reduced to levels which would be

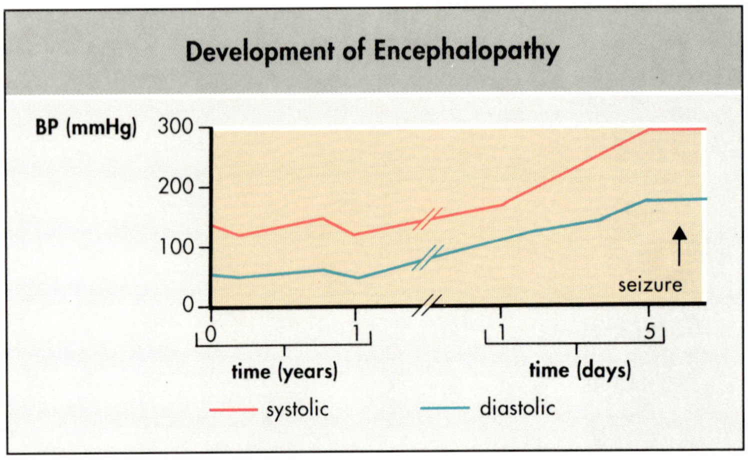

Fig. 4.30 Encephalopathy occurred in this patient with scleroderma and rapidly developing malignant hypertension. Blood pressure, which had previously been normal, rose over a five-day period at the end of which the patient had a *grand mal* convulsion.

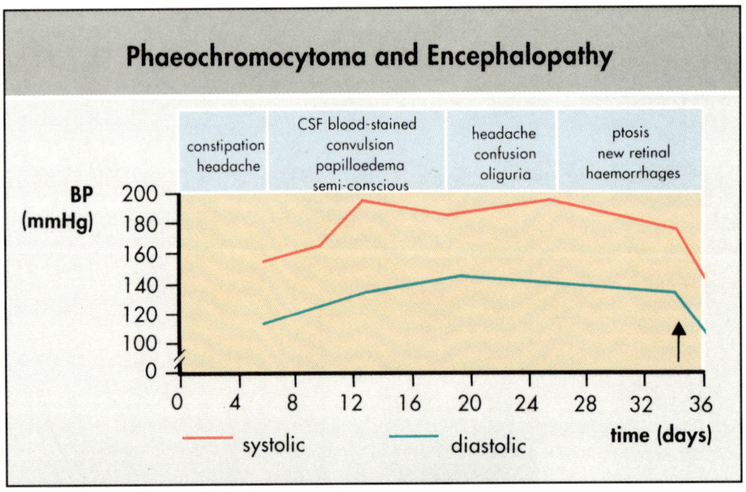

Fig. 4.31 Blood pressure chart of child with phaeochromocytoma. An acute rise in blood pressure was associated with a subarachnoid haemorrhage.

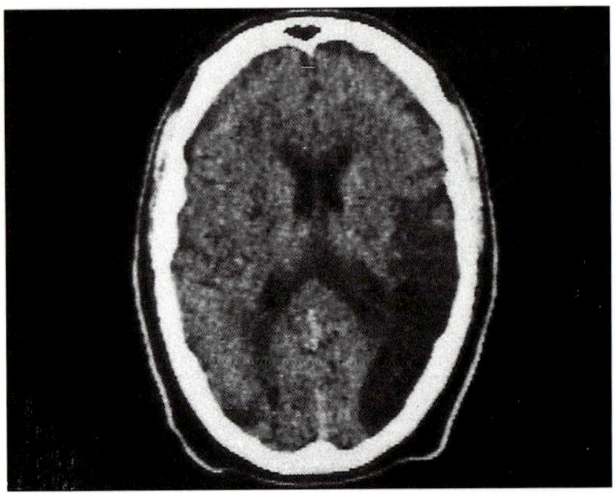

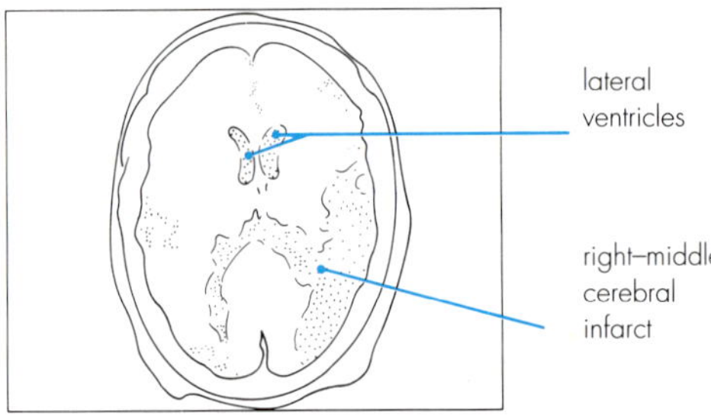

Fig. 4.32 CT scan showing cerebral infarction in a hypertensive patient.

regarded as safe in a normal subject. Caution should thus be exercised when reducing the blood pressure of older patients. In some hypertensive patients cerebrovascular disease manifests itself as a progressive multi-infarct dementia (Fig. 4.33).

Intracerebral Haemorrhage

Intracerebral haemorrhage (Figs. 4.34 and 4.35) in hypertensive subjects usually occurs as a result of Charcot–Bouchard aneurysms (Fig. 4.36). These

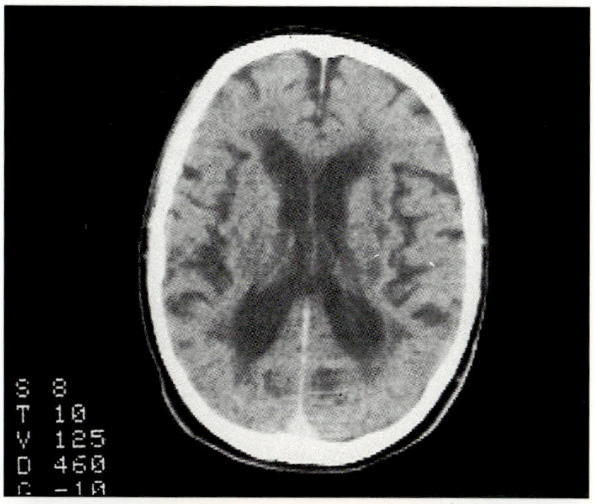

Fig. 4.33 CT scan showing multi-infarct syndrome in a hypertensive patient.

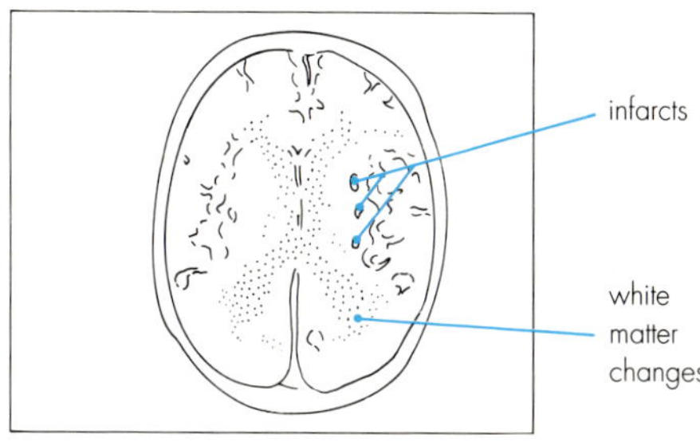

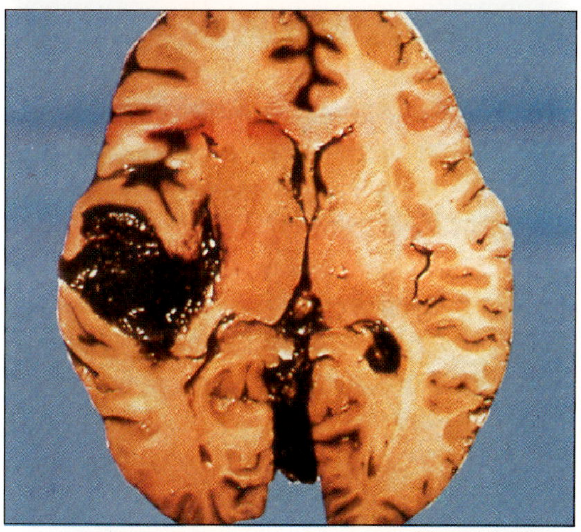

Fig. 4.34 Postmortem specimens showing intracerebral haemorrhage.

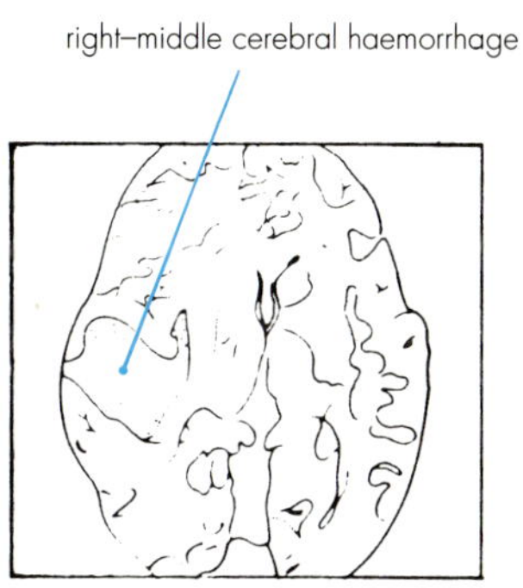

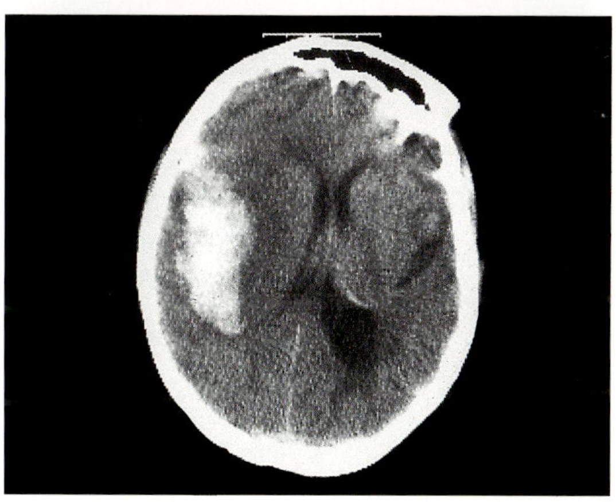

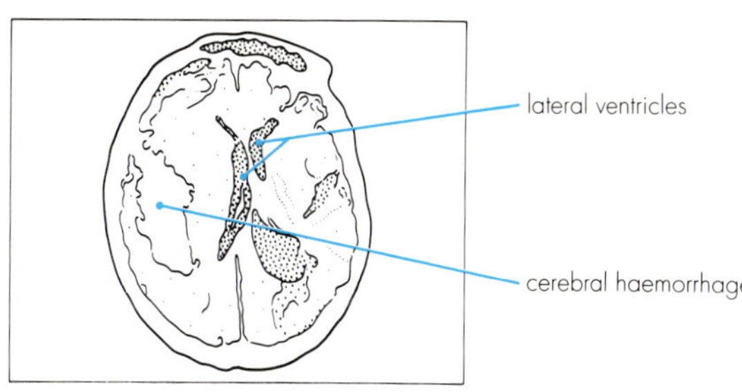

Fig. 4.35 CT scan of a hypertensive patient with extensive intracerebral haemorrhage.

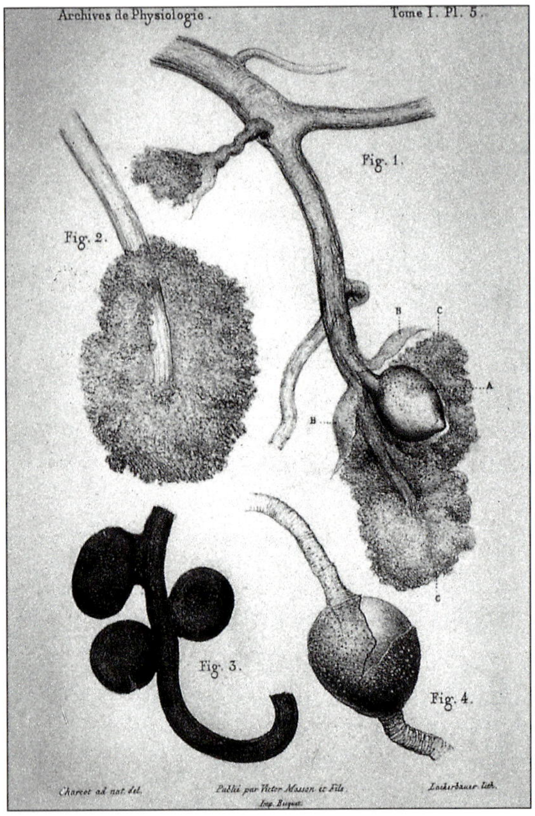

Fig. 4.36 Charcot's original diagram showing Charcot–Bouchard aneurysms.

were originally described in 1868 in sixty patients who had died of cerebral haemorrhage. This finding was neglected, however, until Russell rediscovered the lesions in 1963. Charcot–Bouchard aneurysms occur particularly in the small perforating arteries in the region of the basal ganglia, thalamus and internal capsule (Fig. 4.37). At the site of the aneurysm there is a vascular defect associated with hyaline degeneration of the media. A close correlation exists between blood pressure and the frequency of aneurysms (Fig. 4.38). Their frequency also increases with age. These two factors act synergistically so that Charcot–Bouchard aneurysms are most frequent in elderly hypertensive subjects.

Lacunar Infarctions

Charcot–Bouchard aneurysms are also associated with lacunar infarctions of the brain. These are observed as small cavities and are most frequent in the basal ganglia, pons, cerebellum, and posterior limb of the internal capsule. They appear to be the result of a thrombotic occlusion of small arteries and are usually accompanied by minor strokes which give rise to focal signs suggestive of

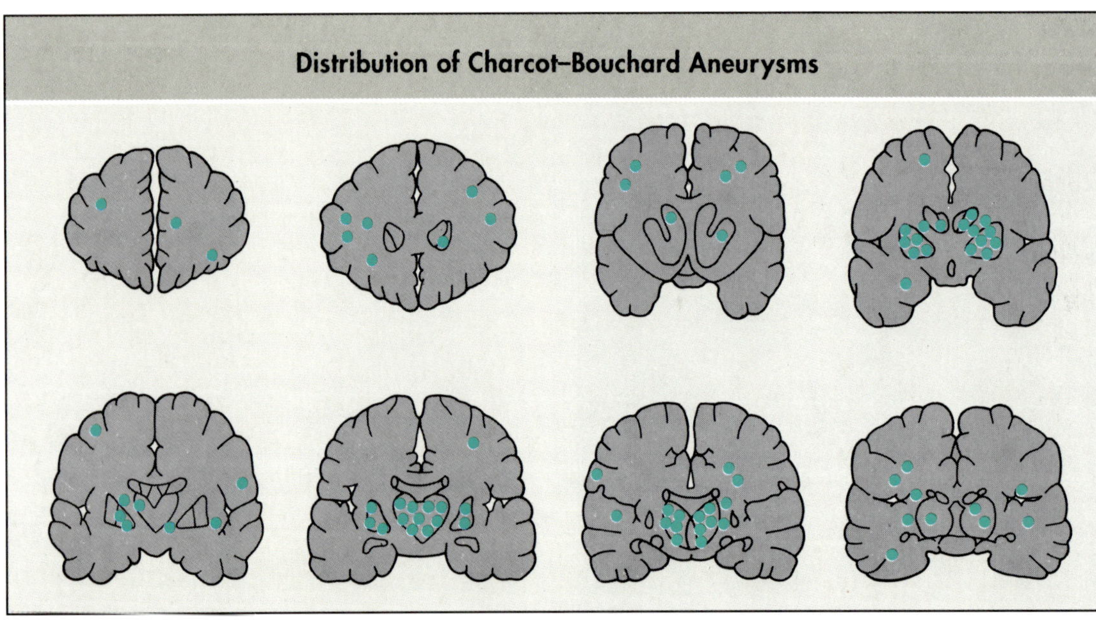

Fig. 4.37 Distribution of Charcot–Bouchard aneurysms in hypertensive patients. Note the predominantly subcortical distribution.

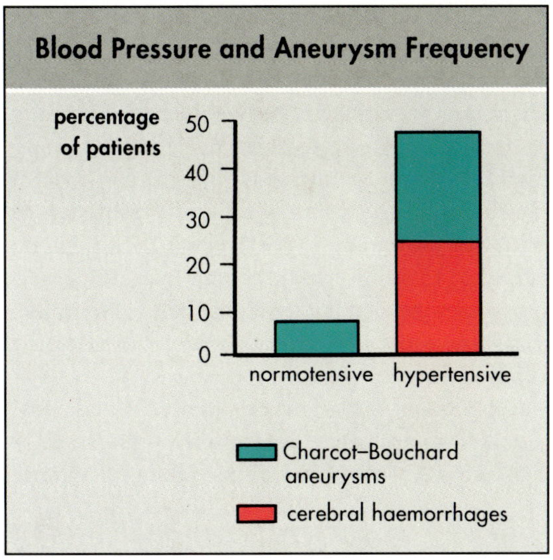

Fig. 4.38 At postmortem, Charcot–Bouchard aneurysms are much more common in patients who are known to have been hypertensive. A substantial proportion of patients die of cerebral haemorrhage.

lesions in the internal capsule, thalamus, or pons. In some cases a 'lacunar state' may be produced by multiple lacunar infarctions of the brain. This causes progressive dementia, pseudobulbar palsy and upper motor neurone lesions of the limbs.

Subarachnoid haemorrhage

Subarachnoid haemorrhage is a less common complication of hypertension. The sites for such haemorrhages are berry aneurysms occurring at the junction of vessels belonging to the circle of Willis and developmental absence of the media appears to be responsible (Figs. 4.39 and 4.40). Such berry aneurysms occur with increased frequency in polycystic renal disease, aortic coarctation and hypertension.

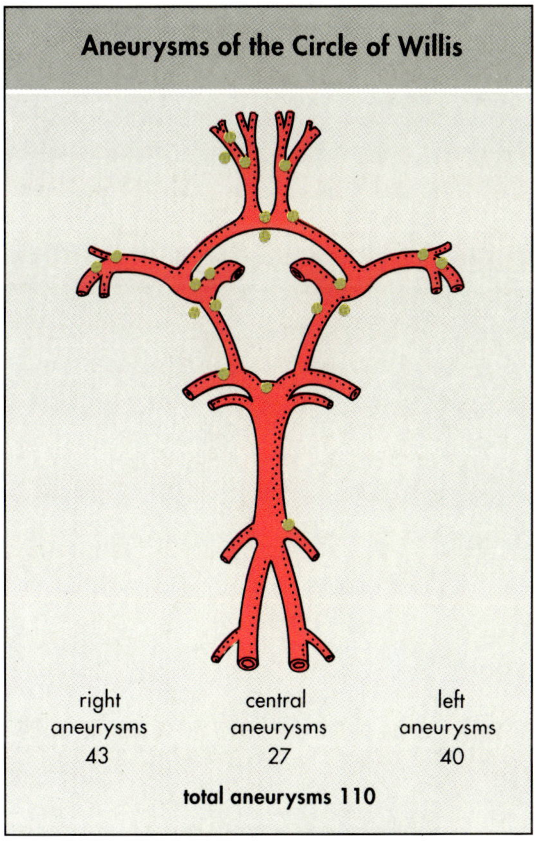

Fig. 4.39 Distribution and frequency of aneurysms of the circle of Willis.

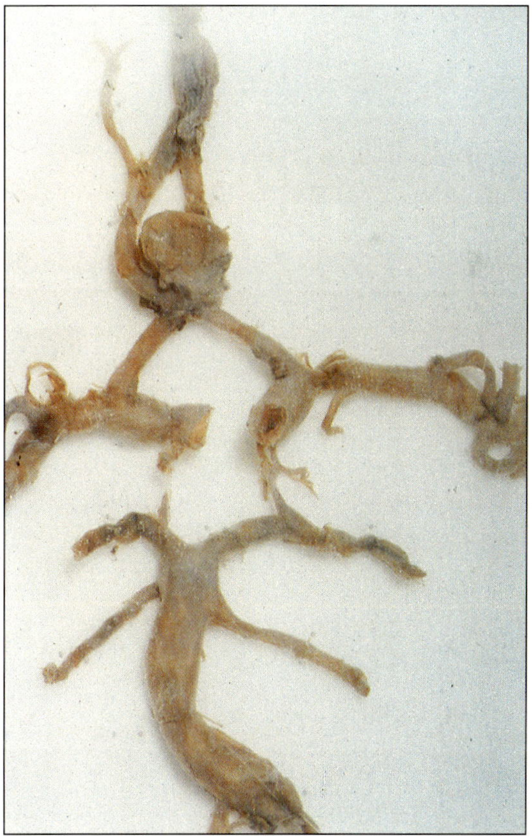

Fig. 4.40 Gross pathological specimen of the circle of Willis showing a berry aneurysm of the anterior communicating artery.

HYPERTENSIVE EFFECTS ON THE KIDNEY

Essential hypertension is associated with an increase in renal vascular resistance with a consequent reduction in renal plasma flow. However, the glomerular filtration rate (GFR) is well preserved so that the fraction of renal plasma filtered at the glomerulus is increased (Fig. 4.41). Macroscopically, the kidneys are normal or only slightly reduced in size and have a slightly granular appearance (Fig. 4.42). Microscopically, the vessels show benign nephrosclerosis with hyalinization of the afferent arteriolar wall, beginning in the subendothelial region and extending to the media (Fig. 4.43). This is a patchy process which may occur in the elderly even in the absence of hypertension. Besides causing an alteration in renal haemodynamics, nephrosclerosis has been implicated in two renal functional changes which are frequently observed in hypertension. These are the reduction in urate clearance (with resulting hyperuricaemia) and the subnormal response of plasma renin to stimulation by salt restriction or diuretics ('low-renin hypertension'). There is no evidence to suggest that benign nephrosclerosis progresses to renal failure. Renal failure becomes a problem only if malignant hypertension or extrarenal complications supervene.

In malignant hypertension, both GFR and renal blood flow are almost invariably reduced (Fig. 4.44). This is associated with moderate proteinuria

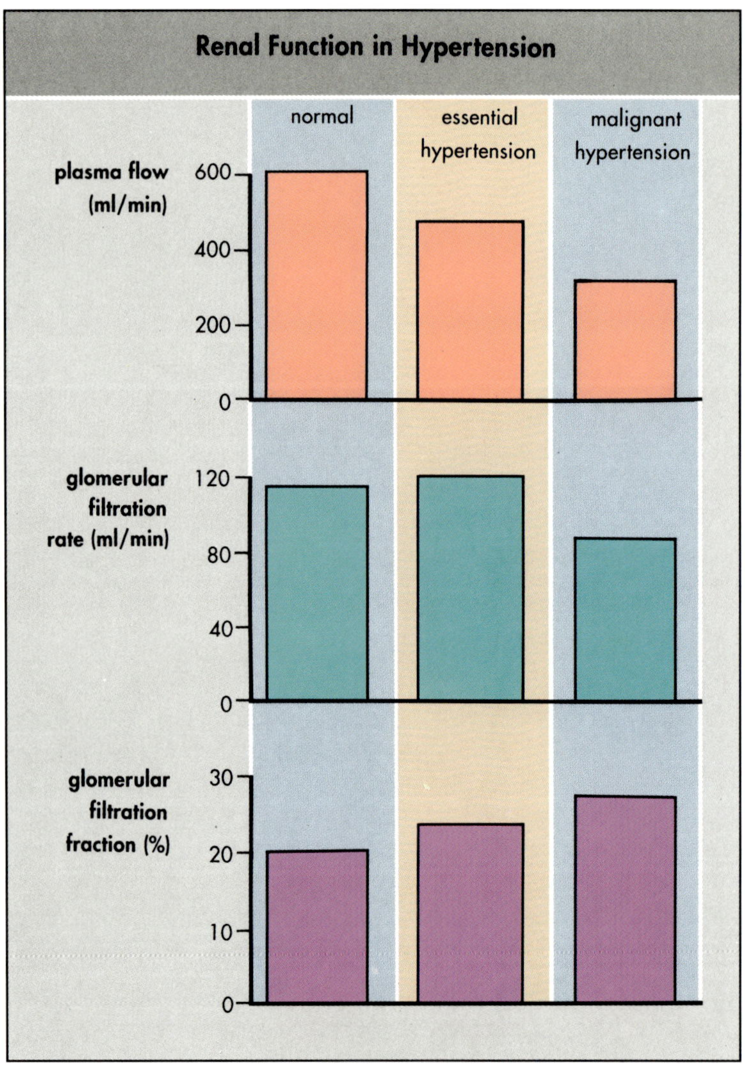

Fig. 4.41 Renal function in hypertension. While renal plasma flow is reduced, glomerular filtration rate is maintained so that filtration fraction is increased. In malignant hypertension, both renal plasma flow and glomerular filtration rate are reduced.

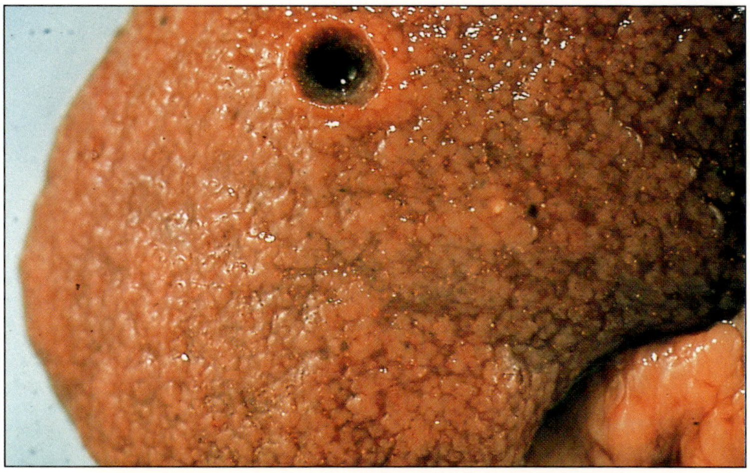

Fig. 4.42 Macroscopic view of a kidney from a patient with essential hypertension. The size of the kidney is normal but there is an adherent capsule with a slightly granular appearance.

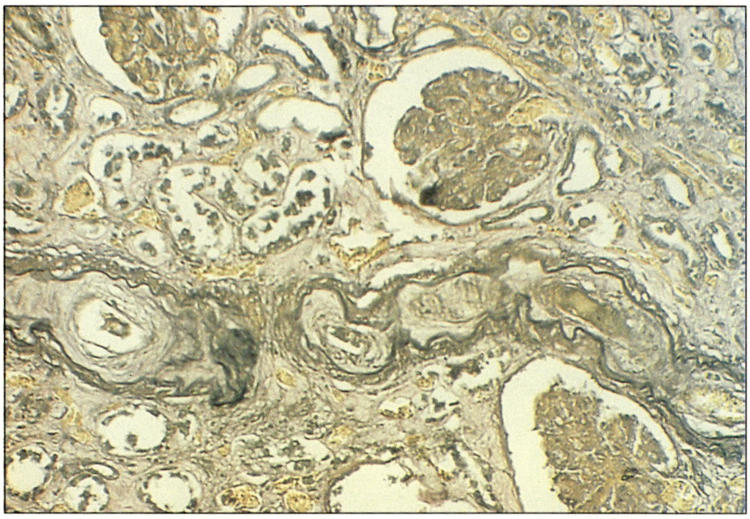

Fig. 4.43 Histology of a glomerulus from a patient with essential hypertension showing benign nephrosclerosis with hyaline change: this is particularly marked in the afferent arteriole (stained yellow).

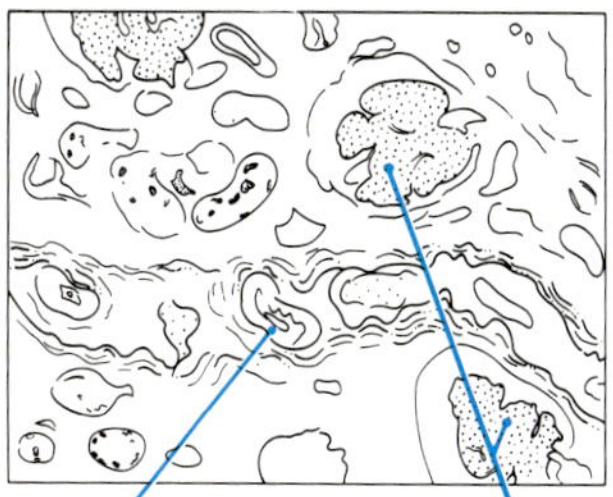

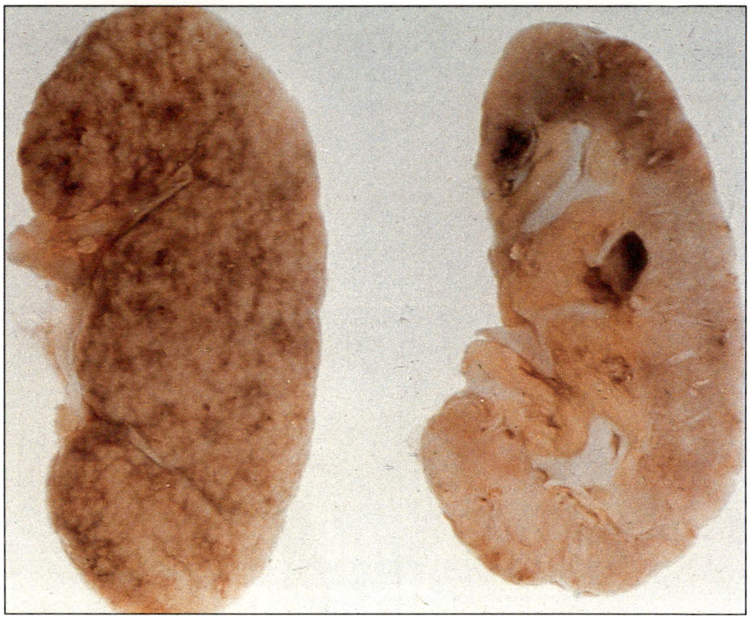

Fig. 4.44 Macroscopic view of a kidney from a patient with malignant hypertension. It is of normal size but there are numerous small surface haemorrhages.

(1–2g/day) and microscopic haematuria. Renal failure may become clinically important and occasionally acute renal failure may develop (Fig. 4.45). However, so long as the deterioration in renal function is not too far advanced, it is reversible by active antihypertensive therapy.

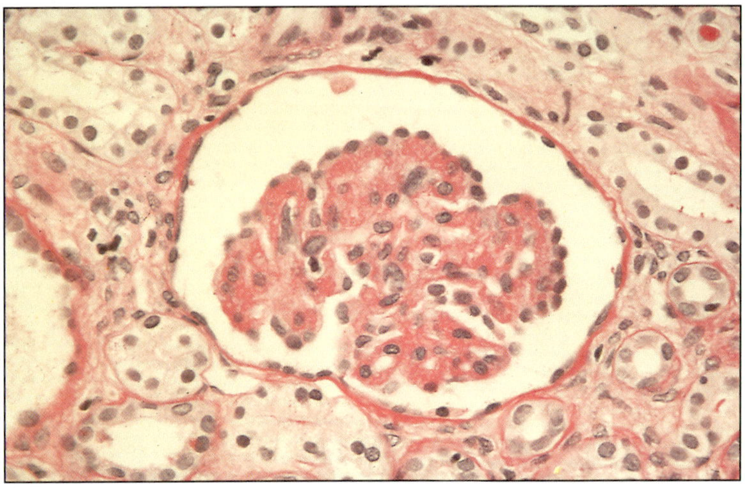

Fig. 4.45 Histology of a glomerulus from a patient with malignant hypertension showing extensive fibrinoid necrosis of the glomerular vessels.

CHAPTER 5

Known Causes of Hypertension

INTRODUCTION

Blood pressure control is achieved by a combination of a number of factors. The relative importance of each factor varies, depending on the haemodynamic state. When any one factor plays a dominant role it may become an identifiable cause of hypertension.

Many of the causes are identified with disease of particular organs or (occasionally) systems, but this does not necessarily identify the precise mechanisms by which the blood pressure remains elevated – although short-term control of blood pressure is under the influence of baroreceptors in the carotid sinus and aortic arch, these can rapidly reset to higher pressures giving the opportunity for sustained hypertension (Fig. 5.1). This chapter considers some of the most important conditions that can cause hypertension.

Presumably high blood pressure has had no major evolutionary consequences because any untoward effects on organ function are of a delayed nature and do not affect reproductive capacity.

MECHANISMS OF HYPERTENSION

Richard Bright (1789–1858) was the first to notice a connection between albuminous urine, various types of nephritis (including glomerulonephritis – Fig. 5.2), and the common finding of hypertrophy of the heart without valvular disease (particularly in the left ventricle). At that time, blood pressure could not be measured in humans. Nonetheless, Bright commented that 'This [finding] naturally leads us to look for some less local cause for the unusual efforts to which the heart has been impelled'. He further suggested '...that it so affects the minute and capillary circulation, as to render greater action necessary to force the blood through the distant subdivisions of the vascular system'. This proposed increase in peripheral resistance is now known to be associated with most forms of chronic hypertension.

Much of the increased resistance is related to vascular hypertrophy, but in the process leading up to this state the renin–angiotensin system does seem to play a dominant role in some cases, although it is of uncertain significance in others.

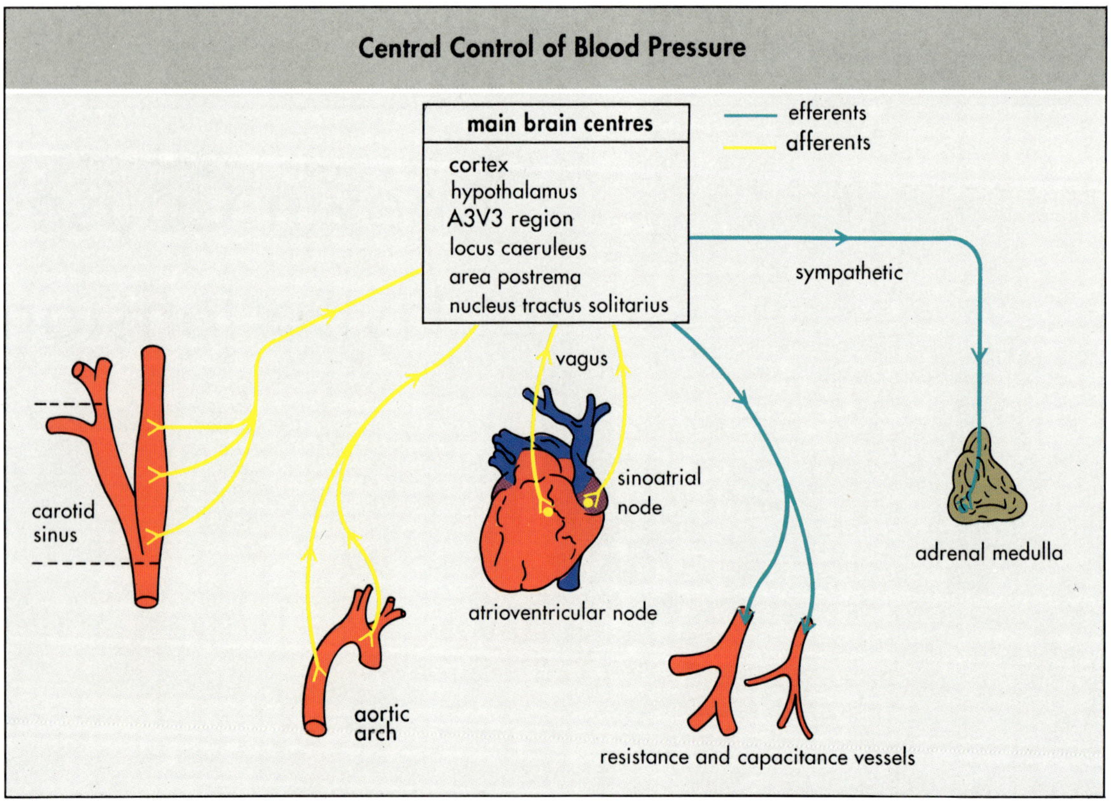

Fig. 5.1 Diagram illustrating the central control of blood pressure.

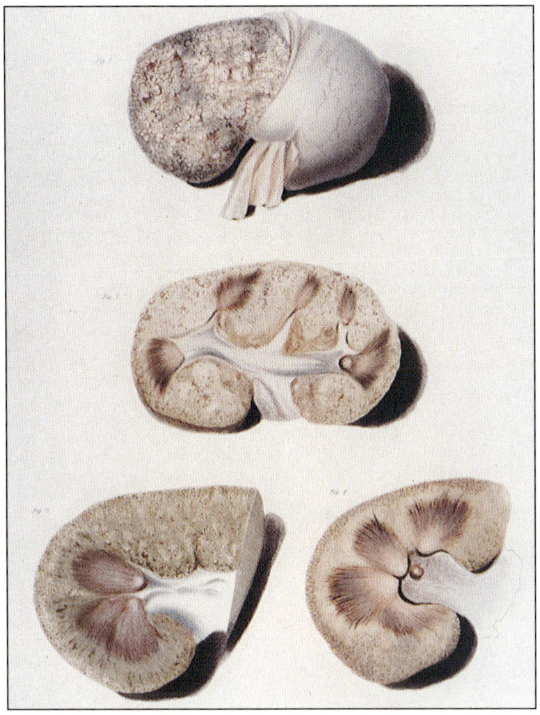

Fig. 5.2 Coloured lithograph of kidneys from a patient with chronic glomerulonephritis, used to illustrate Richard Bright's first description of the disease (1827). He also noted the presence of left ventricular hypertrophy in such patients, which he correctly attributed to increased resistance in the blood vessels.

The presence of hypertension is undoubtedly linked to the type of glomerular lesion. It is uncommon in minimal change glomerulonephritis, even with marked proteinuria, but is nearly always present with proliferative and extracapillary (crescentic) glomerulonephritis (see Fig. 5.24), especially if corticosteroids are used therapeutically. As renal deterioration progresses, sodium and water retention may develop. The end-stage of all types of severe renal failure is associated with hypertension. At this stage dialysis with sodium and water withdrawal results in a lowering of blood pressure. This can usually be maintained so long as a low-sodium diet is followed. There are the rare occasions, however, when blood pressure rises as sodium is removed – this points to a high renin level (which is increased by dialysis) and suggests a major role for renin in the maintenance of hypertension. In such cases blood pressure may actually be reduced by giving sodium and water. This approach requires great care if overloading is

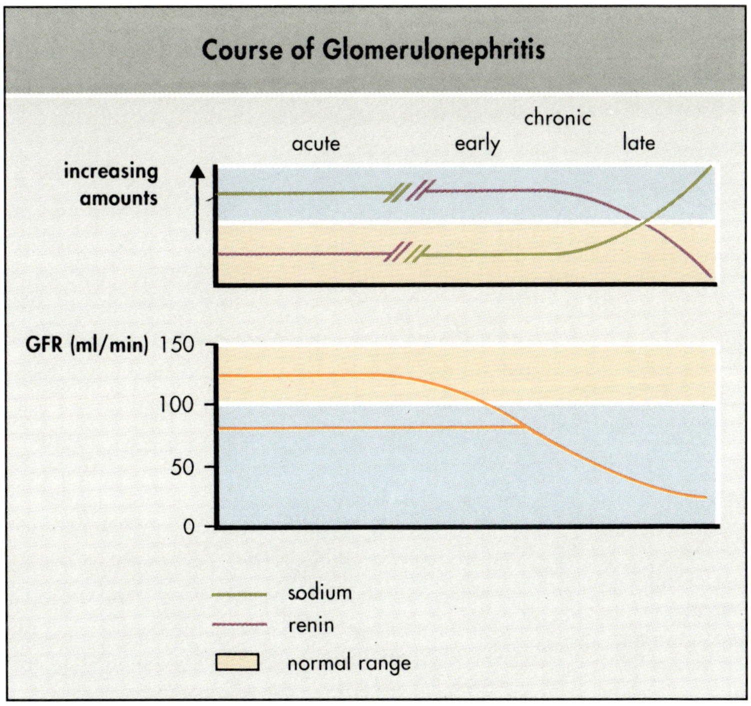

Fig. 5.3 In acute glomerulonephritis, hypertension is associated with sodium retention and a normal plasma renin. In the earlier stages of chronic glomerulonephritis hypertension is usually associated with a high plasma renin. As the disease progresses, sodium- and water-retention become progressively more important in maintaining blood pressure.

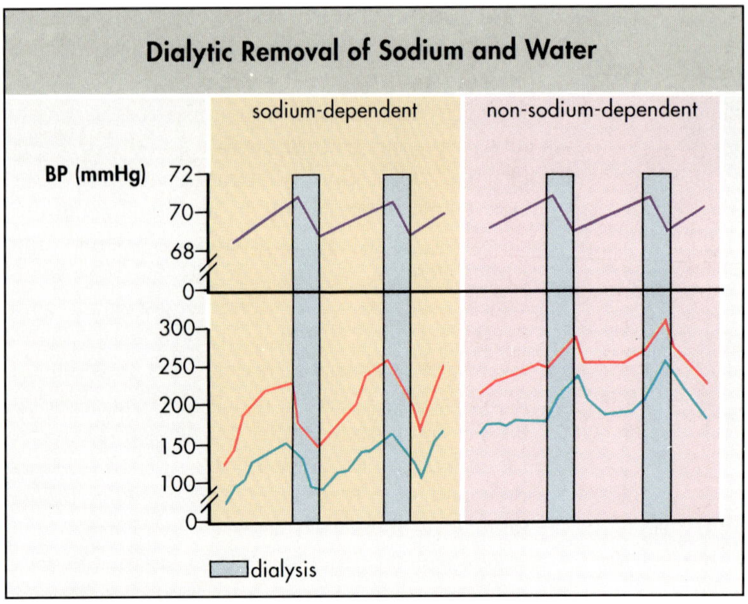

Fig. 5.4 In most patients with advanced chronic renal failure, hypertension is associated with sodium overload and is therefore relieved by the dialytic removal of sodium and water. In a minority of patients (usually with a high plasma renin) removal of sodium does not lower blood pressure, which may even rise during dialysis.

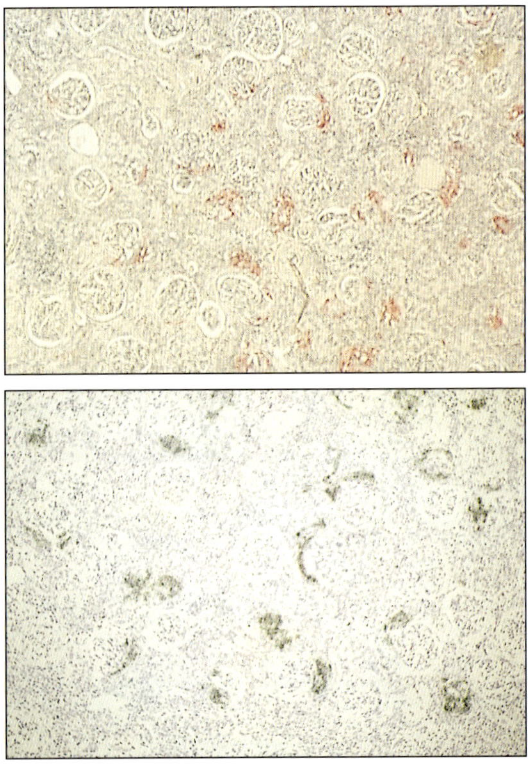

Fig. 5.5 Top: Immunohistochemical appearance of end-stage renal disease showing renin (pink) in the juxtaglomerular region and in the efferent arterioles. Note the tubular atrophy and the crowding of glomeruli in various stages of obsolescence. These are typical features of severe renal ischaemia. Bottom: The same region of the kidney in which in situ hybridization has been carried out with a marker for renin mRNA showing the sites of renin production. Both slides courtesy of Dr M. Taylor.

to be avoided (Figs 5.3 & 5.4). Removal of the kidneys at this stage may also reduce the pressure, as the kidneys may contain large amounts of renin produced in the afferent arterioles as well as in the juxtaglomerular apparatus (Fig. 5.5).

Renal Hypertension

Kidneys showing ischaemic change were all originally believed to cause hypertension via the renin–angiotensin system. In many of the cases of renal artery stenosis with high levels of renin and angiotensin in the circulation, this is certainly true – it is demonstrated by the fall in blood pressure, sometimes precipitous, produced by blockade of the system with converting enzyme inhibitors (Fig. 5.6). This theory was lent further weight by observations of the effects of certain rare tumours, usually of vascular origin, called haemangiopericytomata. These tumours are usually small, situated on the outer part of the cortex and contain large amounts of renin. Patients with such tumours have high peripheral blood levels of renin; following removal, the blood pressure falls (Fig. 5.7). It is likely that the rare mesoblastoma of infancy is, occasionally, a renin-producing tumour; both renin and renin mRNA have been shown in vessel walls within the tumour, and removal of the kidney leads to cure of the hypertension (Fig. 5.8).

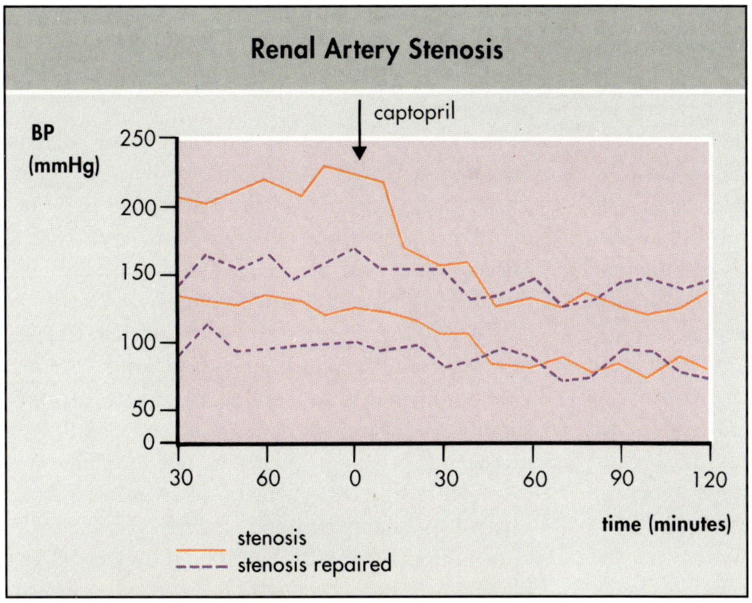

Fig. 5.6 The fall in blood pressure due to 50μg captopril in a patient with severe hypertension caused by a renal artery stenosis. Following repair of the stenosis, captopril was without significant effect.

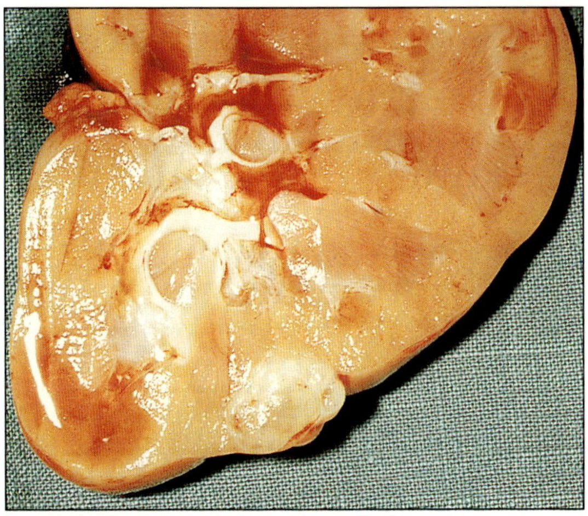

Fig. 5.7 Kidney removed at operation from a hypertensive child with a renin-secreting haemangiopericytoma. These lesions are small and often difficult to demonstrate radiologically.
Courtesy of Dr J. J. Brown.

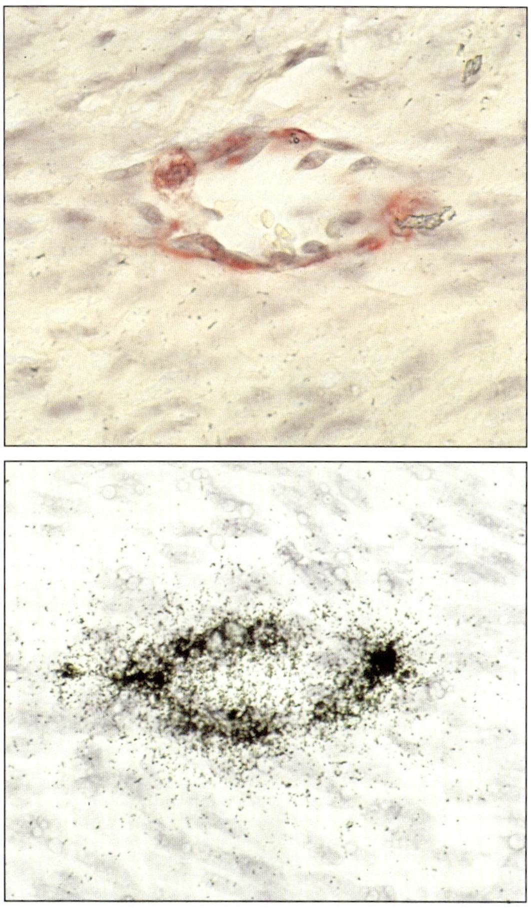

Fig. 5.8 Identical retin and mRNA distribution shown by immuno-histochemistry (top) and by *in situ* hybridization (bottom) in a vessel in a congenital mesoblastic nephroma. Note the absence of renal cortical structure Courtesy of Dr M. Taylor.

In many cases of hypertension-associated renal artery stenosis and unilateral renal disease, correction of the stenosis or removal of the kidney leads to a fall in blood pressure. The contribution of the renin–angiotensin system here is not clear. This particularly applies to those cases where blockade of the renin–angiotensin system does not cause a fall of blood pressure; the immediate pressor effects of the system are ruled out, but the induction of other mechanisms, particularly in the nervous system, remains a distinct possibility.

The precise involvement of the nervous system in the pressor action of angiotensin is unclear, and there remain many questions about the site of action, both in the central nervous system and the periphery. It is certain, however, that sympathetic vasoconstriction in the hand is centrally induced.

In some situations the renin–angiotensin system may not be involved at all. This probably applies to those cases of renal artery stenosis or unilateral renal disease where the levels of renin and angiotensin in the circulation are not high. Increased sensitivity of the adrenal cortex to normal levels of angiotensin, as shown by increased aldosterone release in sodium deprivation, has not been demonstrated for the pressor effects, but even there, pharmacological blockade of the system should still reveal it readily.

The nervous system has been invoked as the predominant cause of hypertension at all stages of experimental renal artery stenois. However, both the severity and extent of the nervous lesions which reverse the hypertension require careful examination.

In all forms of hypertension the hypothesis created by Borst and refined by Ledingham, Floyer, and Guyton indicates a sequence of sodium and water retention, increased plasma volume and cardiac output and increased blood pressure and peripheral resistance. The model proposes a cardinal role for the kidney, which is believed to require a higher pressure to excrete the same sodium and water load as a normal kidney at lower pressure.

This hypothesis can be modified to fit various pathological renal conditions. However, when stages of the hypothesis have been tested in different clinical conditions, discrepancies have arisen. For example, sodium- and water-retention is not the rule in most cases of hypertension, only in acute glomerulonephritis and terminal renal failure. Equally, cardiac output and plasma volume are not raised except in similar, extreme conditions. It is obviously not usually possible to follow the precise sequence of events in human diseases, but certain elements carry support from experimental approaches in man – the observations of Borst, using the sodium and water retaining compound glycyrrhizic acid (liquorice), remain the most convincing.

Hypertension always leads ultimately to vascular damage in the kidney. This damage is sometimes severe (Fig. 5.9) and particularly affects the afferent arterioles and glomeruli. Atheroma, particularly that in the renal artery and aorta, is increased by hypertension and may therefore accelerate the process. For these reasons some believe that most forms of hypertension may involve a renal component.

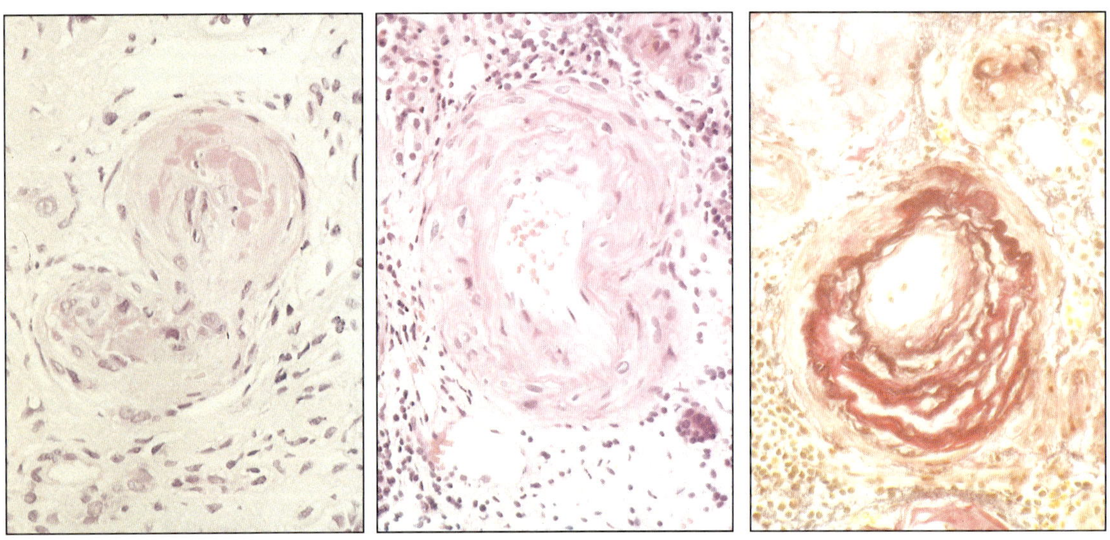

Fig. 5.9 Left: Malignant hypertension with fibrinoid necrosis. Haematoxylin and eosin stain. Centre: Severe hypertension with muscular hypertrophy and hyaline change. Haematoxylin and eosin stain. Right: Severe hypertension showing duplication of the internal elastic lamina. Haematoxylin and van Gieson's stain.

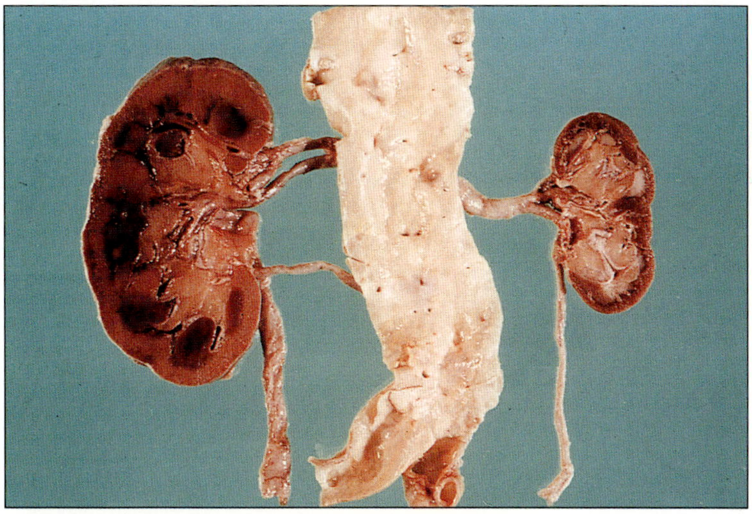

Fig. 5.10 Renal artery stenosis discovered post-mortem in a hypertensive patient. The aorta is grossly atheromatous and the renal artery is narrowed by atheroma resulting in renal ischaemia on the left with a small shrunken kidney.

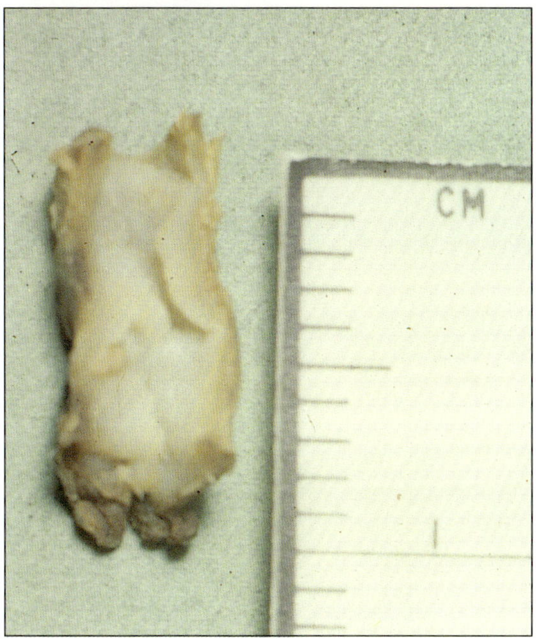

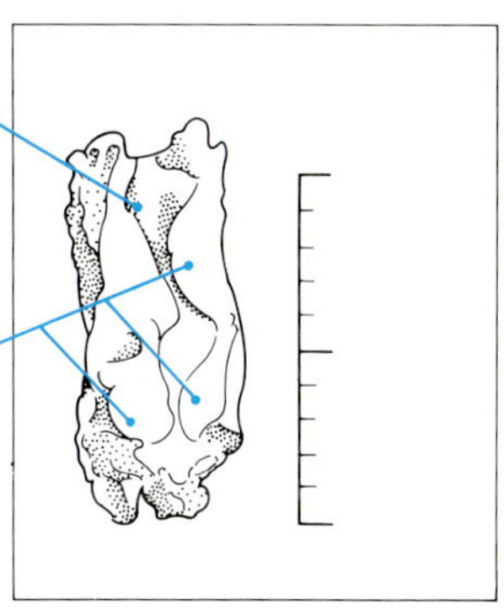

Fig. 5.11 Fibromuscular dysplasia. The renal artery has been opened longitudinally to show the lumen obstructed by a series of collagen protrusions.

THE KIDNEY

Diseases of this organ are common causes of hypertension. The key factor is usually ischaemia produced either by preglomerular arterial narrowing or by direct pathological involvement of the glomeruli or their blood supply by scar tissue (secondary, for example, to pyelonephritis).

Renal artery stenosis (Fig. 5.10) is a typical example of the former; correction of the stenosis by surgery or angioplasty (dilatation by balloon catheter) leads to cure.

Arterial Dysplasia

Arterial dysplasia is the most common form of renal artery stenosis in the younger age group (32% in one series).

Intimal fibroplasia is one of the rarest forms of dysplasia (1%) and occurs as a circumferential, annular, or eccentric thickening of the intima of the main renal artery. Perimedial fibroplasia occurs in about 20% of cases of dysplasia, and is the result of a replacement of the circumference of the outer half or two-thirds of the media by dense collagen tissue. This may vary in thickness, so that beading may be observed on the angiogram. Medial fibromuscular dysplasia (Fig. 5.11) is the commonest form (64% in one series). The distal two-thirds of the main renal artery and its branches show intermittent fibromuscular ridges separated by thin segments of vessel wall, giving the characteristic 'string of onions' angiographic appearance. The disease is frequently bilateral and involves other vessels, such as the mesenteric, iliac or carotid arteries (Fig. 5.12), much less frequently.

Although the cause is unknown, the fact that it is often progressive and appears later in life in the opposite artery clearly indicates either a continuing local stimulus, or a growth or differentiation factor with a long latent period. Any explanation must also take account of the fact that fibromuscular dysplasia characteristically presents predominantly in women in their second and third decade.

Atheroma

Atheroma is the most common cause of renal artery stenosis in the older age group (63% in one series). It is often associated with atheroma elsewhere, particularly in the distal parts of the aorta (see Figs 5.10 & 5.13). The most frequent site is at the mouth of the renal artery – distal to the narrowing the renal artery is dilated, often with a very thin wall which may become aneurysmal.

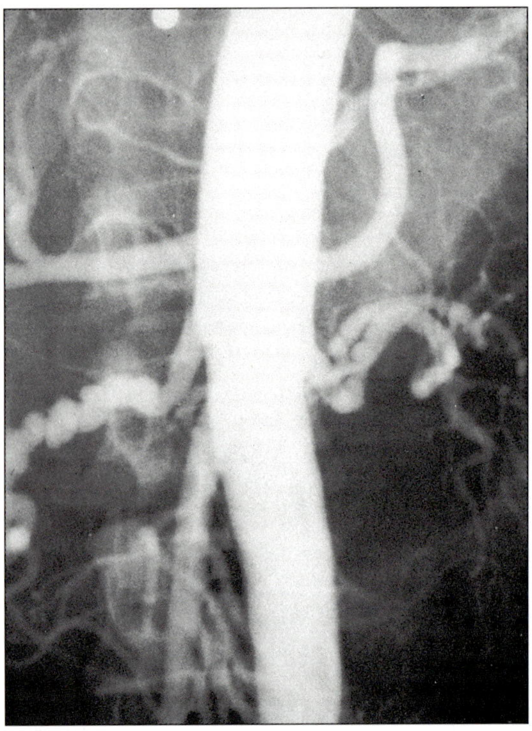

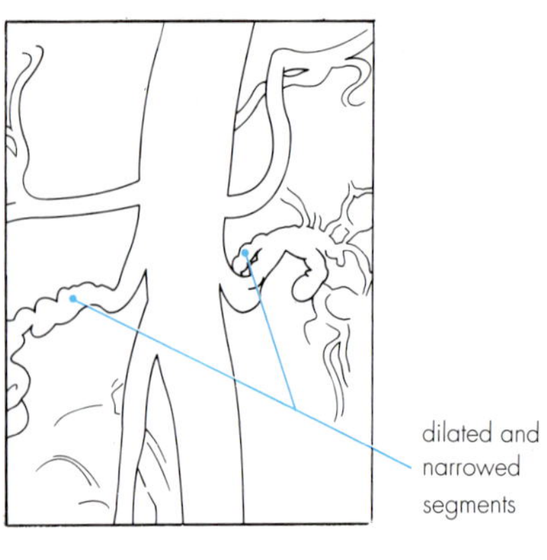

Fig. 5.12 Arteriogram from a patient with bilateral fibromuscular dysplasia. The renal artery shows a characteristic 'corkscrew' or 'string of onions' appearance with alternate areas of narrowing and dilatation.

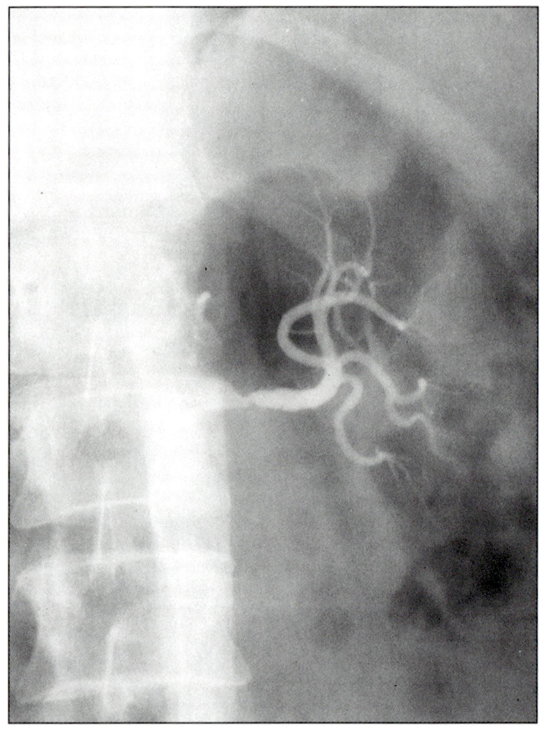

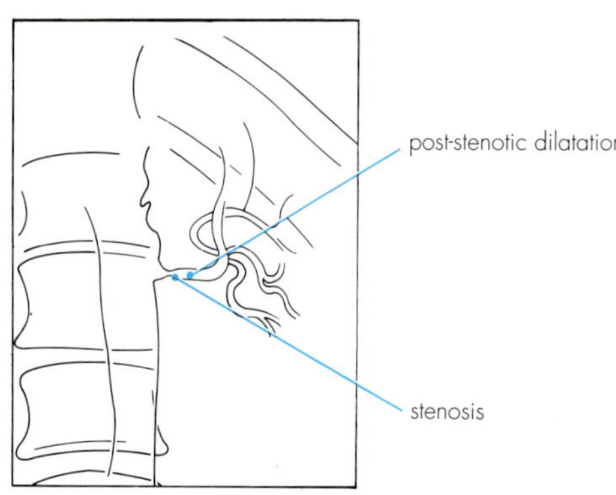

Fig. 5.13 Arteriogram showing a tight renal artery stenosis on the left with post-stenotic dilatation of renal artery.

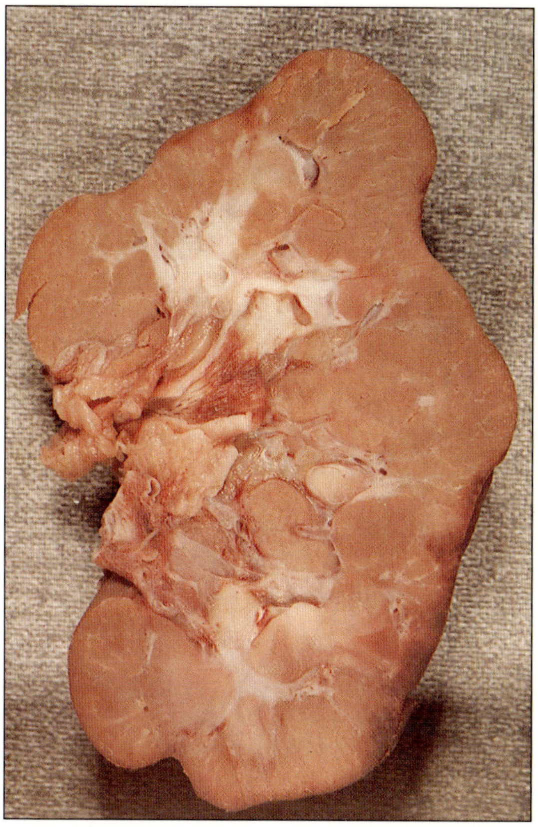

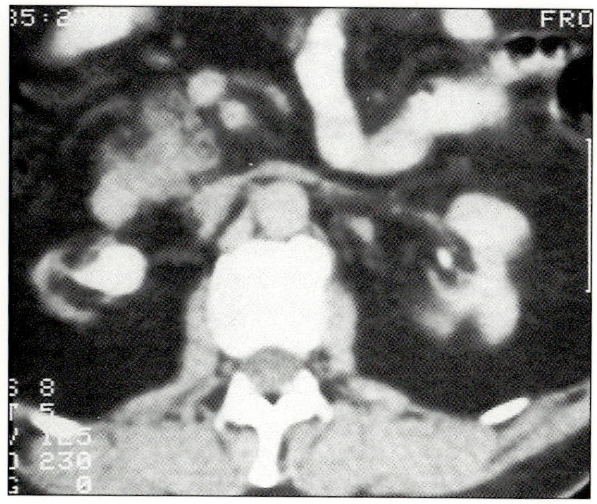

Fig. 5.14 Above: Multiple infarcts in kidney due to emboli (cardiac fibrillation). Top right: CT scan of the upper abdomen showing infarcts in the left kidney due to emboli from renal artery stenosis.

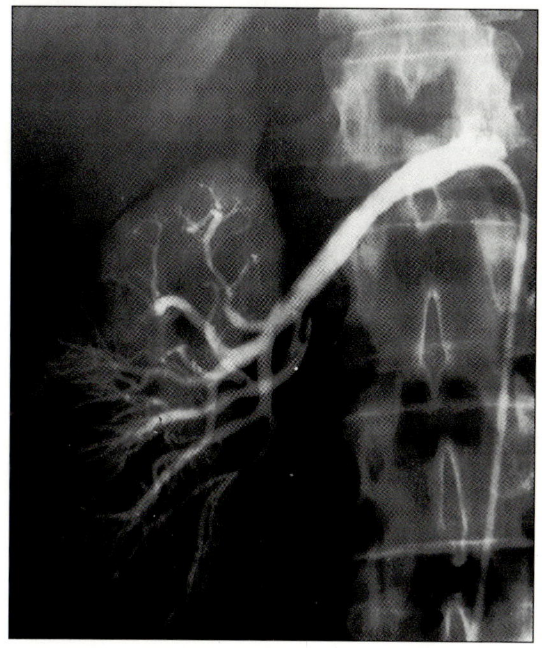

Fig. 5.15 Renal artery dissection. This is seen at the origin of the branch to the lower pole just below the main renal artery.

Other Causes of Arterial Narrowing

Occasionally narrowing is caused by an external fibromuscular band or by tumours such as phaeochromocytomata. Neurofibromatosis can cause multiple narrowings in the branches of the renal artery by nodular neural compressions. Emboli arising from the proximal renal artery or from the fibrillating heart (Fig. 5.14), particularly if associated with mitral stenosis, may also be a cause of hypertension. Presumably, it is the ischaemic areas around the small infarcts which are responsible. A rare but important cause occurs in neonates, where umbilical artery catheterization leads occasionally to retrograde embolization of the renal artery with eventual stenosis. Another important cause, due to the frequency of abdominal trauma in car accidents, is dissection of the renal artery (Fig. 5.15).

Hypernephroma

Tumours may also cause renal ischaemia by growth within the kidney, so that hypernephroma is an occasional cause of hypertension which may be cured by nephrectomy. There is no evidence of a hormonal basis arising from the tumour itself in these cases; this is in contrast to the specific renin-producing tumours considered later (see Fig. 5.27).

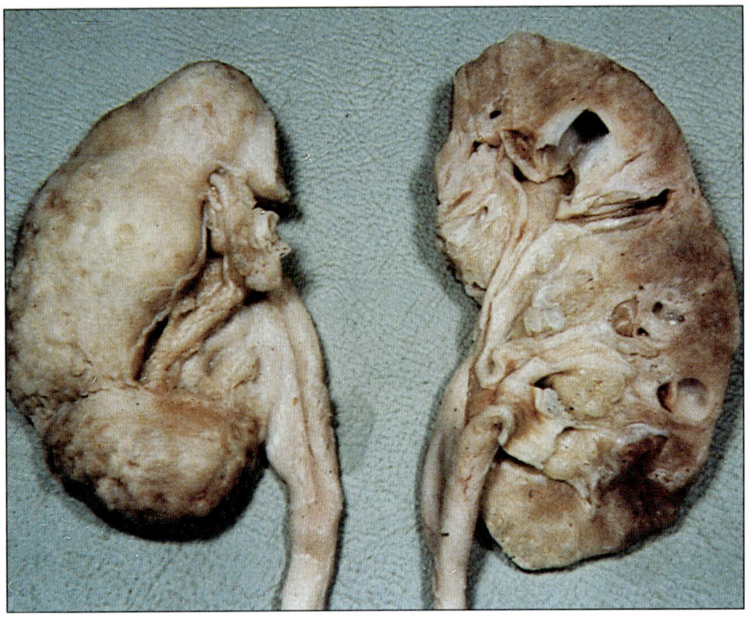

Fig. 5.16 Bilateral chronic pyelonephritis causing hypertension. The kidney are characteristically scarred and shrunken. Courtesy of Dr P. N. Cardew.

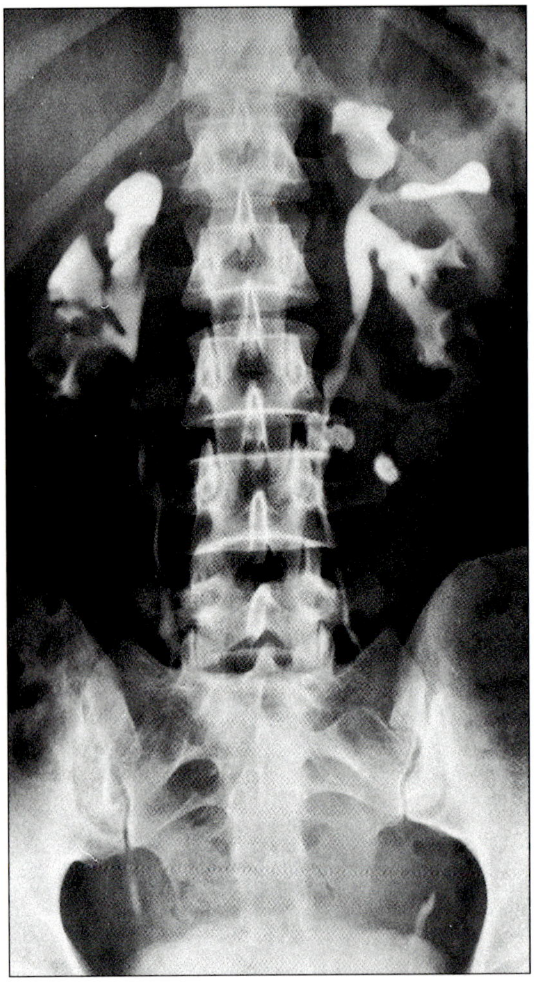

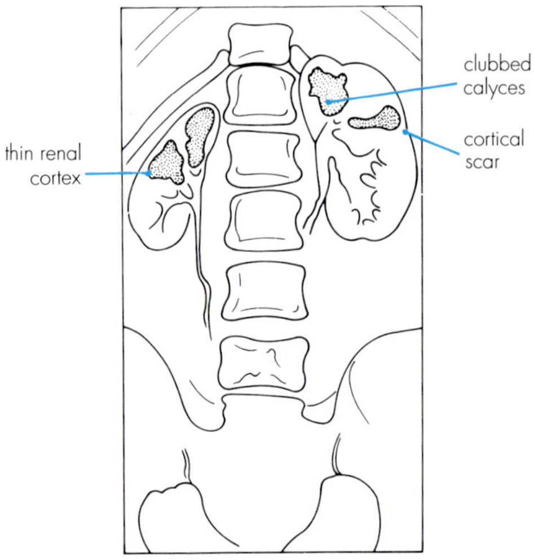

Fig. 5.17 Pyelographic appearances in a patient with bilateral chronic pyelonephritis. The calyces are clubbed and the overlying cortex is thin. Courtesy of Dr D. Finlay and Dr D. James.

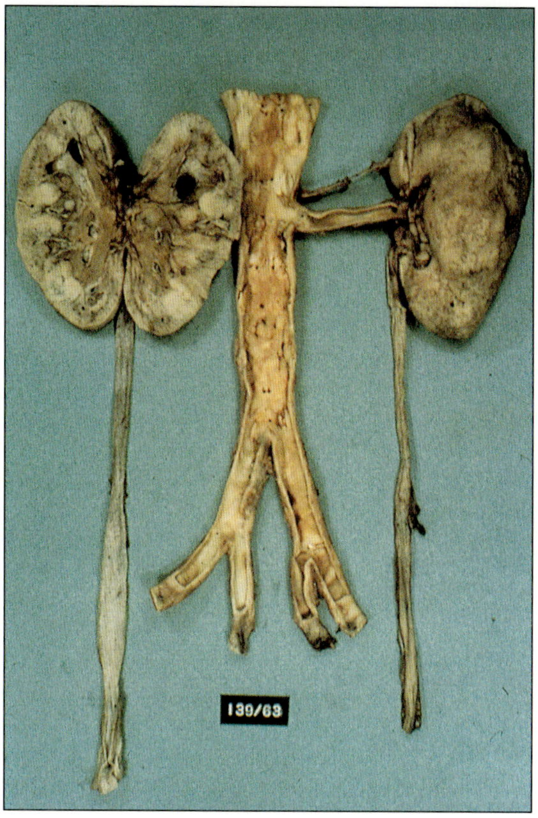

Fig. 5.18 Kidneys from a patient with analgesic nephropathy. Courtesy of Professor P. Kincaid-Smith.

Pyelonephritis

Reflux pyelonephritis, where associated with infection acquired in childhood, often shows no obvious symptoms. It leads first to scarring, either on one kidney or on both, and subsequently to hypertension, which can be relieved by unilateral nephrectomy (Figs 5.16 & 5.17). Interestingly, obstruction to the urinary tract with hydronephrosis is not usually associated with hypertension, and it may be that it is the cortical scarring associated with pyelonephritis which is important in its initiation.

Analgesic Nephropathy

Analgesic abuse, with or without infection, leads to considerable scarring of the kidney as well as papillary loss, tubular damage and sometimes hypertension (Figs 5.18 & 5.19). As in pyelonephritis, the branches of the renal artery going through the medulla are often affected and show intimal thickening and fibrosis, so the basis here may also be ischaemic.

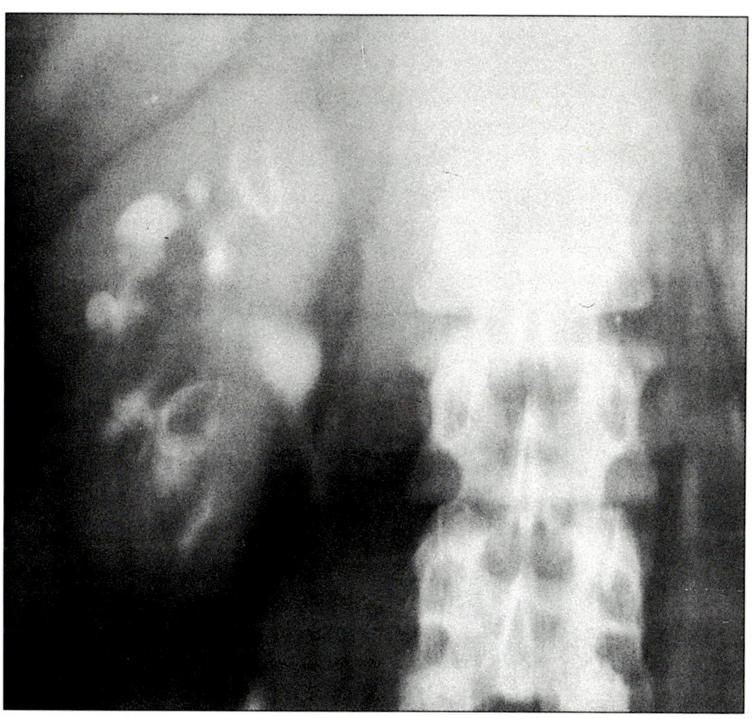

Fig. 5.19 Pyelogram in analgesic nephropathy. The calyces are distorted and necrotic papillae cause characteristic 'ring' shadows.

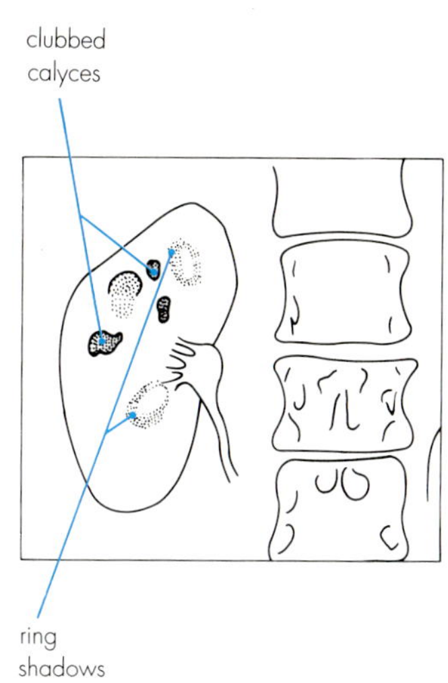

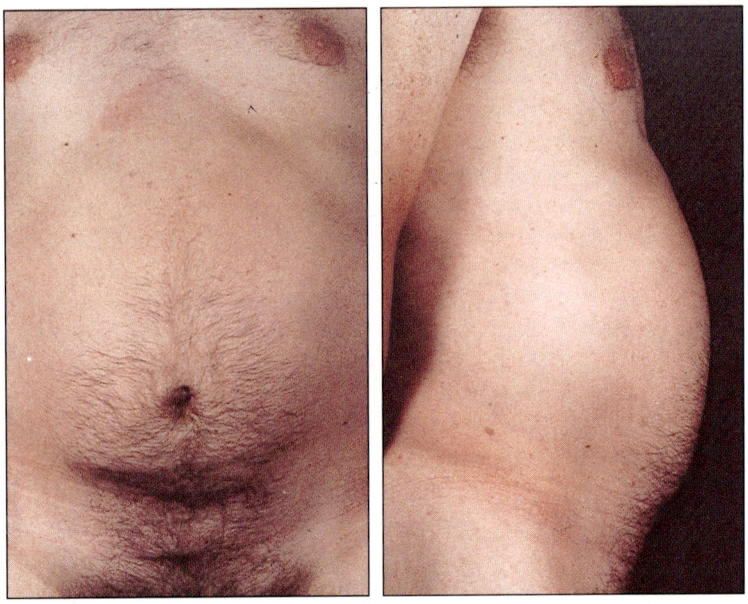

Fig. 5.20 Abdominal masses caused by polycystic kidneys.

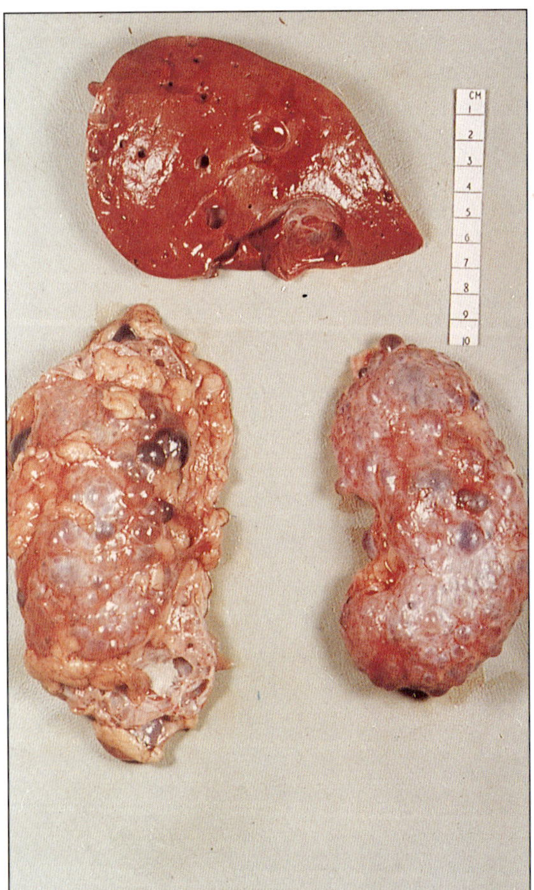

Fig. 5.21 Enormous polycystic kidneys. Haemorrhage has occurred into some of the cysts. Cysts also involve the liver. Courtesy of Dr P. N. Cardew.

Polycystic Disease

This may initially appear predominantly in only one kidney. It is inherited as a dominant genetic fault and usually causes mild to moderate hypertension, which may appear quite early in the course of the cystic development. (Figs 5.20, 5.21, 5.22 & 5.23). Although ischaemia due to local pressure is possible, puncturing the major cysts has not proved to be effective in halting the progression of the disease.

Glomerulonephritis

In most cases this disease has an immunological basis. In former times, pathogenesis involved the haemolytic streptococcus; in developed countries this factor seems to have been superseded by conditions like Berger's disease, where IgA deposits occur in the glomerular basement membrane (Fig. 5.24). Some hereditary conditions such as Alport's syndrome, associated with deafness and occasionally retinal disease, also cause glomerulonephritis. The clinical classsification (acute, subacute and chronic) is helpful in the context of hypertension, as it draws attention to the different haemodynamic states that are encountered. In the more severe cases of acute nephritis, where the glomeruli are swollen and filtration is markedly reduced, oliguria or even anuria can develop. This is characteristically associated with generalized

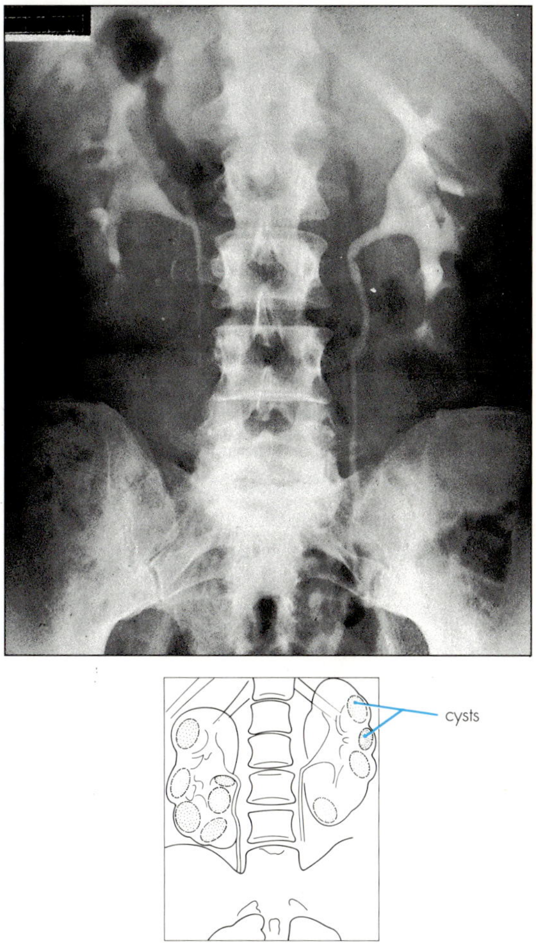

Fig. 5.22 Pyelogram of a patient with polycystic kidneys. The kidneys are enlarged and the calyces drawn out around large cysts.

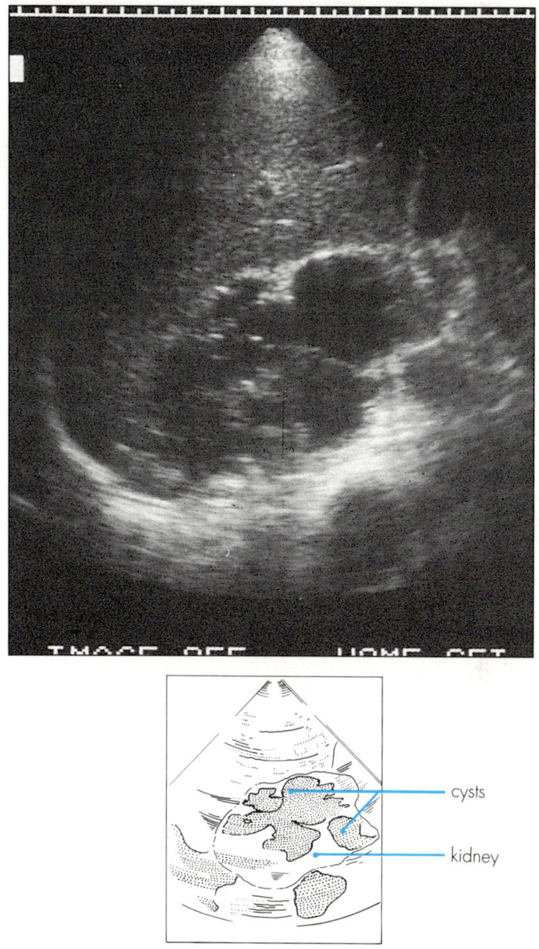

Fig. 5.23 Ultrasound scan of the abdomen showing trans-sonic renal cysts as black spaces in a patient with polycystic renal disease.

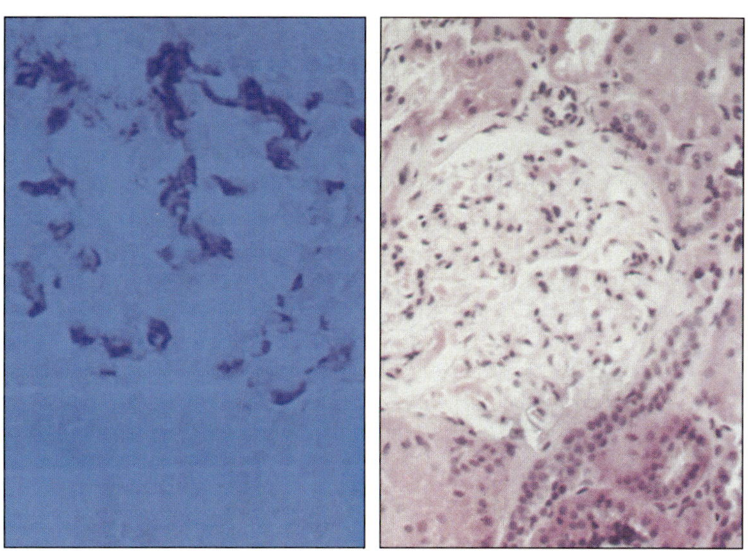

Fig. 5.24 Renal biopsy of a patient with Berger's nephritis. Left: Normal appearance of glomerulus. Haematoxylin and eosin stain. Right: Deposits of IgA in the same glomerulus. Immunoperoxidase stain.

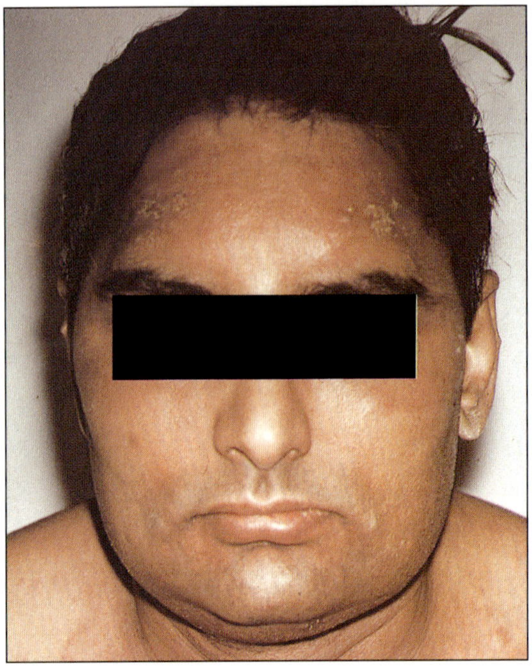

Fig. 5.25 Acute facial oedema in a patient who developed acute glomerulonephritic syndrome following penicillin. In acute glomerulonephritis, oedema is characteristically periorbital, while in chronic renal failure it is characteristically dependent.

oedema particularly noted in the face, hands and feet, and it is highly likely that the capillaries are leakier than usual (Fig. 5.25). Since fluid intake is usually maintained there is the added factor of a positive water and electrolyte balance, which adds to the oedema. At this stage the blood pressure may rise to quite high levels, and may lead to pulmonary oedema with severe dyspnoea, or cerebral oedema with fits. In the acute phase the plasma volume may be high, with a high cardiac output contributing to the hypertension; peripheral resistance is not usually elevated. The plasma renin is not raised in most cases. Following the diuresis which signals recovery, the blood pressure falls to normal. However, if the glomerular lesions do not heal completely and a subacute or chronic course occurs, with crescent formation in Bowman's capsule and (finally) glomerular obliteration, the blood pressure may not subside and may even rise further, together with a rise in plasma renin activity (Fig. 5.26). There is sometimes a long period of apparent quiescence before pressure begins to rise, signalling the chronic phase with contracted kidneys and impaired function.

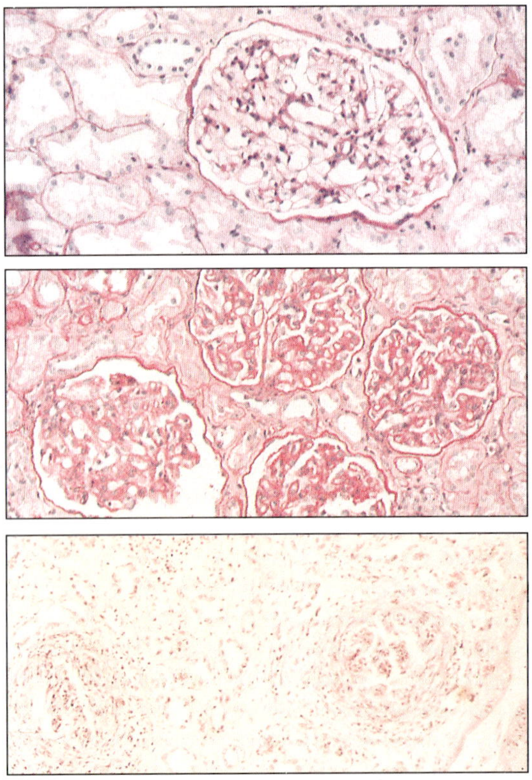

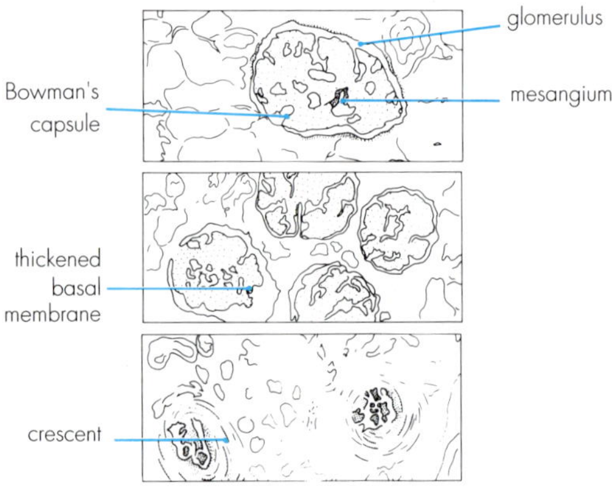

Fig. 5.26 A range of pathological appearances is seen in glomerulonephritis. Top: In minimal change glomerulonephritis associated with nephrotic syndrome, hypertension is rare. Middle: It is more common in the more severe types of glomerular change encountered in membranous glomerulonephritis. Bottom: It is very common in proliferative glomerulonephritis. Courtesy of Prof. K. Porter and Prof. J. R. Tighe.

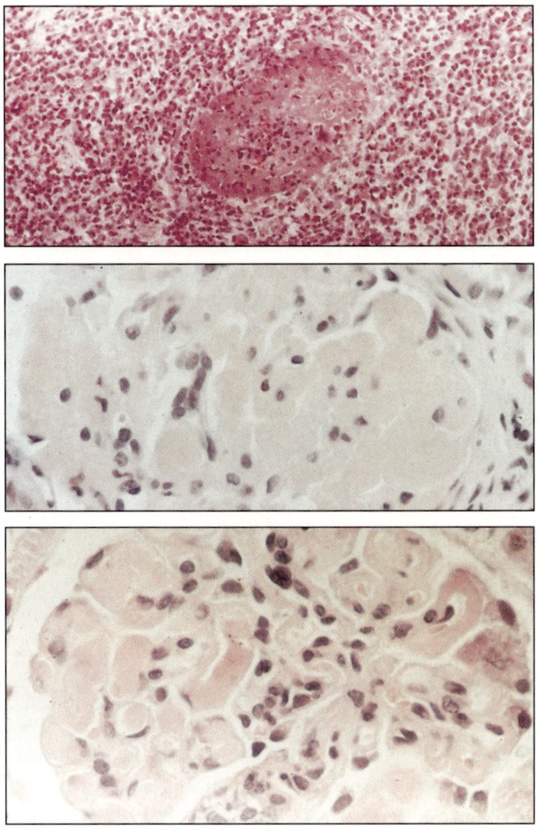

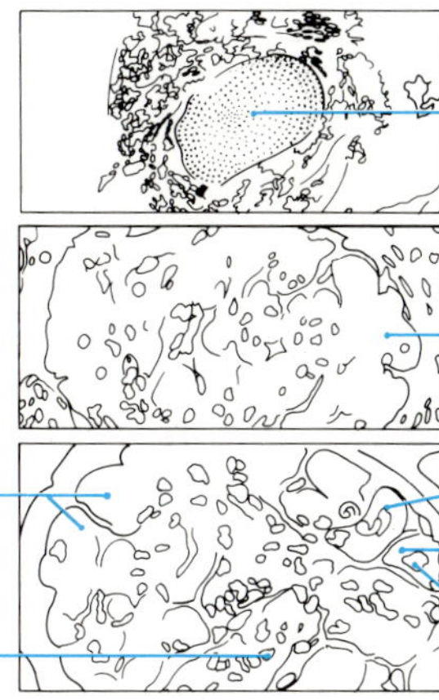

Fig. 5.27 Top: Renal biopsy from a patient with hypertension due to polyarteritis nodosa. The vessels show cellular infiltration and fibrinoid necrosis with extensive infiltration of the interstitial tissues. Middle: Scleroderma with widespread fibrinoid necrosis. Bottom: Disseminated lupus erythematosus showing a focal glomerulonephritis with extensive focal thickening of the glomerular capillary walls ('wire loop' lesion). Courtesy of Prof. K. Porter and Prof. J. R. Tighe.

Other Diseases

Glomerular lesions and hypertension are often encountered in polyarteritis and scleroderma. Disseminated lupus is more frequently associated with the nephrotic syndrome (Fig. 5.27). Scleroderma is sometimes associated with exceptionally rapid and severe hypertension. Another curious feature observed in scleroderma is that fibrinoid necrosis, the characteristic arteriolar vascular change of malignant hypertension, may appear in the afferent glomerular arteriole before hypertension develops.

In diabetes, hypertension may be related either to atheromatous vascular obstruction in the renal arteries or to glomerular lesions, as are seen in the Kimmelstiel-Wilson syndrome (Fig. 5.28). Renal involvement can be shown at an early stage by the presence of small but excessive albuminuria (microalbuminuria).

Other infiltrating diseases of the glomerulus such as amyloidosis seem to produce heavy proteinuria without hypertension until the final stages of renal failure occur.

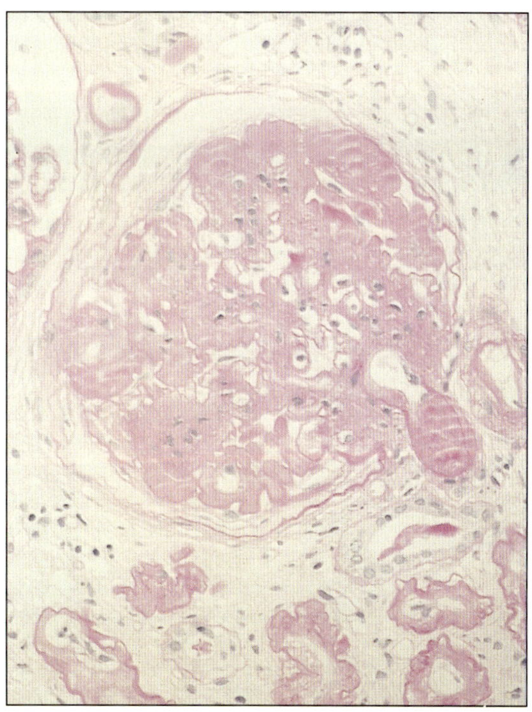

Fig. 5.28 Kimmelstiel–Wilson Syndrome. Courtesy of Dr T. Book.

NERVOUS SYSTEM

This always plays a major role in the control of cardiac output, peripheral resistance and capacitance vessels.

In most types of hypertension this influence may be regarded as permissive (without evidence of hyperactivity) but in some cases a primary role has been suggested. For example, paroxysms of hypertension likened to 'hypothalamic epilepsy' are claimed to emanate from this important centre of sympathetic nervous control; certainly in bulbar poliomyelitis hypertension is seen. Whether this is a mixed response to respiratory depression and anoxia as well as stimulation of sympathetic pathways is not known. The rise of pressure seen with intracranial haemorrhage or head injury may be a consequence of hind brain compression, and therefore again of mixed cause.

The rise of pressure seen in patients with acute pulmonary oedema and anoxia may also depend on afferent signals from the lungs, subsiding when the oedema is relieved. The importance of inhibitory pathways is perhaps best revealed in patients with complete transection of the spinal cord at a level between C3 and C5. The afferent stimuli caused by a full bladder or by tapping the suprapubic region results in a considerable rise of blood pressure which only subsides when the bladder is empty or the stimulus is stopped. The inhibition's precise origin and pathway are unknown, but there is good evidence that spinal sympathetic reflexes are involved in the pressor response (Fig. 5.29).

It has long been accepted that the sympathetic system plays a dominant role in anxiety, fear and rage reactions. However, its role in the development of prolonged hypertension remains uncertain. It is embodied in the concept of labile blood pressure leading to labile hypertension, and then on to more fixed hypertension. Nevertheless, there is evidence that sympathetic innervation is necessary for vascular hypertrophy to occur – sympathetic denervation of one territory in the development of experimental hypertension prevents the vascular hypertrophy normally seen. This implies that vascular hypertrophy and increased vascular resistance could be due to sympathetic overactivity.

The ability of drugs affecting the sympathetic nervous system to control high blood pressure does not necessarily point to overactivity, since removal of a major controlling factor in the circulation could effectively lower the pressure, leaving the original causal factor still operative. The case for a major role for the sympathetic pathways in the development of hypertension must therefore be regarded as unproven, albeit suspicious.

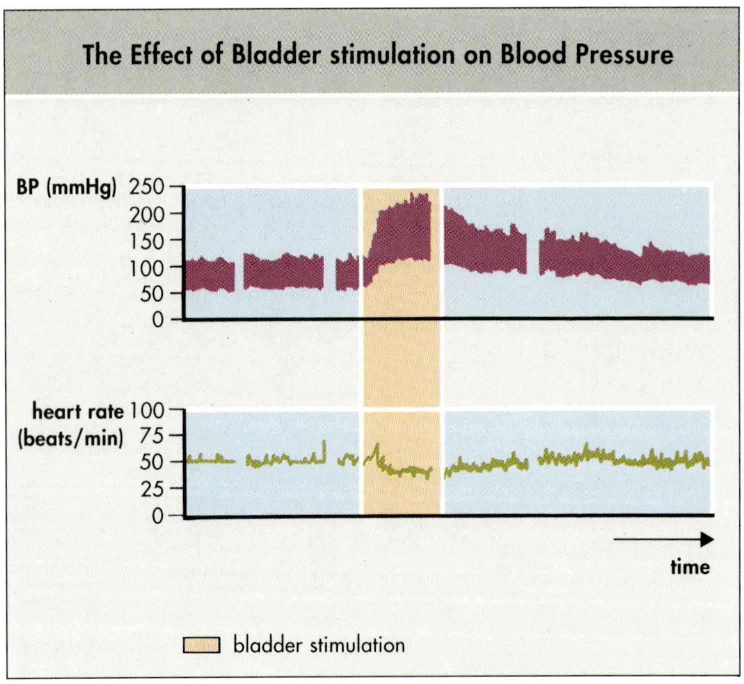

Fig. 5.29 The effect of bladder stimulation (by suprapubic tapping of the anterior bladder wall) on blood pressure and heart rate in a chronic tetraplegic. There is a rapid rise in blood pressure. Heart rate may rise initially, presumably as a result of sympathetic stimulation. Blood pressure gradually falls to basal levels after the stimulus has been withdrawn. The breaks in the record indicate where blood has been withdrawn. Courtesy of Dr J. Kooner.

Hypertension and the Endocrine System	
site	**disorder**
pituitary	acromegaly, Cushing's syndrome
thyroid	myxoedema, hyperthyroidism
adrenal cortex	adenoma, multinodular hyperplasia, Cushing's syndrome
adrenal medulla	phaeochromocytoma
parathyroid	hyperparathyroidism
kidney	renal tumours e.g. haemangiopericytoma
gonads	inborn errors of metabolism abnormalities of sexual steroid production

Fig. 5.30 Hypertension and the endocrine system.

THE ENDOCRINE SYSTEM

Endocrine disease can have a considerable effect on blood pressure (Fig. 5.30) and diseases of the adrenal gland (Fig. 5.31) are particularly important.

Structurally and biochemically the adrenal gland has two major components, the cortex (consisting of the zonae glomerulosa, fasciculata and reticularis) and the medulla.

The adrenal cortex can induce hypertension through excessive secretion of corticosteroid hormones – hyperactivity or tumours of the zona glomerulosa may result in excessive production of aldosterone and the zonae fasciculata and reticularis may give rise to excessive glucocorticoid production. The most common mineralocorticoid hormones, such as deoxycorticosterone and 18-hydroxydeoxycorticosterone, may occasionally be implicated. Excess quantities of these mineralocorticoids can be secreted either in isolation or as part of the adrenal cortical hyperactivity observed in Cushing's syndrome; in this case the steroid pattern responsible for hypertension is still uncertain. Severe hypertension is uncommon in Cushing's syndrome even though the clinical and more obvious biochemical features do not distinguish those with or without it.

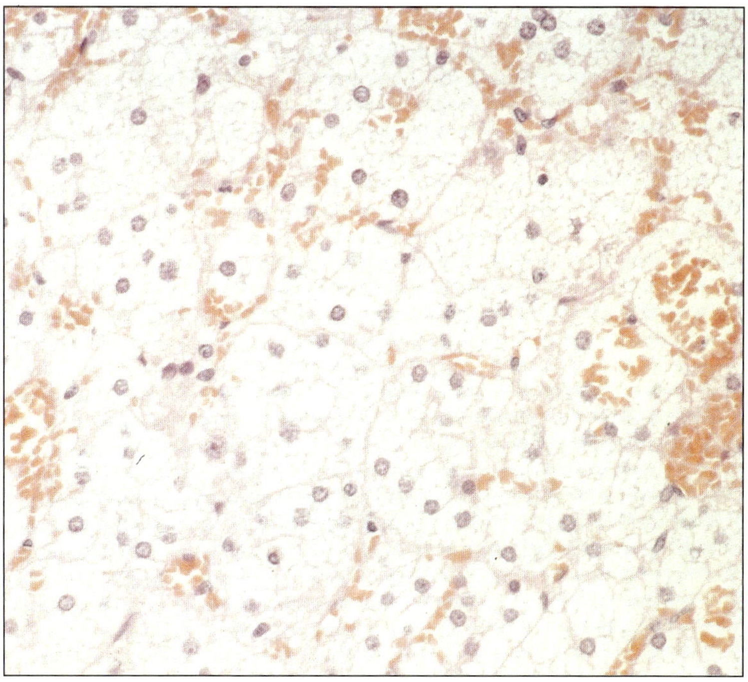

Fig. 5.31 Clear cells in an adrenal adenoma from a case of Conn's syndrome.

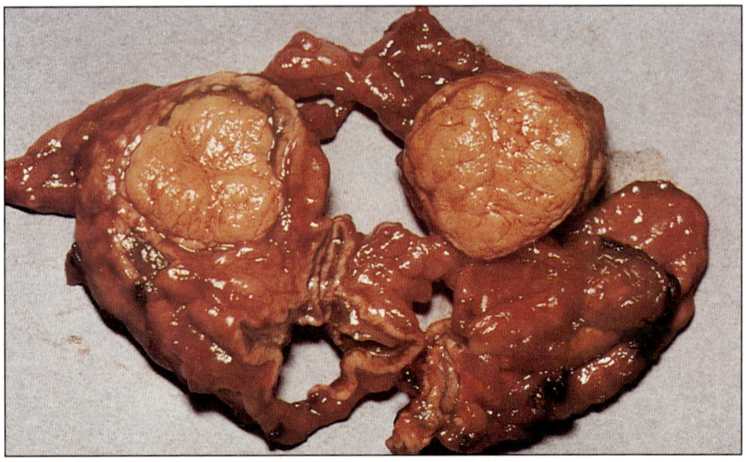

Fig. 5.32 An adrenal adenoma causing primary aldosteronism (Conn's syndrome). This was removed from a hypertensive patient with hypokalaemia. Courtesy of Dr P. N. Cardew.

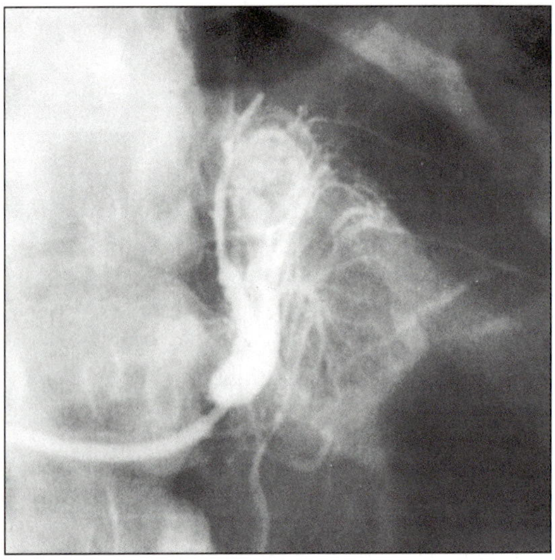

Fig. 5.33 Adrenal phlebogram showing an adrenal adenoma as a discrete vascular mass.

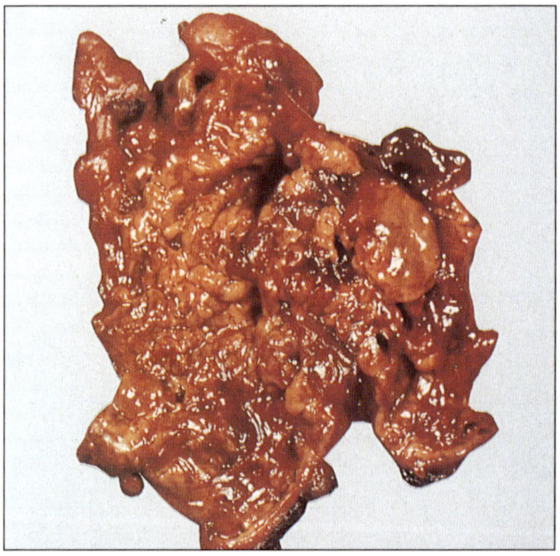

Fig. 5.34 Hyperplastic adrenal gland from a patient with primary aldosteronism. Multiple small nodules are seen in an enlarged gland (multinodular hyperplasia). Courtesy of Dr P. N. Cardew.

Primary Aldosteronism

There are two common forms of primary aldosteronism: adrenal adenoma (see Figs 5.31, 5.32 & 5.33) and multinodular hyperplasia (Fig. 5.34). The stimulus which causes the (slightly less common) hyperplasia is unknown, but the end result in both cases is similar, in that hypertension is associated with hypokalaemic alkalosis. The clinical and biochemical manifestations of aldosterone-secreting adenomata are, as a rule, more pronounced than the manifestations of multinodular hyperplasia. An adenoma and bilateral hyperplasia can often, but unfortunately not always, be differentiated by an adrenal scan using radiolabelled cholesterol (cholesterol is the substrate utilized in the production of adrenal steroids). The isotope is concentrated in the adrenal glands and detected by external scanning. Adenomata are seen as areas of increased activity on only one side, while bilateral increased activity can be seen in patients with multinodular hyperplasia (Figs 5.35 & 5.36).

Congenital Hyperplasia

Congenital adrenal hyperplasia is due to an inborn error of steroid metabolism and is a rare form of mineralocorticoid hypertension. Two enzyme defects may cause hypertension (Fig. 5.37).

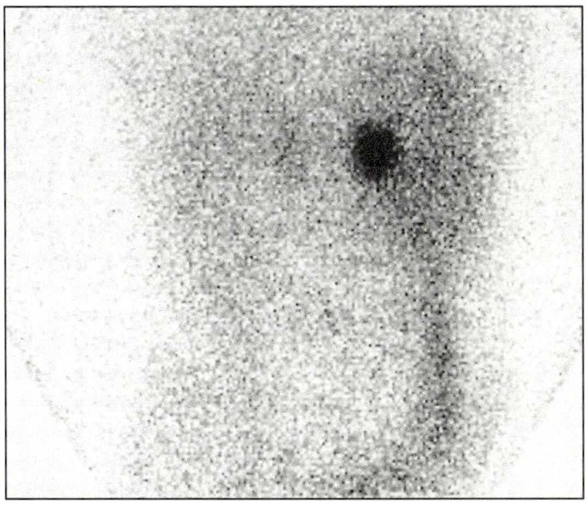

Fig. 5.35 Adrenal adenoma in Conn's syndrome. The tumour on the left is shown by a ^{75}Se-methionine scan. The patient presented with hypertension and low plasma potassium and renin. Removal of the tumour led to correction of both biochemical findings and blood pressure.

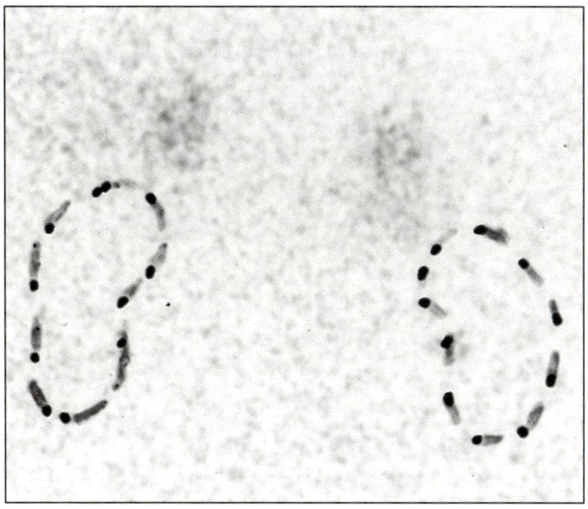

Fig. 5.36 Bilateral adrenal hyperplasia demonstrated by ^{75}Se–methionine uptake. The renal outlines are drawn in by hand from a separate renal scan using ^{99}Tc-DTPA. The patient presented with hypertension, low plasma potassium and low plasma renin.

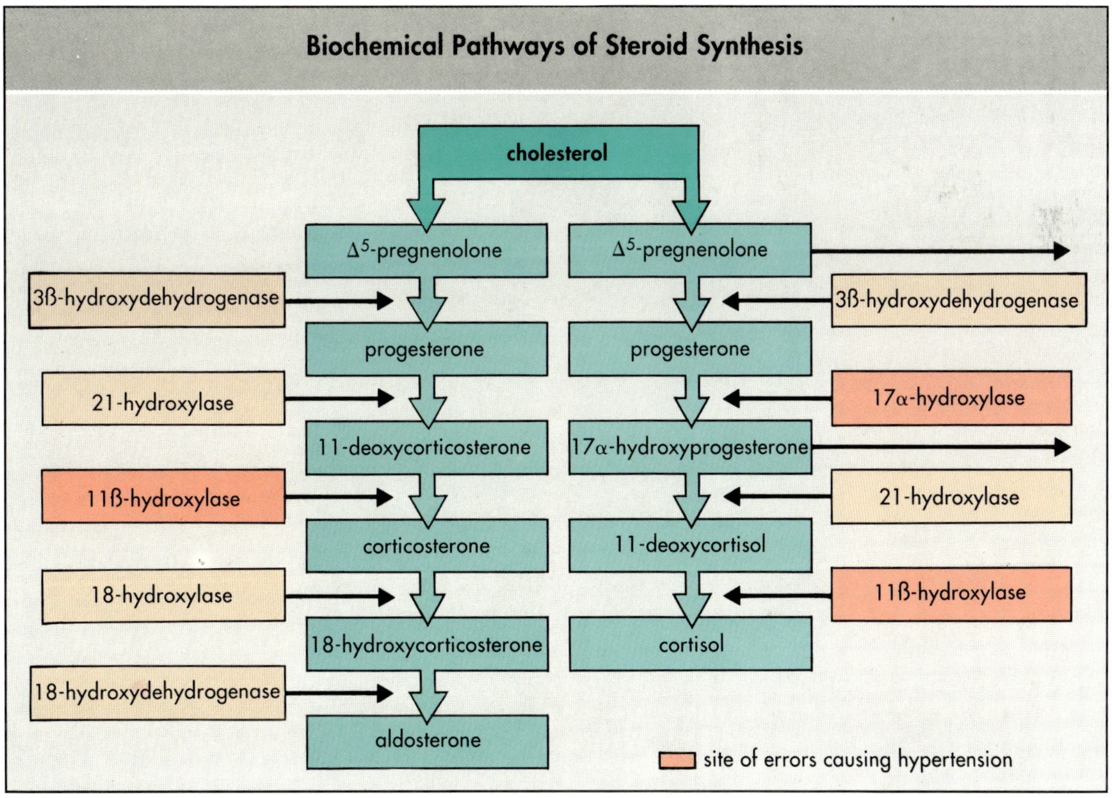

Fig. 5.37 Biochemical pathways of steroid synthesis. Enzyme deficiencies result in accumulation of precursors with mineralocorticoid activity. Inhibition of cortisol synthesis prevents feedback inhibition of ACTH secretion. Pathways leading to synthesis of sex steroids (arrows to right) are preserved, unless there is a separate block in these pathways.

- A defect in 11-hydroxylation causes a decrease in cortisol production. This results in stimulation of ACTH secretion with accumulation of the mineralocorticoid hormones 11-deoxycorticosterone and 11-deoxycortisol. Increased androgen synthesis gives rise to virilization or female pseudohermaphroditism (Fig. 5.38).
- The much rarer defect in 17-hydroxylation is also associated with high ACTH levels and hypersecretion of mineralocorticoid precursors. In this case, however, there is also a block of gonadal synthesis of oestrogens and androgens and the patients fail to develop secondary sexual characteristics. In addition, there is primary amenorrhoea.

The mechanism by which glucocorticoid hormones produce hypertension is uncertain. While glucocorticoids enhance synthesis of renin substrate, hypertension in Cushing's syndrome is not usually associated with hyperactivity of the renin–angiotensin system (Fig. 5.39). ACTH readily produces hypertension in sheep, but even here it is not clear precisely which hormonal response is causative.

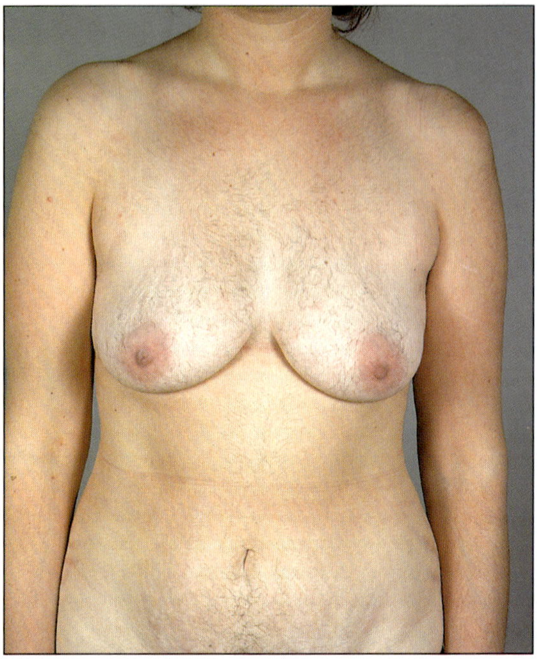

Fig. 5.38 Hirsute female. High ACTH levels in some patients with inborn errors of steroid metabolism may result in excessive production of sexual steroid. A more likely cause of hirsutism in a hypertensive patient is treatment with potent vasodilators (diazoxide or minoxidil). Courtesy of Dr P. N. Cardew.

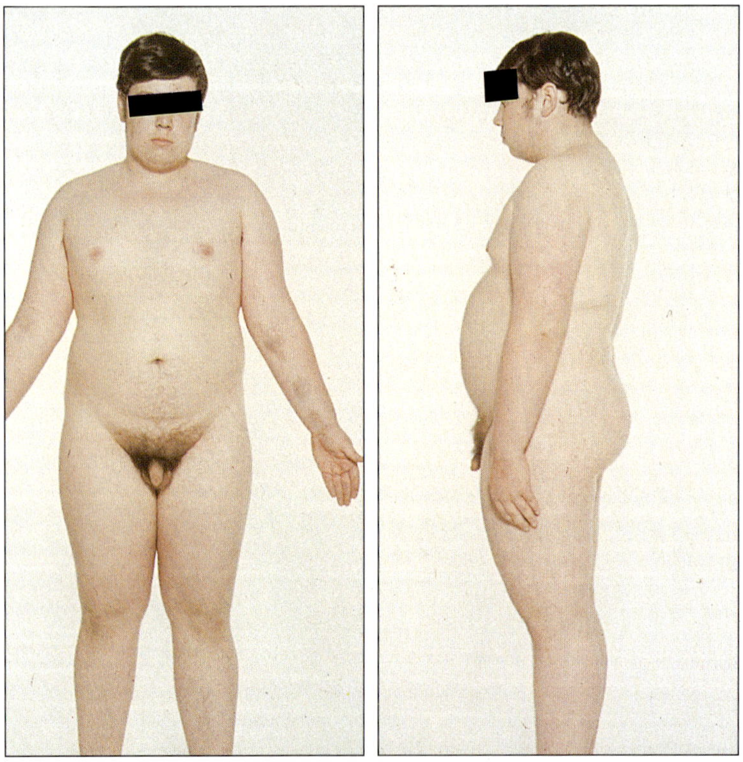

Fig. 5.39 A man with hypertension associated with Cushing's syndrome. Obesity is largely truncal in types with a 'buffalo' hump. The face is rounded and the patient bruised readily.

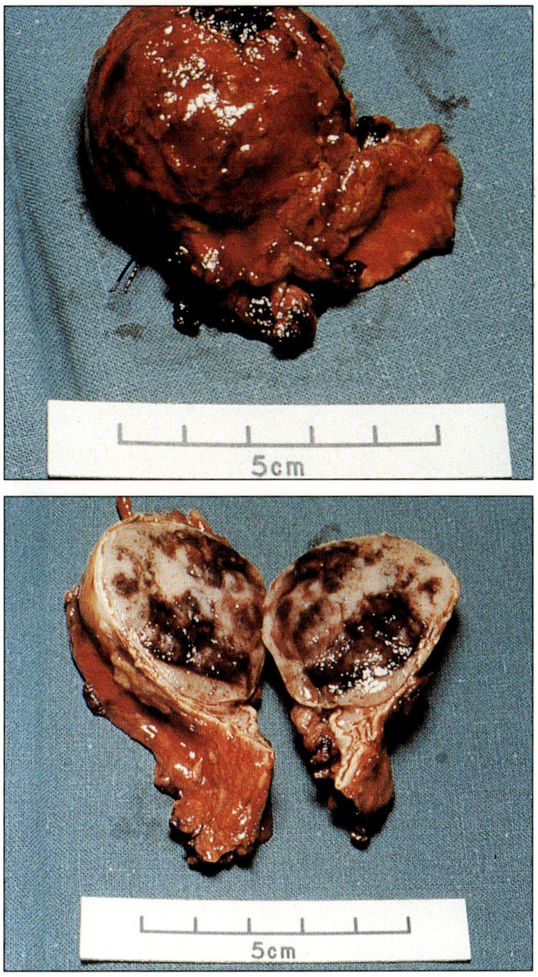

Fig. 5.40 Large haemorrhagic phaeochromocytoma removed from a hypertensive patient at operation.

Phaeochromocytoma

Hypertension in phaeochromocytoma (Fig. 5.40) is the result of hypersecretion of catecholamines (Fig. 5.41). These tumours synthesize either predominantly norepinephrine, or both epinephrine and norepinephrine, depending upon the activities of the biosynthetic enzymes present in the tumour tissue. The majority of tumours are situated in the adrenal medulla (Fig. 5.42). Occasionally, however,

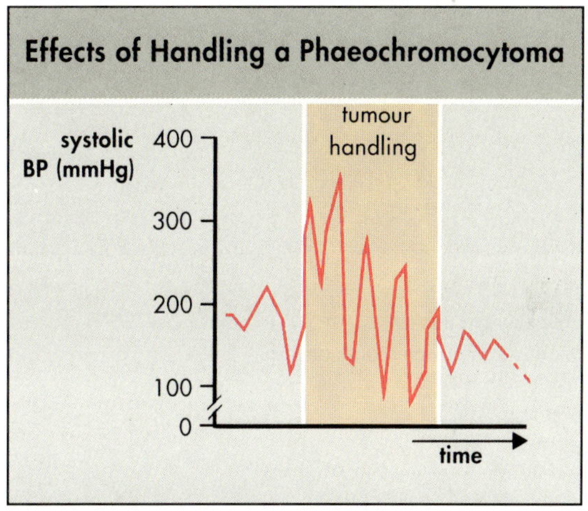

Fig. 5.41 Blood pressure changes occurring during tumour handling at operation on a patient with phaeochromocytoma who has received inadequate α- and β_1-receptor blockade. Wild fluctuations in blood pressure were only eliminated when the adrenal blood supply was occluded.

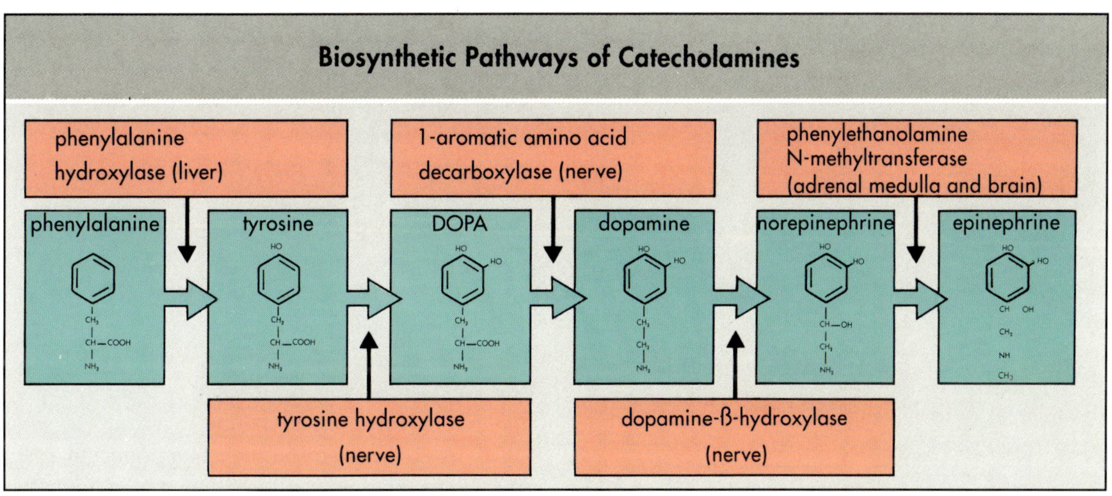

Fig. 5.42 Biosynthetic pathways of catecholamines by the adrenal gland. Tumours may synthesize both norepinephrine and epinephrine although norepinephrine is usually released in larger quantities. Rarely, DOPA or dopamine may be released.

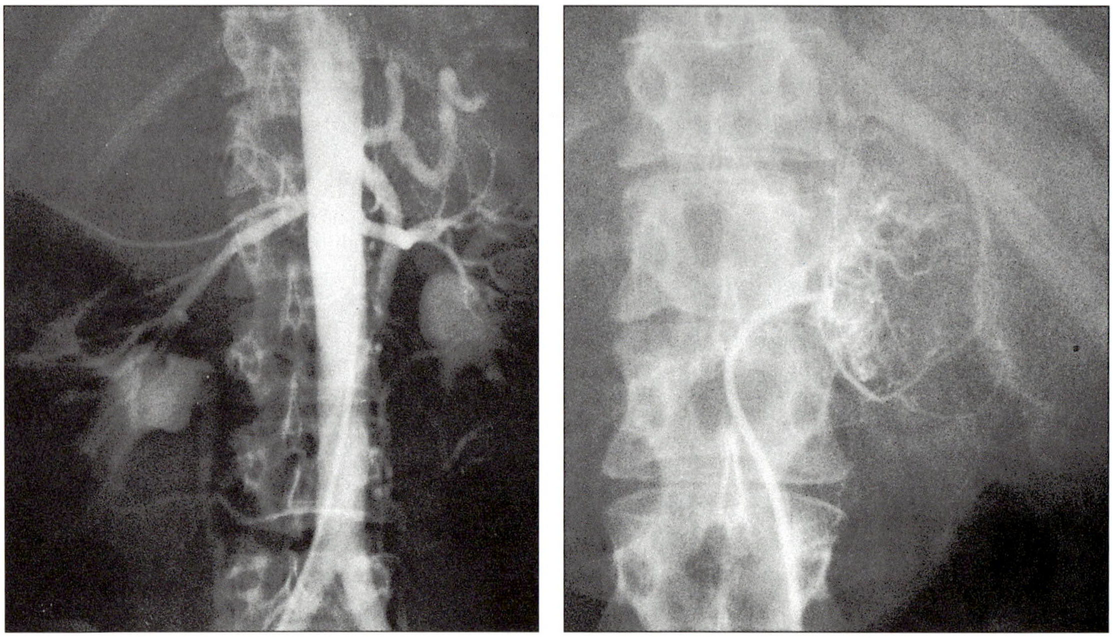

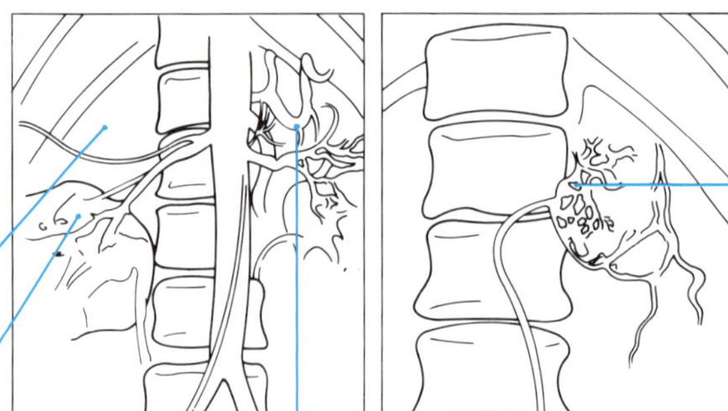

Fig. 5.43 Arteriography in a patient with bilateral phaeochromocytomata. A discrete lesion with a tumour circulation is best seen with selective arteriography.

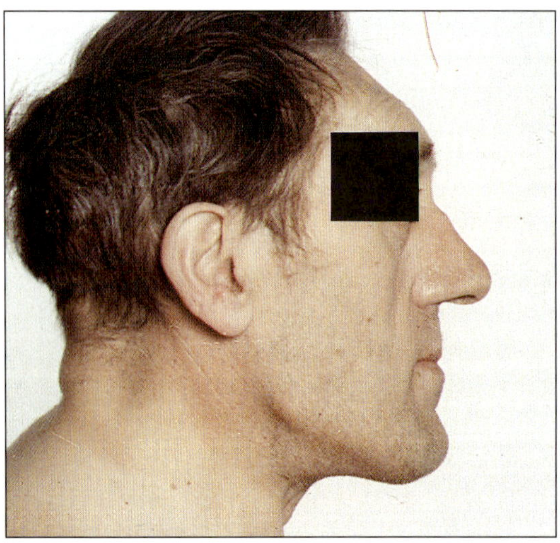

Fig. 5.44 Acromegaly – typical lantern jaw, large nose and prominent supraorbital ridges. Such patients sometimes present with hypertension. Courtesy of Dr P. N. Cardew.

phaeochromocytomata occur in the thorax, the urinary bladder, the organ of Zuckerkandl, the liver hilum, and other intra-abdominal sites (Fig. 5.43). Most of these tumours secrete norepinephrine almost entirely; the predominant secretion of epinephrine suggests an adrenal rather than an extra-adrenal site. The important clinical characteristic of a phaeochromocytoma is paroxysmal hypertension (40–50% of patients) which is associated with other evidence of catacholamine over-activity. Although the majority of patients (90%) are hypertensive at all times, the blood pressure profiles may be variable or truly paroxysmal, with blood pressure falling to normal or even lower levels between attacks. Hypertension may be precipitated by abdominal palpation, by unusual or stressful situations and by micturition, defecation or parturition. When the tumour is

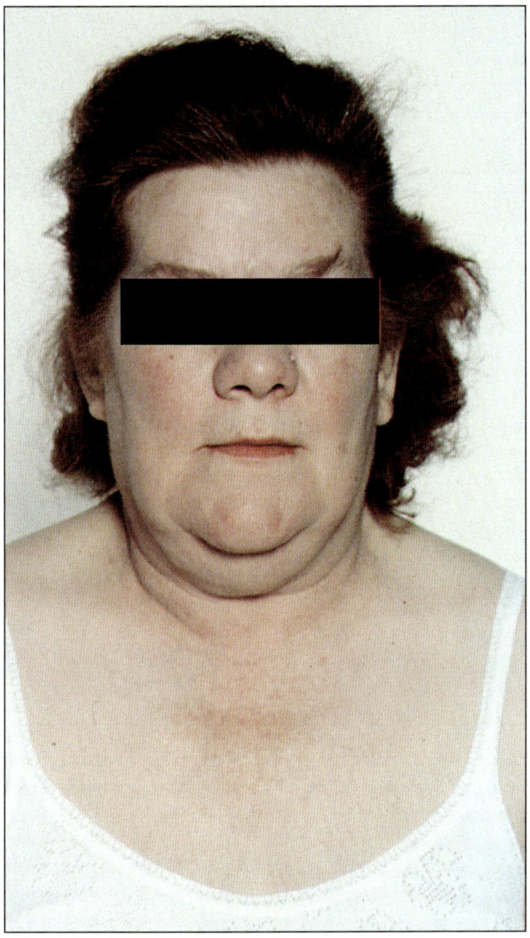

Fig. 5.45 Myxoedema and hypertension. The face is puffy and the skin characteristically coarse. There is a suggestion of malar flush. Courtesy of Dr P. N. Cardew.

being manipulated before surgical removal, very severe hypertension may occur if the patient has not previously received adequate α- and ß-adrenoreceptor blocking agents (see Fig. 5.41).

Acromegaly

Hypertension is seen in about one-third of patients who have acromegaly (Fig. 5.44) and this is sometimes (but not always) reversed by surgical or bromocriptine treatment. Mild hypertension is frequently seen in myxoedema (Fig. 5.45) and may be associated with increased plasma noradrenaline levels. Treatment with thyroxin often results in a lowering of blood pressure. Labile blood pressure with definite hypertensive episodes occurs in hyperthyroidism. Hyperparathyroidism is also associated with high blood pressure.

COARCTATION

Uncomplicated coarctation often presents as mild hypertension in childhood or early adulthood (Fig. 5.46). It is often asymptomatic and only picked up on routine screening (Fig. 5.47). The initial elevation of blood pressure is caused by the resistance to flow offered by the coarctation, which is usually a short localized obstruction just below the origin of the left subclavian artery. Hypertension can become self-perpetuating with advancing years and may persist in patients who are operated upon in adulthood. This is possibly due to vascular changes in the vessels of the upper part of the body, including perhaps the collateral vessels. In addition, the operation carries a high mortality rate in adults. For this reason, it is preferable to operate in early childhood even when there are no clinical symptoms.

Coarctation

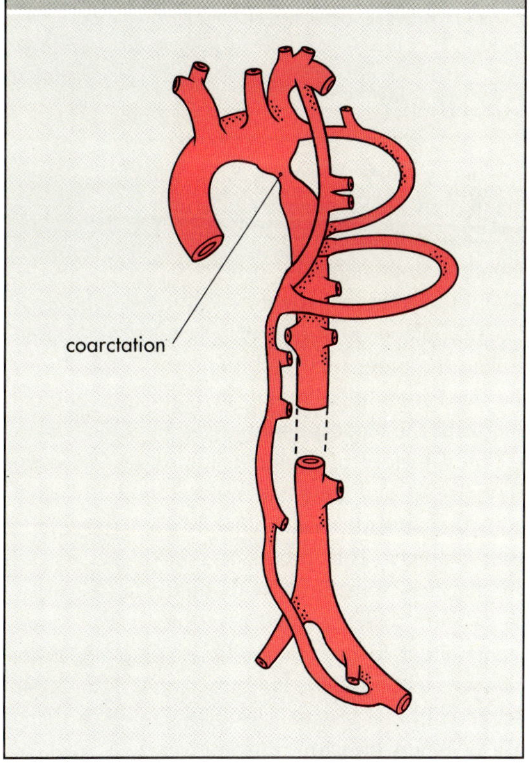

Fig. 5.46 Uncomplicated coarctation is a narrowing of the aorta distal to the origin of the left subclavian artery. Prominent collateral vessels bypass the obstruction.

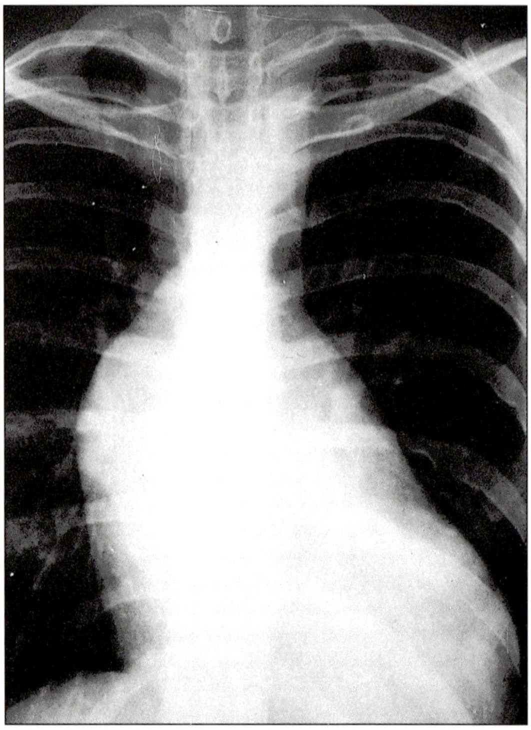

Fig. 5.47 Coarctation presenting as hypertension in a young woman. The ascending aorta is dilated and the collateral vessels produce 'notching' of the undersurface of the ribs.

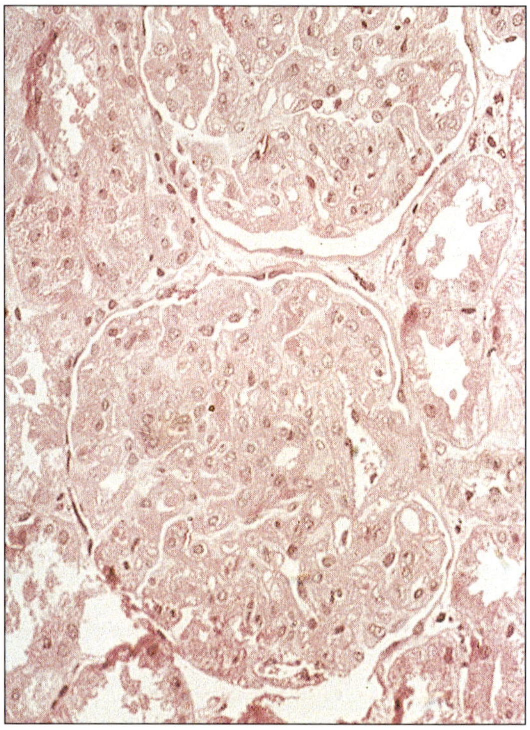

Fig. 5.48 Renal histology in pre-eclamptic toxaemia. The glomeruli are enlarged and the capillary lumina reduced by cytoplasmic swelling of the endothelial cells.

PREGNANCY

Pregnancy may be associated with significant changes in blood pressure (see chapter 6 & Fig. 6.17). In normal pregnancy the blood pressure usually drops slightly from the third to the seventh month. In patients with underlying renal disease, blood pressure may rise at any time during the pregnancy and often does so at about the third month. Following delivery or intrauterine death the blood pressure falls. In women with a family history of hypertension, blood pressure may rise at any time but more commonly rises from the seventh month onwards and then falls after delivery. This process recurs in successive pregnancies, sometimes with increasing severity. In patients with essential hypertension, pressure seems either to rise markedly early in the pregnancy or, occasionally, fall only to rise again after delivery. In first pregnancies there may be a sharp rise of blood pressure after the thirtieth week of gestation together with proteinuria and oedema (pre-eclamptic toxaemia). This does not necessarily indicate an underlying cause or a familial trait.

Pathologically, the characteristic lesion in pre-eclamptic toxaemia is cytoplasmic swelling of the glomerular endothelial cells (Fig. 5.48). However, this lesion is by no means specific and can be reproduced by low grade intravascular coagulation. Physiologically, the woman with pre-eclamptic toxaemia has evidence of fluid retention greater than would be expected in a normal pregnancy. Plasma levels of renin, angiotensin II, and aldosterone are usually lower than in normal pregnancy; this may reflect the effects of sodium and water retention. The pathogenesis of both the renal lesion and the hypertension are unknown. Fluid retention may be partly responsible for the elevated blood pressure, but there is also evidence to suggest that the blood vessels of the pre-eclamptic patient are unduly sensitive to the vasoconstrictor action of angiotensin II.

The pathogenesis of hypertension during pregnancy remains one of the great unsolved mysteries in the field, although in eclampsia a major clue lies in the fact that intrauterine death leads to reduction of the hypertension.

DRUGS AND INGESTED COMPOUNDS

The Contraceptive Pill

There is uncertainty about the mechanism by which the contraceptive pill raises blood pressure. A minor rise in blood pressure is seen in most women receiving oestrogen-containing contraceptive pills (Fig. 5.49). In some cases a very marked rise in blood pressure can occur with the development of accelerated hypertension (Fig. 5.50) and, in some of these, underlying renal disease such as glomerulonephritis is revealed. Cessation of the drugs leads to a fall of pressure. There is less evidence concerning the progestagen-only contraceptive pill, but recent studies suggest that this may cause a lesser degree of hypertension.

Oestrogens cause an increased synthesis of renin substrate by the liver and this results in the generation of increased quantities of angiotensin II *in vivo*. There is, however, no correlation between increased activity of the renin–angiotensin system and hypertension caused by the contraceptive pill; nor can hypertension be related to sodium- or water-retention; overall the mechanism remains obscure. There is evidence pointing to a family history of hypertension in the women with the largest response to the contraceptive pill (oestrogen and progestogen).

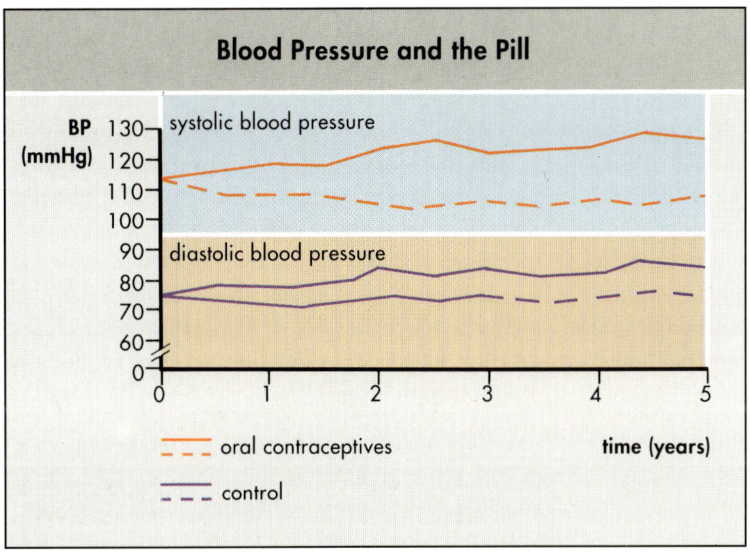

Fig. 5.49 Blood pressure changes in a group of women receiving the oestrogen-containing contraceptive pill. Both systolic and diastolic blood pressure rose gradually over the five years of treatment.

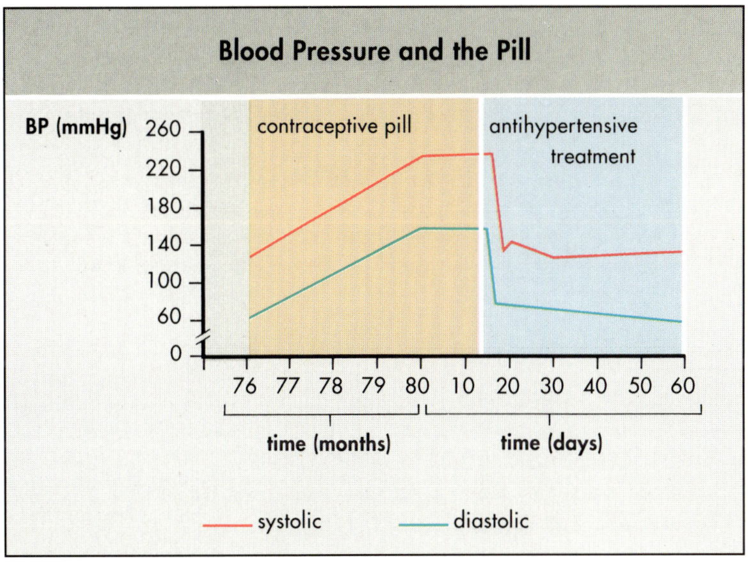

Fig. 5.50 Blood pressure in a woman who developed malignant hypertension during four years on the contraceptive pill. Emergency antihypertensive treatment was required as well as withdrawal of the pill. After two months it was possible to stop the antihypertensive treatment and blood pressure remained normal. Underlying renal disease should always be suspected and sought.

Other Drugs

In addition to the contraceptive pill and corticosteroids, several other drugs cause hypertension. These can be classified according to the different changes associated with raised blood pressure.

Expansion of Extracellular Fluid and Sodium Space

- Sodium-containing compounds (particularly in renal failure).
- Sodium-retaining drugs:
  carbenoxolone;
  glycyrrhyzinic acid;
  mineralocorticoids and anabolic steroids;
  NSAIDs (non-steroidal anti-inflammatory drugs).

Carbenoxolone and glycyrrhizinic acid (the active principle of liquorice) are structurally similar to aldosterone and have a similar effect upon distal tubular sodium reabsorption (Fig. 5.51). Clinically, therefore, they may give rise to a picture resembling primary aldosteronism with hypokalaemic alkalosis and hypertension. Sodium retention and blood pressure elevation can also be produced by NSAIDs (such as indomethacin) and by sodium-containing compounds (such as some indigestion mixtures and sodium-phase resins) when administered to patients with advanced renal failure.

Drug Actions and Interactions Mimicking Sympathetic Nervous System Overactivity

- Direct and indirect sympathomimetic drugs.
- Monoamine oxidase inhibitors and tyramine-containing foods.
- Clonidine withdrawal reaction.
- Ketamine hydrochloride.
- ß-adrenergic receptor blockers used alone in some patients with phaeochromocytoma.
- Intravenous post-ganglionic adrenergic neurone blocking drugs – first dose effect (for example guanethidine) – rarely used now.

Severe paroxysmal hypertension can be produced by the combination of monoamine oxidase inhibitors (such as phenelzine and tranylcypromine) and tyramine-containing foods such as mature cheese. Amphetamine and monoamine oxidase inhibitors will have the same effect. Both tyramine and amphetamine cause the release of stored norepinephrine from sympathetic nerve terminals. The effect of this process is enhanced when the normal degradative enzyme, monoamine oxidase, is inhibited. The abrupt withdrawal of clonidine is also associated with severe paroxysmal hypertension and evidence of excessive sympathetic nervous activity (Fig. 5.52). This appears to be related to the withdrawal of the central effects of clonidine upon sympathetic outflow from the brain.

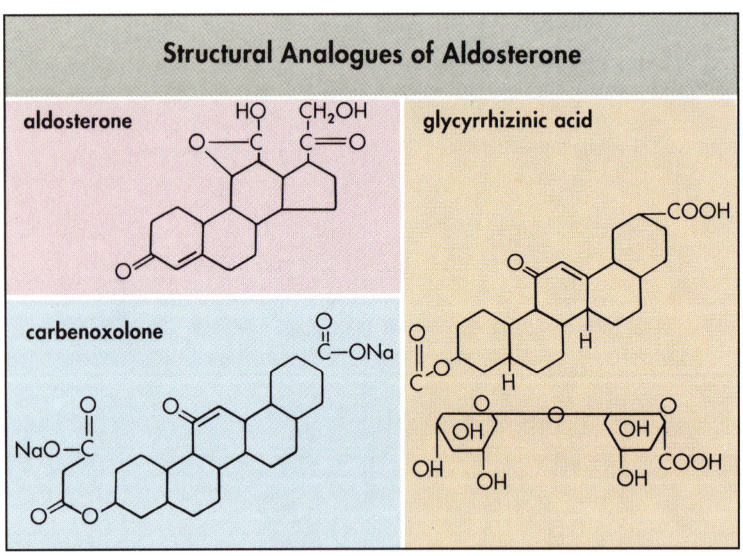

Fig. 5.51 Both glycyrrhizinic acid and carbenoxolone have a mineralocorticoid-like action and may cause a clinical picture resembling primary aldosteronism.

Drugs Interfering with Anti-Hypertensive Medication

- Sympathomimetic agents, interfering with postganglionic adrenergic neurone blockers.
- Tricyclic antidepressants, interfering with postganglionic adrenergic neurone blockers.
- Prostaglandin inhibitors, such as indomethacin, interfering with ß-adrenergic receptor blockers.

A number of agents can cause hypertension by interfering with the action of antihypertensive drugs. Thus, postganglionic adrenergic blocking drugs must be taken up by the norepinephrine pump of the nerve fibre and stored within the nerve terminal for their inhibitory effect to occur. Certain drugs interfere with the uptake of these agents and so may block their antihypertensive action acutely. It is often forgotten that cough mixtures and nasal decongestants usually contain synthetic sympathomimetic agents and may interfere with antihypertensive treatment (Fig. 5.53).

Drugs with Direct Vascular Action

- Ergot alkaloids.
- Phenylephrine.

These drugs increase blood pressure through their direct action on the muscular coats of arteries and arterioles. Phenylephrine, a direct vasoconstrictor, also interferes with uptake mechanisms.

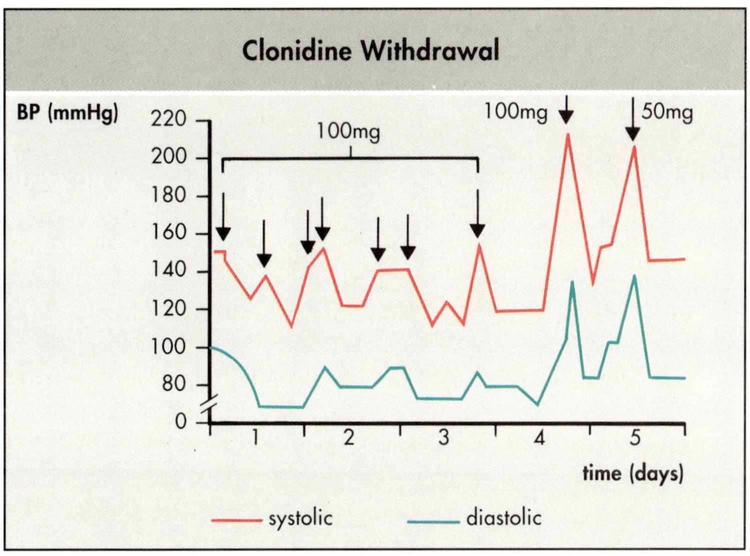

Fig. 5.52 Effect of abrupt withdrawal of clonidine. Severe acute hypertension was associated with evidence of sympathetic overactivity with profuse sweating and tachycardia. Administration of clonidine temporarily reversed these features.

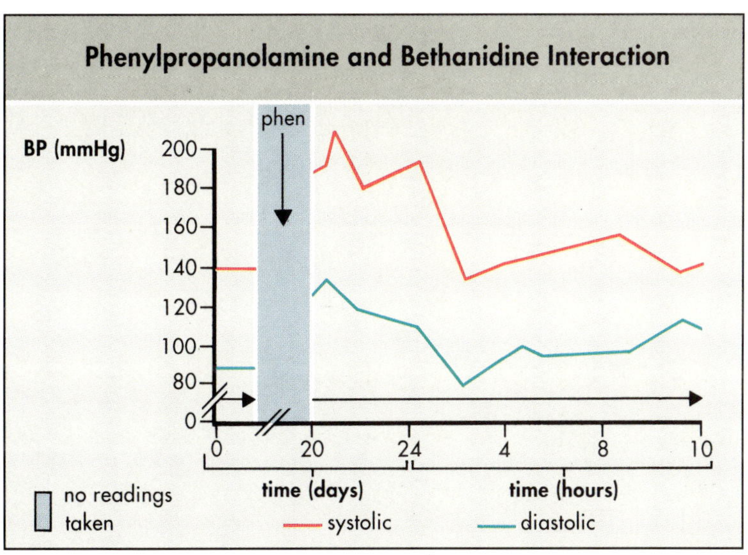

Fig. 5.53 Effect of the sympathomimetic nasal decongestant phenylpropanolamine upon the blood pressure of a hypertensive patient receiving bethanidine. By displacing bethanidine and thereby preventing its neuronal uptake, phenylpropanolamine inhibits its therapeutic action. Although bethanidine is no longer in use, this example serves to emphasize the need to always consider possible drug interactions.

CONCLUSIONS

Hypertension of definite cause is not common in unselected patients whose blood pressure is found to be elevated on routine screening. Probably less than 1% of hypertensive patients have a demonstrable renal cause, although the incidence of renal hypertension is much higher in special centres where selective referral of patients occurs. Patients with phaeochromocytoma and hypertension due to adrenal cortical disease are rarer still, with an incidence of probably less than 1 in 1,000 unselected hypertensive patients. Numerically, pregnancy and the contraceptive pill are more frequent causes of high blood pressure than any other condition known to cause it.

CHAPTER 6

Clinical Subgroups

Hypertension poses particular problems in certain specific groups of patients. These clinical subgroups will be discussed in detail in this chapter.

HYPERTENSION IN CHILDHOOD

Measurement

Children present two clinical problems in the assessment of blood pressure. Firstly, complete cooperation may be difficult to achieve in younger children. Secondly, small arm size creates technical difficulties when using conventional sphygmomanometers.

If a small cuff is used, blood pressure can be measured in children of normal stature using a mercury sphygmomanometer (Fig. 6.1). The recommendations for cuff size in children are similar to those for adults – the width of the inflation bag of the cuff should cover at least two-thirds of the length of the upper arm and the length of the cuff should be at least three-quarters of the circumference of the upper arm. Cuff sizes varying between 4.0 × 13.5cm and 6.6 × 15.5cm are advised for children up to the age of eight years, after which it may be possible to use an adult cuff. Conventional methods of indirect blood pressure measurement are more difficult in children below the age of five (three years according to some groups) since the small size of the brachial artery renders the Korotkoff sounds difficult to distinguish. The most popular alternative method, used in several epidemiological studies, utilizes the Doppler effect upon an ultrasound beam reflected by the movement of red blood cells within the brachial artery (Fig. 6.2). This provides a system for detecting the pulse which is occluded in the usual way by a proximally situated sphygmomanometric cuff. This system therefore only measures systolic blood pressure. Direct comparison of systolic pressures in infants using a Doppler system and a direct intra-arterial measurement have demonstrated fairly poor correlations however. Nevertheless this technique has been extensively used in epidemiological studies of the evolution of blood pressure in neonates and infants.

Children are more likely than adults to show a stress-induced elevation of blood pressure. Particular care must therefore be taken to ensure that the child is not crying or resisting when blood pressure measurement is attempted (Fig. 6.3).

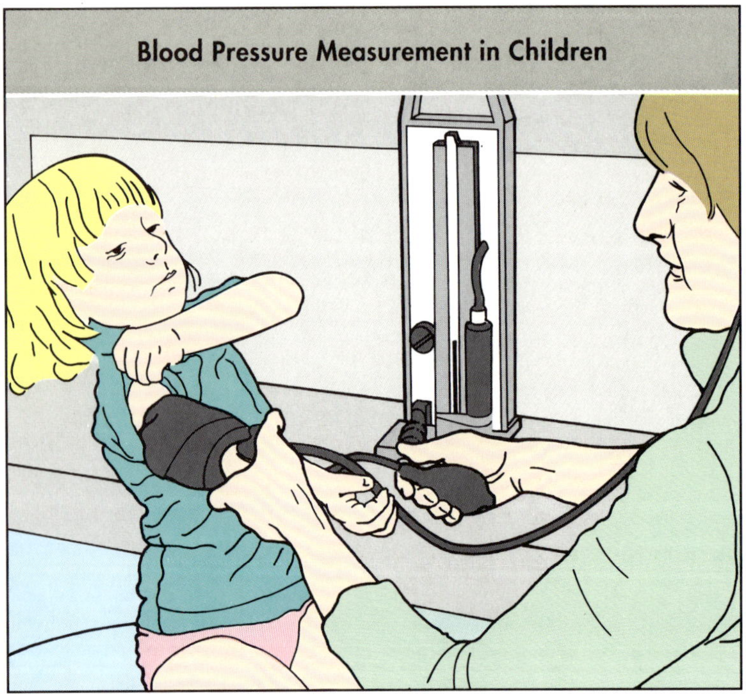

Fig. 6.1 Blood pressure can usually be measured in a child of more than five years of age with the normal sphygmomanometer so long as a small arm cuff is used.

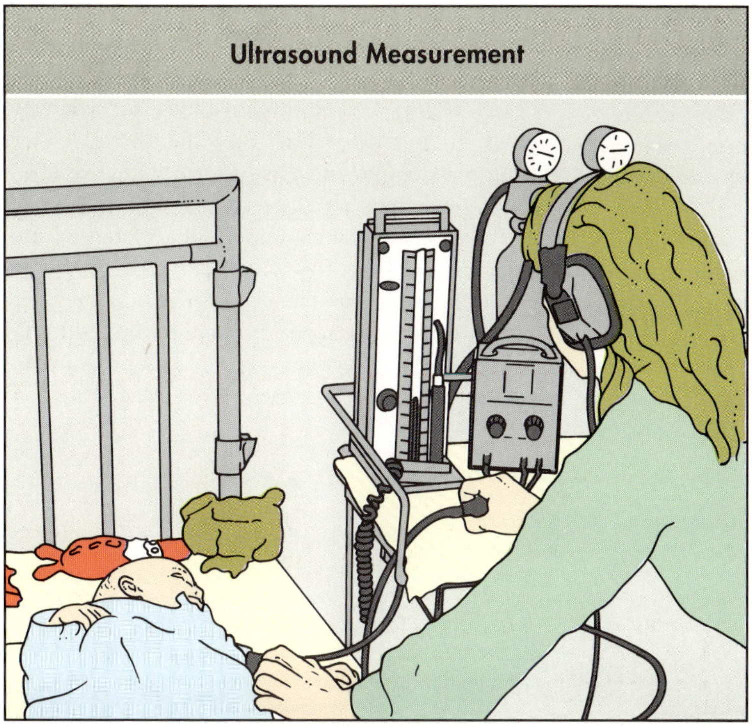

Fig. 6.2 Below the age of five years, special systems are required. The most popular system is the Parkes–Doppler ultrasound system.

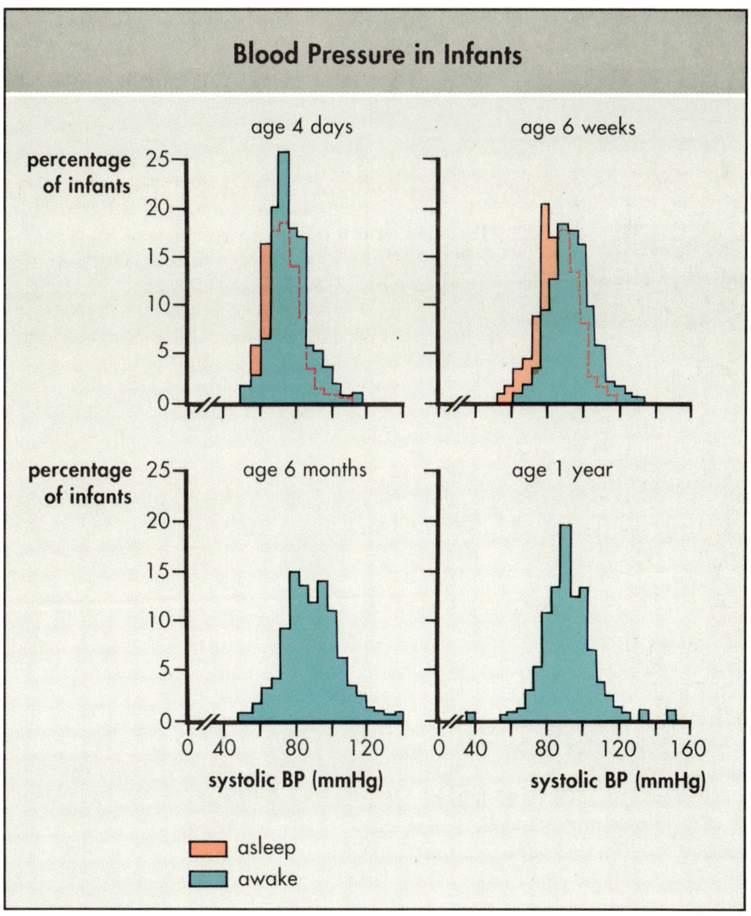

Fig. 6.3 Although mean blood pressure rises over the first year of life, the same unimodal distribution can be seen in infants as has been described in adults. Blood pressures measured during sleep show less variability than conscious blood pressure in infants.

Evolution of Blood Pressure in Children

Blood pressure rises rapidly in the first few days of life, slightly more slowly over the next few weeks and then shows little change between six weeks and six years of age, when blood pressure again begins to rise slowly (Fig. 6.4).

The criteria used to define hypertension in adults clearly cannot be applied to children. The distribution of blood pressure by percentiles offers the best basis for classification of children as hypertensive. The Task Force on Blood Pressure Control in Children has recommended that sustained blood pressure levels (obtained at least on three separate occasions) above the 95th percentile for age should be considered abnormal. Values obtained from the Brompton Study for younger children and from the Task Force for Older Children are shown in Figure 6.4. Other studies have yielded rather discrepant results (Fig. 6.5). The reasons for such important differences are probably multiple. One factor is the use of single or multiple measurements. When blood pressure measurements are repeated for the same individual there is a tendency for blood pressure to regress towards a mean, with a resulting reduction

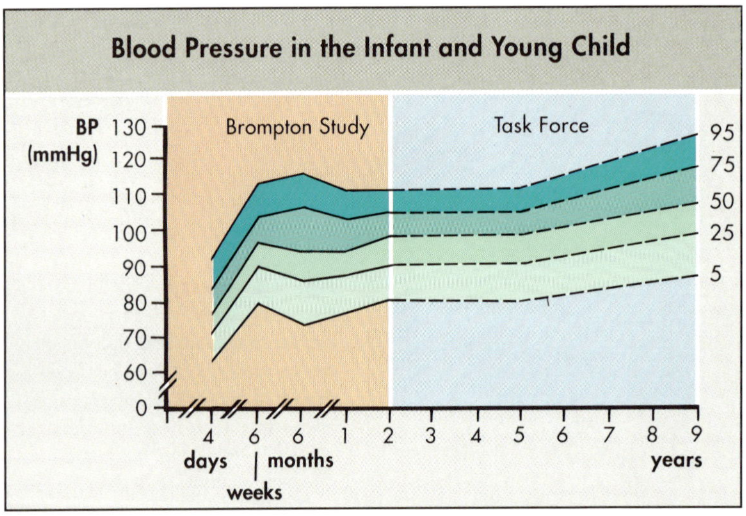

Fig. 6.4 Percentile distribution of blood pressure during infancy and childhood: the sharpest rise is seen in the first six weeks of life. [Modified from De Swiet, M. *et al.* (1980) *Brit Med J*, **280,** 1567–1569 and from Task Force on Blood Pressure Control (1977) *Paediatrics*, **59** (Suppl.), 797–820.]

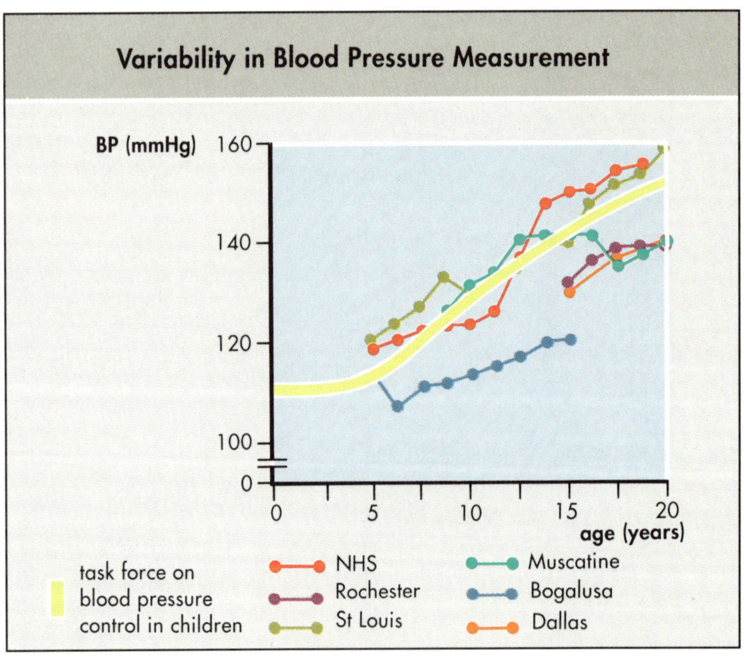

Fig. 6.5 95th percentile values for systolic blood pressure of children vary between studies. [Modified from Fixler, D.E. *et al.* (1980) *Hypertension*, **2**, I-3–I-7.]

in apparent variability in blood pressure in the population studied and a tendency for the 95th percentile to be lower. Variation in measurement techniques, insufficiently large sample sizes and genuine differences in the population sampled probably also contribute to the discrepancies.

Blood pressure in children is correlated with height (Fig. 6.6) and weight. Obesity in children, just as in adults, is associated with higher blood pressure levels (Fig. 6.7). Blood pressure is also related to maturity: children who mature when relatively young have a higher blood pressure initially , although the pressure of later maturers tends to catch up'. Indices of maturation are cumbersome to use in routine clinical practice and blood pressure values are usually related to the child's age. However, the relation to height and weight remains the best criterion up until puberty.

The blood pressure of children tends to resemble that of their parents. Such familial aggregation of blood pressure could of course reflect both environmental as well as genetic factors. This difficult problem can be approached by examining blood pressures in adopted children and step-children and in monozygotic and dizygotic twins (see chapter 1). Such studies suggest that in children as

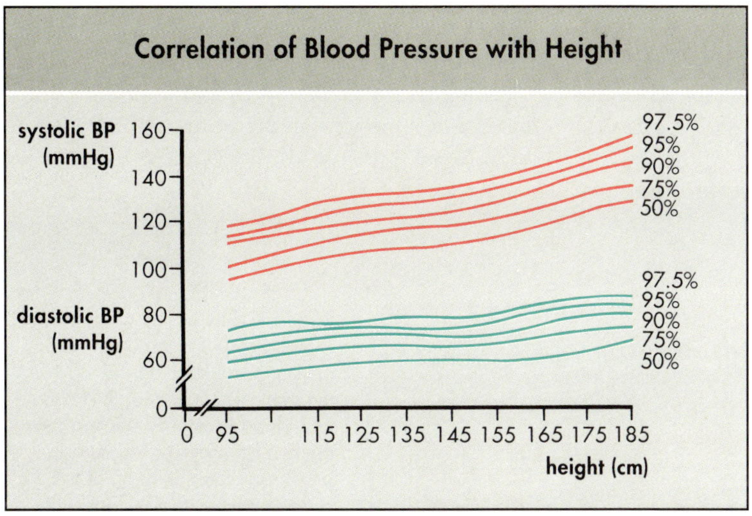

Fig. 6.6 Normal values of blood pressure are correlated with height. Blood pressures, for boys, are expressed in percentiles for age; values were recorded in a health centre, in supine position, in 17,067 children. The fifth Korotkoff sound was used for diastolic pressure. [Modified from Andre, J.L. *et al.* (1980) *Arch Fr. Pediatric,* **37**, 477–482.]

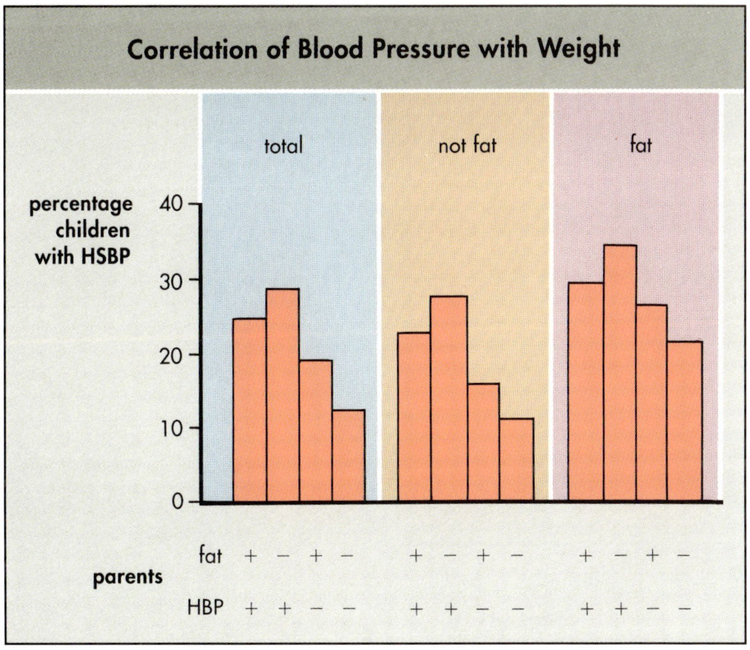

Fig. 6.7 This study showed a correlation between obesity and blood pressure in children. Obesity and blood pressure in the parents also seem to be important factors. [Modified from Higgins M. W. *et al* (1980) *Hypertension*, **2**, I-117–I-123.]

young as six months of age, genetic factors are important contributors to familial similarities in observed blood pressure.

Blood pressure of course shows day-to-day variability. Like height, it tends to be a particular characteristic of the individual. In children this is expressed as the tendency for an individual to remain in the same position within the blood pressure distribution over a period of time. Thus, individuals with a high normal blood pressure in childhood continue to show a high normal blood pressure in later years. The ability of childhood blood pressure to predict blood pressure at a later age is measured by the tracking coefficient (Fig. 6.8). Several longitudinal studies have assessed the tracking coefficients of blood pressure in children. These are in general lower than the corresponding coefficients in adults, and coefficients for diastolic blood pressure are lower than those for systolic pressure. This may reflect greater difficulty in measuring diastolic blood pressure precisely, or the fact that diastolic blood pressure in children appears to be influenced by environmental factors more than is systolic blood pressure. Predictions of future blood pressure based on current measurements improve in accuracy after the age of (about) twenty. In some studies, measurements taken during the first few days of life have failed to show any correlation with blood pressures in childhood: this is probably due to the influence of height and weight up to puberty, and to additional factors thereafter.

Although tracking is of epidemiological significance, the relatively low values of tracking coefficients in childhood mean that it is impossible to predict future hypertension with any degree of accuracy by selecting children in the top percentiles for blood pressure. Nevertheless, children with higher blood pressures and a strong family history of hypertension are at the greatest risk of high blood pressure during adolescence and as young adults.

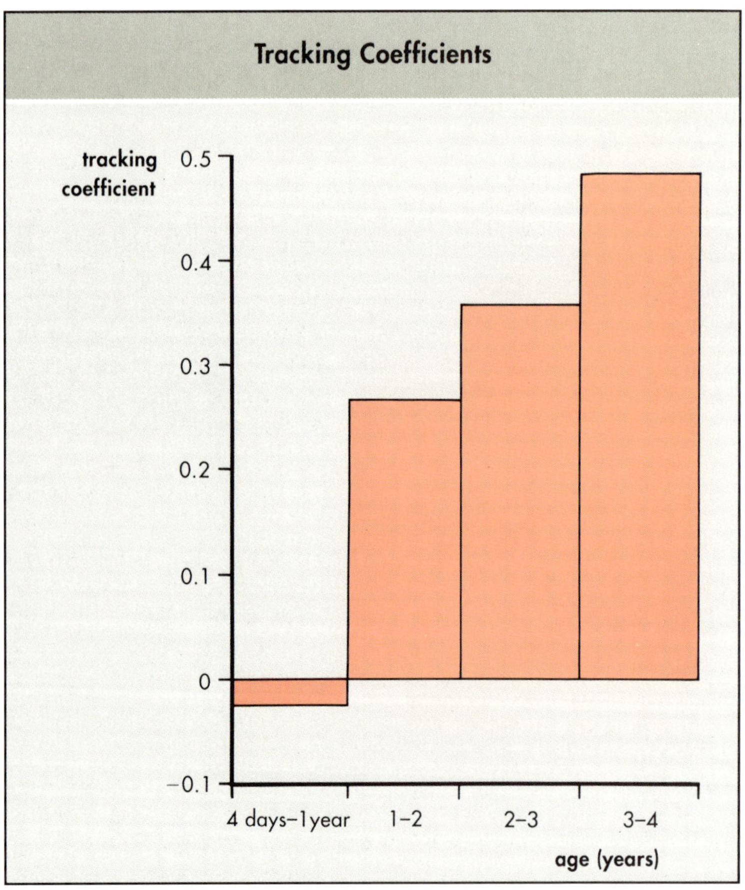

Fig. 6.8 The ability of measured blood pressure to predict blood pressure at a later age is shown by the tracking coefficient. It is clear that blood pressures measured in the first few days of life do not predict the later position of the child in the percentile distribution. From the first year onwards, children tend to remain within the same percentile. Courtesy of Dr M. de Swiet.

Prevalence of Primary and Secondary Forms of Hypertension in the Young

author, year and country	number of patients	age range (years)
Singh and Page (1967) USA	22	<23
Breckenridge *et al.* (1967) Britain	229	12–40
Loggie (1969) USA	15	14–15
Ooi *et al.* (1973) Singapore	13	<20
Londe *et al.* (1973) USA	74	4–18
Loggie *et al.* (1973) USA*	47	2–15
Loggie (1975) USA*	29	12–18

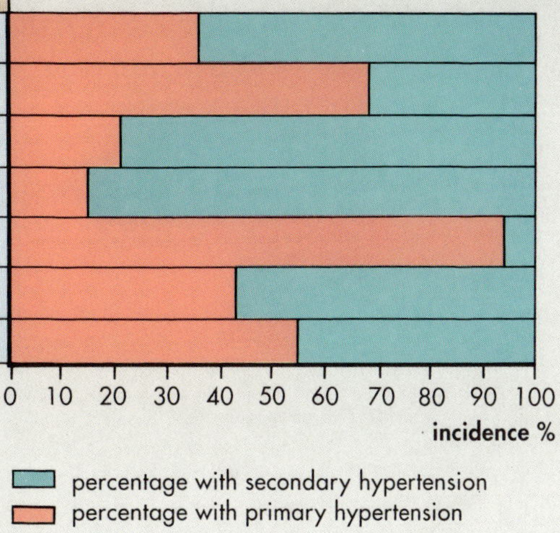

* unpublished data

Fig. 6.9 The relative prevalence of essential (primary) and secondary hypertension in children is entirely dependent upon the composition and source of the population studied.

Hypertension in Neonates

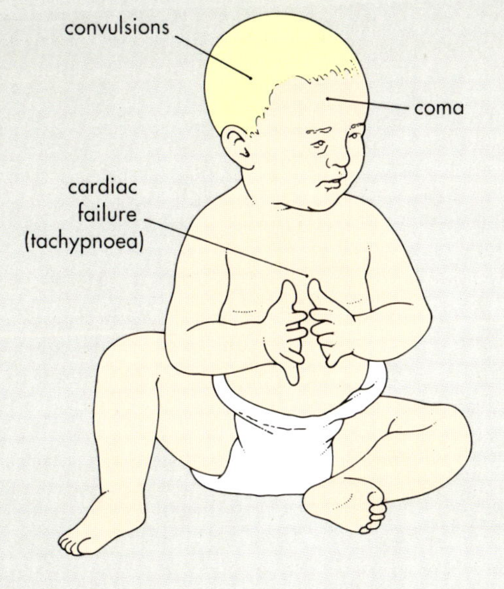

Fig. 6.10 Features of hypertension in neonates.

Causes of High Blood Pressure in Childhood

Secondary hypertension is more common in children than in adults, although its incidence falls with increasing age. Essential hypertension in children is more common than was once thought. There is wide variation in the estimated prevalence of primary and secondary forms of hypertension in children, depending upon the definition of elevated blood pressure and the source of the population studies (Fig. 6.9).

In neonates, coarctation of the aorta is the most common cause of hypertension. Renal ischaemia secondary to renal artery thrombosis (often as a complication of umbilical artery catheterization in exchange transfusion of neonates) is also seen occasionally. Hypertension may also accompany increased intracranial pressure as a result of intracranial haemorrhage during birth. It may present in neonates as congestive cardiac failure, tachypnoea, coma or convulsions (Fig. 6.10).

Renal disease, renovascular disease and essential hypertension become more common as causes of high blood pressure with increasing age (see Figs 6.11–6.16). Acute glomerulonephritis is becoming

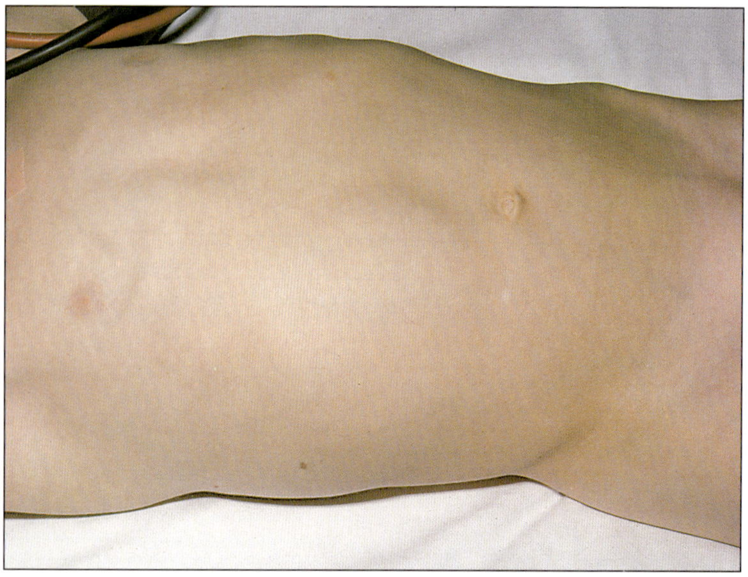

Fig. 6.11 Child with Wilm's tumour. Notice the prominent renal mass. Courtesy of Dr H. J. Whitely.

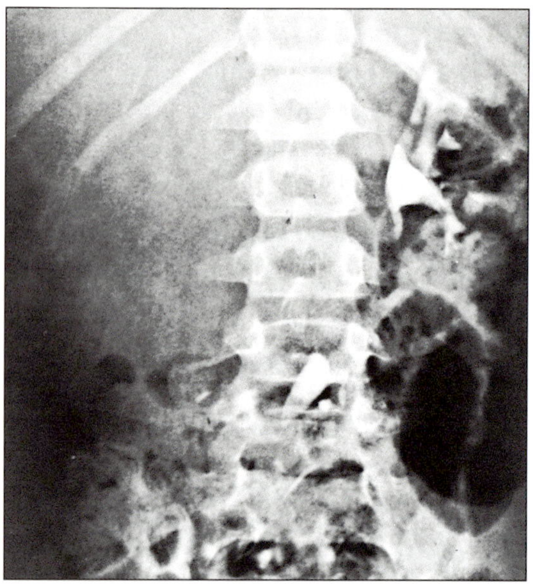

Fig. 6.12 IVP from the same patient. Notice the gross displacement of the right renal calices. Courtesy of Professor T. Sherwood.

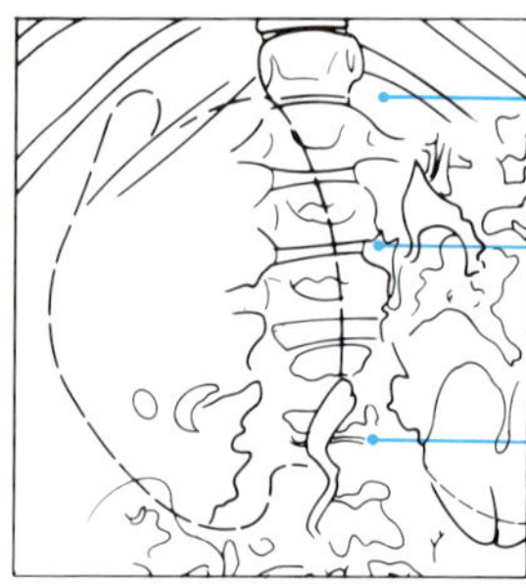

less common in Westernized cultures, although it is still a major problem on the African continent. In older children and adolescents essential hypertension is probably the major cause, although secondary hypertension is still rather more prevalent than in adults.

In children just as in adults, high blood pressure may be detected on routine examination. However, very severe hypertension may present with acute cerebrovascular disturbances suggestive of encephalopathy, including headache, transient neurological signs, vomiting or fits. Occasionally it may present with acute cardiac failure. Although the dangers of severe hypertension in childhood are fully recognized as matters of clinical experience, there is comparatively little known otherwise about the natural history of high blood pressure in childhood. There is, however, no reason to believe that there is any qualitative difference in the overall risks and dangers to children compared with the risks to which hypertensive adults are exposed, although the frequency of various forms of target organ damage, such as ischaemic heart disease, is clearly lower.

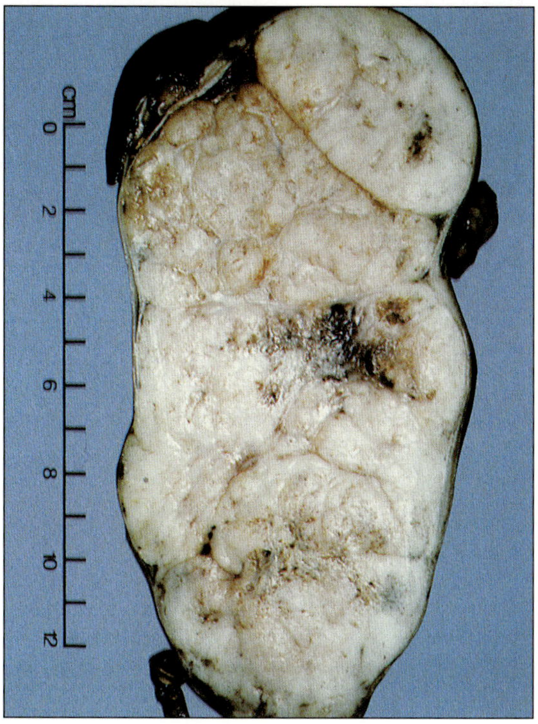

Fig. 6.13 Kidney from the same patient showing replacement of normal tissue by tumour tissue. Courtesy of Dr H. J. Whitely

Hypertension in Neonates and Infants
neonates
coarctation (aorta)
intracranial haemorrhage
renovascular disease
infants <2 years
neuroblastoma
coarctation
renovascular disease (stenosis)
renal cysts
hydronephrosis
pyelonephritis
Wilm's tumour

Fig. 6.15 In neonates and young infants, hypertension is usually secondary to other diseases.

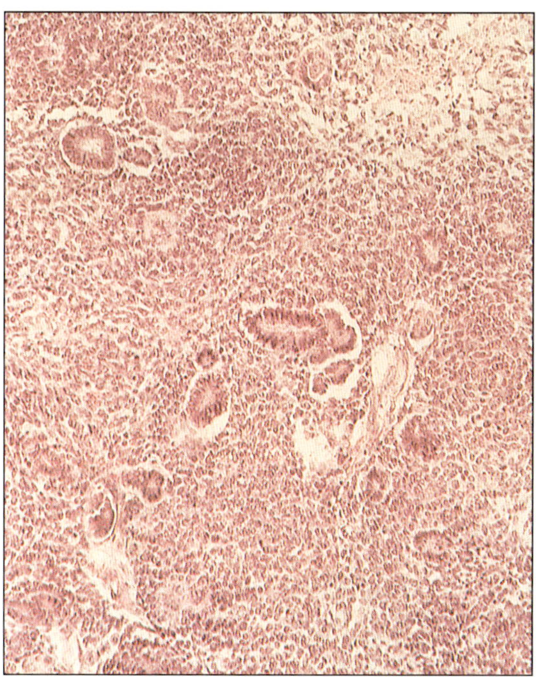

Fig. 6.14 Histology of the kidney illustrated in Figure 6.13. The kidney tissue is largely replaced by tumour cells. Courtesy of Dr H. J. Whitely

Secondary Hypertension in Children and Adolescents
younger children (2–8 years)
renovascular disease
renal cystic disease
pyelonephritis
coarctation
older children and adolescents
renovascular disease
cystic disease
chronic pyelonephritis
chronic glomerulonephritis
collagen diseases
essential hypertension

Fig. 6.16 Secondary hypertension is still relatively common in older age groups.

HYPERTENSION IN PREGNANCY

Definition

Hypertension frequently complicates pregnancy and pregnancy frequently worsens pre-existing hypertension. The constraints which naturally apply to investigating pregnant women and the frequent absence of information about pre-gestational blood pressure have led to considerable confusion in classification. The simplest approach is to define four classes, as follows:

- pre-eclampsia and eclampsia;
- chronic hypertension (primary or secondary);
- chronic hypertension with superimposed pre-eclampsia;
- late transient 'gestational' hypertension.

Although theoretically all cases of hypertension can be classed under one of the above groups, in practice the cause of hypertension remains debatable in a substantial number of pregnant women.

Criteria for hypertension have also been debated extensively. The most widely accepted value at present is a blood pressure equal to or above 140/90mmHg. The position in which blood pressure is taken may also have a greater influence upon observed readings in pregnant women than in other subjects. Significant differences have thus been recorded in the supine, left lateral recumbent and sitting positions, particularly in late pregnancy when the gravid uterus may restrict venous return to the heart and hence reduce blood pressure in the supine position. In addition, the point of disappearance of the Korotkoff sounds (Phase V) may be much lower than the point of muffling and, indeed, Korotkoff sounds may be audible down to zero pressure; the use of Phase IV is essential in such cases.

Epidemiology

The prevalence of hypertension in pregnancy differs widely from one study to the next, with a range of 2–10% or even greater. Whilst undoubtedly much of the discrepancy is due to the use of different criteria for hypertension, there are probably also genuine differences in the populations studied. Thus, pregnancy-induced hypertension shows genuine differences in incidence in different geographical and racial groups. It is more common in the lower socioeconomic classes, in Blacks and in the Far East.

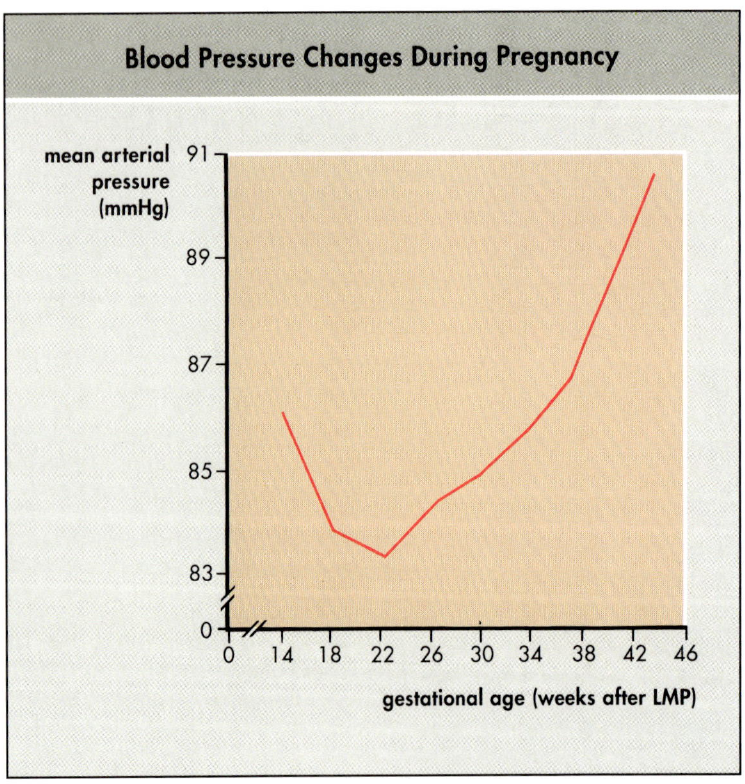

Fig. 6.17 Blood pressure decreases in early pregnancy, then increases from 22 weeks onwards. These data were gathered from white nulliparous women, aged 25–34 years, in the San Francisco–East Bay area between 1959 and 1967. [Modified from Neuman *et al.* (1979) *Obstet and Gynae*, **53**, 50s–55s.]

Normal Pregnancy

Blood pressure decreases in early pregnancy, reaching its nadir at weeks 20–22 and gradually increasing thereafter (Fig. 6.17). Towards term, in normal pregnancy pressure approaches the non-pregnant values (Fig. 6.18). The first haemodynamic change in pregnancy is a reduction in peripheral resistance, particularly involving vasodilatation in the kidneys, liver and breasts. This change is associated with an increase in cardiac output of 20–50% in the first six to ten weeks. In the last trimester of pregnancy cardiac output is high in the lateral recumbent position, but decreased in the supine position. Uteroplacental blood flow increases from about 50ml/minute in the tenth week to 700ml/minute at term.

Plasma renin activity, renin substrate and angiotensin II are all elevated during pregnancy (Fig. 6.19). However, healthy pregnant women are resistant to both the pressor effect and the renal effects of infused angiotensin II. This seems to be a specific receptor-mediated response since there is no decreased sensitivity to other pressor hormones. In addition there are kinetic differences in the reaction between renin and substrate in plasma from pregnant women, probably reflecting differences in the circulating forms of substrate and the presence of greater than normal levels of inactive renin. There is also increased synthesis of vasodilator prostaglandins, which may account for resistance to angiotensin II since indomethacin restores sensitivity to normal in resistance vessels obtained from the omentum at caesarean section.

Although the renal capacity to excrete sodium is not impaired in pregnancy, plasma volume is increased by approximately 50% by the 32nd week of pregnancy.

Normal Pregnancy Haemodynamics and Fluid Volumes	
cardiac output	↑
peripheral resistance	↓
renal blood flow	↑
plasma volume	↑
extracellular fluid volume	↑

Fig. 6.18 Changes in haemodynamics and fluid volumes in normal pregnancy.

Normal Pregnancy Hormonal Factors	
renin	↑
renin substrate	↑
angiotensin II	↑
vascular reponsiveness to angiotensin II	↓
oestrogens	↑
progestagens	↑
vasodilator prostaglandins (urinary PGE_2)	↑

Fig. 6.19 Changes in hormonal factors which may be relevant to blood pressure control in normal pregnancy.

Pre-eclampsia

Classical pre-eclampic toxaemia (Fig. 6.20) presents with proteinuria, oedema and blood pressure which rises around the 30th week of a first pregnancy. All these features disappear with delivery (see Fig. 6.21).

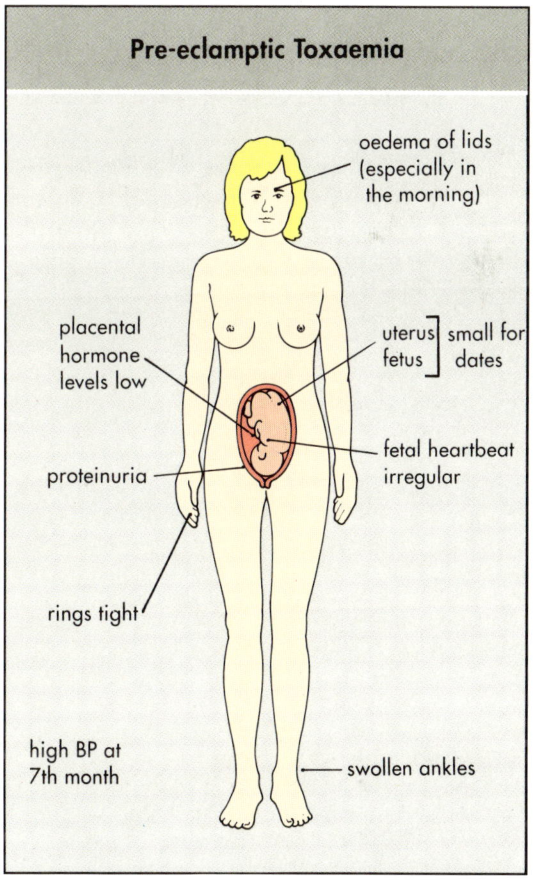

Fig. 6.20 Clinical features of pre-eclamptic toxaemia.

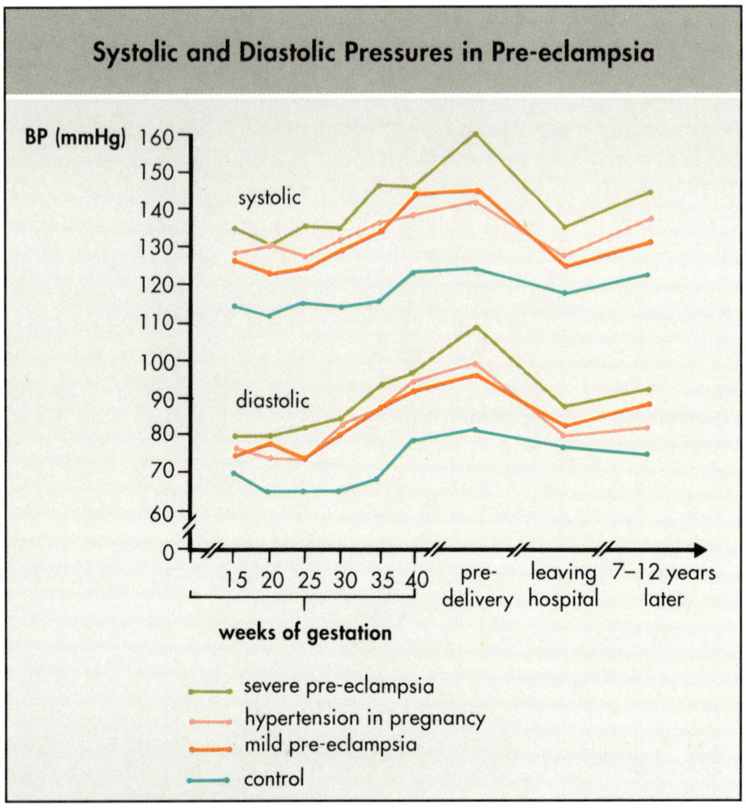

Fig. 6.21 The high systolic and diastolic blood pressures associated with pre-eclamptic toxaemia present at around the 30th week of a first pregnancy and delivery. [Modified from Svensson, A. (1985) *Acta Med Scand (Suppl.)*, **695**, 1–50.]

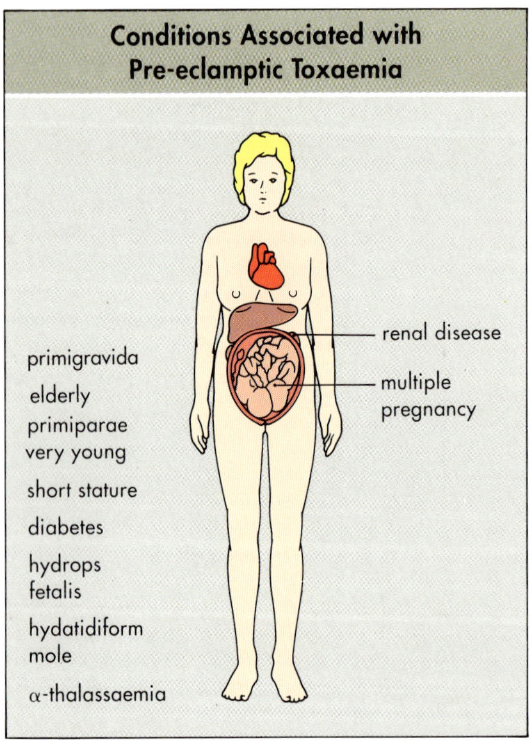

Fig. 6.22 Conditions in which pre-eclamptic toxaemia is prevalent.

Slight elevation of blood pressure in the first trimester may be the first danger signs heralding later toxaemia. The normal circadian rhythm of blood pressure is often lost or even reversed in pre-eclamptic toxaemia. Whilst in the past considerable importance was attached to oedema, it is now recognized that in about 40% of pregnancies women may have varying degrees of oedema at some stage, although oedema tends to be worse in pre-eclamptic toxaemia.

Pre-eclamptic toxaemia is seen particularly in first pregnancies, elderly primiparae and in very young pregnant women, individuals of short stature and in association with multiple pregnancies, diabetes, pre-existing hypertension and renal disease. It is also seen in hydrops fetalis, α-thalassaemia and in women with hydatidiform moles (Fig. 6.22). 'True' pre-eclampsia probably carries no implications for future blood pressure, whereas pre-existing hypertension does. The controversy surrounding the long-term outcome of pre-eclampsia is attributable to the difficulty in distinguishing clinically between pre-eclampsia and pre-existing hypertension. Thus, where the diagnosis of pre-eclamptic toxaemia has been confirmed by renal biopsy (see below), there has been no increased incidence of hypertension in later life.

Hypertension in pre-eclampsia is associated with an increase in peripheral resistance and a decrease in plasma volume relative to normotensive pregnancies, although extracellular fluid volume is expanded (Fig. 6.23). Renal blood flow and glomerular flow rate are likewise reduced in comparison with normotensive pregnancies. Serum urate measurements (which reflect proximal tubular function) provide a good index of pre-eclampsia in this context. Even in the first trimester of pregnancy when angiotensin II is infused into pregnant women there is an increased pressor response in those who are later to develop pre-eclamptic toxaemia (Fig. 6.24). This relative hypersensitivity can also be demonstrated in isolated resistance vessels from women with pre-eclamptic

Pre-eclampsia Haemodynamics and Fluid Volume	
cardiac output	↓
peripheral resistance	↑
renal blood flow	↓
plasma volume	↓
extracellular fluid volume	↑

Fig. 6.23 Changes in haemodynamics and fluid volumes in pre-eclamptic toxaemia compared with changes observed in normal prenancy.

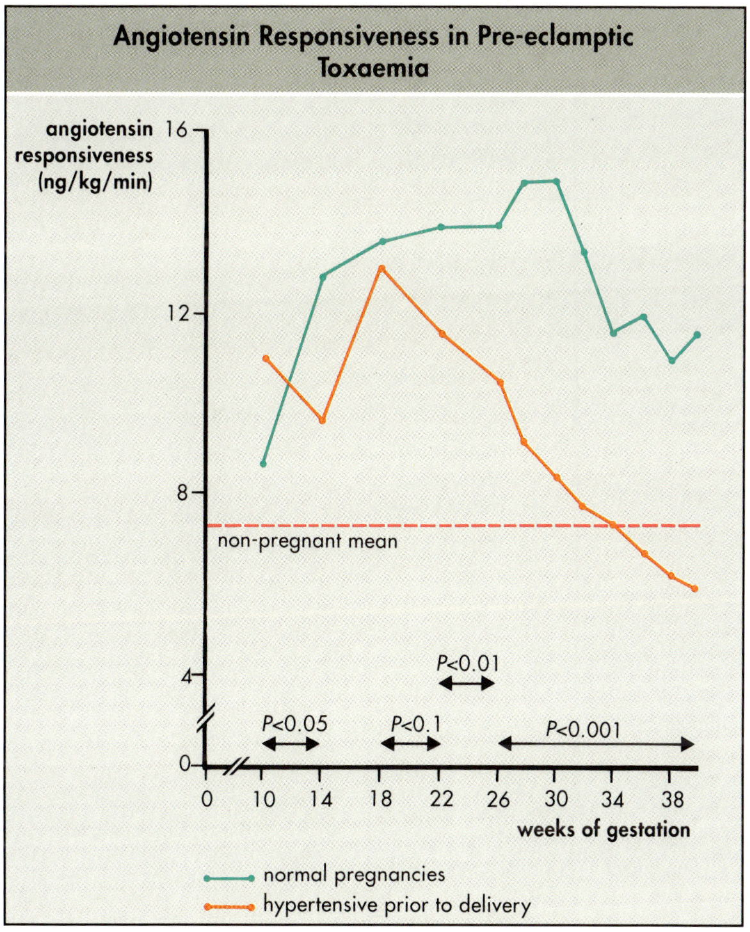

Fig. 6.24 Angiotensin responsiveness. Women who develop pre-eclamptic toxaemia show an increased responsiveness to angiotensin II. This is shown here by the smaller infused dose of angiotensin II required to raise blood pressure by a specified amount. [Modified from Gant, N. F. *et al.* (1973) *J Clin Invest*, **52**, 2682–2689.]

toxaemia. Circulating renin and angiotensin II are lower in pre-eclamptic toxaemia than in normotensive pregnancy. Active (ouabain-sensitive) leucocyte sodium pumping is also reduced (Figs 6.25 & 6.26). This has been attributed by some to the presence of a circulating inhibitor of sodium–potassium ATPase. This remains unconfirmed, and its significance is unclear.

Proteinuria is due to the presence of IgG, albumin and transferrin. Where dip-stick testing reveals proteinuria, quantitative measurement is important; more than 500mg/day is significant, and heavy proteinuria suggests a glomerular lesion. Renal biopsies usually reveal a characteristic abnormality termed glomerular endotheliosis (Fig. 6.27). This is manifest as a swelling of endothelial and mesangial cells which encroaches upon the capillary lumina of the glomerulus, accounting for the fall in glomerular filtration rate and renal blood flow. The pathogenesis of this swelling is unknown.

The cause of pre-eclamptic toxaemia is equally uncertain. A number of suggestions (which are not mutually exclusive) have been made.

- A fairly slow development of intravascular coagulation could be induced by the release of thromboplastic material into the circulation, thus increasing platelet aggregability and consumption. There are reports of decreased production of stable metabolites of prostacyclin and increased production of thromboxane. Loss of the vasodilator action of prostacyclin may contribute to the elevation of blood pressure in this situation. Further, drugs known to inhibit platelet thromboxane production (such as low-dose aspirin or specific thromboxane antagonists)

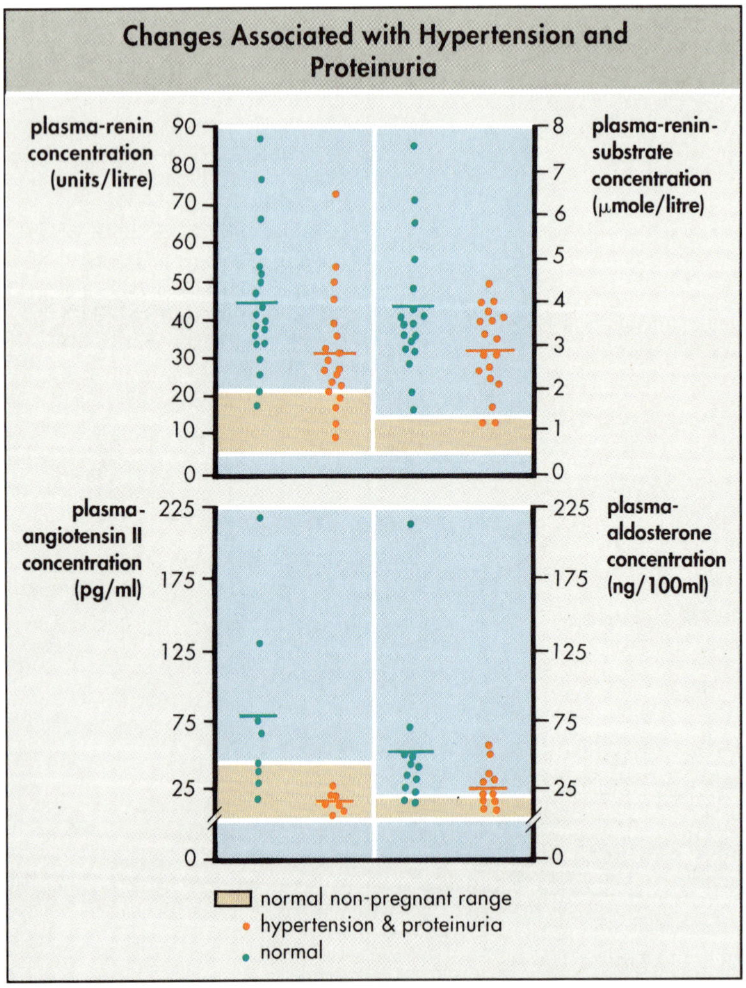

Fig. 6.25 Levels of circulating renin, renin substrate, angiotensin II and aldosterone are lower in pregnancies associated with hypertension and proteinuria. [Modified from Weir *et al.* (1976). In *Hypertension in Pregnancy*. Edited by Lindheimer *et al.* New York: John Wiley and Sons.]

have exerted a beneficial effect in some trials.

- Uteroplacental ischaemia could lead to decreased uterine release of prostaglandin-like materials. Some studies have demonstrated that constriction of the aorta or the uterine arteries in pregnant animals produces renal lesions resembling those seen in pre-eclamptic toxaemia.
- A failure of the maternal immune response to the fetus. There is a tendency for pre-eclamptic toxaemia to occur where there is higher similarity than usual between fetal and maternal antigens. This is also consistent with the fact that pre-eclamptic toxaemia usually only involves the first pregnancy.
- Familial aggregation of predisposition to pre-eclamptic toxaemia suggests a genetic factor. Family studies have indicated an autosomal recessive mode of inheritance (Fig. 6.28).

Hormonal Factors in Pre-eclampsia	
renin	↓
renin substrate	↓
angiotensin II	↓
vascular responsiveness to angiotensin	↑
vasodilator prostaglandins (urinary PGE_2)	↓
? circulating Na^+-K^+ ATPase inhibitor	↑

Fig. 6.26 Changes in hormonal factors in pre-eclamptic toxaemia compared with normal pregnancy.

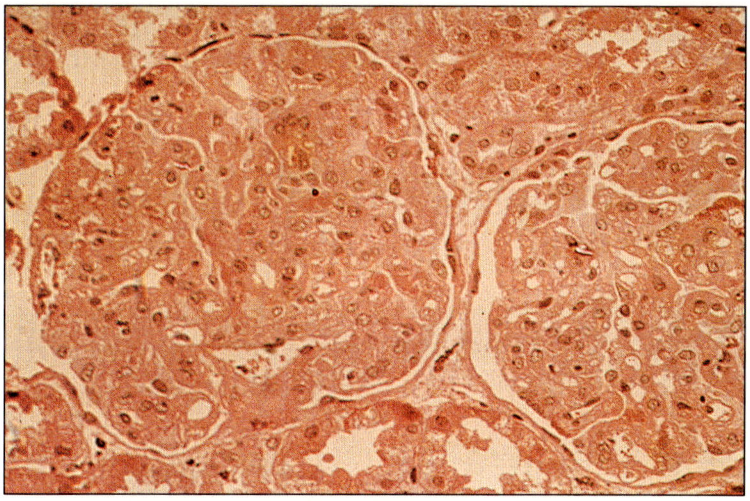

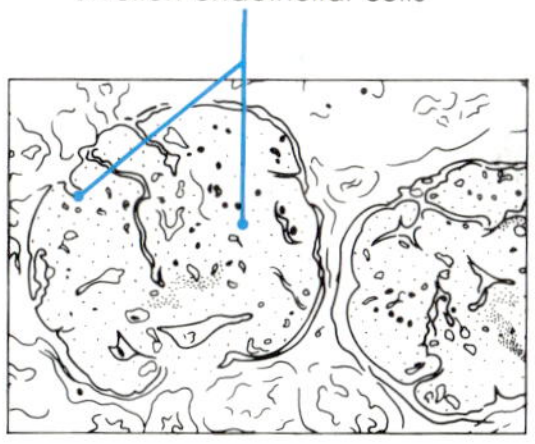

Fig. 6.27 Renal histology in pre-eclamptic toxaemia. The glomeruli are enlarged and the capillary lumina reduced by cytoplasmic swelling of the endothelial cells. Courtesy of Professor P. Kincaid-Smith.

Pre-eclampsia or Eclampsia in Relatives of Eclamptics			
relationship	number	pre-eclampsia or eclampsia during first pregnancy	
		expected*	observed
sisters	147	58.0	55
daughters	187	48.9	48
one daughter	72	18.4	18
two daughters	28	12.5	13
three to five daughters	12	8.3	8
daughters-in-law (controls)	75	4.9	6

* predicted numbers if caused by single recessive gene

Fig. 6.28 Pre-eclampsia or eclampsia in relatives of eclamptics. Observed numbers conform closely to those predicted by a single recessive mode of inheritance. [Modified from Chesley, L.C. (1980) *Kidney International*, **18**, 234–240.]

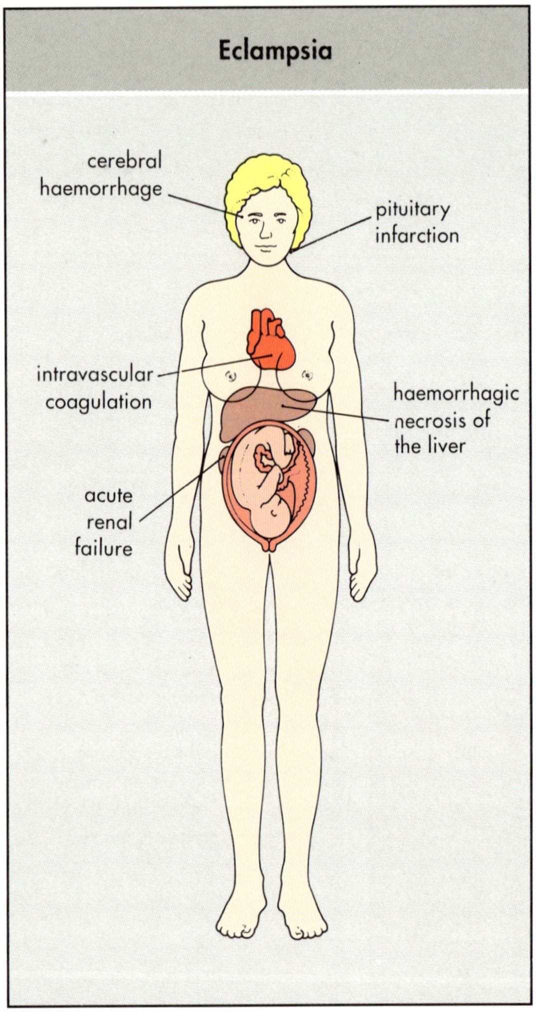

Fig. 6.29 Clinical features of eclampsia.

Eclampsia

Eclampsia is recognized by the presence of generalized seizures not caused by any lesion of the central nervous system in a patient who has previously had pre-eclampsia (Fig. 6.29). Eclamptic convulsions may occur either during pregnancy, during delivery or during the first postpartum day. Eclampsia is usually associated with a rapid rise in blood pressure. It may therefore be a manifestation of hypertensive encephalopathy with a failure of cerebral vascular autoregulation (see chapter 3). It is also often associated with evidence of disseminated vascular coagulation with thrombocytopaenia, deformed red cells (Fig. 6.30) and a high titre of fibrin degradation products in the plasma and urine (Fig. 6.31). Whether the presence of fibrin clots within the cerebral microcirculation contributes to the fits is debatable. Multiple placental infarction frequently occurs (Fig. 6.32). Impairment of liver function and subcapsular liver haemorrhage are also occasionally seen in advanced disease. Potentially fatal cerebral haemorrhage occurs less frequently. Eclampsia is now very unusual in developed countries but is still frequent in Third World countries and in women whose antenatal care has been neglected.

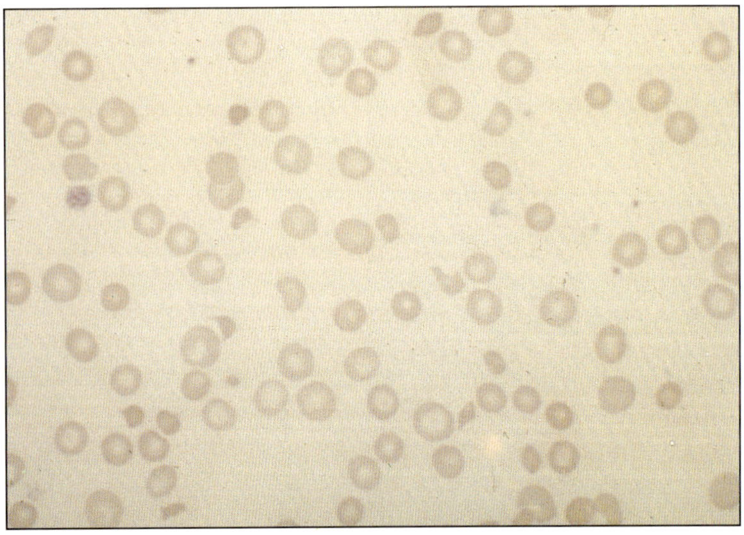

Fig. 6.30 Intravascular coagulation in eclampsia is associated with fragmentation and distortion of the red cells.

Chronic Hypertension First Observed in Pregnancy

Hypertension is often observed in pregnancy, but is not always directly attributable to it. Essential hypertension accounts for the vast majority of cases, but other causes of secondary hypertension (such as renal and renovascular disease, coarctation and phaeochromocytoma, primary aldosteronism and Cushing's syndrome) may occasionally be responsible. Secondary hypertension is not necessarily worsened by pregnancy except in cases of phaeochromocytoma or renal scleroderma where pregnancy may have a devastating effect upon the course of the disease.

Characteristically, patients with chronic hypertension show elevated blood pressures from the very onset of pregnancy. Nevertheless, since many patients with pre-eclamptic toxaemia also show marginal blood pressure elevations early in pregnancy, the distinction between the two forms of hypertension is not easy. Where renal biopsies have been carried out to look for the characteristic lesion of pre-eclamptic toxaemia, clinical diagnosis has been erroneous in a substantial number of patients. The course of chronic hypertension in pregnancy is frequently complicated by other evidence of pre-eclamptic toxaemia later on during pregnancy, further confusing the issue.

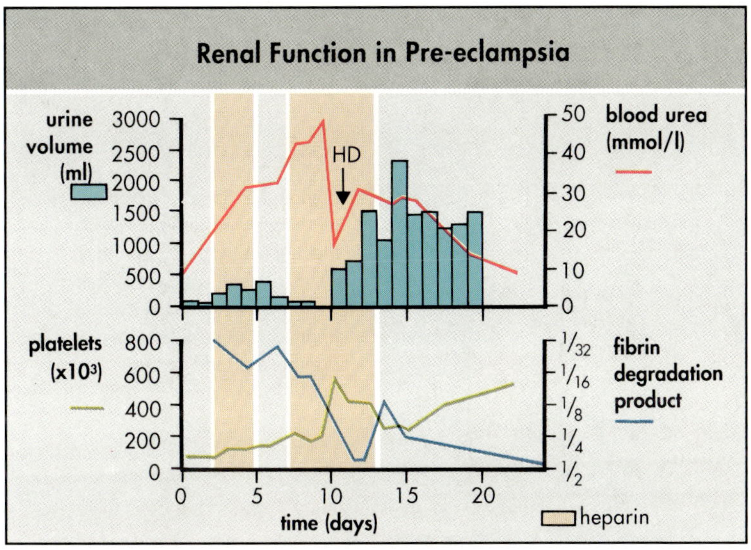

Fig. 6.31 Renal function in a patient who presented with eclampsia at 32 weeks of pregnancy. Oliguria was associated with a low platelet count and a high concentration of fibrin degradation products in the urine. The patient required haemodialysis (HD) and was treated with heparin. The evidence for intravascular coagulation disappeared and renal function returned to normal.

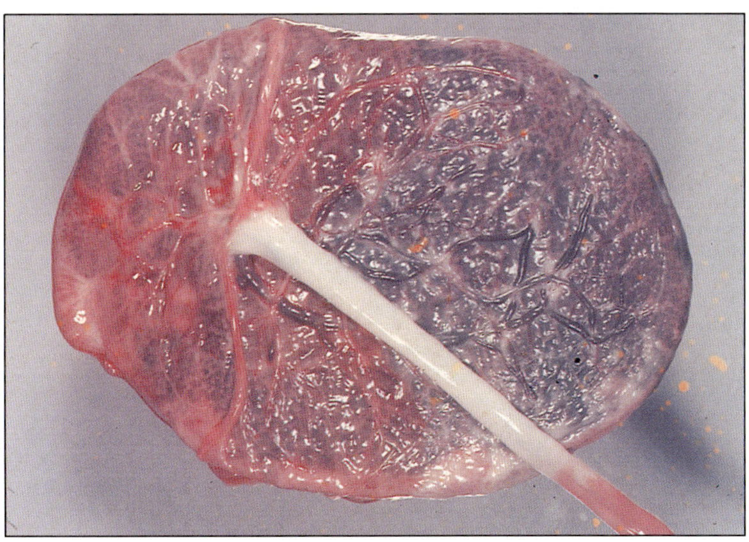

Fig. 6.32 Placental infarction following a history of eclampsia.

Late, Transient or Gestational Hypertension

Occasionally women develop a transient hypertension late in pregnancy or during the puerperium. These patients tend to develop hypertension in later life. It has been suggested therefore that it is an early manifestation of essential hypertension. In addition some patients' blood pressure falls in pregnancy from previous higher levels and postpartum it rises again.

Clinical consequences

The 30–50% reduction in uteroplacental blood flow gives rise to fetal retardation and, in more severe cases, fetal asphyxia and death. In one large study hypertension without proteinuria was associated with a threefold increase in fetal mortality; the presence of proteinuria increased fetal mortality 20-fold. The reduction in placental blood flow may give rise to placental infarction.

Effects of Treatment

Theoretically, reduction in systemic blood flow could give rise to further reduction in uteroplacental perfusion and therefore worsen the fetal prognosis. Only a limited number of studies have been carried out, but there is evidence for an improved prognosis with methyldopa, for instance, where careful blood pressure control improved the outcome in terms of fetal survival (but not fetal size) (Figs 6.33 & 6.34). A follow-up of children whose mothers were treated in pregnancy with methyldopa showed no long-term adverse effects. Studies using atenolol have shown a significant reduction in maternal proteinuria and improved maternal blood pressure control (Figs 6.35 & 6.36).

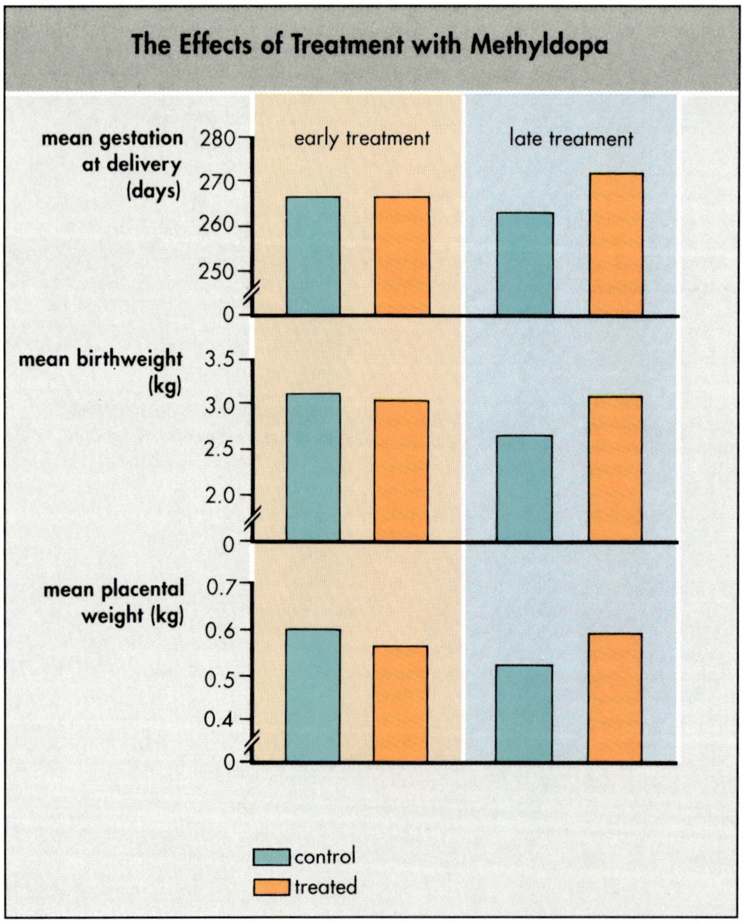

Fig. 6.33 Effect of early and late treatment of hypertension with methyldopa during pregnancy. Although fetal size and placental weight were increased by late treatment, these differences were not significant. [Modified from Redman *et al.* (1976) *Lancet*, **2**, 733–756.]

The Effects of Methyldopa and Oxyprenolol

		oxyprenolol	methyldopa
birthweight	weight (g)	3051	2654
	% of normal for gestational age	95	83
placental weight	weight (g)	534	479
	% of normal for gestational age	85	76
apgar score	at 1 minute	7.8	7.6
	at 5 minutes	9.4	9.2
	intrauterine deaths	0	0
	neonatal deaths	0	2

Fig. 6.34 A comparison of the effects of methyldopa and oxyprenolol upon the outcome of pregnancy. [Modified from Gallery, E. D. M. *et al.* (1979) *Brit Med J*, **1**, 1591–1594.]

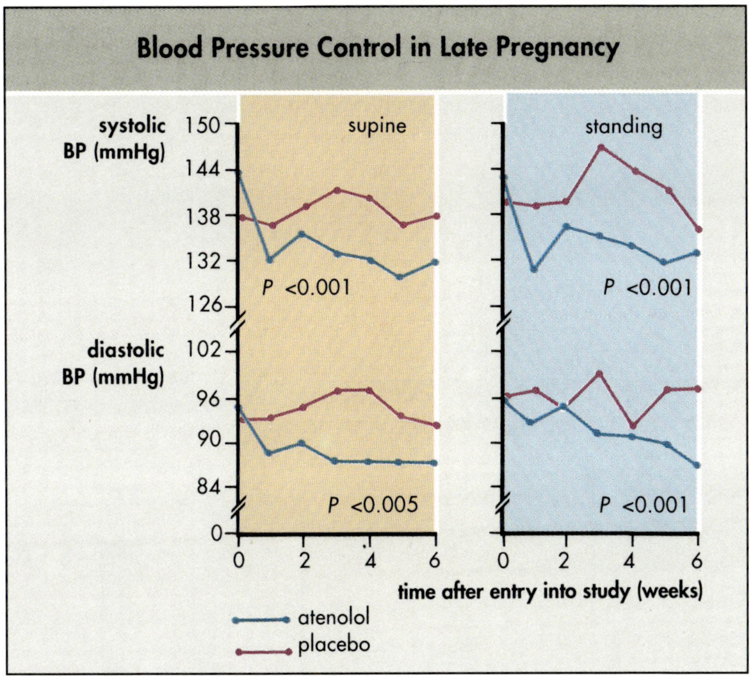

Fig. 6.35 Blood pressure control during late pregnancy in women treated with atenolol compared with those given a placebo. [Modified from Rubin *et al.* (1983) *Lancet*, **1**, 431–434.]

Effects of Treatment of Hypertension of Pregnancy

	placebo	atenolol
neonatal weight (g)	3017 ± 586	2961 ± 614
apgar (5 min)	9	9
spontaneous respiration delayed >1min (babies)	6	7
placental weight (g)	608 ± 163	549 ± 145
low weight for length of gestation	7	7
hypoglycaemia	4	1
bradycardia	4	18
respiratory distress syndrome requiring ventilation	1	0
bilirubin >250mmol/litre	4	3
proteinuria (>0.5g/d)	10	3

Fig. 6.36 The effects of treatment of hypertension of pregnancy upon the fetus and upon maternal proteinuria in the study shown in Figure 6.35. Proteinuria is significantly reduced. Apart from causing bradycardia, atenolol had no significant effect upon the fetus.

HYPERTENSION IN THE ELDERLY

Epidemiology

Blood pressure changes with age (see chapter 1). In addition, there are more subtle changes in cardiovascular physiology which play a profound role in the prognosis and treatment of hypertension. Defining the elderly is just as arbitrary as defining hypertensive patients, but clinical trials have employed a cut-off point of either 60 or 65 years to define the elderly population. Intthe wealthy countries, systolic blood pressure rises with age, while diastolic blood pressure shows a steady decline. This decline cannot be wholly explained by selective mortality (patients with highest diastolic blood pressures dying prematurely), and it seems likely that in the population as a whole there is a genuine decline in diastolic blood pressure with advancing age. Because systolic and diastolic blood pressures diverge, isolated systolic hypertension becomes more frequent in the elderly.

In the great majority of elderly subjects indirect auscultatory blood pressure measurement is as accurate as it is in younger individuals. However, spurious elevated blood pressure readings can be observed as a result of rigidity of the brachial artery wall (pseudohypertension). One clue to such a situation is the presence of apparently high blood pressure without any other evidence of target organ damage such as left ventricular hypertrophy or retinopathy. Additional help may be given by the presence of Osler's sign (that is, the presence of a palpable radial artery after the pulse has been occluded by inflating a sphygmomanometric cuff proximally). Blood pressure in the elderly also tends to be more variable than in younger subjects as a result of the decline in baroreceptor function, so that posture has a greater effect on blood pressure (see below). It is therefore even more important in this group than in others to obtain several readings for proper clinical assessment. It is impossible to obtain a precise figure for the prevalence of hypertension, which varies according to the population studied and the

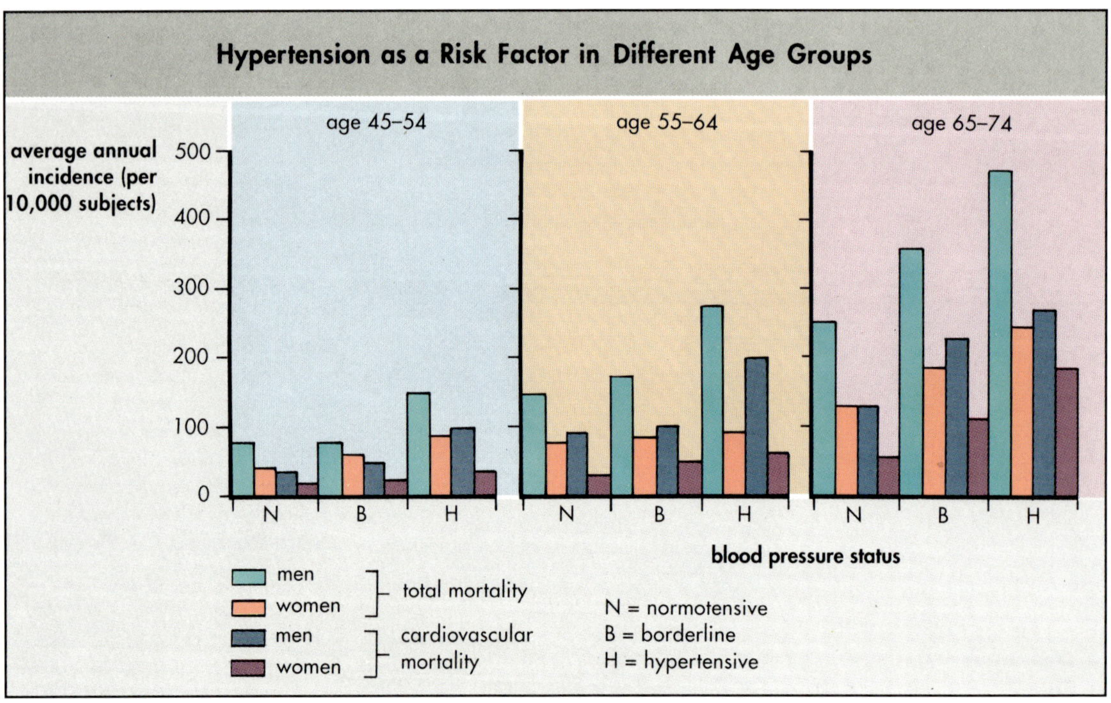

Fig. 6.37 In the Framingham Study, hypertension was just as important a risk factor in the elderly as in the younger age groups. [Modified from Kannel, W.B. (1975) *Angiology*, **26**, 1–14.]

criteria used. In the US National Health Survey, hypertension was defined as a blood pressure equal to or greater than 160/90mmHg – prevalence of systolic and diastolic hypertension combined ranged from 17–24%. However, these data are based upon single readings and because blood pressure usually falls with successive readings, these figures represent a gross over-estimate of the prevalence of hypertension, which is probably only about one-third of these values (6–8%).

Data from both the Framingham study and from life insurance statistics indicate that hypertensive elderly subjects bear an increased risk of death (Fig. 6.37). The 30-year follow-up from the Framingham study indicates that this risk extends beyond the age of 74 into extreme old age. Indeed from these figures, the individual risk of hypertension is greater in the elderly than in younger subjects since strokes and heart attacks are much more common in the elderly (Figs 6.38 % 6.39) and any proportionate increase in risk therefore has much greater absolute effect. Not all studies are in accord with the Framingham and Life Insurance data. Several smaller studies in selected populations have failed to demonstrate a worsening of prognosis in hypertensive subjects. The reasons

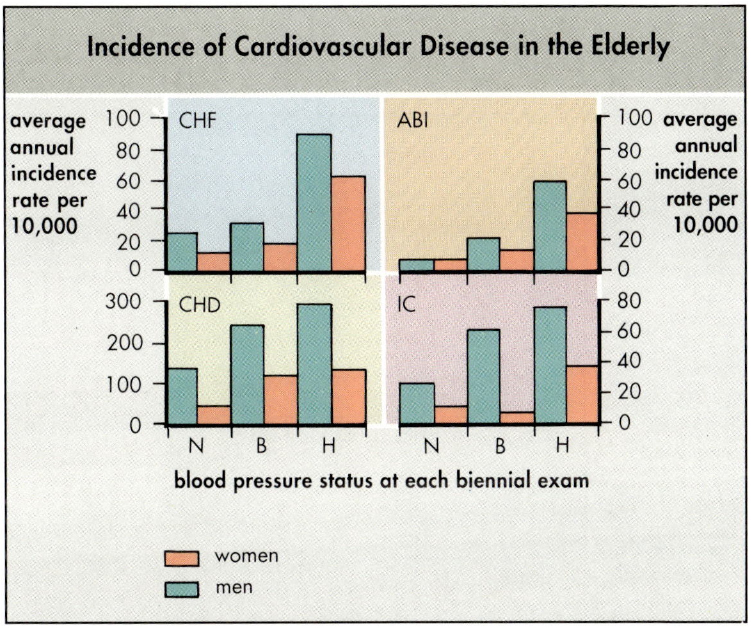

Fig. 6.38 Strokes and heart attacks are more common in the elderly. The average annual incidence of cardiovascular disease is related to blood pressure status (normotensive, borderline or hypertensive) at each biennial examination of men and women aged 55–64 years at entry into the Framingham Study: this is an 18-year follow-up. CHF = congestive heart failure; ABI = atherothrombotic brain infarction; CHD = coronary heart disease; IC = intermittent claudication. (Modified from Framingham Monograph No. 30.)

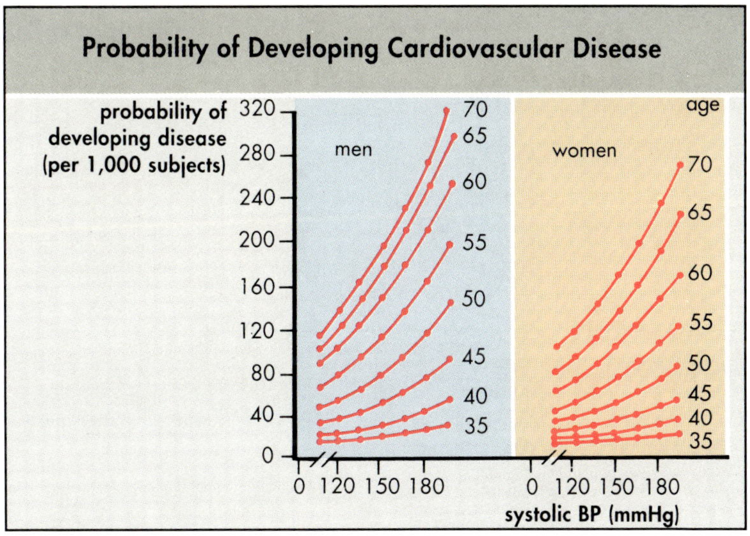

Fig. 6.39 The probability, according to systolic blood pressure, of low-risk persons developing cardiovascular diseasewithin eight years rises with age. Subjects were non-smokers aged 35–70 at the time of entry to the study, with serum cholesterol ≤185mg%, normal glucose tolerance and no ECG–LVH. (Modified from Framingham Monograph No. 28.)

for these discrepancies are uncertain but it seems possible that in some individuals low blood pressure may be a manifestation of serious circulatory or other disease and therefore associated with a worse prognosis.

Pathophysiology

The ageing process has an important effect upon cardiovascular physiology. From the standpoint of hypertension this interaction is relevant at several different sites (Fig. 6.40):

- the large arteries;
- baroreceptor reflexes;
- the heart;
- the kidney.

Deteriorating intellectual capacity may worsen the clinical picture.

Large Arteries

The increase in systolic blood pressure with age is largely due to degenerative changes in the aorta and the large arteries (Windkessel vessels). Contraction of the heart in systole forces blood into these vessels. Since they normally have a substantial content of elastic tissues in their walls they distend (distensibility being measured as 'compliance'). At the end of systole the elastic pressure exerted by the distended vessel wall forces blood down the arterial tree since blood cannot return through the aortic valve (Fig.6.41). As a result of ageing the elastic fibres of the Windkessel vessels uncoil and fracture leaving relatively inelastic collagen. In addition calcium is deposited in substantial quantities in the media. As a result there is a progressive loss of elasticity. The force generated

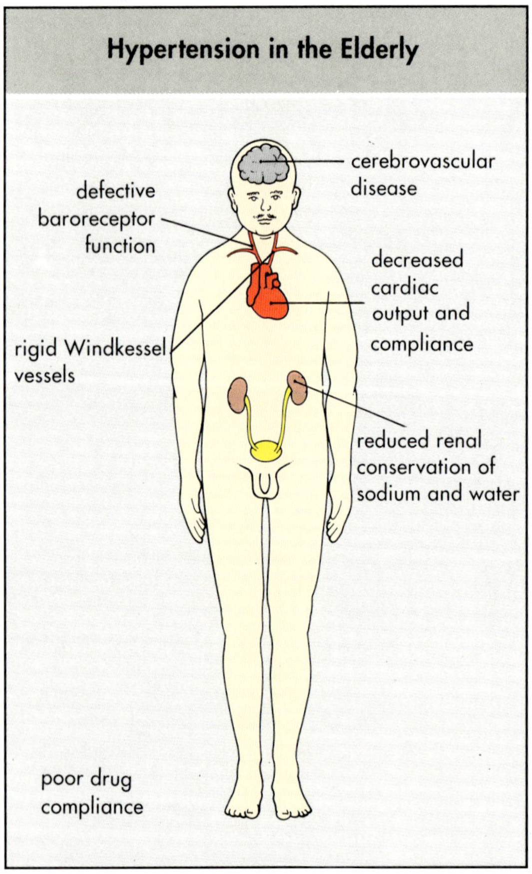

Fig. 6.40 The elderly patient presents particular problems in his response to antihypertensive therapy because of associated cerebrovascular disease, defective baroreceptor function, rigid Windkessel vessels and reduced conservation of sodium and water.

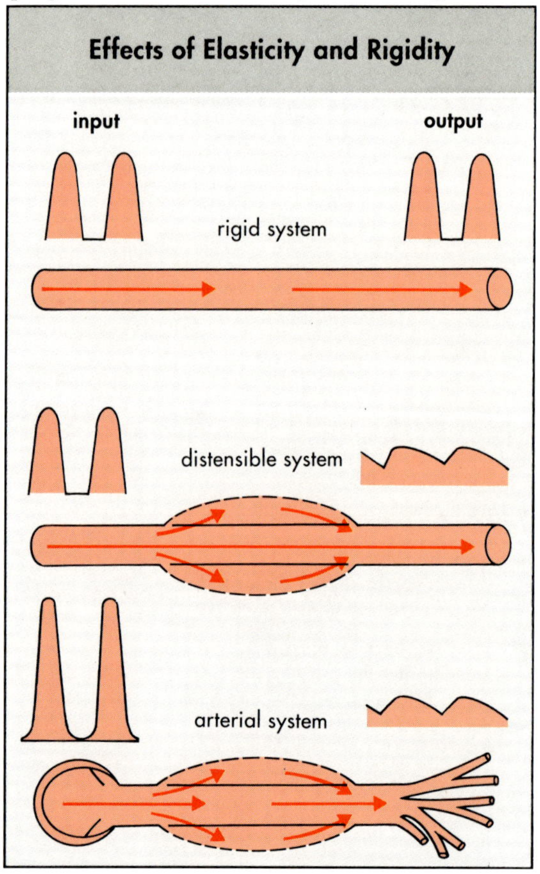

Fig. 6.41 The effect of rigidity and elasticity upon wave transmission in a fluid-filled system. The distensible system dampens the pressure wave which is reduced in amplitude and prolonged in duration.

during systole is therefore transmitted to the more peripheral parts of the arterial tree in a less damped form (Fig. 6.42). A large pulse pressure with high systolic pressure and relatively low diastolic pressure is therefore characteristic of the elderly (Fig. 6.43). This loss of elasticity creates additional problems when hypertension is treated. There may be a disproportionate fall in both diastolic and systolic pressure as a result of using agents which reduce stroke volume (for example diuretics or ß-blockers). Indeed it may be impossible to lower systolic blood pressure to normal levels without producing unacceptable diastolic hypotension – a too enthusiastic pursuit of the ideal may cause a stroke or impairment of consciousness, especially if the pressure falls rapidly.

Baroreceptor Reflexes

Baroreflex sensitivity declines with increasing age (Fig. 6.44). This can be demonstrated by measuring the reflex bradycardia produced when the blood pressure is raised pharmacologically with an agent such as phenylephrine. Alternatively, the tachycardia produced by sodium nitroprusside infusion can be measured. Under these circumstances blood pressure shows a greater fall in elderly subjects than in younger subjects. The loss of baroreceptor function also contributes to the greater variability of systolic blood pressure which has been demonstrated using indirect intra-arterial ambulatory monitoring in elderly patients. The reasons for the loss of baroreflex sensitivity are

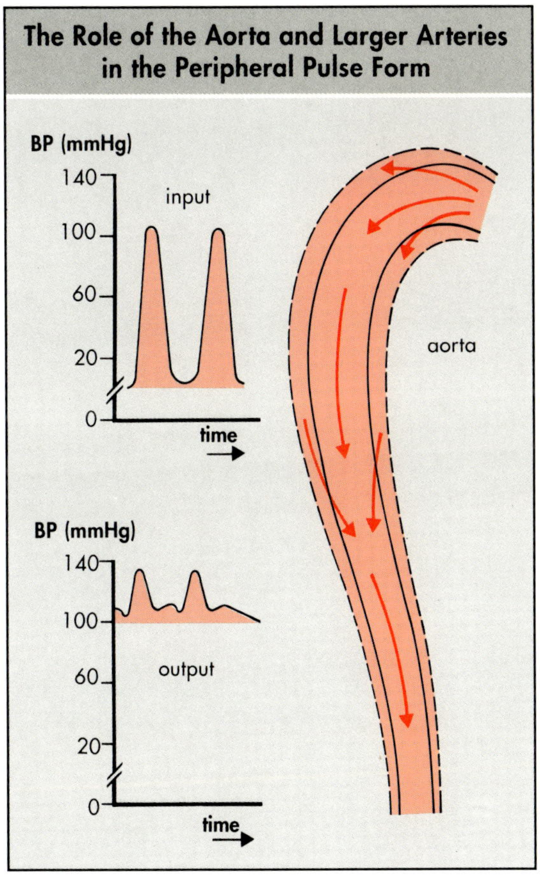

Fig. 6.42 The role of the aorta and larger arteries in determining the wave-form of the peripheral pulse. During systole the aorta is distended, storing energy which is released as kinetic energy in diastole. The net effect is therefore a reduction in systolic blood pressure and an increase in diastolic blood pressure in the peripheral vessels.

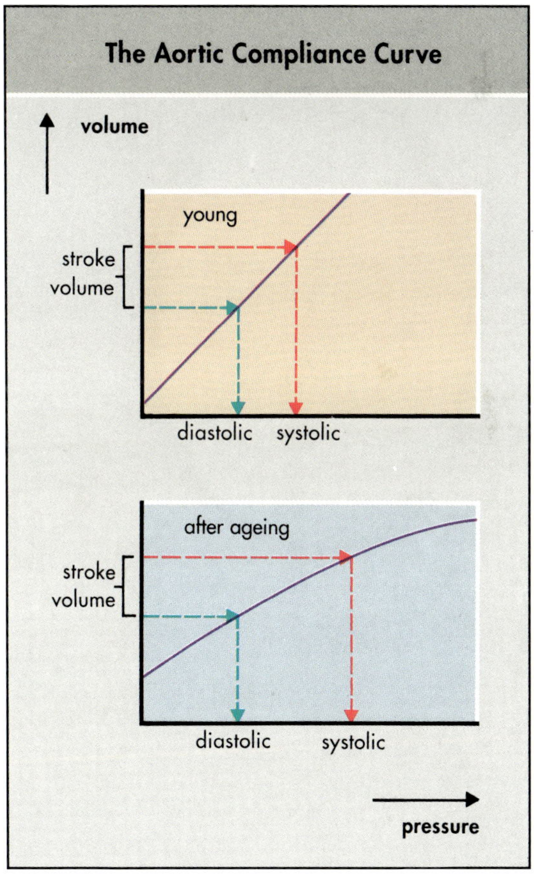

Fig. 6.43 The effect of ageing on the aortic compliance curve. The relationship between the volume of fluid injected into the aorta during systole, and the pressure generated, ceases to be linear (lower graph), so that pulse pressure is increased with a higher systolic and lower diastolic pressure. Reduction of systolic pressure produces a greater fall in diastolic pressure.

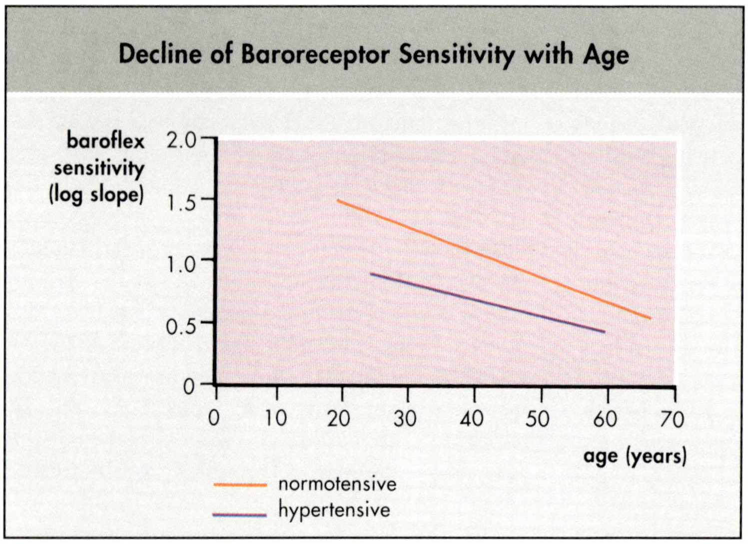

Fig. 6.44 Baroreceptor sensitivity (the slope of the line relating pulse interval and pressure) declines with age.

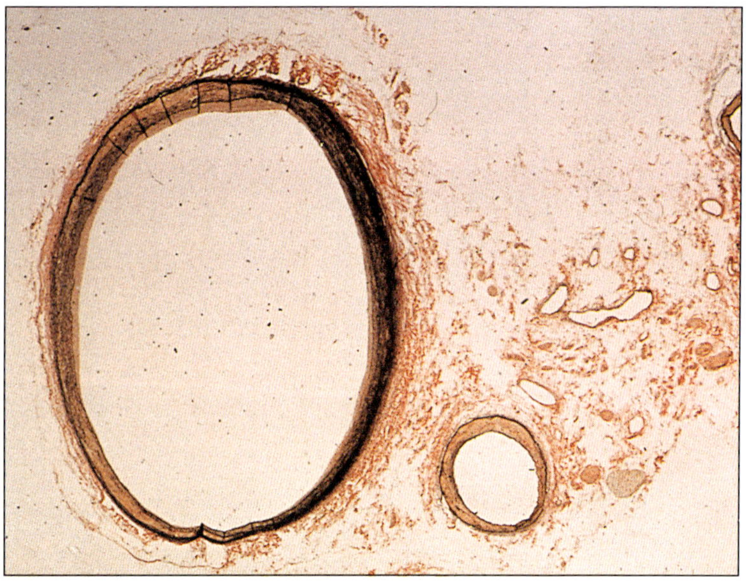

Fig. 6.45 Internal and external carotid artery from a 23-year-old man. Note the comparatively thin arterial wall.

controversial. One contributory factor is probably the increased rigidity of the arterial wall (Figs 6.45 & 6.46) in the region of the carotid and aortic baroreceptor, diminishing its capacity to respond to changes in pressure. There is also, however, a reduction in the response of cardiac ß-receptors to agonists so that the normal tachycardia produced by a fall in blood pressure is attenuated.

The clinical importance of reduced baroreceptor sensitivity is twofold. Firstly, the ability of the circulation to respond to changes in posture may be impaired, causing postural hypotension (Fig. 6.47). Secondly, if blood pressure is reduced excessively as a result of medication, compensatory mechanisms are inhibited (Fig. 6.48). Hypotensive responses to medication are therefore particularly common in the elderly.

The Heart

Left ventricular compliance and cardiac decrease and left ventricular mass increases with ageing. The clinical significance of this is still uncertain, but impairment of the ability to increase cardiac output may contribute to an exaggerated hypotensive response to agents that reduce venous return to the heart, such as diuretics or nitrates.

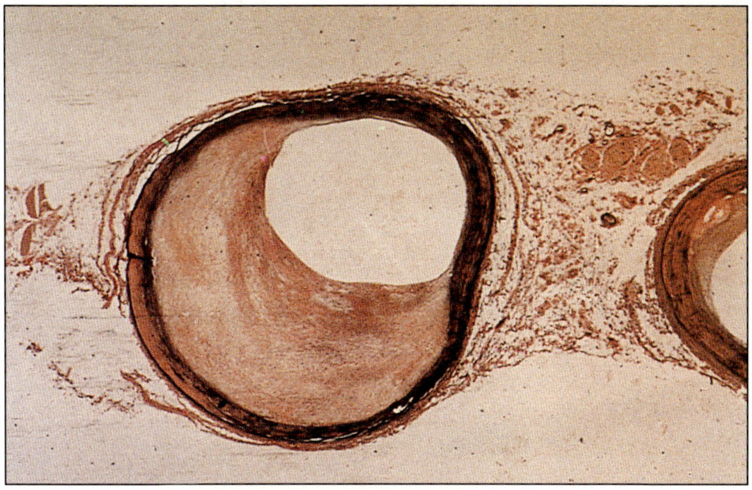

Fig. 6.46 Internal and external carotid artery from an 83-year-old patient. Note the increased thickening of the arterial wall with extensive collagen deposition.

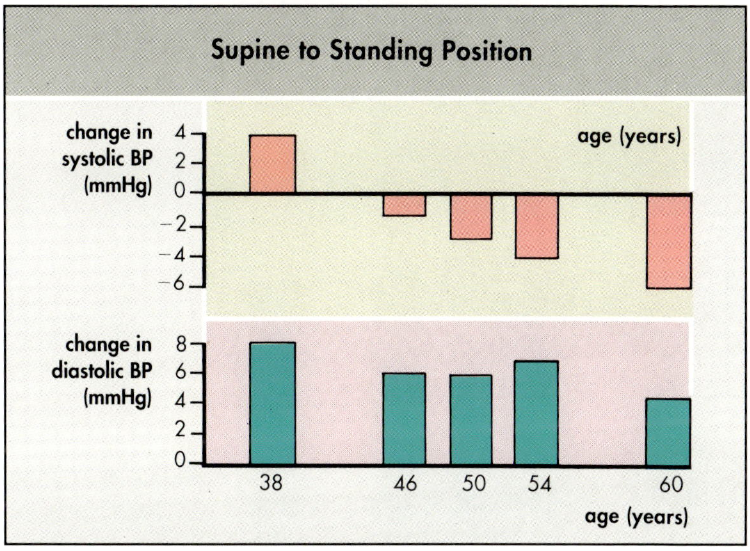

Fig. 6.47 Change in blood pressure produced by moving from the supine to the standing position. Systolic blood pressure falls and diastolic blood pressure rises slightly. The fall in systolic blood pressure is greater in the older age groups.

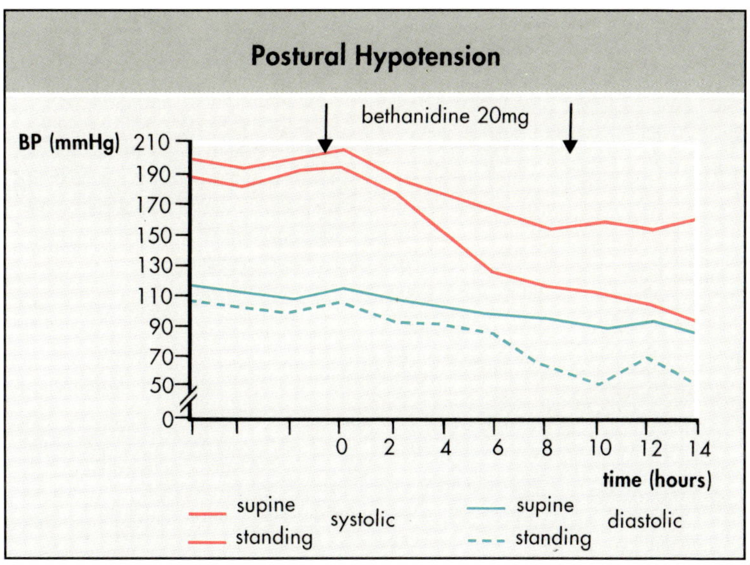

Fig. 6.48 Post-ganglionic adrenergic blocking agents are particulary liable to cause problems in elderly patients. In this patient, the use of bethanidine (two 20mg doses) was associated with incapacitating postural hypotension.

The Kidneys

All aspects of renal function decline with age. In particular, renal blood flow, glomerular filtration rate and urinary concentration, dilution and acidification all show a progressive fall. Histologically the number of hyalinized glomeruli (Fig. 6.49) increases and surviving nephrons show a reduction both in glomerular surface area and tubular volume, perhaps as a result of the decrease in renal blood flow. These changes may have important effects upon the management of hypertension. Thus, renal conservation of sodium in the face of salt restriction is impaired (Fig. 6.50). As a result, when elderly patients are placed on a sodium-restricted diet, urinary sodium takes longer to come into equilibrium than it does in younger patients. Patients thus become more sodium-depleted before finally coming into balance. This may be of importance when treating patients with diuretics or by means of salt restriction.

It is possible that the decline in renal function contributes to the rise in systolic blood pressure observed in the elderly. Alternatively, elevated blood pressure might contribute to deterioration in renal function. There is a significant, albeit

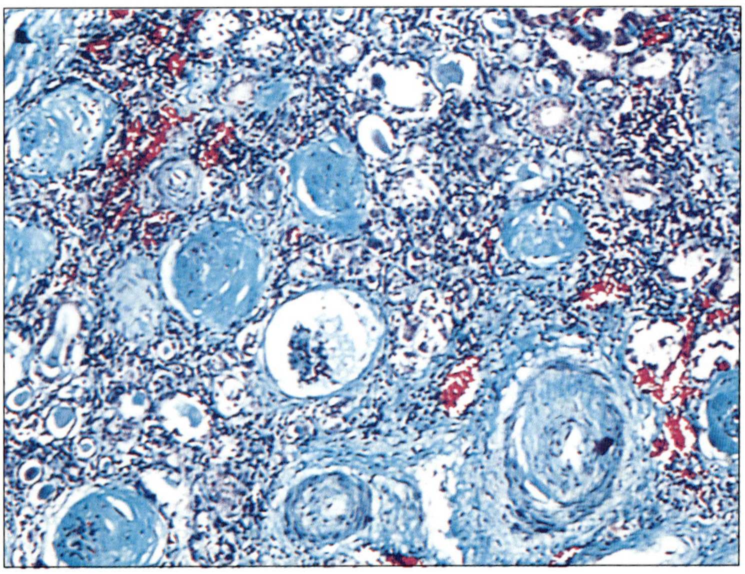

Fig. 6.49 Hyalinized glomeruli in the kidney of an elderly patient.

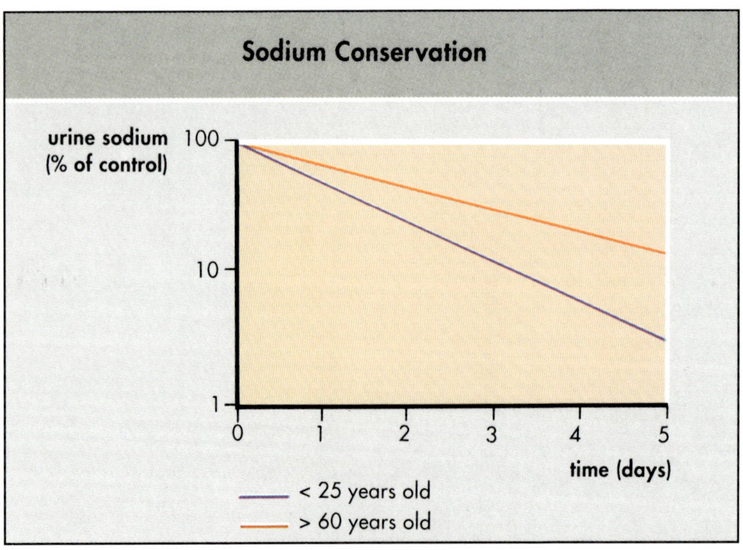

Fig. 6.50 The ability of the elderly patient to conserve sodium is reduced. Thus when subjects were placed on a severely salt-restricted diet, the rate of fall in urinary sodium was less in the elderly patients and as a result intake and output only came into equilibrium at a greater level of body salt depletion.

weak correlation between the change in creatinine clearance with age and the initial blood pressure in elderly hypertensives followed over a period of years (Fig. 6.51). There is, however, no evidence for either sodium retention or elevated plasma renin (see below) in hypertension observed in elderly subjects, and it seems more likely therefore that elevated blood pressure participates in the genesis of chronic renal damage.

The kidney also acts as an endocrine organ through the secretion of renin. Plasma renin levels decrease with age (Fig. 6.52) and the response of plasma renin to such stimulatory manoeuvres as dietary treatment, salt restriction or tilting is also impaired. This phenomenon may be a manifestation of the reduced ß-adrenoceptor responsiveness already mentioned, or it could reflect reduced distensibility of the afferent glomerular baroreceptor. The renin–angiotensin system assumes particular importance in blood pressure maintenance when the circulation is put under stress by postural change, sodium and fluid depletion or haemorrhage. The impaired renin responsiveness could therefore prove additive to the effects of impaired baroreflex control, adrenoceptor sensitivity and reduced capacity to maintain sodium balance.

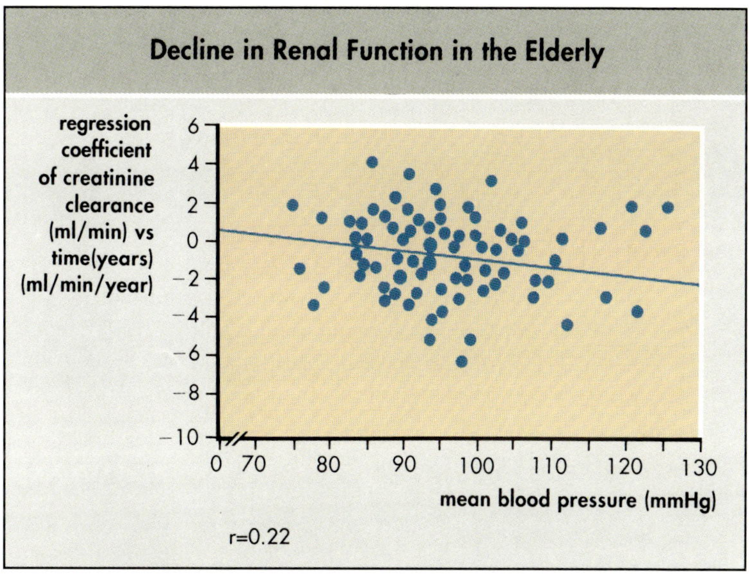

Fig. 6.51 In the elderly the greatest decline in renal function is observed in subjects with the highest blood pressure. These data show regression coefficients, plotting the decline in renal function (change in creatinine clearance vs. time in years) against mean blood pressure in 3,254 normal subjects. [Modified from Lindeman *et al.* (1984) *Kidney International*, **26**, 861–868.]

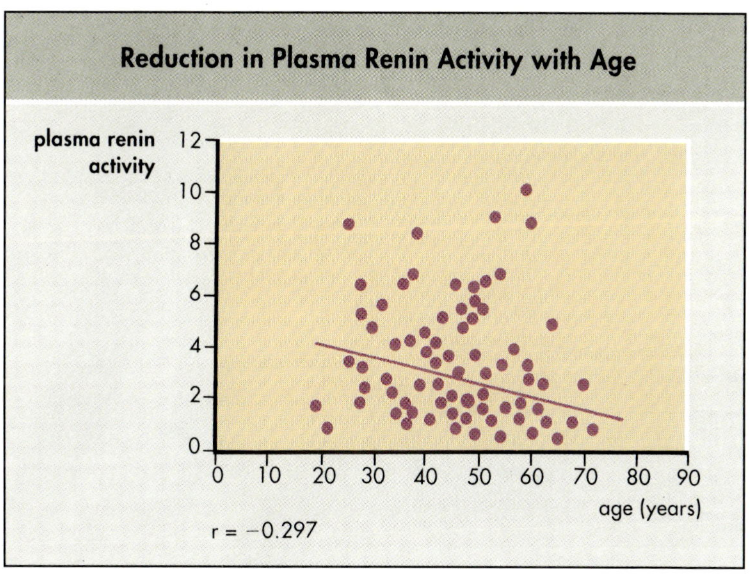

Fig. 6.52 Plasma renin in untreated hypertensive patients falls with age. Thus the proportion of patients with low-renin hypertension tends to increase with age.

Effect of Treatment on the Frequency of Cerebrovascular Events – EWPHE

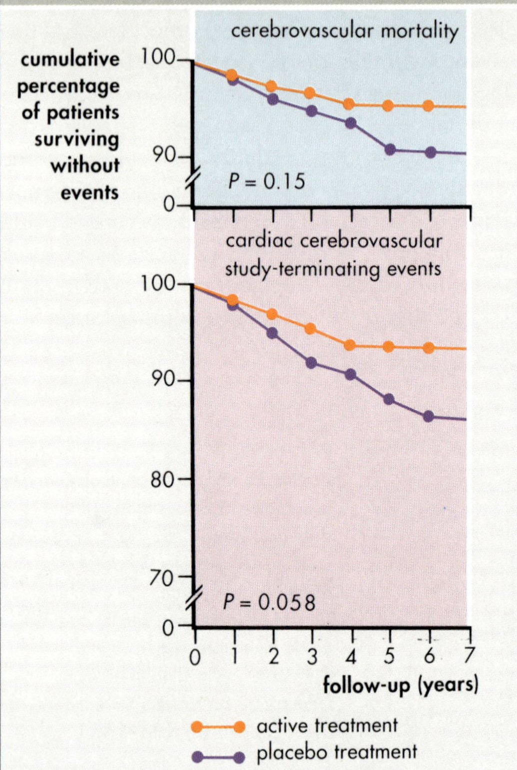

Fig. 6.53 Treatment significantly reduces strokes in patients over 60, as can be seen from the cumulative percentage of survivors without cerebrovascular study-terminating events, calculated for the patients on randomized treatment using the life table method. Cerebrovascular study-terminating events include cerebrovascular deaths, cerebral haemorrhage and retinal haemorrhages, exudates or papilloedema. [Modified from Amery *et al.* (1985) *J Hypertension*, **3**, S501–S508.]

Effects of Treatment

Two large multi-centre trials – the European Working Party on Hypertension in the Elderly (EWPHE) and the Hypertension in the Elderly in Primary Care (HEP) studies – have shown a significant reduction in strokes in patients over 60 using a variety of treatments (Figs 6.53 & 6.54). In the subgroup of patients over 80 years of age in the EWPHE trial benefits of treatment were not evident. Total cardiac mortality was also reduced in EWPHE (Fig. 6.55) although the incidence of myocardial infarction was not affected. Cardiac mortality was not influenced in HEP. Since the incidence of strokes is much greater in the elderly the absolute benefits of treatment to the individual are much greater in this age group. Both these trials are also important in demonstrating that with appropriate care it is possible to maintain good blood pressure control in elderly patients without an unacceptably high withdrawal rate.

Conclusions

The physiological changes produced by ageing (Fig. 6.56) render the elderly patient more susceptible to hypotension as a result of therapy, rapid changes of posture or disease. In addition decline in mental function may impair the individual's capacity to comply with antihypertensive regimes. Drug pharmacokinetics may be altered and as a result adverse effects are more common. The treatment of high blood pressure therefore requires especially careful monitoring, with the avoidance of alterations in drug regimes likely to produce major acute changes in blood pressure.

Effect of Treatment on Stroke in the Elderly – HEP

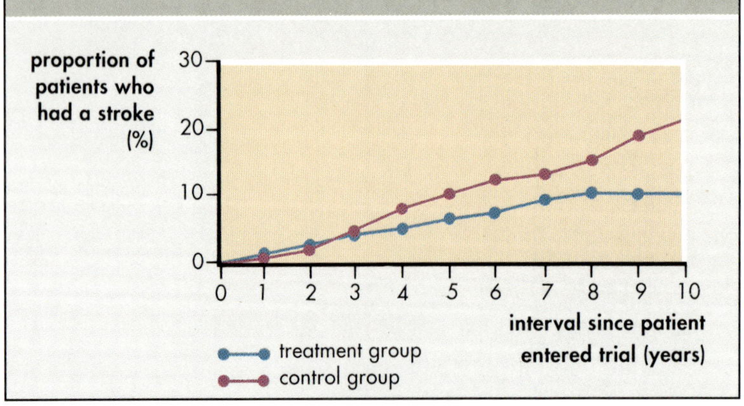

Fig. 6.54 Treatment significantly reduced the proportion of patients who had a stroke (transient ischaemic attack, minor, major or fatal) in the interval since entry to the HEP trial. [Modified from Coope & and Warrender (1986) *Brit Med J*, **243**, 1145–1151.]

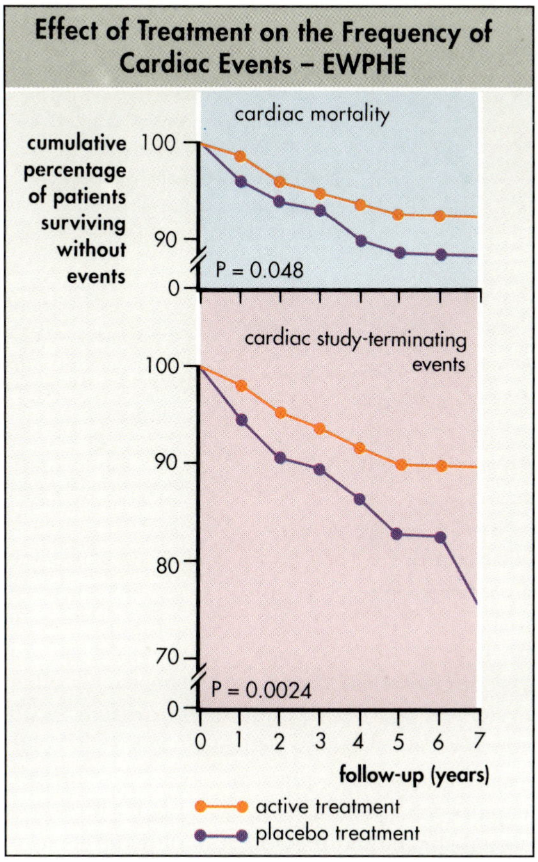

Fig. 6.55 Treatment significantly reduces cardiac deaths and severe congestive heart failure in patients over 50, as can be seen from the cumulative percentage of survivors without cardiac study-terminating events, calculated for patients on randomized treatment, using the life table method. Cardiac study-terminating events include cardiac deaths and severe congestive heart failure in the EWPHE study. [Modified from Amery *et al.* (1985) *J Hypertension*, **3**, S501–S508.]

HYPERTENSIVE EMERGENCIES

The vast majority of hypertensive patients are treated in the office, surgery or clinic. Occasionally however the sequelae of hypertension become life-threatening and immediate emergency treatment is then required. The risks are also high when severe hypertension develops acutely. The likelihood of vascular catastrophe is much greater under these circumstances.

The Malignant Phase of Hypertension

The malignant or accelerated phase may occur in either essential or secondary hypertension. There appear to be two predisposing factors. These are the absolute height of blood pressure and the rate of rise of blood pressure. The latter is particularly important. Thus, malignant hypertension is relatively unusual in coarctation of the aorta, whereas it is relatively common in renovascular hypertension of short duration (see Fig. 6.57). Partial obstruction of the renal artery may however precipitate a rapid rise in blood pressure and malignant hypertension in a patient with pre-existing essential hypertension. Such an acute change in the natural history of hypertension in a particular individual should therefore always indicate the possibility of such an event. Malignant hypertension is more common in males than in females and in Blacks compared with Whites. It most commonly occurs between the ages of 40 and 50, although it is occasionally seen in individuals below the age of 35 or over the age of 60. Patients may be asymptomatic although they more usually complain of early morning or occipital headache, blurring of

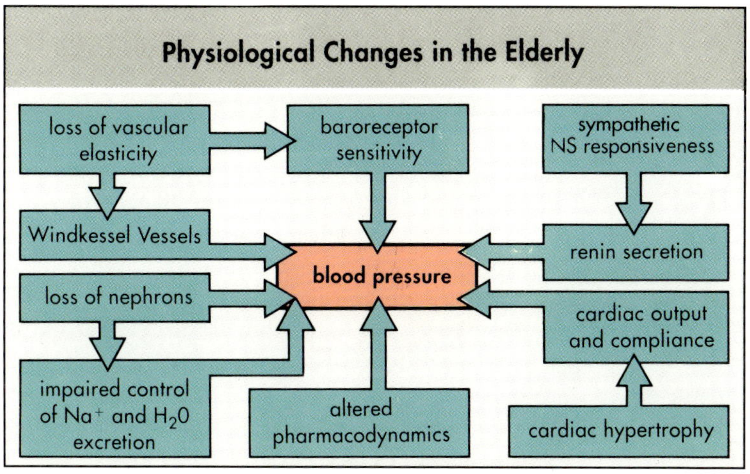

Fig. 6.56 Physiological changes encountered in the elderly that affect blood pressure control.

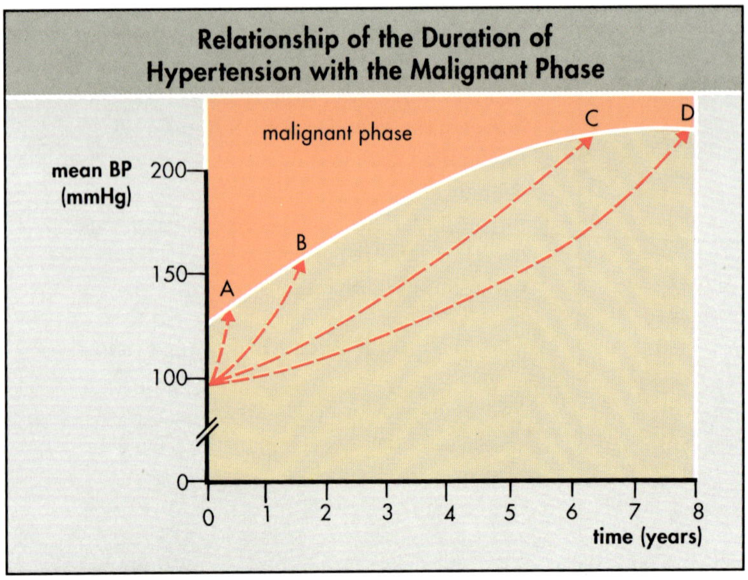

Fig. 6.57 The malignant phase of hypertension tends to supervene at lower blood pressure levels when the duration of hypertension is short (A and B). When the history is prolonged, malignant hypertension usually occurs at higher blood pressure levels (C and D).

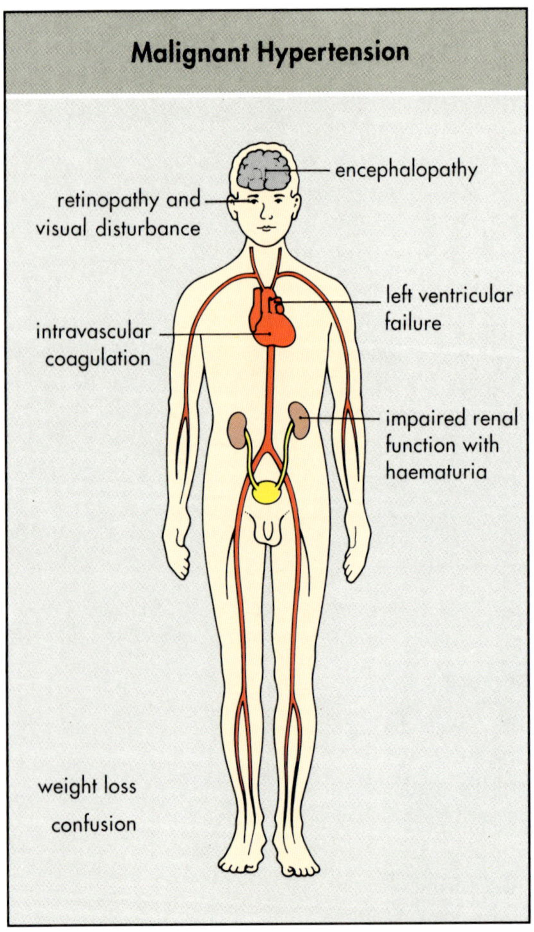

Fig. 6.58 Although malignant hypertension may be asymptomatic, it is frequently associated with clinical features which may suggest the diagnosis.

vision, mental impairment or dyspnoea. On other occasions patients sometimes present with advanced renal failure or weight loss (Fig. 6.58). The characteristic physical signs are fundal. Papilloedema (Fig. 6.59) is associated with raised cerebrospinal fluid pressure. Cotton-wool spots or haemorrhages, even in the absence of papilloedema, convey the same serious prognostic import; it has become customary to regard the presence of any of these abnormalities as indicating the malignant phase of hypertension. The cardinal pathological hallmark is fibrinoid necrosis of the arterioles. The correlation between the presence of fundal changes and fibrinoid necrosis is close but not complete.

Before effective antihypertensive drugs became available the prognosis of malignant hypertension was grave, with most subjects dying within two years of diagnosis. This has now however been revolutionized by the development of effective treatments. The most important prognostic feature is the presence of renal failure. Thus, even when blood pressure is controlled effectively where the patient has significant renal impairment, life expectancy is still reduced (Fig. 6.60). When renal function is not impaired significantly on presentation, medium- and short-term prognosis is excellent. Minor changes in renal function with some proteinuria and haematuria are however seen in the vast majority of patients with malignant hypertension (Fig. 6.61).

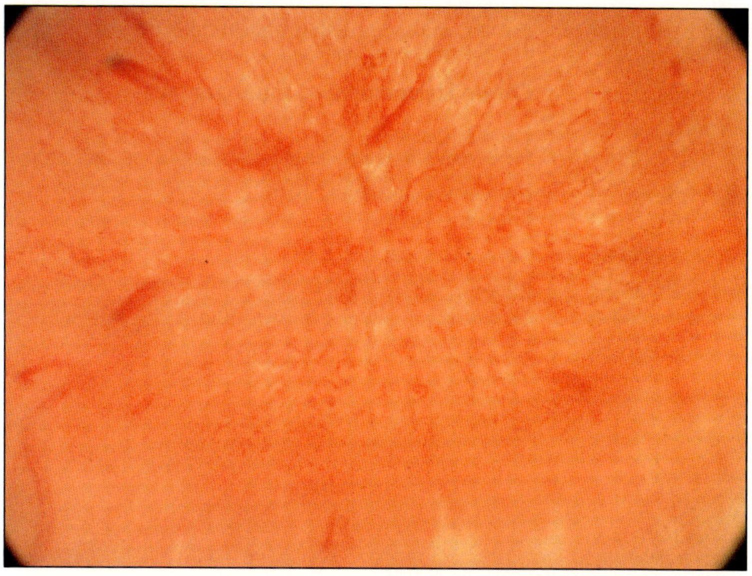

Fig. 6.59 Papilloedema in malignant hypertension. The disc is swollen and pink with the loss of the normal optic cup. The blood vessels are partly obscured as they pass over the borders of the disc.

Life Expectancy with Renal Impairment

	all	grade IV	grade III	IRF	NRF	EHT
n	100	38	62	40	60	68
systolic blood pressure (mmHg)	218 ± 3	217 ± 5	218 ± 5	221 ± 6	215 ± 4	217 ± 4
diastolic blood pressure (mmHg)	128 ± 2	132 ± 4	125 ± 2	131 ± 3	125 ± 3	128 ± 2
serum creatinine > 150 mmol/l (%)	40	50	34	(100)	(0)	28
5-year survival (%)	82 ± 4	73 ± 7	87 ± 4	65 ± 8	96 ± 3	88 ± 4
10-year survival (%)	67 ± 5	65 ± 8	67 ± 6	51 ± 8	81 ± 5	73 ± 5

Fig. 6.60 Life expectancy is reduced in renal impairment, even if blood pressure is controlled. Five- and ten-year survivals of 100 cases of accelerated-malignant hypertension and subgroups according to presence or absence of papilloedema and normal or impaired renal function (means ± s.e.m.). IRF = impaired renal function; NRF = normal renal function; EHT = essential hypertension. [Modified from Bing *et al.* (1986) *J Hypertension*, **4**, S42–S44.]

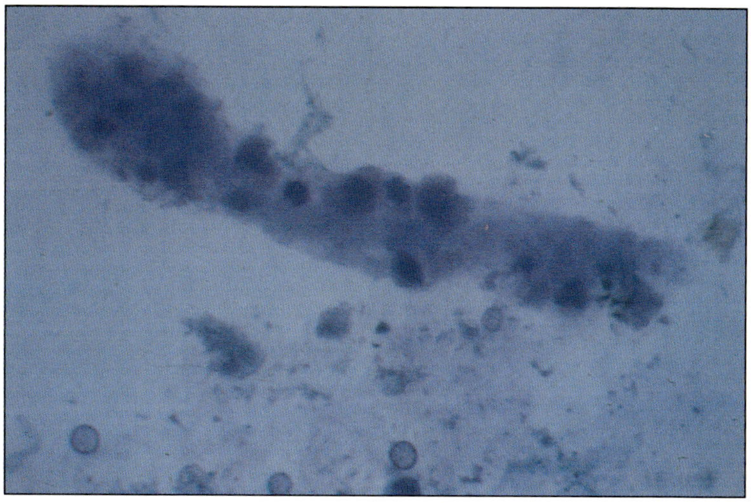

Fig. 6.61 Urine microscopy from a patient with malignant hypertension showing red cells and casts. Courtesy of Professor K. Porter.

In the absence of left ventricular failure or hypertensive encephalopathy patients with malignant hypertension should be treated orally with drugs, as rapid lowering of pressure by intravenous therapy is associated with a substantial risk of brain and retinal infarction. Even vigorous oral therapy may be associated with a temporary decline in renal function (Fig. 6.62) due to a fall in renal perfusion pressure and renal blood low. This change is usually reversed with the passage of time, however, and steady improvement of renal function can be obtained in patients treated for malignant hypertension (Fig. 6.63) as long as renal damage is not far advanced when treatment is begun.

Other Hypertensive Emergencies

Hypertensive left ventricular failure is an important life-threatening condition which merits parenteral therapy to restore blood pressure to normal levels (Fig. 6.64). This is also true of hypertensive encephalopathy, which results from the elevation of blood pressure above the autoregulatory range (which may range up to a mean pres-

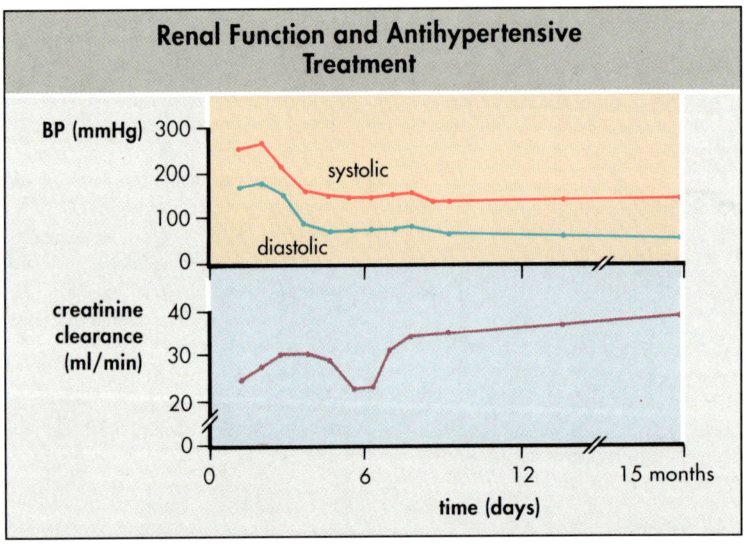

Fig. 6.62 Effect of antihypertensive treatment on blood pressure and renal function of a patient with malignant hypertension. A marked decrease in creatinine clearance occurred at the end of the first week, but renal function then improved progressively as renal hypertensive vascular damage was reversed.

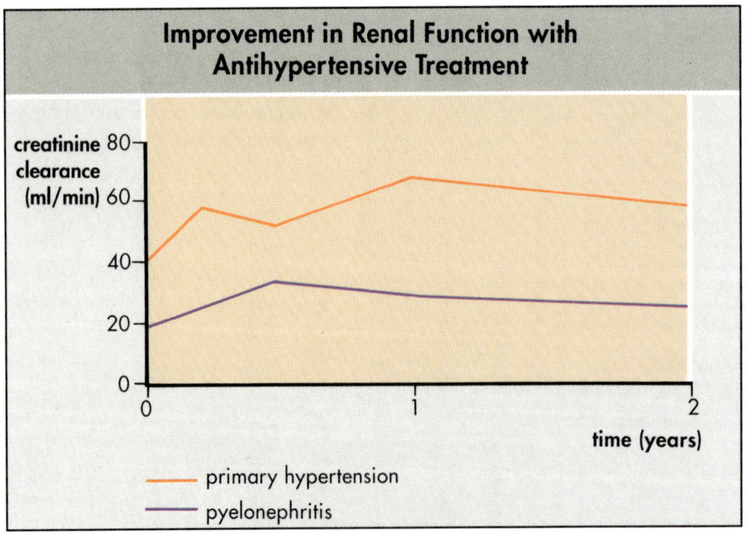

Fig. 6.63 Renal function in a group of patients with malignant hypertension. With intensive treatment of blood pressure a significant increase in glomerular filtration rate was observed. A smaller increase occurred in patients with radiological evidence of chronic pyelonephritis, suggesting that hypertension probably played some role in the renal failure of these patients.

sure of 200mmHg in hypertensive individuals). Although the cardinal features of encephalopathy are transient neurological signs, fits and disturbances in consciousness (including coma) it is often difficult to distinguish between these signs and those due to a cerebrovascular accident, except perhaps retrospectively. Examination of the retina, looking for the presence or absence of papilloedema, haemorrhages and exudates, is often helpful.

Life-threatening hypertension may also develop during the course of several diseases or as a result of adverse drug reactions (Figs 6.65 & 6.66).

Acute Hypertensive Crises
hypertensive crisis
scleroderma eclampsia acute glomerulonephritis phaeochromocytoma
adverse interaction of drugs
withdrawal of clonidine tyramine and monoamine oxidase inhibitors adrenergic neurone blocking drugs and sympathomimetic amines

Fig. 6.65 Hypertension occasionally presents as an acute hypertensive crisis. This can occur during the course of certain diseases or as a result of an adverse drug interaction.

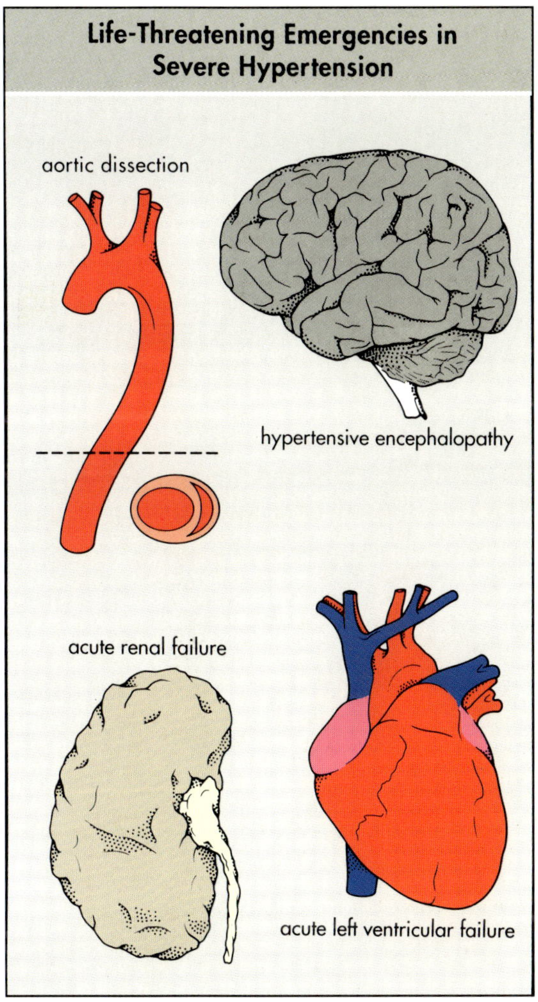

Fig. 6.64 Life-threatening emergencies occurring in severe hypertension.

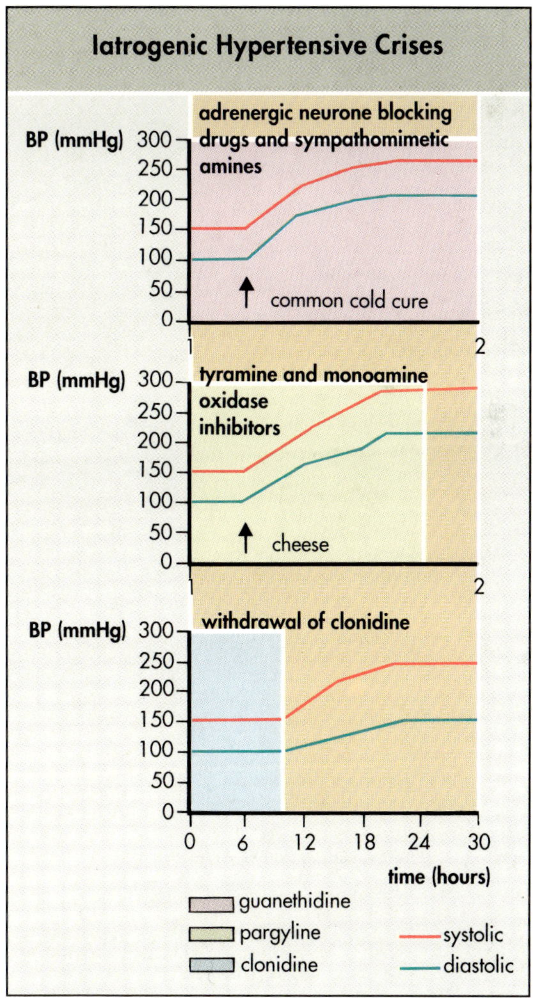

Fig. 6.66 Hypertensive crisis may be iatrogenic. In these three clinical situations, paroxysmal hypertension was associated with evidence of sympathetic overactivity.

FURTHER READING

Chesley, L. C. (1978) *Hypertension in Pregnancy*. New York: Appleton-Century-Croft.

Dyer, A. R. Stamler, J., Skekelle, R.B., Schoenberger, J.A., Farinaro, E. (1977) Hypertension in the elderly. *Medical Clinics of North America*, **61**, 513–531.

Hofman, A. (1984) Blood pressure in childhood: An epidemiological approach to the aetiology of hypertension. *Journal of Hypertension*, **2**, 323–328.

Kotchen, E. (Ed.) (1980) High blood pressure in the young. *Hypertension*, **2**, I-1–I-135.

Svensson, A. (1985) Hypertension in pregnancy. *Journal of Hypertension*, **3**, (Suppl. 3), S395–S403.

Swales, J. D. (1986) Pathophysiology of blood pressure in the elderly. *Advanced Geriatric Medicine*, **5**, 89–96

CHAPTER 7

History and Examination

INTRODUCTION

Raised blood pressure is usually asymptomatic, unless severe, and even malignant hypertension may pass unnoticed by the patient and physician. Many cases are found by chance on routine examination, of which blood pressure measurement should be an integral part (Fig. 7.1).

The most common symptom of hypertension is headache, either early in the morning or at the weekend, when people lie in bed longer than usual. Alcohol may precipitate the headache, the typical site of which is occipital – this can occur even without excessive consumption, probably as a result of raised intracranial pressure. The precipitating diastolic pressure is usually 120mmHg and above, except when the pressure is rising abruptly as it does in eclampsia, acute glomerulonephritis, or phaeochromocytoma, when headache occurs at lower pressures. Less specific types of headache may be related to the anxiety of knowing that blood pressure is raised (Fig. 7.2). In such cases, the patient can usefully be questioned about migraine. Although not directly linked to high blood pressure, migraine may reflect an anxious disposition, causing labile blood pressure, or even indicate an excessive consumption of ergot or analgesics, which can be causally linked to high blood pressure. Epistaxis is not commonly due to a raised blood pressure except in the presence of renal failure.

Visual disturbance is an occasional symptom, frequently presenting as unilateral blurring of vision due to retinal venous obstruction, with haemorrhages and exudates often involving the macula. Arterial obstruction, usually due to emboli from atheromatous carotid arteries, is less common. Even papilloedema may cause little complaint although, in malignant hypertension, blurring occurs with macular changes and retinal oedema. Shortness of breath after effort is also common (Fig. 7.3) and nocturnal dyspnoea occurs at the higher pressures, especially with acute glomerulonephritis, eclampsia, and coronary artery disease. Occasionally, patients present with congestive cardiac failure having had very few symptoms of pulmonary congestion; children with hypertension often present in this fashion.

Angina pectoris is a common condition and may be the presenting symptom in hypertension, as may intermittent claudication due to atheromatous arteries of the leg. Atheromatous vascular disease is a common companion of hypertension, especially in smokers.

Nocturia occurs when the blood pressure rises quickly or when the diastolic pressure reaches

Discovering Hypertension

insurance and employment medicals

screening programmes

case-finding by general practitioners

contraceptive pill ⎤
⎬ routine measurement
pregnancy ⎦

Fig. 7.1 The ways in which high blood pressure is discovered.

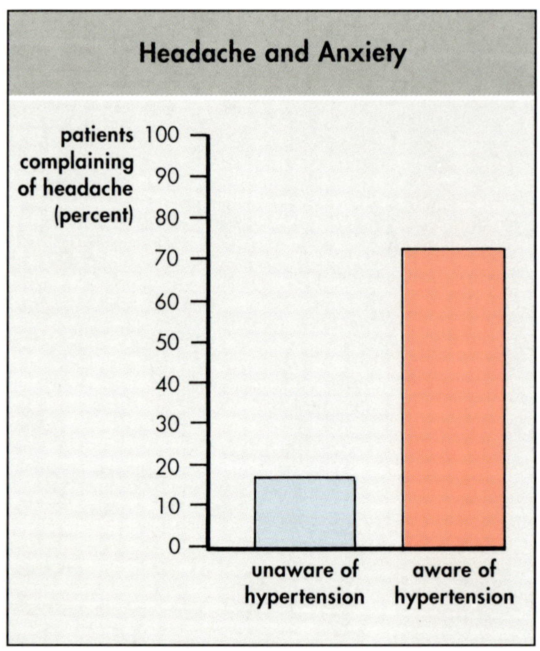

Fig. 7.2 Effect of knowledge of a raised blood pressure on the incidence of headache.

120–130mmHg consistently. This is the so-called 'pressure diuresis' which causes the patient to get up two to three times during the night, and which stops when the pressure is lowered. Occasionally, loin pain with haematuria occurs; while this may sometimes be due to pyelonephritis (especially in women with a previous history of urinary infection and/or diabetes), it may also be the result of a renal infarct secondary to atheromatous renal vascular disease. Frank haematuria occasionally reveals malignant hypertension. Acute glomerulonephritis must always be borne in mind, especially if pulmonary oedema and headache are prominent at lower than expected pressures (180/110mmHg). Similarly, epileptiform seizures are a presentation of acute glomerulonephritis, eclampsia, and of malignant hypertension. In malignant hypertension, admission to a neurological service with a diagnosis of cerebral tumour may occur before the basic cause is discovered, especially if unilateral papilloedema and hypertensive encephalopathy or asymmetrical neurological signs are present.

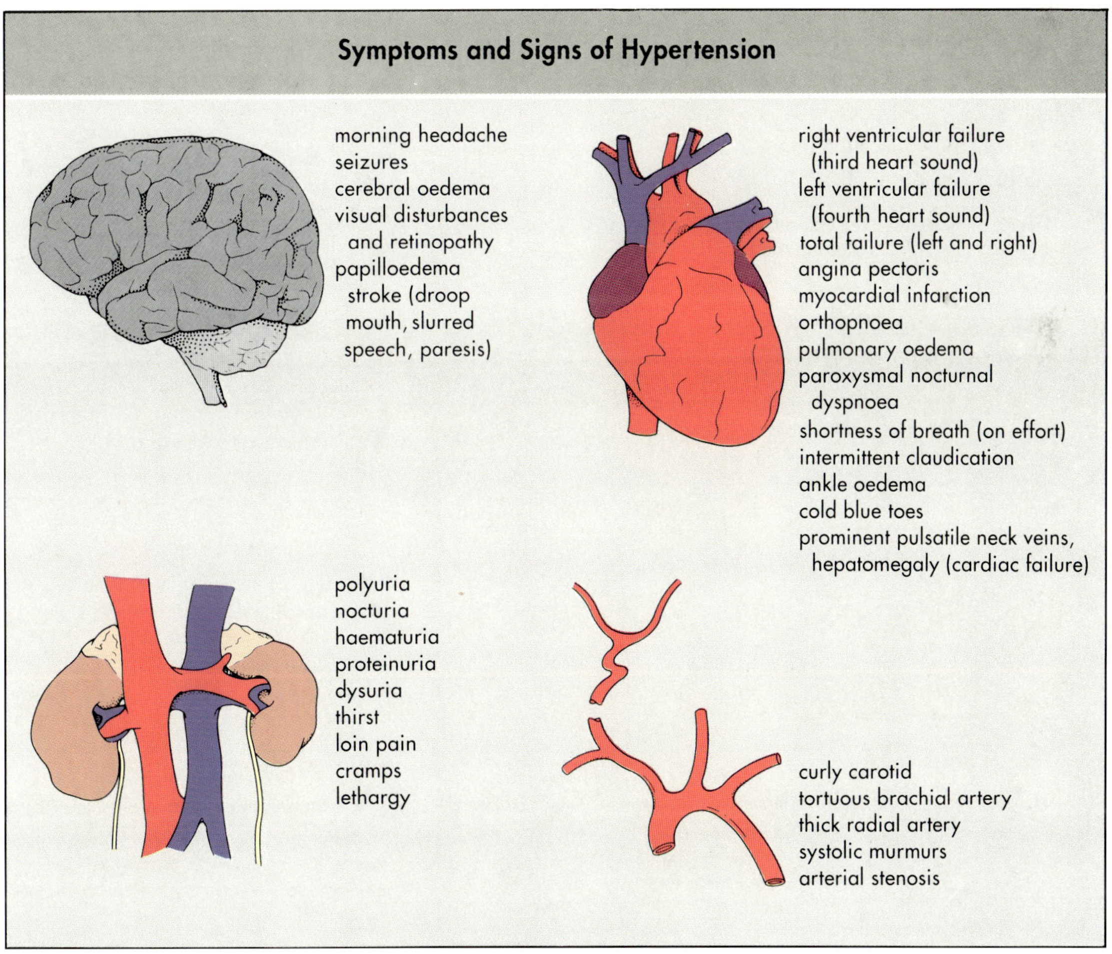

Fig. 7.3 Main cardiovascular, renal, and neurological symptoms and signs associated with hypertension.

Subarachnoid haemorrhage may present as severe headache with unilateral papilloedema and hypertension. In some cases this is a reaction to the event and subsides with recovery, but in others it was clearly present previously. Small or large strokes are one of the most common forms of presentation and are usually accompanied by behavioural disturbances. The small strokes are often progressive, causing the multi-infarct syndrome specially associated with dementia. Most are thrombotic rather than haemorrhagic.

The thirst and cramps of malignant hypertension with polyuria are associated with hyponatraemia and hypokalaemia. In Conn's syndrome, apart from cramps and paraesthesia, there may be a transient muscular paresis due to severe hypokalaemia, which is often exacerbated by diuretics, diarrhoea and vomiting.

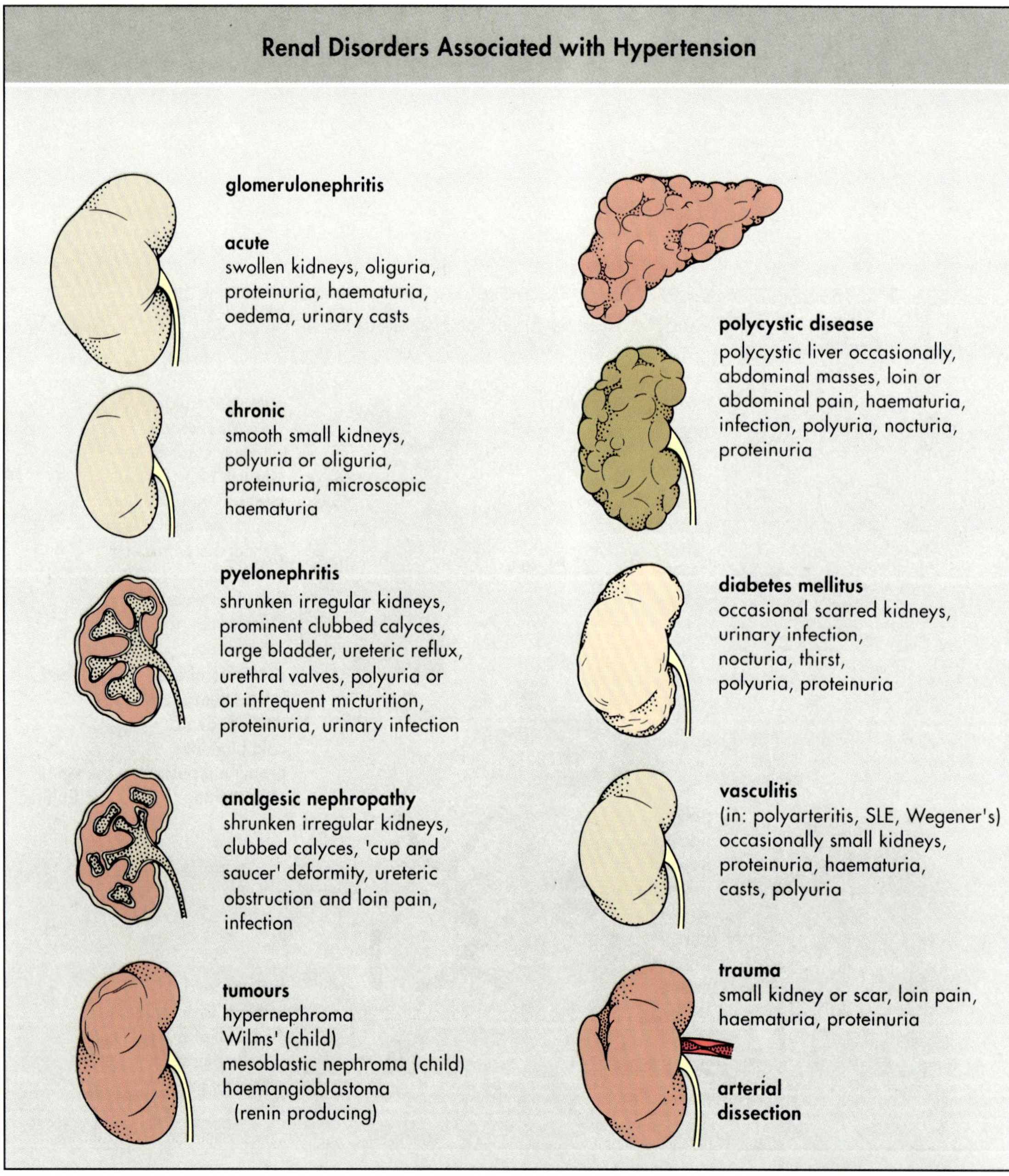

Fig. 7.4 Important renal disorders associated with hypertension.

HISTORY

Medical History

While enuresis is often of psychological origin, it can sometimes be associated with urethral defects such as valvular folds or stenoses and patients may reach adulthood with an enlarged bladder, ureteric reflux and infection (Fig. 7.4). A history of recurrent loin pain with unexplained fevers in childhood may sometimes indicate pyelonephritis and practically all such patients who subsequently have high blood pressure acquire unsuspected kidney scars during this period. Commonly, there is no distinct past history.

Occasionally, nephritis presents with haematuria as a single attack associated with sore throats, oliguria, and puffiness of the face and ankles. The history of Berger's (IgA mediated) nephritis is distinctive: upper respiratory tract or gut infections (as shown by cough and sputum or episodes of diarrhoea) are followed within 24 hours by brisk haematuria. Occasionally, Henoch–Schönlein purpura presents in childhood with a purpuric rash on the buttocks and widespread urticaria. A further helpful symptom is colicky abdominal pain due to oedema of the small bowel. Previous events involving the kidney are important; trauma (followed by haematuria) and irradiation of the abdomen (for Hodgkin's disease, or seminoma of the testis) may both be followed by renal hypertension (see Fig. 7.4). Trauma can affect the kidney directly (by scarring) or indirectly (by vascular damage such as arterial dissection). Radiation causes internal vascular damage (intimal fibrosis). All these processes lead to ischaemia.

Pregnancy history is particularly important (Fig. 7.5). First pregnancies can lead to hypertension at any stage from the third month onward – oedema and proteinuria are common. This does not necessarily indicate either an underlying cause for the hypertension or a family history. Second pregnancies differ in that the earlier in the pregnancy the blood pressure rises, the more likely it is that an underlying cause will be found. With familial hypertension, the blood pressure usually rises towards the end of term: in each successive pregnancy the rise may be slightly more marked.

Family History

A positive family history does not exclude other causes of hypertension and cannot therefore be used as a reason for not investigating the patient fully. Some families have striking histories where polycystic disease is inherited as a dominant characteristic, shown by death from renal failure with hypertension at around fifty years of age in one of the parents and some of the siblings – sporadic cases may live much longer, either untreated or by

Hypertension in Pregnancy

onset in third month, first pregnancy
usually no underlying cause

onset in sixth month, first pregnancy
mild hypertension – often a family trait
severe hypertension – proteinuria; oedema; headache; intrauterine death (often no cause known, but numerous infarcts in small placenta).
usually no recurrence in the second pregnancy.

onset in third month, second pregnancy
underlying cause, such as renal disease, most likely

onset in second and subsequent pregnancies
look at family history; family trait most likely, but this does not exclude the possibility of an underlying cause, such as renal disease.

Fig. 7.5 The important features of hypertension in pregnancy.

means of dialysis or renal transplantion. Some types of glomerulonephritis also run in families – Alport's syndrome is an hereditary condition leading to glomerulonephritis and, sometimes, deafness and retinal deterioration. Diabetes, hypertension, vascular disease and gout run together historically and it is useful to know about this when thiazide diuretics are prescribed, since glucose intolerance and raised uric acid are the most common adverse effects of these drugs. Families in which one or both parents have hypertension often show a variable emergence of this trait in the children (Fig. 7.6). At present, however, it is uncertain whether it is inheritance or environment which causes these differences, and the rise of blood pressure with age may not always occur at a similar time in different families, nor in individuals of similar age within families.

Drug History

This is an important part of the history, with special emphasis on the following:

- nasal drops containing phenylpropanolamine;
- ergot;
- acetylsalicylic, acid phenacetin analgesics;
- laxatives (with particular reference to liquorice which causes sodium and water retention);
- some non-steroidal anti-inflammatory agents (which can raise blood pressure associated with retention of sodium and water), and carbenoxalone, used for peptic ulcers, which behaves like deoxycorticosterone acetate;
- monoamine oxidase inhibitors (occasionally used as antidepressants) can cause a dangerous rise in pressure – if followed by foods with a high tyra-

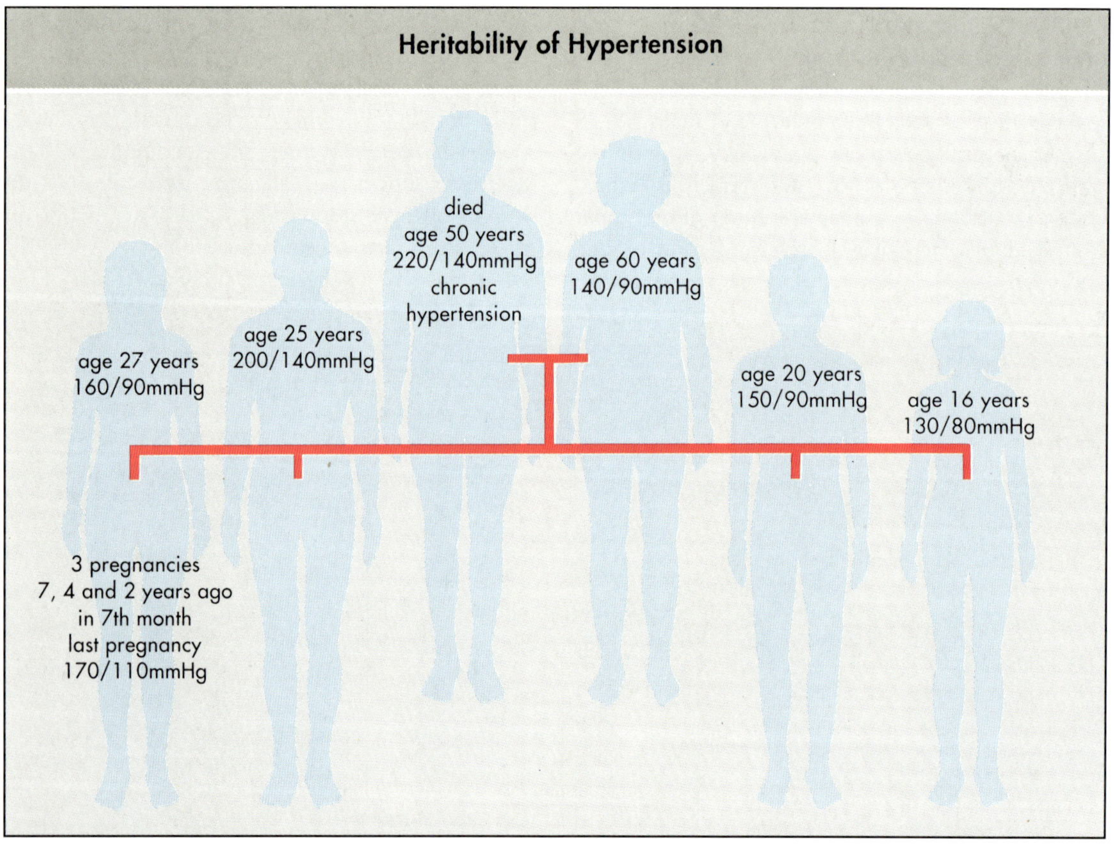

Fig. 7.6 A typical family tree with hypertension in the father (who died of a stroke) showing the variable occurrence of a raised blood pressure in the children, partly dependent upon age but also revealed by pregnancy. Environmental and inheritable factors interact in hypertension.

mine content (such as cheese and red wine) or sympathomimetic drugs; they can even precipitate cerebral haemorrhage;
- isoprenaline and salbutamol, asthma treatments which, if used in excess, may raise both cardiac output and systolic blood pressure;
- corticosteroids such as prednisolone – these may, even in moderate doses, cause hypertension, especially where renal disease already exists.

Enquiries into the use of the contraceptive pill (Fig. 7.7) or hormone replacement therapy in the menopausal female must always be made. Although the significance of the latter is not yet quite clear, the former raises the pressure uniformly in a treated group of women and occasionally causes severe hypertension.

Smoking and alcohol intake are very important parts of the drug history. In both sexes, vascular disease and smoking are closely associated. The history of alcohol intake needs a sceptical ear – if it is thought to play a part in the hypertension then clinical tests should be made. Macrocytosis, raised plasma liver enzymes (especially γ-glutamyl transpeptidase and low blood urea) all reflect high alcohol intake. The frank alcoholic, who shows the biggest withdrawal effects on 'drying out', has the highest blood pressure and therefore the largest fall, and a normal blood pressure may well be maintained with total abstinence (Fig. 7.8). Alcoholics tend to be poor compliers with hypertensive treatment.

Finally, occupational risks due to lead and cadmium must be considered, especially in electric battery workers. While both metals cause renal damage with proteinuria, lead is more likely to cause hypertension and even fits.

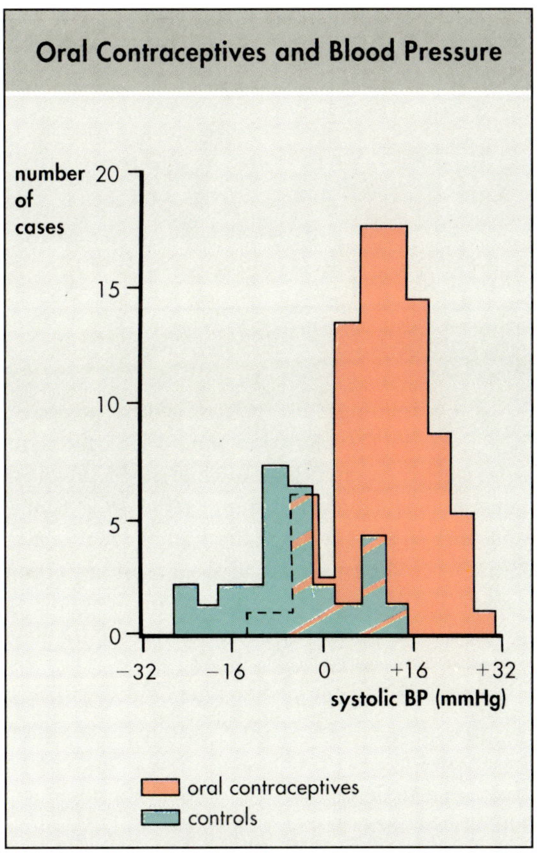

Fig. 7.7 The raised blood pressure in a group of women on an oral contraceptive compared with a group without medication. The whole group is moved to the right, indicating a generalized effect not confined to one segment of the population.

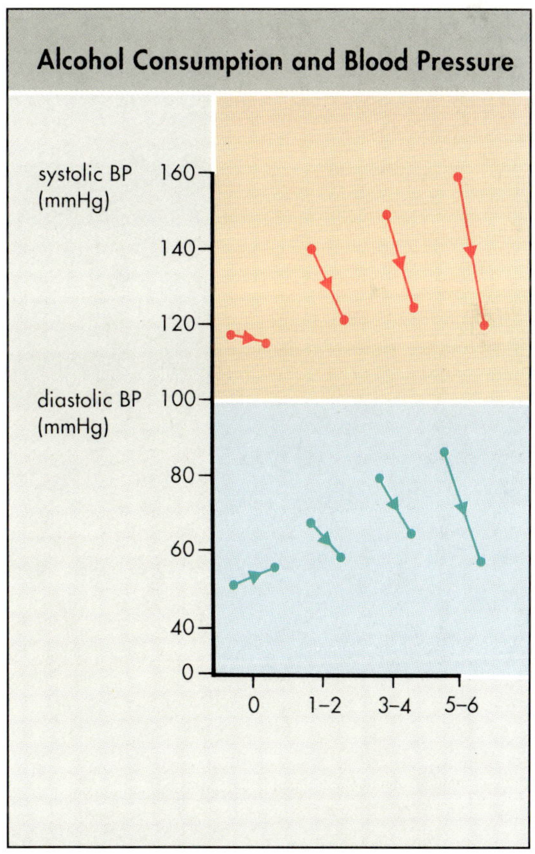

Fig. 7.8 The systolic and diastolic blood pressures in a group of severe alcoholics in relation to the severity of the alcohol withdrawal symptoms. This suggests that the higher initial blood pressures are associated with those showing the greatest withdrawal symptoms.

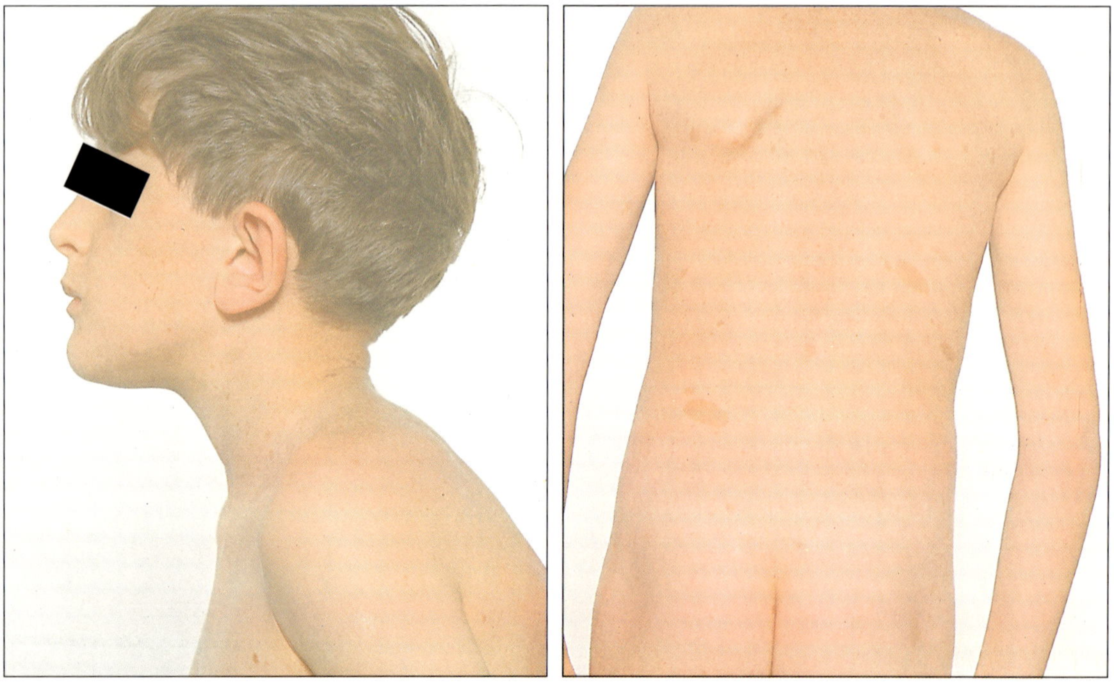

Fig. 7.9 Neurofibromatosis. This shows the low-set ears (left) and the cafe-au-lait spots and winged scalpulae (right) characteristic of the condition.

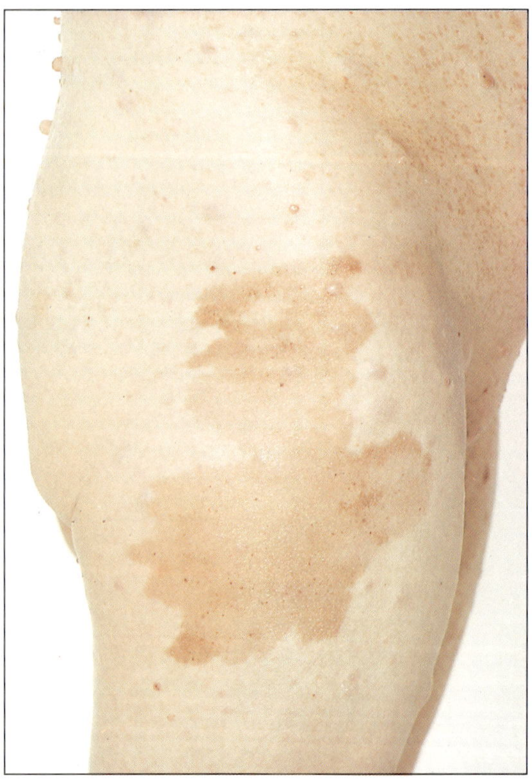

Fig. 7.10 Neurofibromatosis. A large cafe-au-lait blotch with blue-tinted as well as sessile papillomata on the back.

EXAMINATION

Appearance

When examining the patient with suspected hypertension, the physician should look for signs of anxiety associated with a labile blood pressure: general overactivity, blushing, bitten fingernails, and very brisk jerks together with a tachycardia, sweating and tremor. In the absence of important cardiovascular signs, the need for follow-up blood pressure measurements rather than immediate action is indicated.

Thyrotoxicosis should obviously be considered, as must phaeochromocytoma, despite the common nature of these symptoms and signs which can be due to anxiety. Lid-lag and exophthalmos, although common in many patients with thyrotoxicosis, is not always present. The possibility of phaeochromocytoma is raised by the presence of neurofibromatosis, shown by a cafe-au-lait blotch, widespread subcutaneous neuromas, and blue-tinted papillomata in the skin, together with

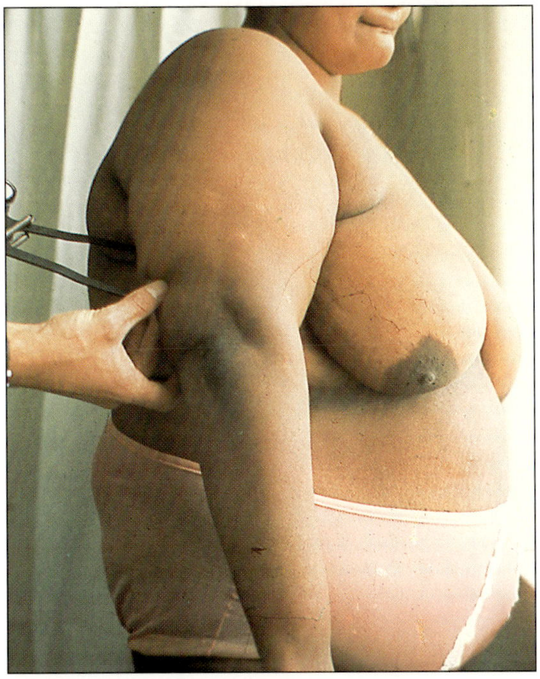

Fig. 7.11 Obesity in gross form. This is associated with high blood pressure; part of the problem is the accurate measurement of pressure in a fat arm using a standard cuff.

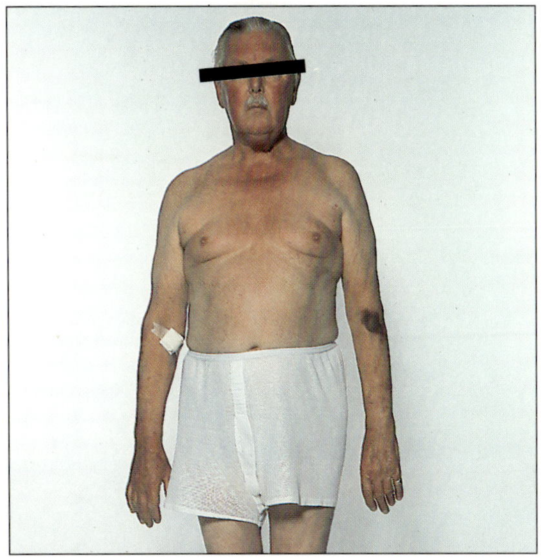

Fig. 7.12 Cushing's syndrome. Typical appearance of a patient with rounded face and increased body fat with wasted limbs. In this case, marked pigmentation is present. Only a few have severe hypertension.

scoliosis and low-set ears (Figs 7.9 & 7.10). Only some of these signs may be present in this rare condition.

Obesity is associated with both hypertension and increased vascular disease. It is, in some cases, an indication of overeating due to some underlying anxiety. Blood pressure is often overestimated if taken from a very fat arm (Fig. 7.11) leading to the somewhat arbitrary use of a wider (thigh) cuff. Weight loss is important since it may cause a reduction in blood pressure in some people.

Rare causes of hypertension, recognisable by appearance alone, include Cushing's syndrome, acromegaly, and hyperthyroidism. In Cushing's syndrome, the typical appearance is of a round pink face, central fat distribution, wasted and weakened peripheral muscles and thinning of the skin leading to purpura and purple striae (Fig. 7.12). The acromegalic patient typically shows coarse facial skin, prominent brows, a large nose, a prognathous lower jaw, widely spaced teeth, a large tongue, and bulky hands and feet (Fig. 7.13).

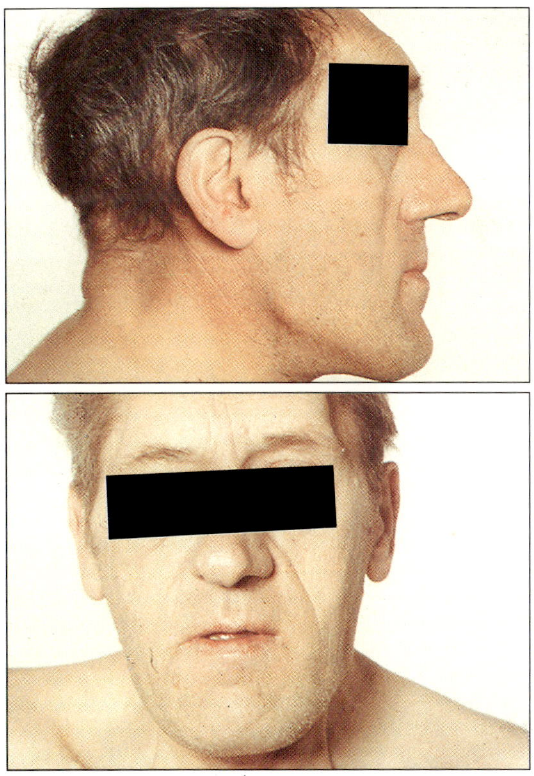

Fig. 7.13 Acromegaly. Typical appearance of the enlarged jaw, nose and supraorbital ridges. Mild-to-moderate hypertension is common, sometimes with glycosuria.

While hyperthyroid patients (Fig 7.14b) do show labile blood pressure readings, the blood pressure is no more labile than in many overanxious patients. Paradoxically, many patients with hypothyroidism (Fig 7.14a) are hypertensive and thyroxine treatment may lower the blood pressure. Atheromatous vascular disease leading to ischaemia in the heart, brain or limbs is possibly more common in myxoedema.

Gouty tophi seen around various joints of the hand (Fig. 7.15), especially in the male, are very rare and association with raised blood pressure is probably coincidental. Hypertension is associated with a higher uric acid level, however, and thiazide treatment is often complicated by gout. A history of the disorder is important in planning the anti-hypertensive treatment, as is a preliminary finding of a high plasma uric acid level.

The puffy face, ankles, and fingers of the pale anaemic patient indicate renal failure (Fig. 7.16), especially when melanin pigmentation of the face, fingers and pressure points is marked.

Excess alcohol may not produce many signs; suspicion is aroused by facial telangiectasia, rhinophyma, marked muscle wasting and weakness, potbelly and Dupuytren's contraction of the hand.

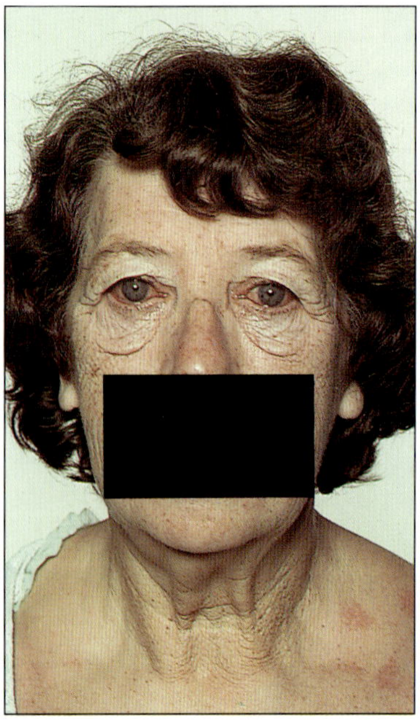

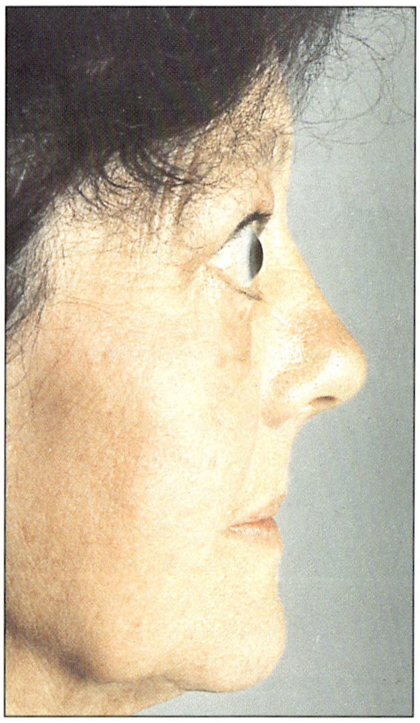

Fig. 7.14a Puffy lids in myxoedema.

Fig. 7.14b Hyperthyroidism. this shows exopthalmos and lid retraction. Systolic hypertension occasionally occurs but is not usually very striking.

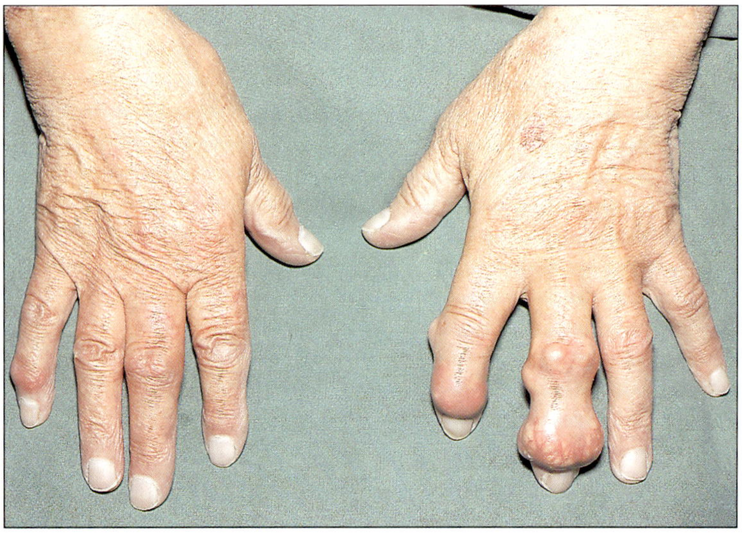

Fig. 7.15 Gouty tophi in the fingers. This severity is uncommon.

Physical Examination

The Cardiovascular System (CVS)

When considering the prognosis of a patient, the vascular pathology is as important as the blood pressure. Examination of the CVS system is first directed towards the presence of all the major arterial, temporal, carotid, radial, femoral, and foot pulses. On rare occasions an absent or delayed femoral pulse in the adult will indicate coarctation or obstruction lower in the aorta (Fig. 7.17). This may be associated with arterial pulsations in collaterals, especially on the posterior surface of the scapula (see Fig. 7.18). The asynchronous arrival of brachoradial or temporal pulses on right and left leads to a search for proximal stenoses in subclavian or carotid arteries.

A conspicuous right carotid artery (known as the 'curly carotid') usually indicates an elongation of the aorta, rather like locomotor brachialis due to the tortuous, lengthened brachial artery. Thickening of the radial artery can often be felt in hypertensive elderly subjects. In a young person this artery is almost impalpable when rolled on the radius.

Symptoms and Signs of Renal Failure

neural	cardio-vascular	gastro-intestinal	renal	other
fatigue	short of breath	nausea	nocturia	pallor (anaemia)
confusion	cardiac asthma	vomiting	polyuria and anuria	wasting
headache	pulmonary oedema	diarrhoea	haematuria	itching
blurred vision	cardiac failure		proteinuria	pigmentation
tremor			oedema	cramps
seizure				

Fig. 7.16 Symptoms and signs of renal failure, which is commonly associated with hypertension when fluid retention occurs.

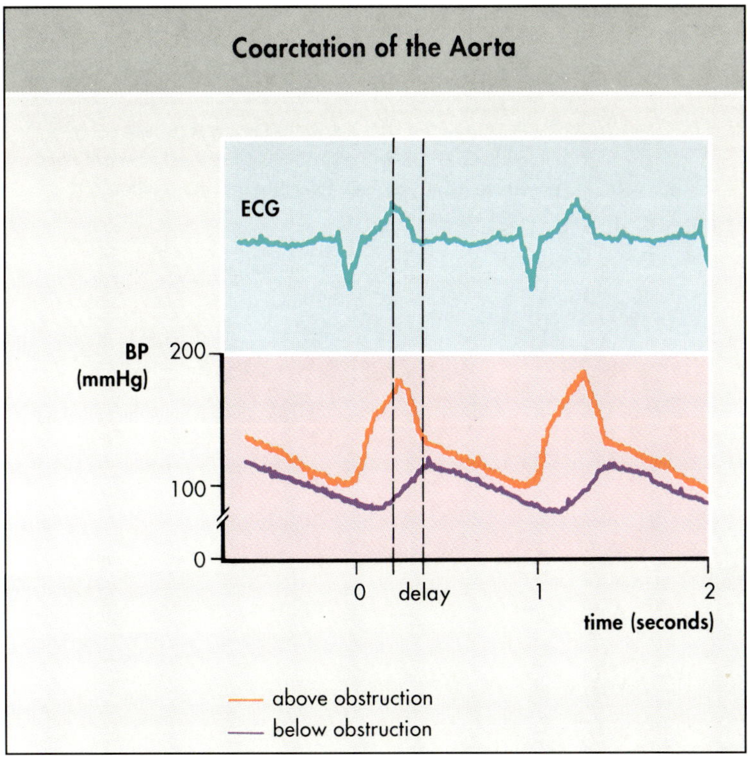

Fig. 7.17 Arterial pulse tracings above and below a coarctation of the aorta, showing the delay to the peak wave form, and the lower pressure below the obstruction.

Signs and Symptoms of Coarctation	
systolic murmur over back and collaterals	arterial neck pulsation
large left ventricle	radial/femoral delay
rib notches (on x-ray)	cold feet
claudication	

Fig. 7.18 Major symptoms and signs in coarctation of the aorta.

Auscultation

Auscultation of the main arteries in the neck, epigastrium and over the course of the iliac and femoral arteries may reveal systolic murmurs that suggest stenoses (which may themselves be asymptomatic). In children, murmurs in the abdomen are common and are not necessarily of pathological significance. In the adult not all epigastric murmurs are of certain origin. However, the long high-pitched murmurs going outwards towards the hypochondria often indicate renal artery stenosis – a diastolic component supports the presence of an organic stenosis. Palpation and

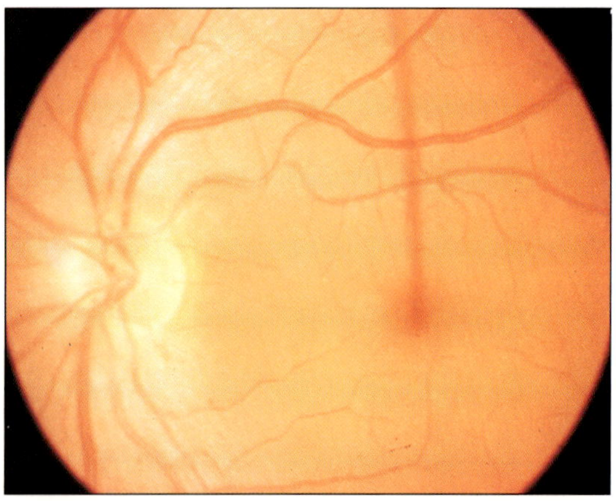

Fig. 7.19 Irregularity in calibre of the arteries, especially the superior and inferior temporal.

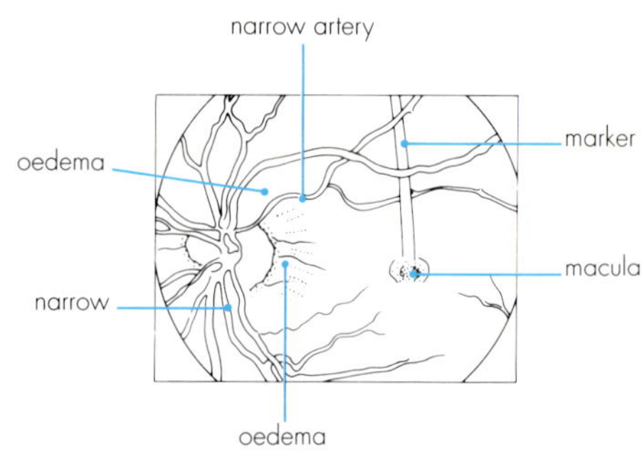

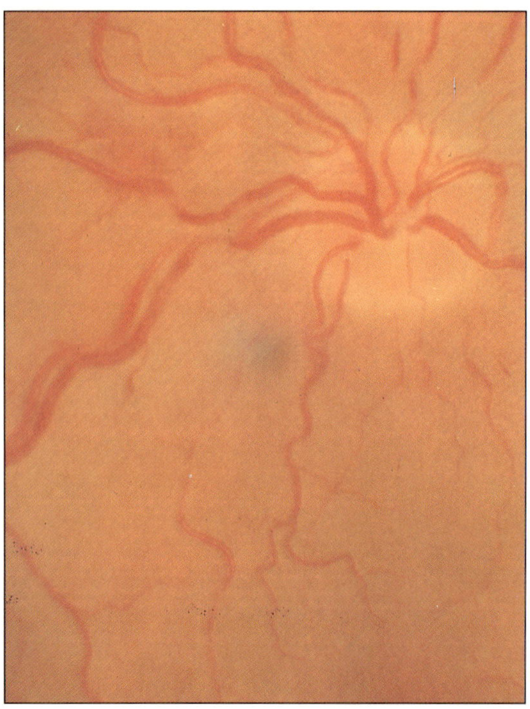

Fig. 7.20 Marked arteriovenous nipping, clearly shown in the vessels just above the disc and at the lower margin of the disc. Irregularity of arterial calibre is also marked, as is the oedema of the disc and adjoining retina. Haemorrhages present to the nasal side of the disc and more diffusely above the disc.

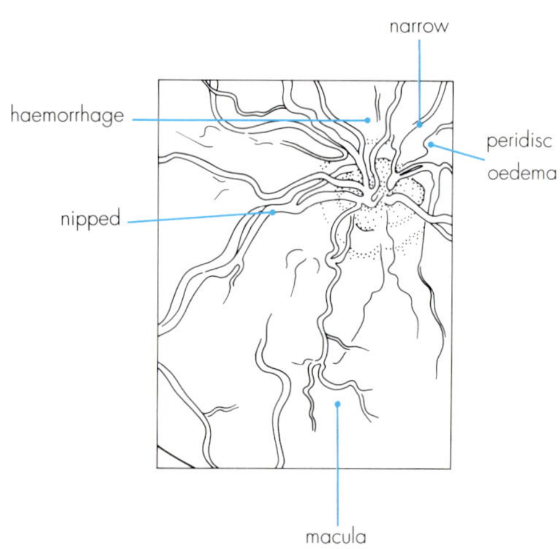

use of the stethoscope are of the greatest importance in cardiovascular examination, and guide sensible requests for further investigations.

Retinal Examination

When examining the retina, particular attention should be paid to irregularity in the calibre of the arteries (Fig. 7.19). Tortuousness alone is not important, since many thin, straight arteries are diseased. Similarly, arteriovenous nipping has to be extreme to be a reliable sign (Fig. 7.20). The distinct pathological signs of malignant hypertension are linear blot- and flame-shaped haemorrhages (Fig. 7.21), and exudates of the clear, small, salt-grain type between the disc and macula, or cotton-wool spots due to arteriolar block. All of these are more florid in renal failure (Fig. 7.22); malignant hypertension is typically associated with oedema between the fibres, leaving the macula relatively spared though redder in appearance. This gives the fan or star figure (see Fig. 7.23). Papilloedema may exist alone, but is more commonly associated with the vascular changes, exudates and haemorrhages (see Figs 7.21 & 7.22). The oedema typically starts at the edge of the disc, giving a blurred appearance, especially on the medial border. Diabetes causes larger, clear-cut, rather geomet-

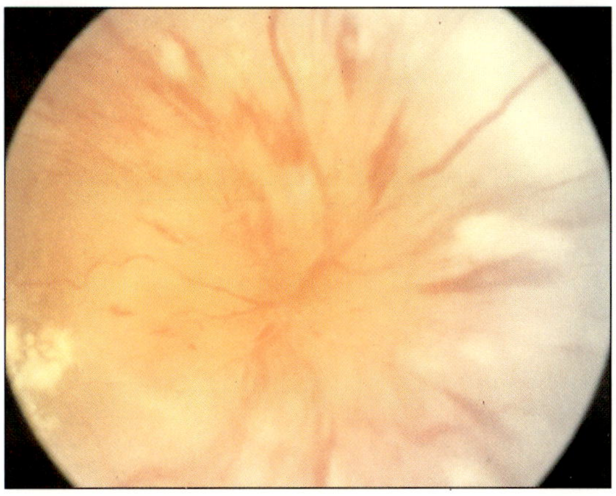

Fig. 7.21 Malignant hypertension. Gross papilloedema with the vessels on the disc obscured. Flame haemorrhages, cotton-wool exudates and retinal oedema at all areas.

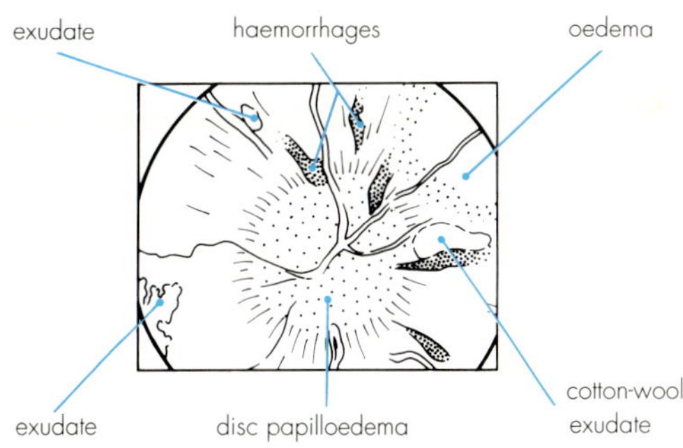

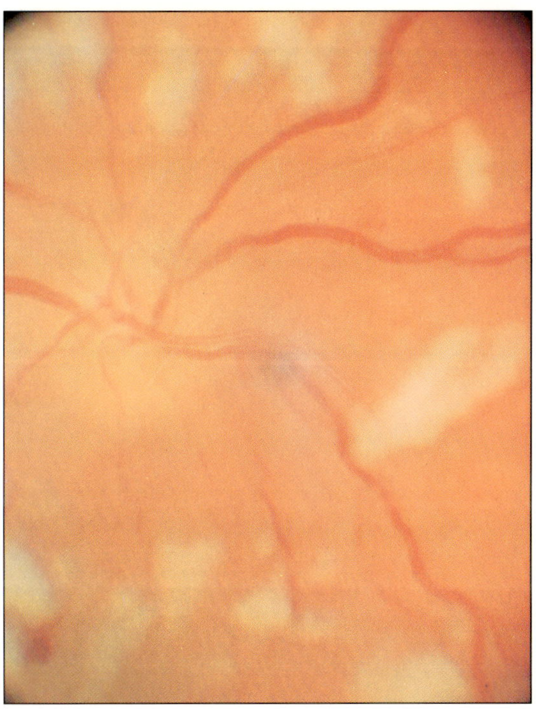

Fig. 7.22 Malignant hypertension and renal failure. Papilloedema and numerous cotton-wool exudates at all areas with a solitary haemorrhage.

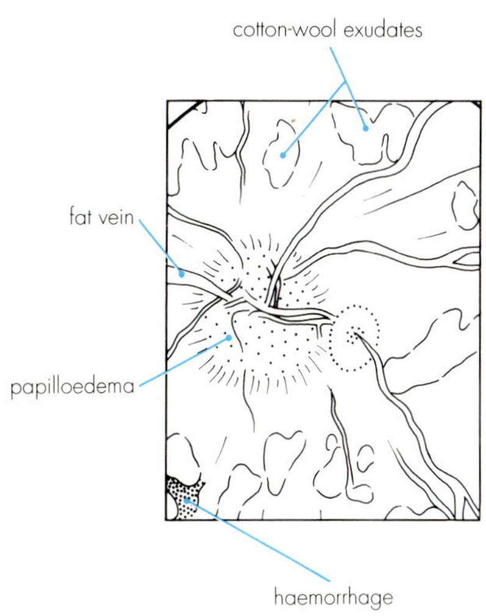

rical white or yellow exudates (Fig. 7.24), as well as the typical capillary microaneurysms most marked at the periphery. Dilated veins are common in the diabetic fundus and in hypertension, and are often associated with sub-hyaloid (Fig. 7.25) or vitreous haemorrhage. Organisation of the haemorrhage in diabetes leads to proliferative retinopathy which is a most serious, sight-threatening complication (Fig. 7.26). One of the most common retinal changes associated with hypertension is venous obstruction, either segmental (Fig. 7.27) or central. The former seems to be distal to an arteriovenous crossing point and fluorescein studies show that the vein is rarely completely thrombosed (see Figs 7.28 & 7.29): the underlying cause is presumably a rise of venous pressure from partial thrombotic obstruction leading to capillary haemorrhage. Fluorescein studies, which show blood flow block and abnormal leakage, have contributed greatly to our understanding of the retinal circulation (see Fig. 7.30).

Other causes of visual disturbance are hemianopia, due to damage secondary to vertebrobasilar disease, and external ocular muscle paralysis, possibly due to ischaemia of the nerve, especially the sixth (see Fig. 7.31).

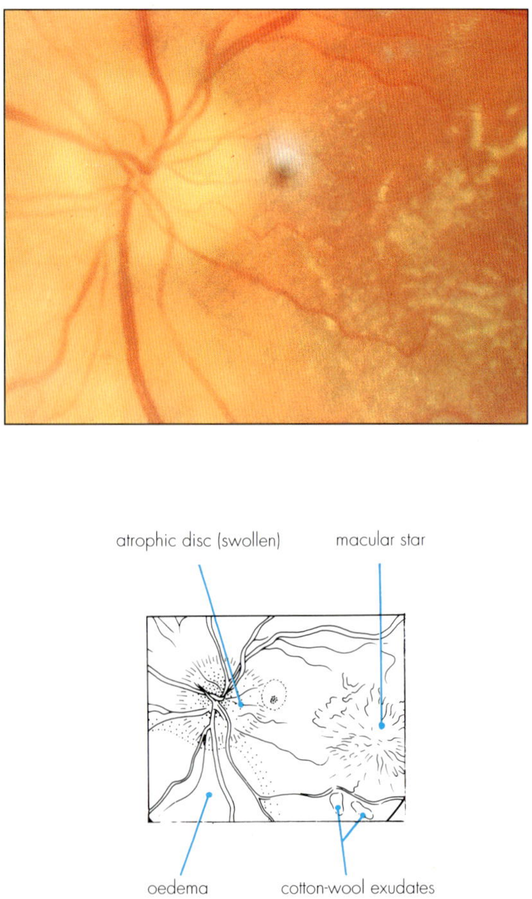

Fig. 7.23 Malignant hypertension. Papilloedema going on to a white atrophic appearance of the disc. A striking macular star figure with a red, rather haemorrhagic appearance at the centre, which is the macula. Retinal oedema is present, particularly below the disc. The arteries are very narrow.

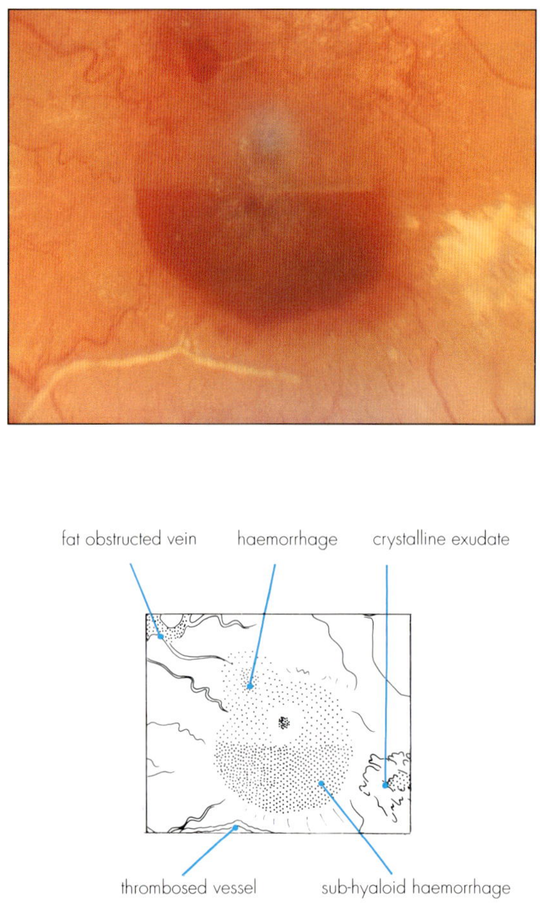

Fig. 7.24 A large sub-hyaloid haemorrhage with a typical straight upper and curved lower margin, like a cup. There are clear-cut, rather crystalline exudates on its outer side, the type often seen in diabetes (which this patient had). Below the haemorrhage is a white thrombosed vessel.

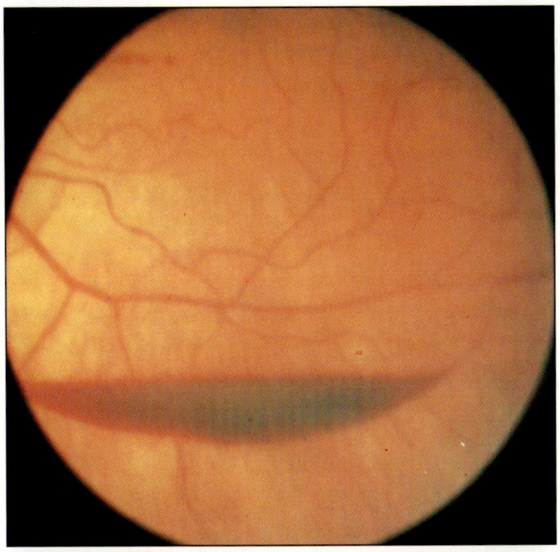

Fig. 7.25 Sub-hyaloid haemorrhage in a patient with hypertension. These are often secondary to venous obstruction but not obviously so here.

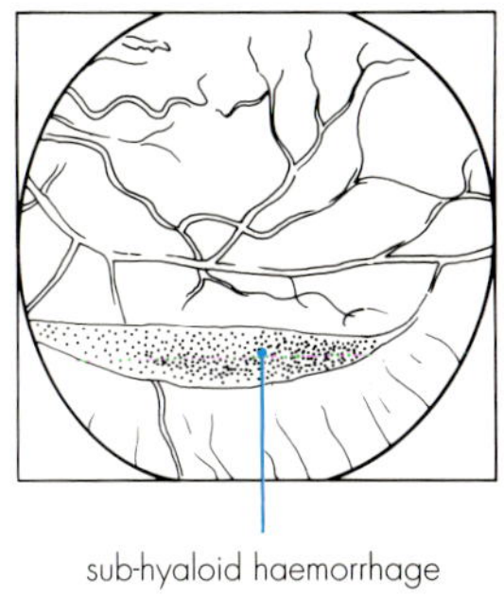

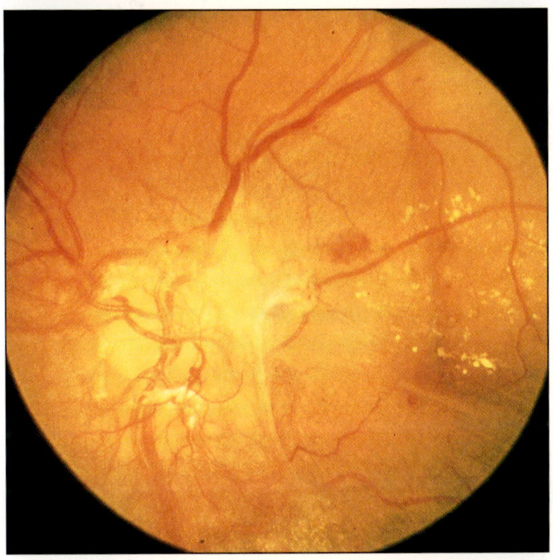

Fig. 7.26 Diabetes with hypertension. An example of an organized haemorrhage in front of the disc with neovascularization. At the upper part of the retina from 10 to 12 o'clock there are microaneurysms, typical of the diabetes underlying these appearances.

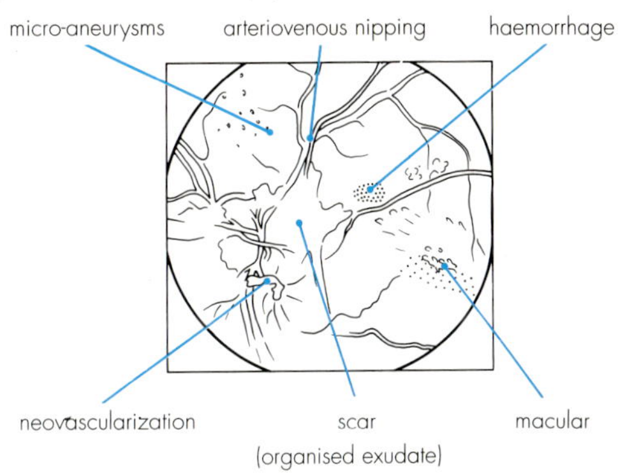

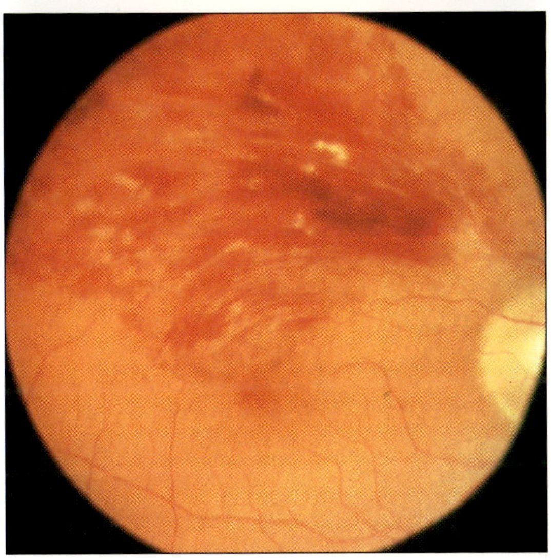

Fig. 7.27 Segmental venous obstruction, typically starting from an arteriovenous crossing point close to the disc with the haemorrhage confined to one segment. Swelling of the retina, shown by the bulge, is also present. The patient had hypertension.

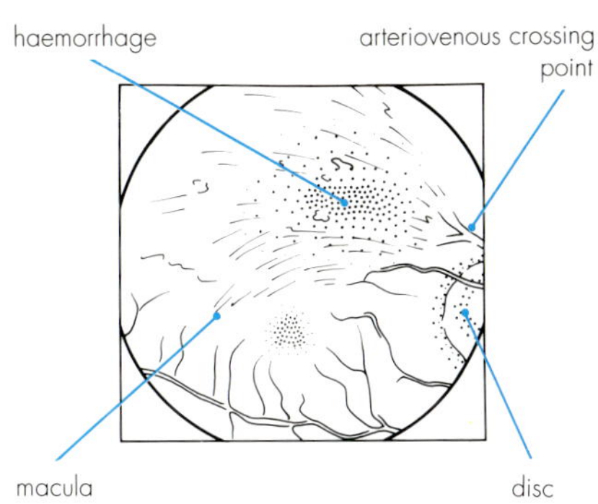

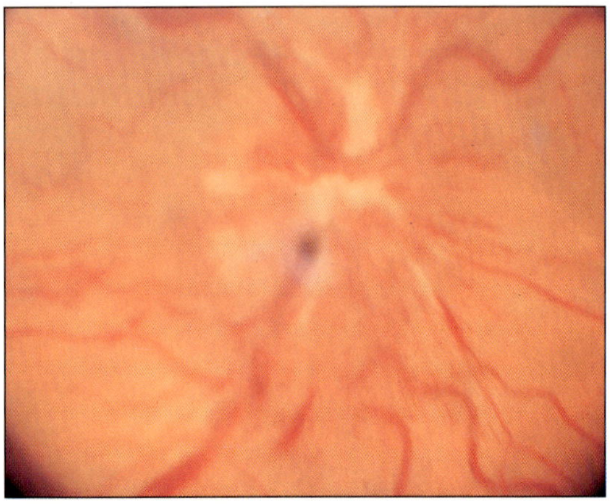

Fig. 7.28 Central retinal venous obstruction. Marked papilloedema with haemorrhages and exudate, radiating from the disc. The veins, especially the superior and inferior temporal, are grossly dilated.

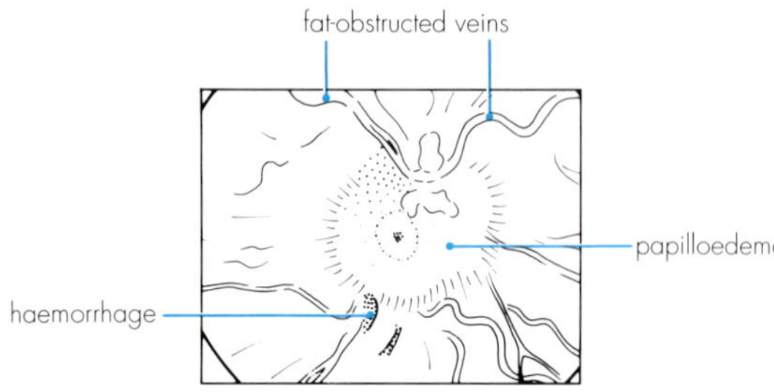

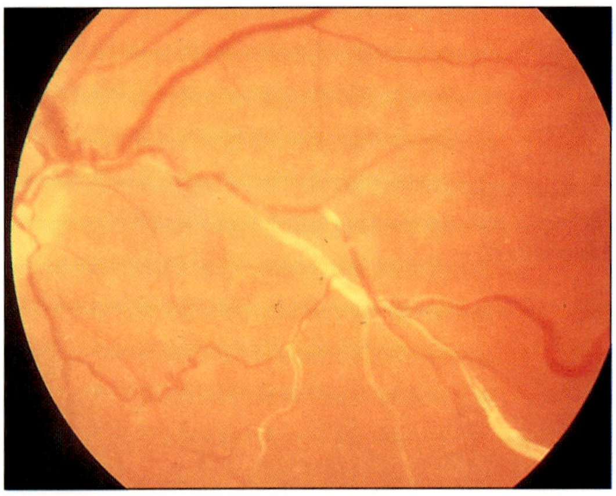

Fig. 7.29 Sheathing of the veins is common in diabetes, even though it occurs in other, especially older, patients. The vein here is thrombosed both proximally and distally. The accompanying artery in the centre has a probable shining embolus just above a bifurcation.

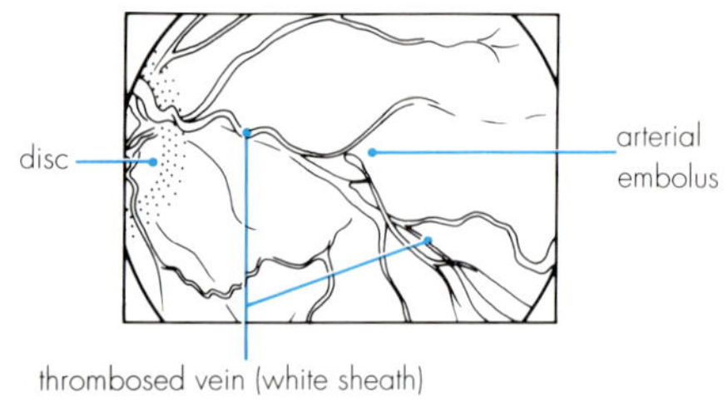

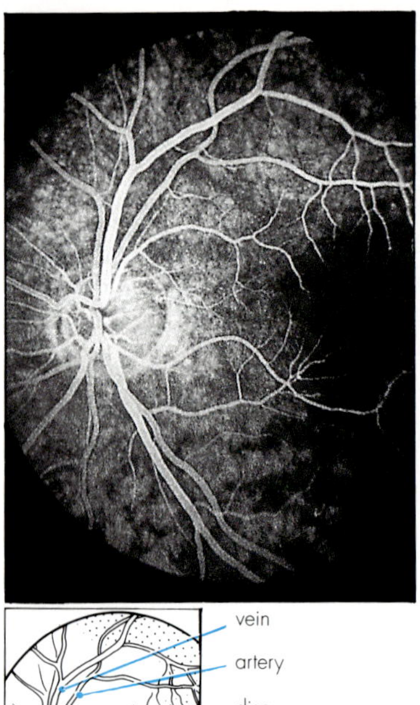

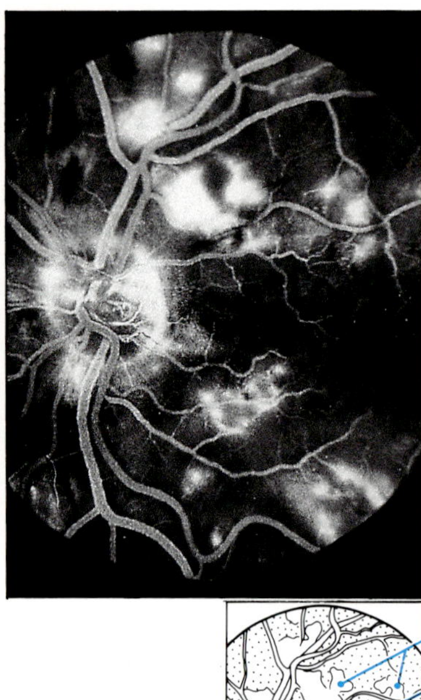

Fig. 7.30 Top: A normal fluorescein picture of the retina. The macular region is usually dark at this stage of perfusion, showing the narrower arteries and fatter veins, with capillary filling between the branches. Bottom: A fluorescein study of a diabetic fundus at a later phase, with more fluorescein in the fatter veins than in the narrower arteries of irregular calibre. Abnormal capillary leakage is shown on and around the disc and in various patches close to the visible blood vessels. The dark areas are due to abnormal capillary occlusion.

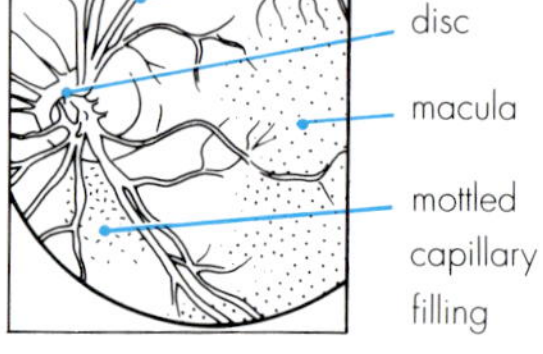

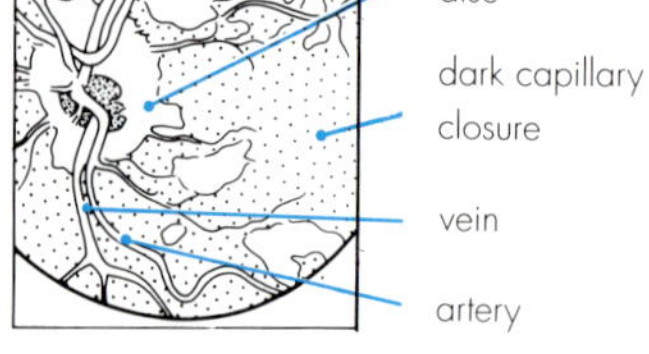

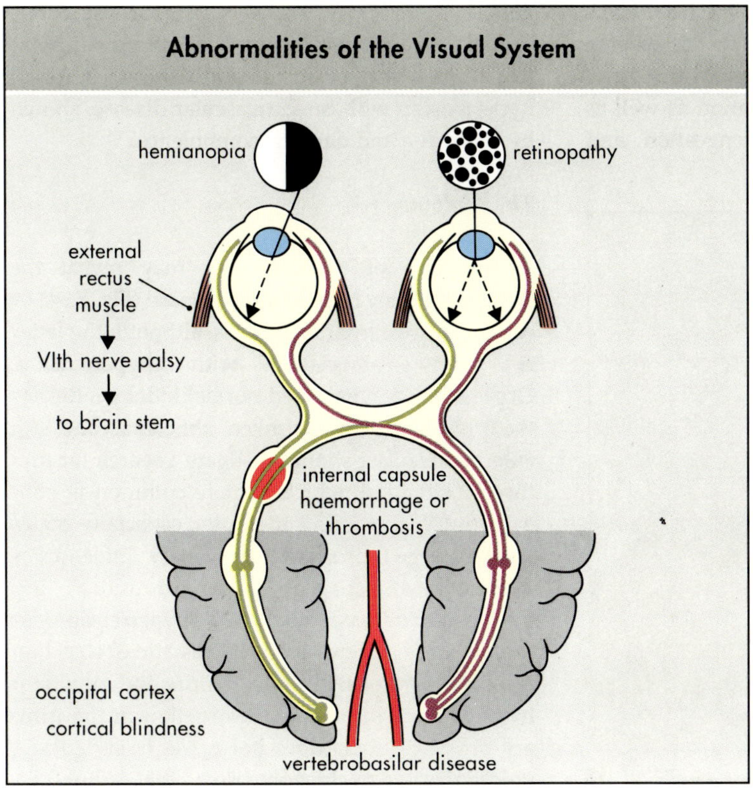

Fig. 7.31 Possible abnormalities of the visual system in hypertension. Retinopathy due to vascular abnormalities, diplopia due to ophthalmoplegia (especially the external rectus muscle), and interference with the optic radiations leading to hemianopias of different degree or more rarely, in vertebrobasilar disease, cortical blindness.

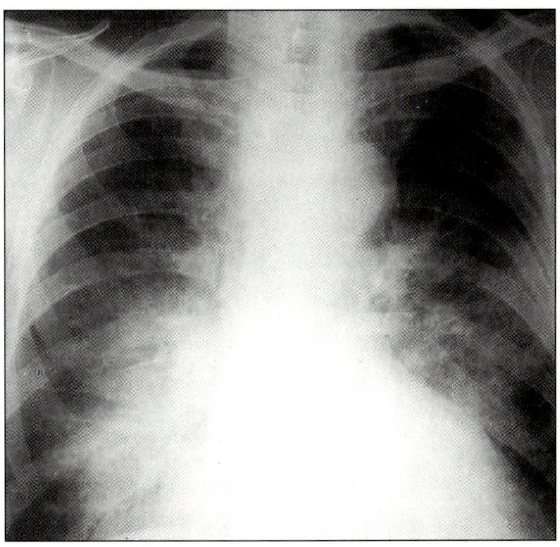

Fig. 7.32 Typical appearances of pulmonary oedema in severe hypertension with left ventricular failure. The bilateral butterfly pattern is typical, even though unilateral oedema may occur.

The Heart

Demonstration of left ventricular hypertrophy by movement of the ribs well beyond the midclavicular line is only common in severe hypertension, and ribs are readily moved by the heart in children and thin anxious adults. Failure to detect cardiac enlargement clinically in hypertension is common.

Auscultation is important principally in picking out the fourth heart sound, which is very prominent in moderate-to-severe hypertension. A loud third sound occurs when congestive failure supervenes. Severe cases are associated with fine crackles in the lung bases due to raised pulmonary venous pressure and oedema (Fig. 7.32) and/or congestive cardiac failure, the usual signs of which are peripheral oedema, raised pulsatile neck veins (Fig. 7.33) and an enlarged liver. In the elderly, ventricular failure is also associated with symptoms of night cough and disorientation as well as dyspnoea, due to pulmonary congestion and anoxia. Peripheral oedema is also a conspicuous sign. Sleep apnoea with marked snoring all point to the possibility of anoxia and the association of hypertension with cerebrovascular disease, shown by confusion and daytime somnolence.

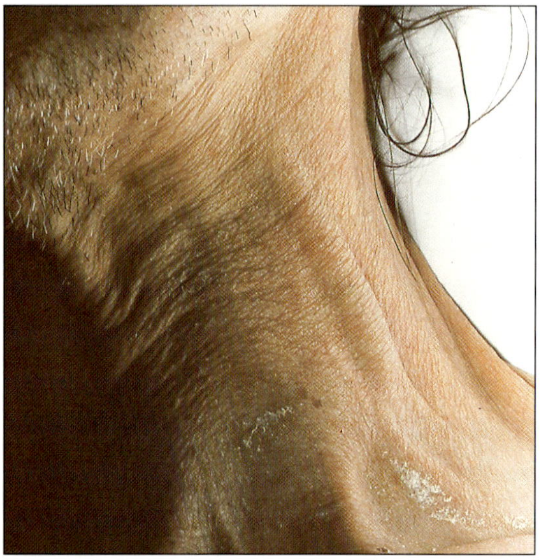

Fig. 7.33 Raised pulsatile external jugular veins in congestive failure complicating hypertension.

The Abdomen

Examination of the abdomen may reveal the enlarged kidney of polycystic disease (Fig. 7.34) or occasionally of hydronephrosis, although the latter is rarely associated with hypertension. Occasionally, an enlarged normal kidney indicates the presence of a shrunken abnormal one. An enlarged bladder should instigate a search for urethral obstruction, which is more common in children but is also found in adults, especially males with enlarged prostates. If urinary infection is demonstrated, it may point to reflux and pyelonephritis associated with hypertension, or the presence of renal stones. Prostatic obstruction can lead insidiously to renal failure and attendant hypertension. In general, obstruction in the urinary drainage tracts does not cause hypertension, unless there is pyelonephritis or renal failure of a severe degree.

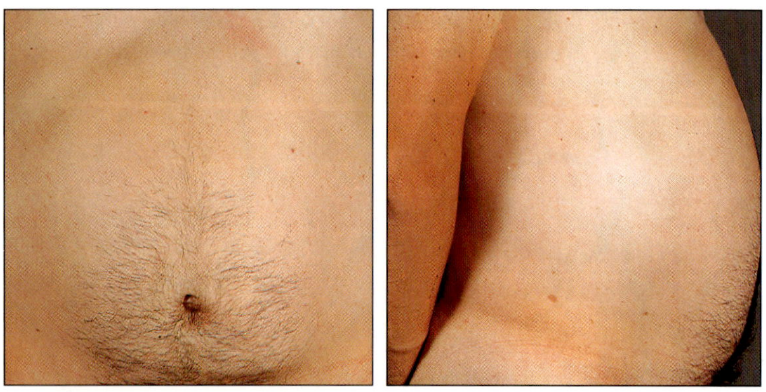

Fig. 7.34 The swelling of the abdomen due to large bilateral polycystic kidneys.

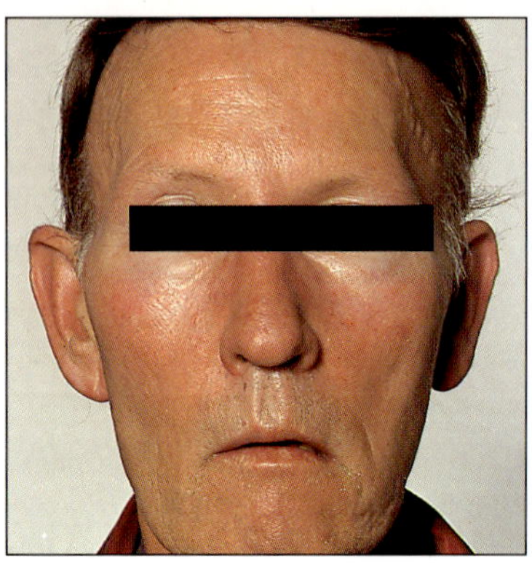

Hypertensive Brain Damage

personality change
memory loss
seizures
droop mouth
dysphasia
dysarthria
weakness
clumsiness

Fig. 7.35 Symptoms and signs of brain damage common in severe hypertension with vascular changes.

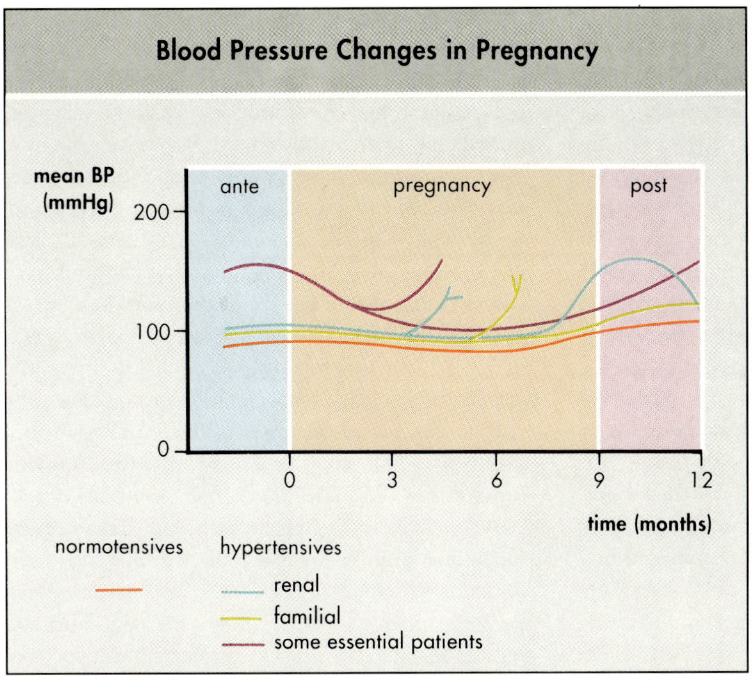

Fig. 7.36 Blood pressure changes in normal and abnormal pregnancy. In normal pregnancy blood pressure usually falls, while in patients with renal disease blood pressure often rises during early pregnancy. Patients with essential hypertension either show an earlier rise in blood pressure, or a blood pressure fall for the duration of the pregnancy. Women with a family history of hypertension or with pre-eclamptic toxaemia most often show a rise in blood pressure in the last trimester. In all cases, blood pressure may rise shortly after the third month.

Pre-Eclampsia and Toxaemia

headache	uterus and fetus small for dates
fits	proteinuria
oedema of lids	fetal heartbeat irregular
BP at 7th month high (150/100mmHg)	oedema rings tight ankles swollen face puffy
amniotic fluid excess	
placental hormone levels low	uric acid high

Fig. 7.37 The clinical picture in pre-eclampsia and severe 'toxaemia' of pregnancy.

The Central Nervous System

In the nervous system, particular attention must be paid to signs of brain damage (Fig. 7.35), starting with mental performance (which can be impaired in severe hypertension without paresis) and other signs of patchy cerebral ischaemia (multiple infarct syndrome). In the elderly, cerebral ischaemia is often revealed by inadequacies of the upper motor neurone and visual system. These can range from quadrantic hemianopia to clumsiness of a hand or foot or slurring of speech, even without a history of a definite attack. It should be remembered that hypertension does not exclude subdural haematoma or tumour, and the possibility of emboli from the heart or extracranial vessels must always be considered.

Pregnancy

It is during the middle to end of pregnancy that the problems due to hypertension usually occur (Fig. 7.36). In severe cases (eclampsia) the patient complains of headache; oedema may rapidly become marked and is associated with proteinuria (Fig. 7.37). It is in these patients that the pressure rises quickly, with papilloedema and pulmonary oedema; convulsions may occur at lower pressures (180/110mmHg) than those in uncomplicated hypertension. At all stages lesser degrees of oedema of the hands, feet and face are a feature. Varying degrees of proteinuria will also be present and a small foetus can usually be detected crudely from measurements of uterine height, or more precisely with ultrasound. Foetal monitoring may show an irregular heart rate which probably reflects poor placental function, as does a low level of placental hormones in the maternal blood. The maternal uric acid level, low in pregnancy, is high.

Urine

Examination of the urine is as important as any physical examination and ideally should be carried out by the doctor personally. While most patients have no change in urine content, those with severe hypertension may have proteinuria, excess of red cells, or diabetes with glycosuria. Proteinuria, even without excess cells, may point to underlying glomerulonephritis, a silent renal stone, inactive pyelonephritis, and even renal artery stenosis. Small amounts of albumin (microalbuminuria) first reported in excess in diabetics, may also indicate important renal involvement in hypertension. Patients with Cushing's syndrome may show glycosuria. This is rarer in attacks due to phaeochromocytoma, but common in patients treated with corticosteroids, which may induce hypertension, especially where there is an underlying renal disease. The red-brown urine due to excess urobilin points to excess alcohol, a close associate of hypertension.

Measurement of Blood Pressure

It is naturally better to take a blood pressure reading under quiet conditions in a patient who has not rushed to an appointment. However, there are many emotional associations connected with the measurement of blood pressure and the patient, without showing it, may be very frightened. A single reading of blood pressure in most ordinary clinical circumstances cannot therefore be used as a basis for judgement without supporting evidence and further readings. The efficiency of the apparatus itself is of the greatest importance. The cuff must extend along two-thirds of the upper arm (Fig. 7.38); small cuff sizes must be available for children (Fig. 7.39) and larger ones for fat people (see chapter 1). Special techniques are needed for babies (Fig. 7.40). The ordinary mercury manometer still remains the best choice. The more convenient aneroid type must be standardized regularly. The cuff must cover the inner aspect of the arm over the artery, and must be inflated

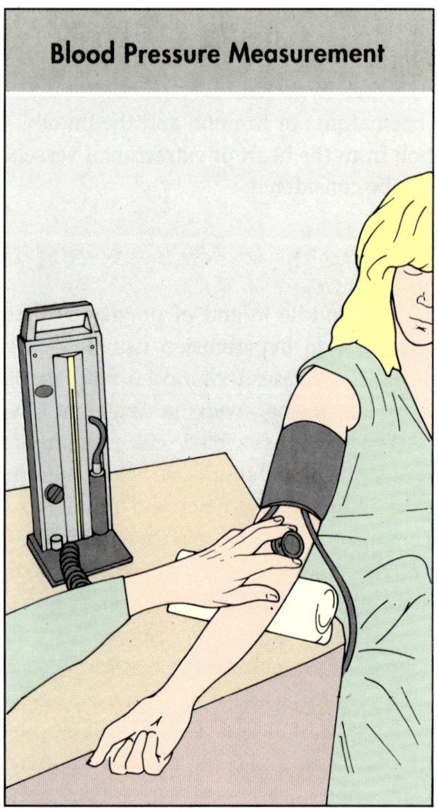

Fig. 7.38 Blood pressure measurement. Note the correct placing of the cuff and its length in relation to the length of the arm. A random zero machine is shown.

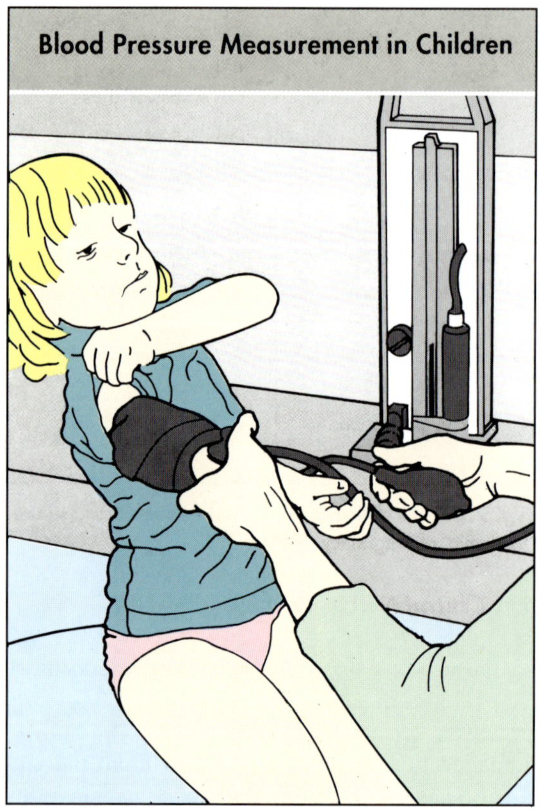

Fig. 7.39 Blood pressure measurement in a child, emphasising the size of cuff needed.

steadily. It is safer to check the point at which the radial pulse disappears as a guide to the systolic pressure, and then to raise the level of cuff pressure 10mmHg above this while listening over the brachial artery. The pressure should be released steadily at a rate of about 5mmHg per second while listening for the Korotkoff sounds. If there is considerable pulsation on the mercury column or oscillations on the aneroid, and there are no sounds heard through the stethoscope, then the observer is in the 'silent gap' and has probably missed the top pressure. The cuff must therefore be reinflated until pulsation stops. In some patients the systolic sounds may only be heard over a narrow range of 5–10mmHg. This, of course, will lead to an underestimation of pressure if the reappearance sounds are mistakenly thought to be at systole. The point of disappearance of the sounds (Korotkoff phase V) is a better measure of diastolic pressure than the point of muffling (Korotkoff phase IV). In children and in anxious, thyrotoxic, anaemic or febrile patients, the sounds may persist to zero and the diastolic pressure is therefore uncertain. Another approach to the measurement of blood pressure involves a semi-automatic machine with recording on tape (Fig. 7.41). There is now considerable movement towards 24-hour measurements by machine, using a tape-recording to identify those subjects that have raised pressure frequently and who therefore deserve treatment (in contrast to those who may only show it in the clinic).

For research purposes, intra-arterial pressure measurements are undertaken with an indwelling

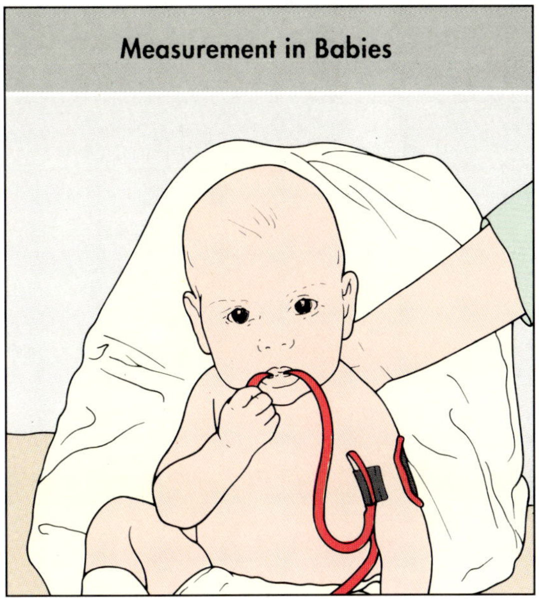

Fig. 7.40 Measurement of blood pressure in babies is best done using a flush method, which gives the sytolic pressure when blood reenters the arm as the pressure in the cuff is lowered.

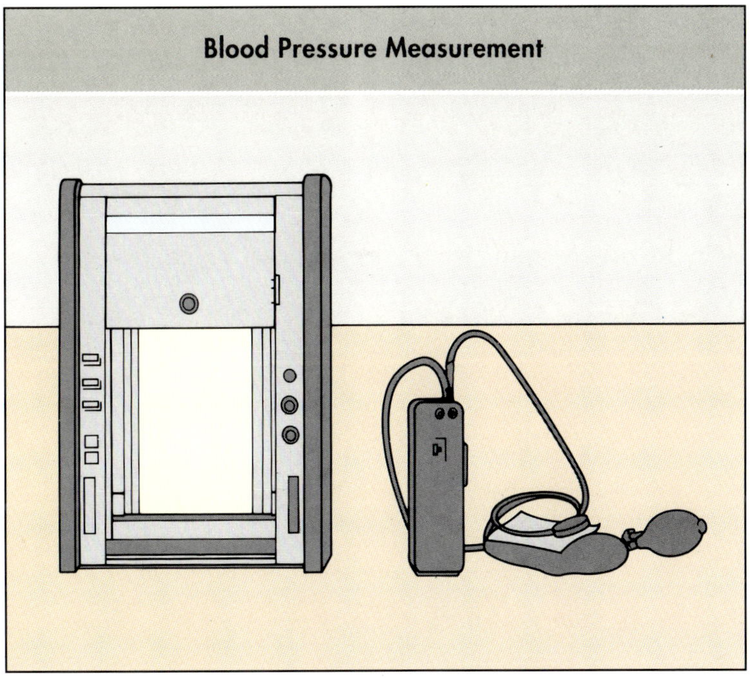

Fig. 7.41 A Remler portable blood pressure machine, showing the cuff and bulb for inflation on the right. The black container in the centre holds the pressure transducer and cassette tape. The tape reader is shown on the left. The pressures are read off on the graph paper.

polythene catheter and a strain gauge manometer recording on to tape (Fig. 7.42). To avoid observer error, a 'zero muddler' sphygmomanometer is the most convenient instrument and is frequently used in drug trials (Fig. 7.43). This cannot exclude the anxiety response however and is one of the reasons for the fall of mean pressure observed with further readings in such trials.

CONCLUSION

The importance of history and examination cannot be emphasized too strongly, since it is the key to further investigation and possible treatment. Especially in symptomless subjects with labile blood pressure, the basis for converting them into patients must be very clearly established.

Intra-arterial Measurement

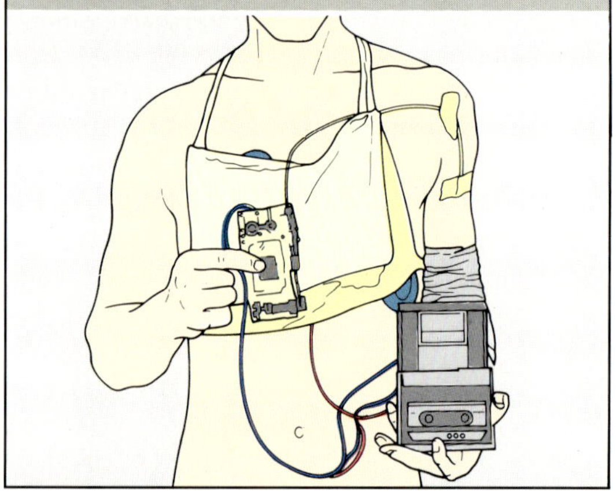

Fig. 7.42 A portable intra-arterial pressure measurement system. The polythene catheter is taped to the arm and enters the brachial artery under the bandage at the left elbow. Patency is maintained by a small heparin pump (held for demonstration in the right hand). Pressure recordings are made on the cassette tape (held in the left hand for demonstration).

Blind Blood Pressure Measurement

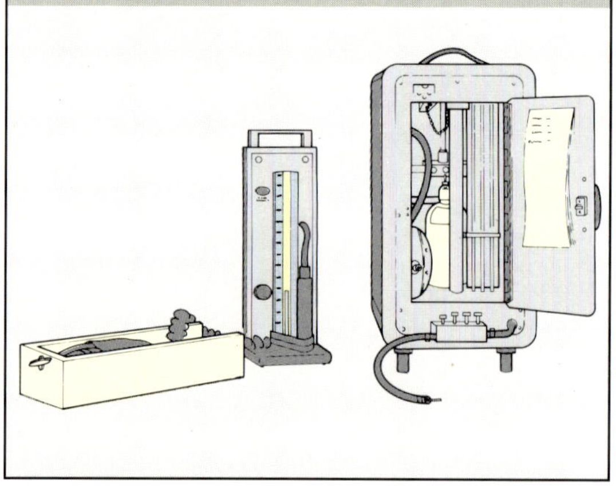

Fig. 7.43 Two types of 'blind' blood pressure machines. On the left, the random zero, where the position of the zero is altered by manipulation of the screw to the left of the figures, giving a value which is unknown to the observer until the end of measurement. On the right is the Rose (London School of Hygiene and Tropical Medicine) manometer, where the cuff is inflated and deflated semi-automatically and the mercury in the different columns is stopped by pressing a button for systolic and diastolic pressures, and the values are read subsequently.

CHAPTER 8

Investigation of the Patient

INTRODUCTION

Once it has been firmly established that a patient has high blood pressure, consideration should be given to the type of investigation required. The essential question for the doctor to ask himself is 'Am I looking for a cure?' If the answer is 'Yes', then tests should be made to discover whether or not the condition can be relieved by surgery or other invasive methods. If the answer is 'No', however, then only those routine tests which may show unsuspected causes or reveal the degree of target organ damage are indicated (Fig. 8.1). Further investigation along similar lines is often justified in patients already being treated for hypertension, whether or not the condition is resistant to therapy.

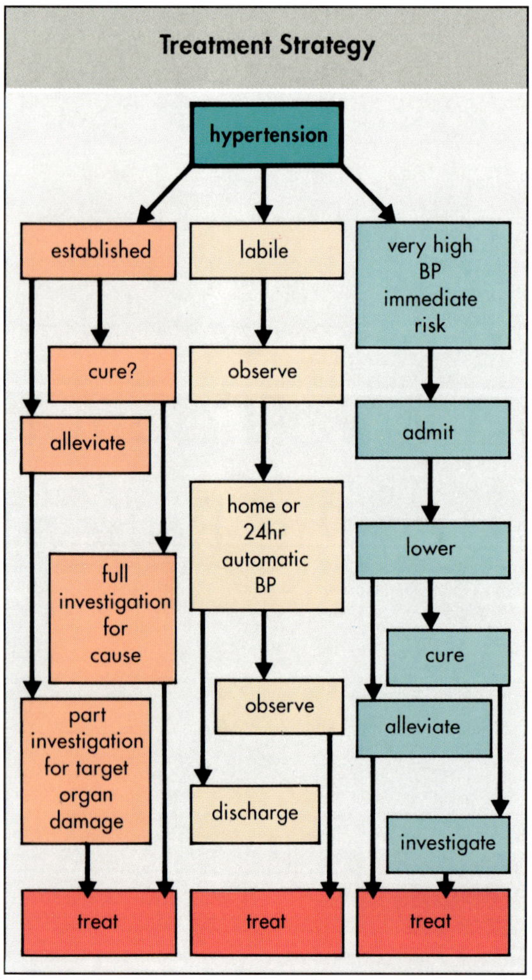

Fig. 8.1 Decision and actions in clinical assessment of patients with raised blood pressure.

INVESTIGATIONS

Urine

Cells and Casts

Examination of the urine under a light microscope is of great importance in detecting haematuria and provides confirmatory evidence for the very sensitive dip-stick tests now available. It also enables a differentiation to be made between renal and lower tract bleeding. With renal bleeding, the red cells are usually deformed or broken and red cell or granular casts may be present in abundance (Fig. 8.2) in contrast to the appearance if bleeding occurs further down the urinary tract. Berger's (IgA) nephritis, for example, may present with

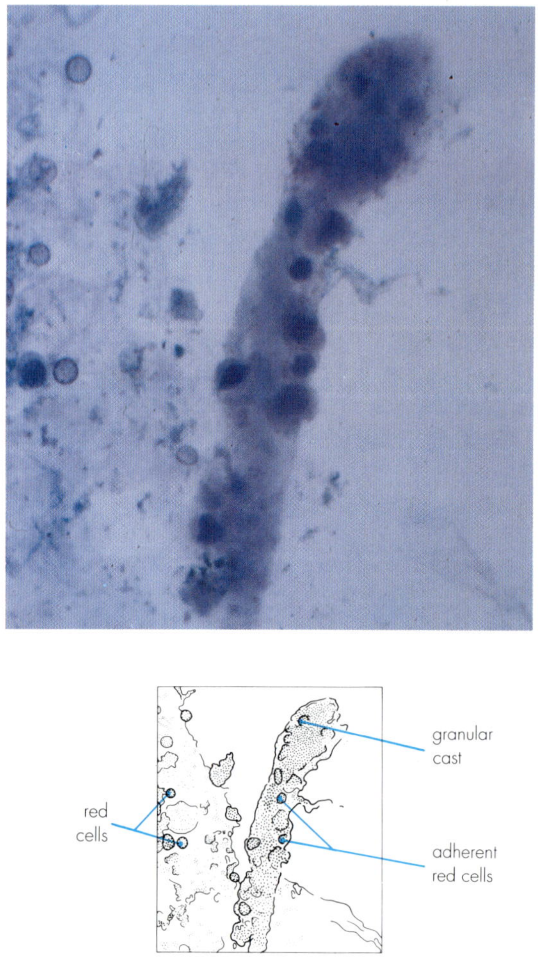

Fig. 8.2 Granular cast with adherent cells and neighbouring red cells in urine from a patient with severe hypertension.

only an excess of red cells, as in malignant hypertension; renal biopsy may then be needed as it is in other forms of nephritis or renal vasculitis where unexplained microscopic haematuria and/or proteinuria is found (lupus erythematosus and polyarteritis nodosa for example – see chapter 5 & Fig. 8.3). Any excessive motility of cells and debris, as well as the presence of pus cells, is indicative of bacilluria. Chronic infection is often symptomless and even a large staghorn calculus may only be revealed by the finding of proteinuria, pus cells and a proteus infection.

Proteinuria

Proteinuria, especially if heavy, indicates the possibility of glomerulonephritis and diseases which damage or infiltrate the glomerulus such as diabetes, vasculitis, scleroderma, amyloidosis, and severe hypertension itself.

Tuberculosis of the kidney and renal tract, as well as renal stone, may present with a symptomless haematuria and proteinuria. Microalbuminuria, the presence of a very small excess of albumin compared to normal, is typical of early diabetic renal involvement and of hypertension itself.

Glycosuria

Glycosuria, while typical of diabetes, may indicate renal glycosuria with a low threshold, occasional tubular defects (Fanconi syndrome), lead and cadmium toxicity, or rarely phaeochromocytoma (with raised plasma glucose). In the treatment of hypertension, thiazide diuretics may sometimes induce diabetes with glycosuria, especially in the long-term therapy of the elderly. In such cases nocturia is common. Regular urine tests for all patients treated for hypertension are mandatory.

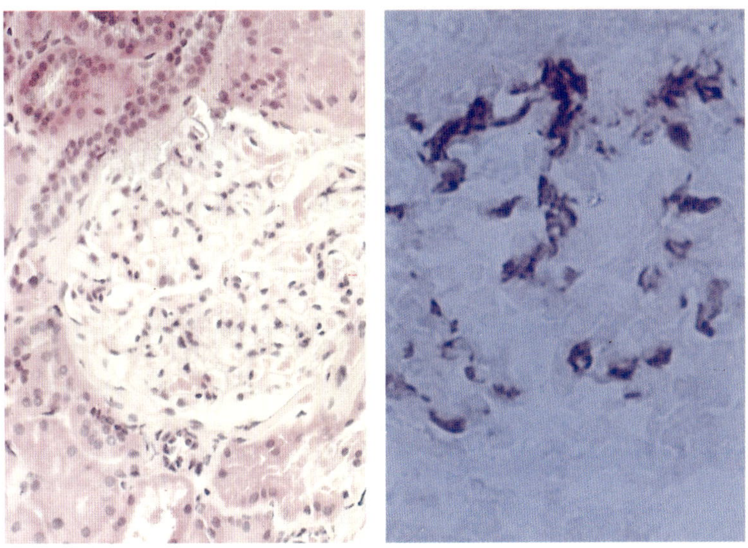

Fig. 8.3 Renal biopsy of a patient with Berger's nephritis. Left: The normal appearance of a glomerulus. Haematoxylin and eosin stain. Right: Deposits of IgA in the same glomerulus. Immunoperoxidase stain for IgA.

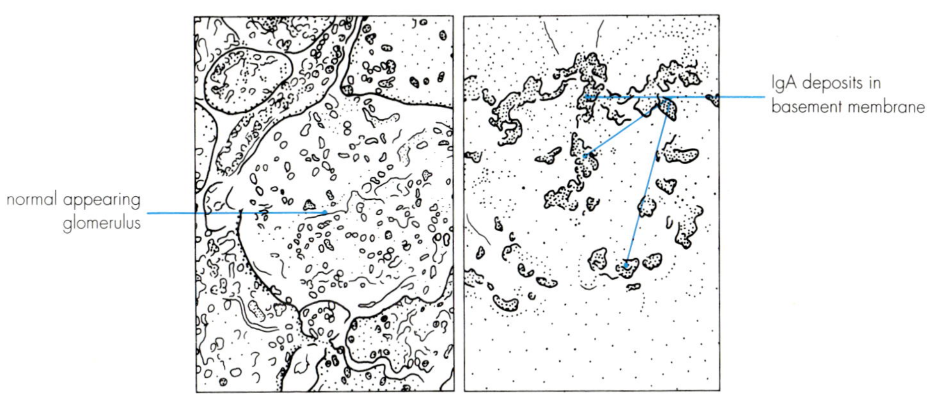

Plasma and Urine Electrolytes

	Na^+ (mmol/l)	normal range	K^+ (mmol/l)	normal range
plasma	132	136–142	3.0	3.5–5.5
urine	150	100–200	80	25–50

Fig. 8.4 Typical plasma and urine electrolytes in a severe form of malignant hypertension. Note the low plasma sodium and potassium in the face of relatively high urinary sodium and potassium. Plasma renin is very high and secondary hyperaldosteronism is present in such patients.

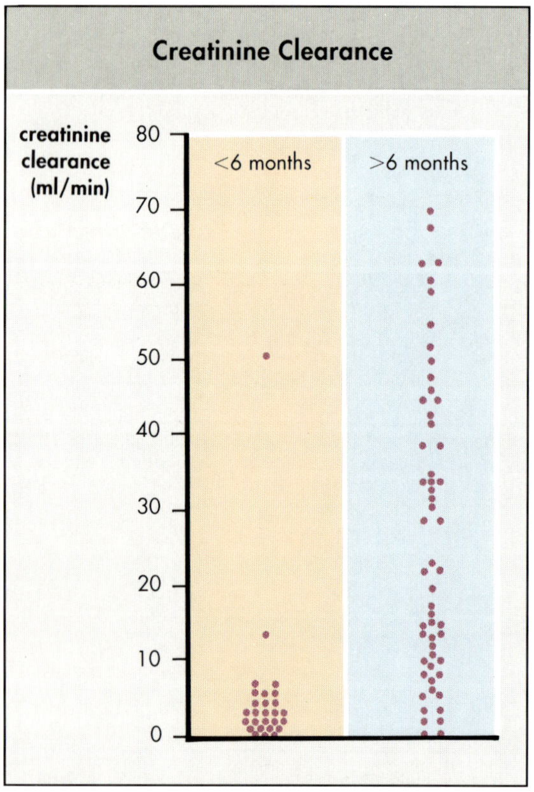

Fig. 8.5 Fate of severely hypertensive patients with low creatinine clearances (left), showing that most survived less than six months from the time of diagnosis, compared with the group with mostly higher creatinine clearances (right) who survived longer.

Urinary Electrolytes

Urinary electrolytes are most helpful in detecting hyperaldosteronism, when an alkaline urine is associated with hypokalaemia and a relatively high urinary potassium, although thiazide diuretics have similar effects.

In malignant hypertension with hyponatraemia, both urinary sodium and potassium are high and the latter may be due to the associated secondary hyperaldosteronism (Fig. 8.4).

Catecholamines

The measurement of free catecholamines and their O-methylated metabolites in urine (the metanephrines) has improved diagnostic precision in phaeochromocytoma.

Urinary vanillylmandelic acid (VMA) excretion is an unreliable indicator of excessive catecholamine secretion by chromaffin tissue. Catecholamines in phaeochromocytomas are metabolized predominantly by catechol-O-methyl transferase (O-methylation) rather than monoamine oxidase (deamination). Regrettably, VMA excretion is still widely used as a relatively inexpensive screening test. It should be abandoned.

Blood

Renal Function

Routine assessment is best made by considering creatinine clearance, while additional information can be gained by a measurement of blood urea. These two measurements provide an extremely reliable chemical assessment of renal function. Incomplete urine collection gives spurious clearance results and the plasma levels are therefore an important guide. Blood urea is influenced not only by renal performance but also by protein intake, diuretic use and the state of hydration; it is therefore not as useful as creatinine in assessing renal function. A marked reduction in creatinine clearance in hypertensive subjects suggests a poor prognosis due to the presence of an underlying or associated condition, such as glomerulonephritis or diabetes, with progressive lesions (Fig. 8.5). Fortunately, extreme renal vascular damage due to hypertension is not a common cause of severe renal failure. Nonetheless, even in well treated hypertension, a falling creatinine clearance should lead to a search for deteriorating renal artery stenosis (which is often bilateral) and urinary tract obstruction. These conditions may be reversible and offer a real therapeutic opporunity. Active hypotensive treatment, especially in malignant hypertension, may lead to improvement in creatinine clearance as the acute arteriolar damage heals. However, a sudden decline in creatinine clearance is also seen in some patients with renal artery stenosis shortly after initiating treatment with converting enzyme inhibitors. This probably reflects the marked reduction of systemic pressure, augmented at the kidney by the stenosis, together with the removal of the postglomerular resistance due to angiotensin II.

Plasma Electrolytes

A raised plasma sodium (147mEq/litre) and lowered potassium (3mEq/litre) with a raised bicarbonate (35mEq/litre) and very low plasma renin point to primary hyperaldosteronism (Fig. 8.6). On the other hand, a lowered plasma sodium (125mEq/litre) with lowered potassium (3mEq/litre) and very high plasma renin point to malignant hypertension (see Fig. 8.27), which is sometimes the result of underlying renal disease (such as unilateral renal artery stenosis). Similar figures would of course be obtained from some (especially more elderly) patients with mild hypertension, or even without hypertension, taking thiazide diuretics.

Other Plasma Changes

The diagnosis of primary hyperaldosteronism is supported by the finding of high plasma aldosterone levels, which are usually higher than those encountered in bilateral nodular hyperplasia together with raised urinary metabolites. High plasma levels of norepinephrine and/or epinephrine, whether recumbent or standing, point to a phaeochromocytoma.

A raised fasting level of glucose is seen not only in diabetes, but also in Cushing's syndrome, acromegaly, patients on thiazides or corticosteroids and occasionally patients with phaeochromocytoma.

A definitive diagnosis of Cushing's syndrome is provided by finding an altered circadian rhythm of plasma cortisol with a high midnight level equal to that of the early morning (see chapter 5).

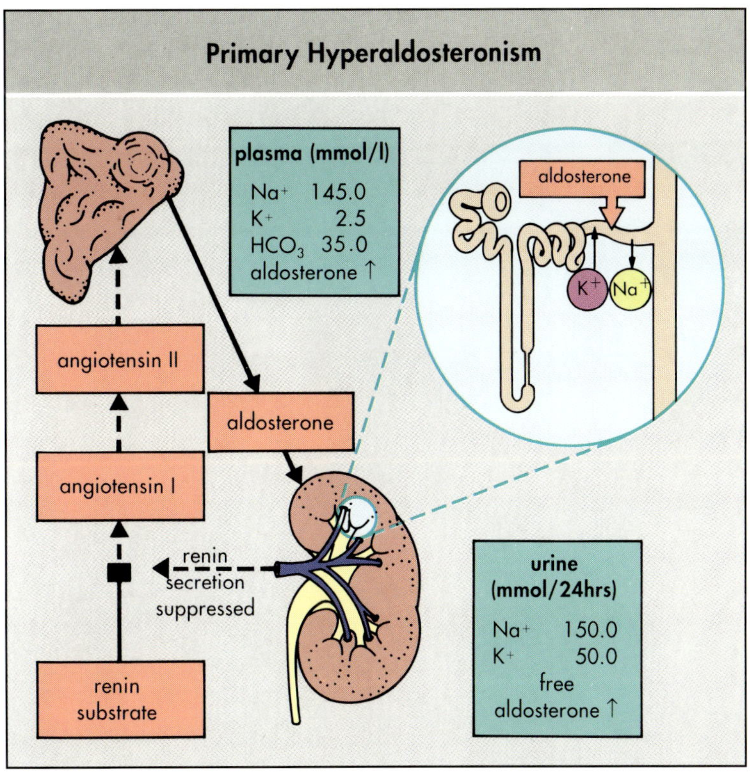

Fig. 8.6 In primary hyperaldosteronism, aldosterone reduces sodium excretion and increases potassium excretion by action on the distal tubule. This causes increased plasma sodium and lowered plasma potassium with alkalosis. Release of renin is inhibited and very low plasma renin activity is observed. The patient remains in sodium balance, with sometimes elevated total body sodium and, usually, lowered total body potassium.

Chest X-Ray

Cardiac enlargement is only detected in severe hypertension (unless cardiac failure is present) and is a late sign of hypertension (Fig. 8.7), unless cardiac failure is associated with acute glomerulonephritis, coronary artery disease or eclampsia. Rib notching is typical of coarctation, as is a small aortic knuckle. Pulmonary oedema is common in acute hypertension, particularly when associated with acute glomerulonephritis or coronary artery disease. Chest radiographs of patients with typical pulmonary oedema show the so-called Kerley's B lines over the lower lobes (Fig. 8.8), or the bat's

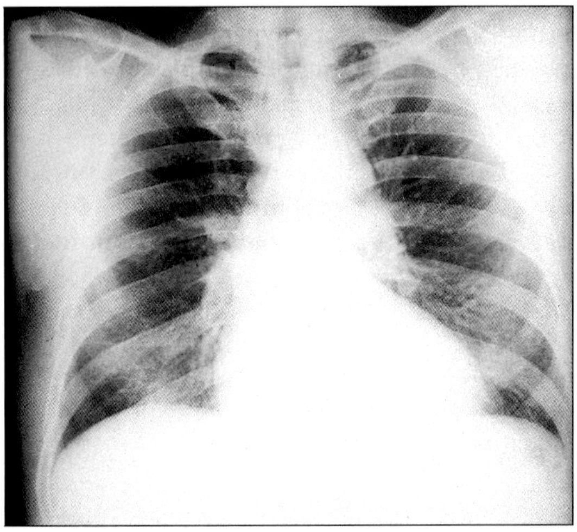

Fig. 8.7 A large heart due to left ventricular hypertrophy in a hypertensive patient.

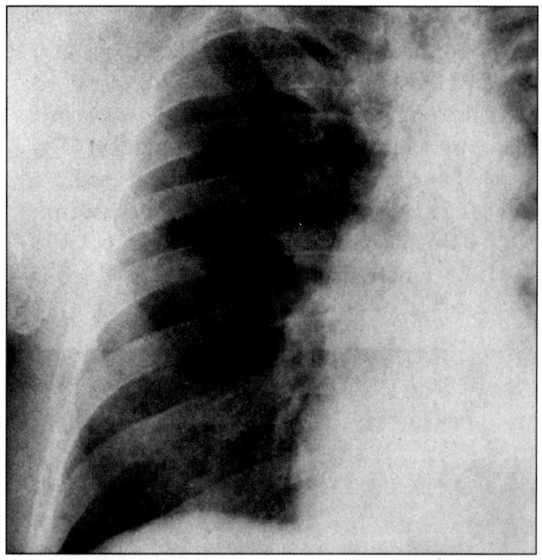

Fig. 8.8 Right: Oedema of the right lower lobe with transverse lines of interseptal oedema or engorged lymphatics known as Kerley's lines. Below left: Dilated heart with typical bat's wing hilar shadows of pulmonary oedema, in a patient with hypertension and renal failure. Below right: Unilateral pulmonary oedema, probably caused by the position of the patient during its development.

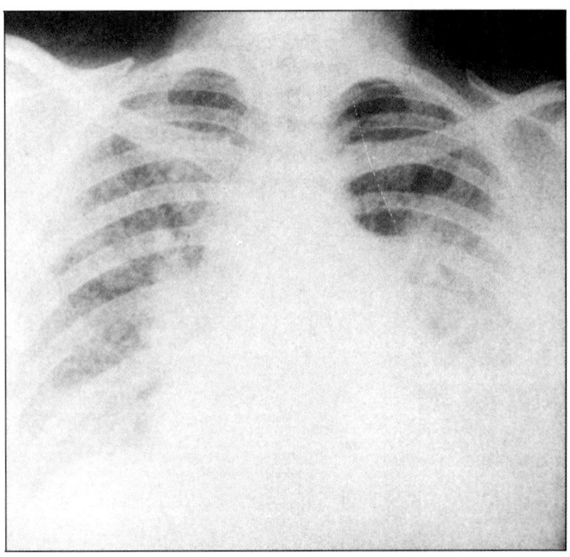

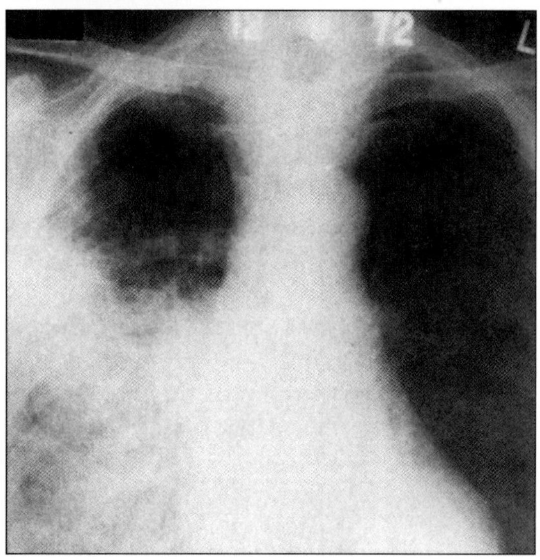

wing hilar shadows of severe hypertensive left ventricular failure, especially in renal deterioration (see Fig. 8.8) with uraemia. Pulmonary oedema is sometimes unilateral, probably due to the position in which the patient has been lying (see Fig. 8.8).

Electrocardiography

Electrocardiographic (ECG) readings are of great importance in first revealing myocardial ischaemia, which governs the approach to hypertension at all levels. Without ischaemic change, ECG readings are only really helpful in cases of severe hypertension. Although the term 'left ventricular strain' is commonly used for the usual pattern, it lacks precision in pathological terms. Severe hypertension usually produces a large R wave and ST depression with T wave inversion in tracings from the left ventricular leads (V4–6 – Fig. 8.9). A large R wave can also occur, however, with an active heart in anxious patients, especially with a thin chest wall (such as in children). Left axis deviation in the limb leads is also common in moderate or severe hypertension. These changes can be reversed by successful treatment of the hypertension. Ischaemic change with ST depression especially in the LV leads is common because of the connection of hypertension with coronary atheromatous disease.

A peaked P wave is present with a high pulmonary artery pressure and a large right atrium, secondary to the left ventricular failure of systemic hypertension.

Hypokalaemia may occasionally be detected by a large U wave after the T, but may also occur with a normal plasma potassium.

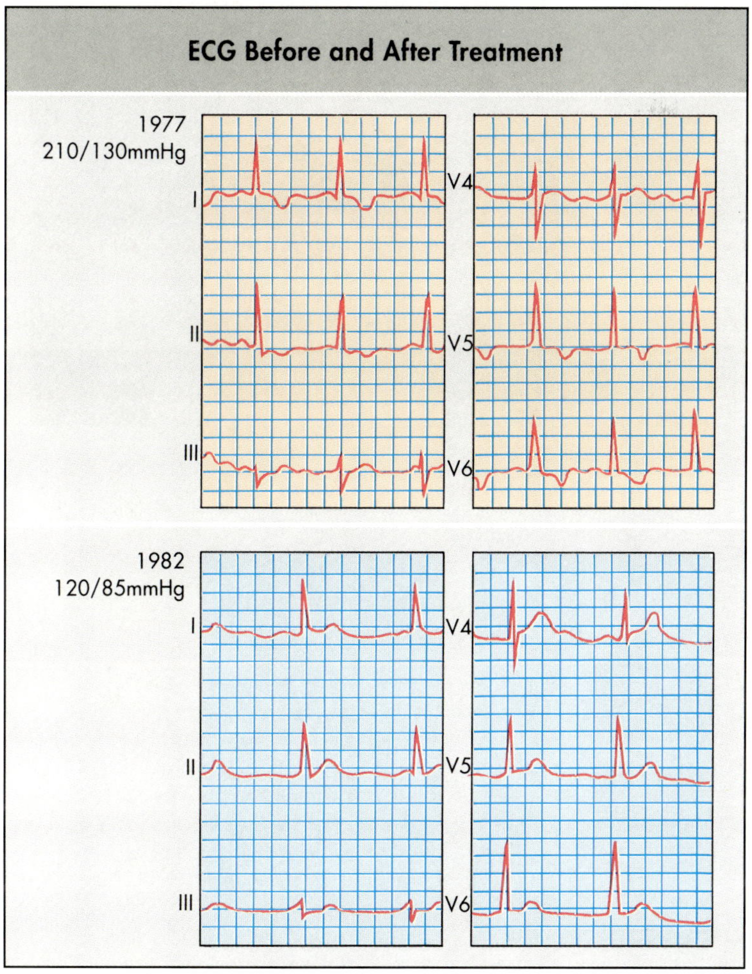

Fig. 8.9 Electrocardiogram of a hypertensive patient before (above) and after (below) treatment. Note the left axis deviation initially, with deep T wave inversion in lateral chest leads. All changes were reversed after successful treatment.

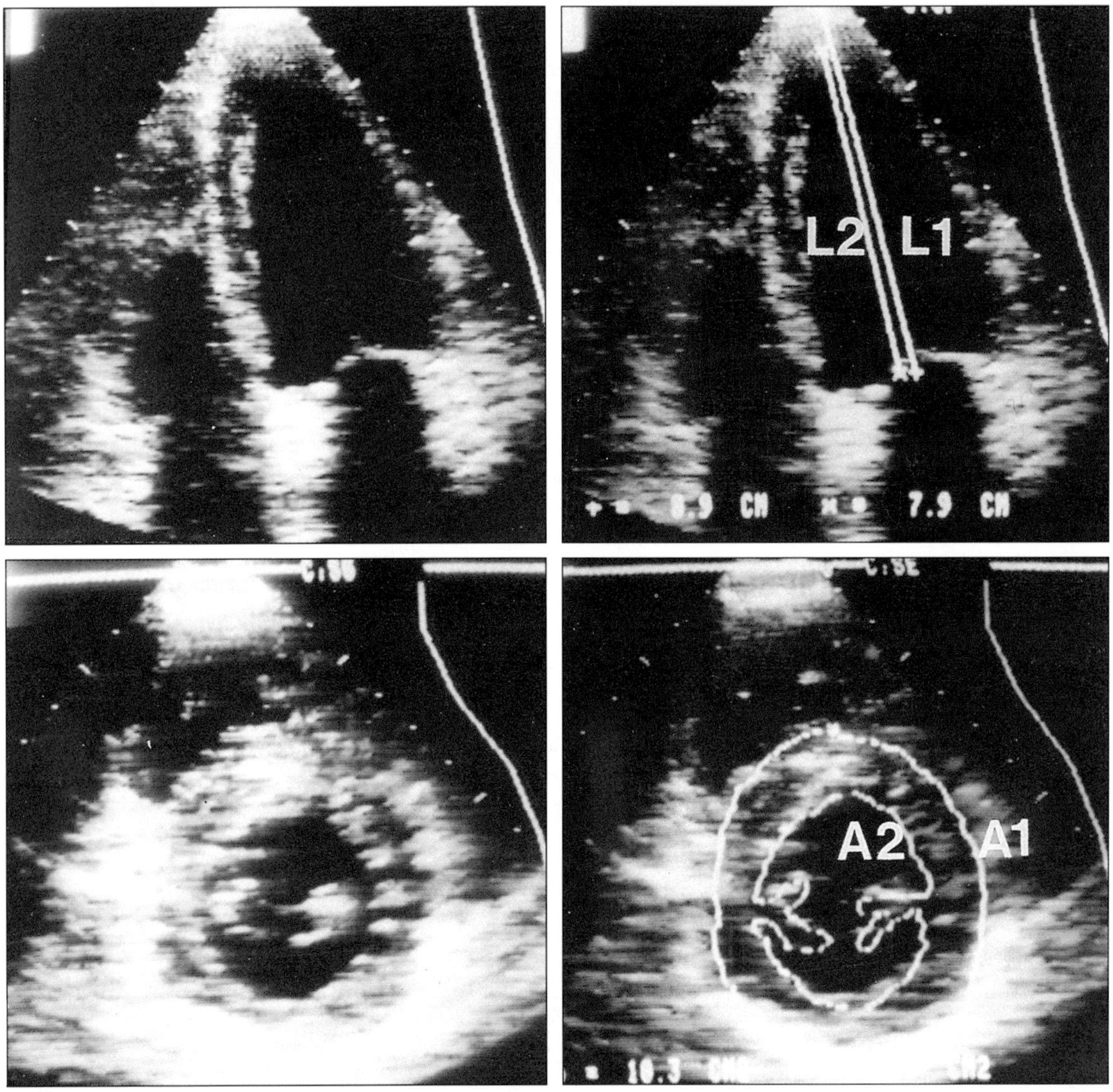

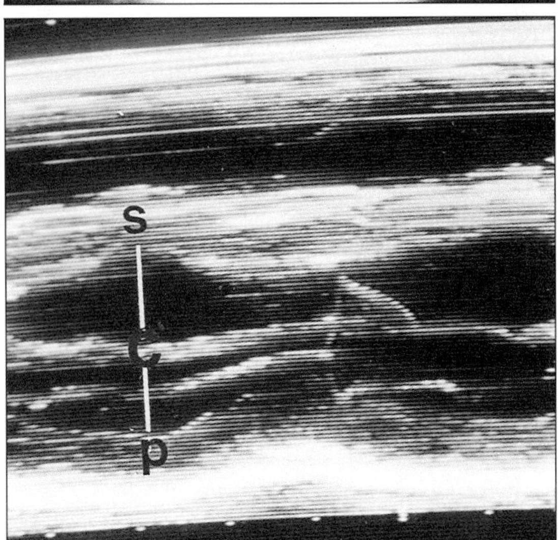

Fig. 8.10 Two-dimensional technique for the determination of left ventricular mass. Upper left: Apical four chamber view. Upper right: Length of left ventricle from mitral annulus to epicardial (Ll) and endocardial (L2) borders. Centre left: Parasternal short axis view.
Centre right: Planimetered epicardial (A1) and endocardial (A2) areas. Calculation for left ventricular mass:
$1.04\ [(5/6 \times A1 \times L1) - (5/6 \times L2 \times A2)]$.
Bottom left: M mode technique for the determination of left ventricular mass. Calculation for left ventricular mass:
$1.04[(\text{septum}(S) + \text{posterior wall}(P) + \text{cavity}(C))^3] - \text{cavity}(C)^3$

Ultrasound

Left ventricular hypertrophy has been recognized as an independent risk factor for cardiovascular morbidity and mortality in hypertensive patients. Its assessment has traditionally relied on clinical examination, chest X-ray and 12-lead electrocardiography, but these methods are limited by their lack of sensitivity. Recently, echocardiography has been used as a non-invasive technique for the accurate measurement of cardiac structure and function. It has been shown to be far superior to the electrocardiogram in detecting left ventricular hypertrophy and also gives information on the type of hypertrophy – concentric, eccentric or apical. A value for left ventricular mass can be obtained from measurements obtained from either M Mode or 2D echocardiography using anatomically validated algorithms. The progression or regression of left ventricular hypertrophy can thus be objectively documented (Fig. 8.10).

The combination of Doppler ultrasound with echocardiography also allows assessment of cardiac function. There is increasing awareness that one of the earliest cardiac manifestations of systemic hypertension is an abnormality of left ventricular diastolic function. This abnormality has been observed not only in patients with left ventricular hypertrophy but also in patients with mild or borderline hypertension. However, its importance as a possible precursor of left ventricular systolic failure or as an independent factor in the stratification of risk in hypertension is as yet undetermined.

Elsewhere in the body, ultrasound is useful for assessing renal size and shape and for demonstrating cysts and tumours in the kidney matrix, obstruction to the renal tracts from the bladder upwards, the presence of renal stones and the size and structure of the aortic wall. It is quick, non-invasive and in experienced hands reduces the need for more complex tests.

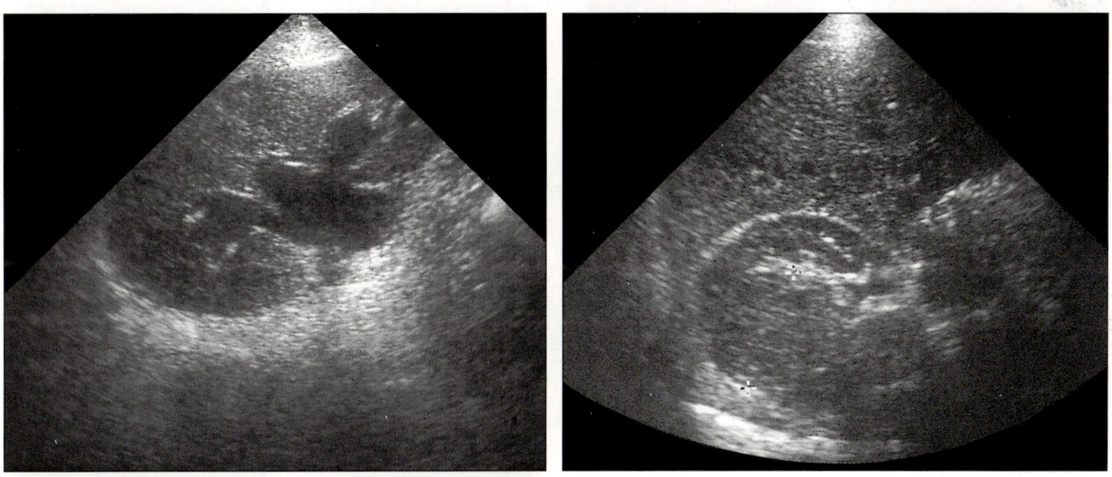

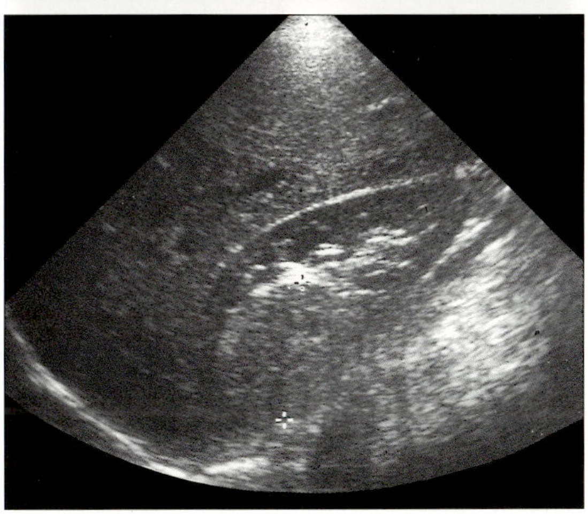

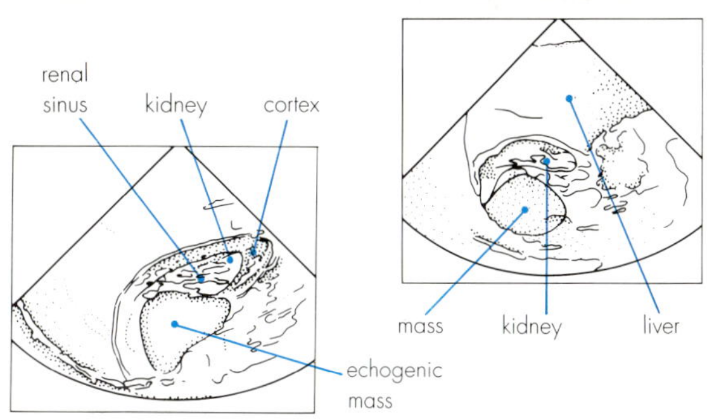

Fig. 8.11 The uses of ultrasound. Upper left: Hydronephrosis. Upper right: Transverse section through the upper pole showing a tumour. Left: Longitudinal section through the left kidney, showing a mass that turned out to be an adenocarcinoma.

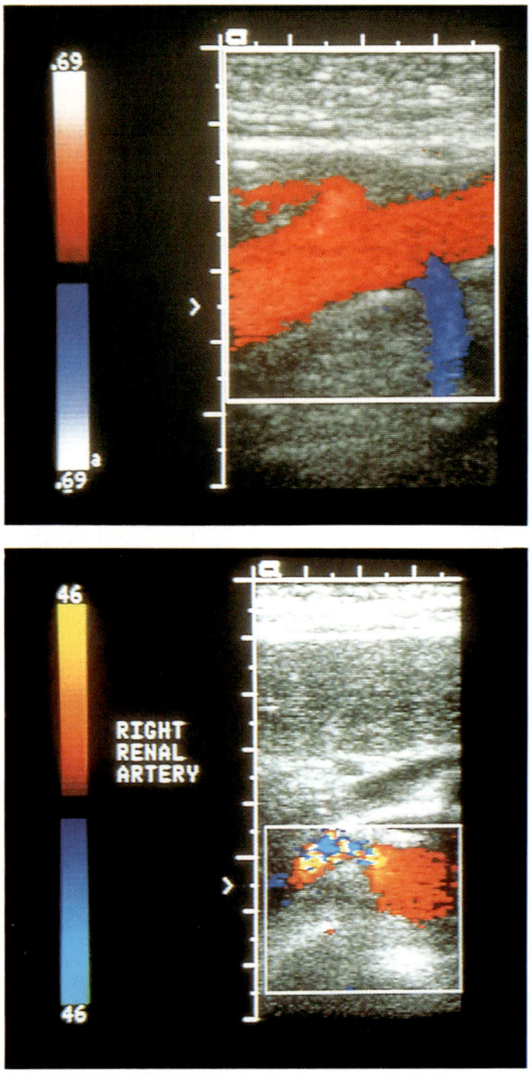

Fig. 8.12 Colour doppler imaging. Top: Aorta and normal right and left renal artery origins in coronal section. Bottom: Transverse scan of aorta and right renal artery origin, demonstrating a right renal artery stenosis. The narrowed segment shows increased colourflow velocities with flow disturbance. Images courtesy of Acuson.

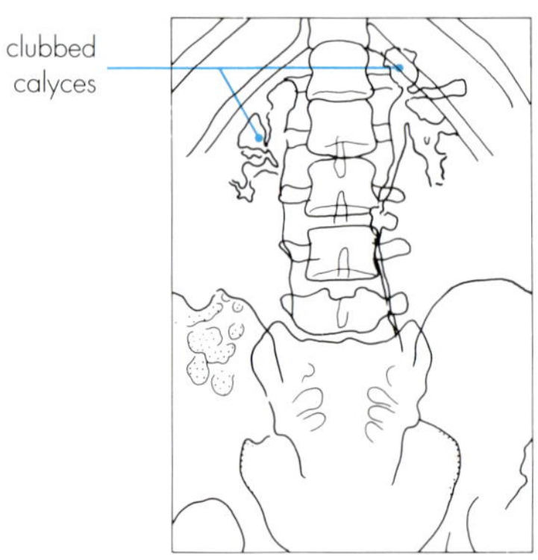

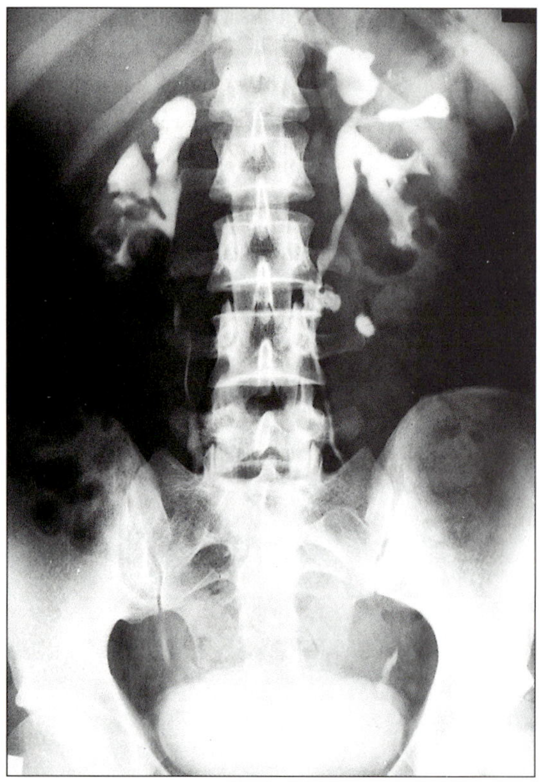

Fig. 8.13 Intravenous pyelogram showing distortion of the cortex and clubbing of calyces in a patient with chronic pyelonephritis.

Pulsed Doppler Ultrasound

This is now applied to show not only the anatomy of accessible blood vessels, including the renal, but also rate of blood flow, for example across arterial stenoses (Fig. 8.12).

Intravenous Pyelography

Intravenous pyelography is principally useful in providing a crude estimate of renal function and the anatomy of its collecting system. Cortical scarring and filling defects may be readily delineated when pyelography is combined with tomography (Fig. 8.13 & 8.14).

Although the yield of surgically correctable conditions is low in the less selective studies made outside hospitals, a pyelogram is helpful once the decision has been made to investigate an individual patient; it provides a well tried method for obtaining relevant information about renal form and function, as well as the lower urinary tract and bladder. For example, the appearance in renal tuberculosis is characteristic, with pooling of dye in small cystic abscesses (Fig. 8.14). Ultrasound removes, in many cases, the need for pyelography.

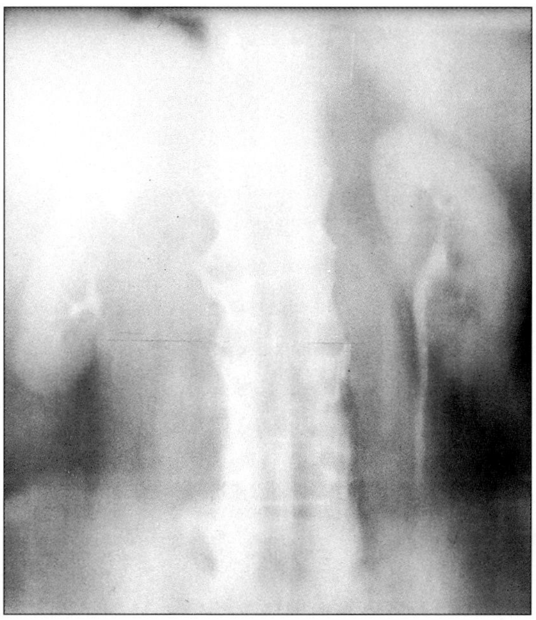

Fig. 8.14 A nephrotomogram illustrates the clarity with which the renal outlines are shown so that any scars in the cortex may be seen.

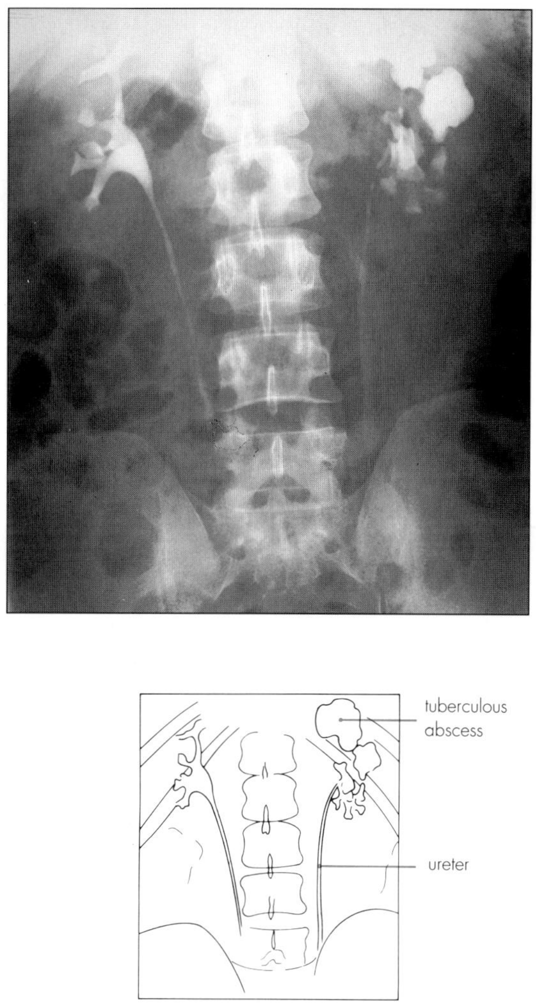

Fig. 8.15 Intravenous pyelogram of a tuberculous kidney showing typical excavated calyces and abscesses of the left kidney.

Radioisotope Scanning

Kidneys

Valuable anatomical and functional data can be obtained from radioisotope scans. The choice of radioisotope will determine the type of information obtained.

Technetium diethylenetriamine penta-acetic acid (DTPA) shows the rate at which blood enters and is cleared from each kidney, allowing the filtration rate to be estimated (Fig. 8.16). The early entry (within the first minute) is the best indication of blood flow, but interpretation must take account of the effect of differing renal size.

Dimercaptosuccinic acid (DMSA) provides a clearer indication of tubular function and mass and cortical structure (Fig. 8.17), as does ^{123}I-sodium-O-iodohippurate (Fig. 8.18).

Adrenals

Extremely clear pictures of the adrenals can be obtained using ^{75}Se-cholesterol. There is an increased uptake of cholesterol by cortical tumours in the adrenal glands so that adenomas in Conn's or Cushing's syndrome may be shown, as well as bilateral adrenal hyperplasia (Fig. 8.19).

MIBG (^{123}I-metaiodobenzylguanidine) has been used successfully to localize both intra- and extra-adrenal phaeochromocytomas. The iodinated compound is taken up by chromaffin tissue (Fig. 8.20). However, small tumours may escape detection using this technique.

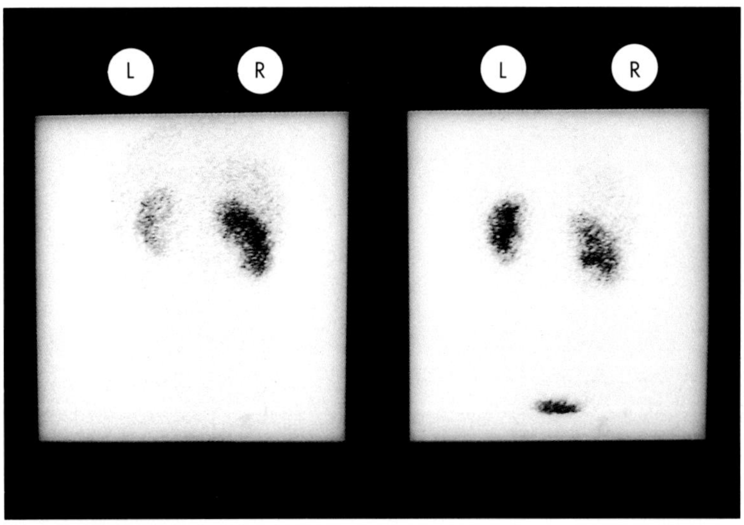

Fig. 8.16 DTPA scans at two minutes (left) and eight minutes (right), showing delayed entry into left kidney. DTPA is excreted by glomerular filtration.

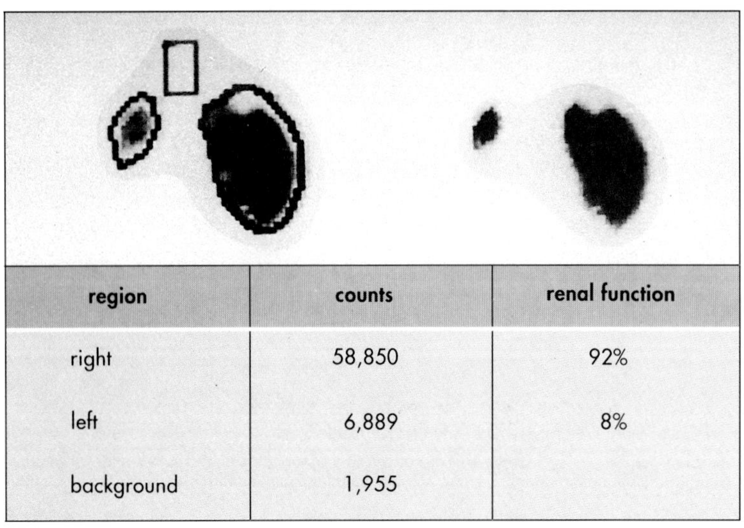

region	counts	renal function
right	58,850	92%
left	6,889	8%
background	1,955	

Fig. 8.17 DMSA scan showing cortical anatomy with a small left renal cortex. Comparison of counts from delineated renal areas shows the right kidney to have 92% of the total and the left 8%. (This substance enters the tubules and is only slowly released).

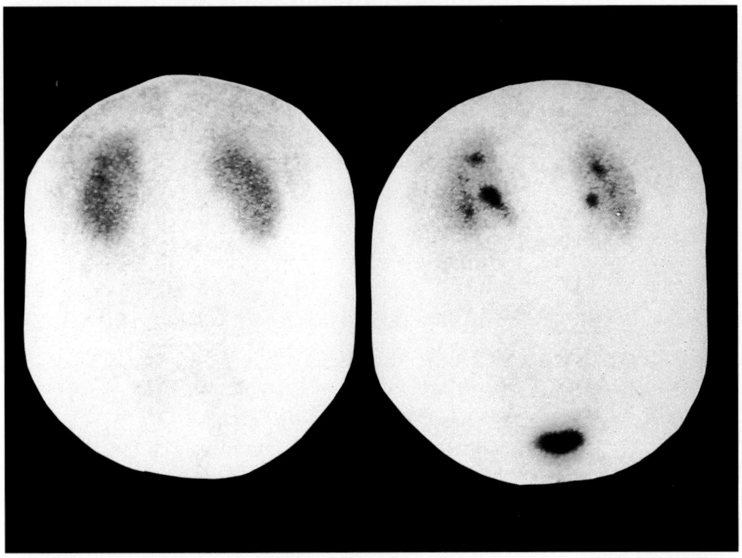

Fig. 8.18 ^{123}I-sodium-O-iodohippurate renal scan showing the symmetrical cortical uptake (left), and the even transfer to the collecting system and bladder (right) in a patient with essential hypertension.

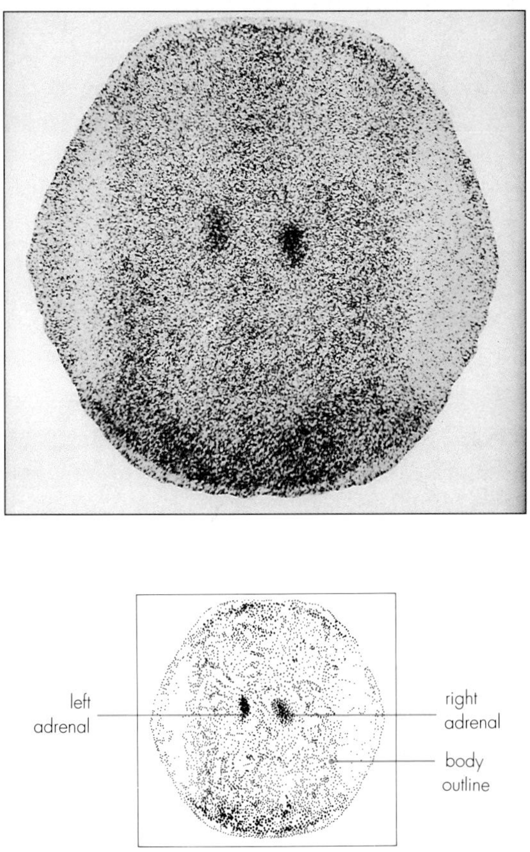

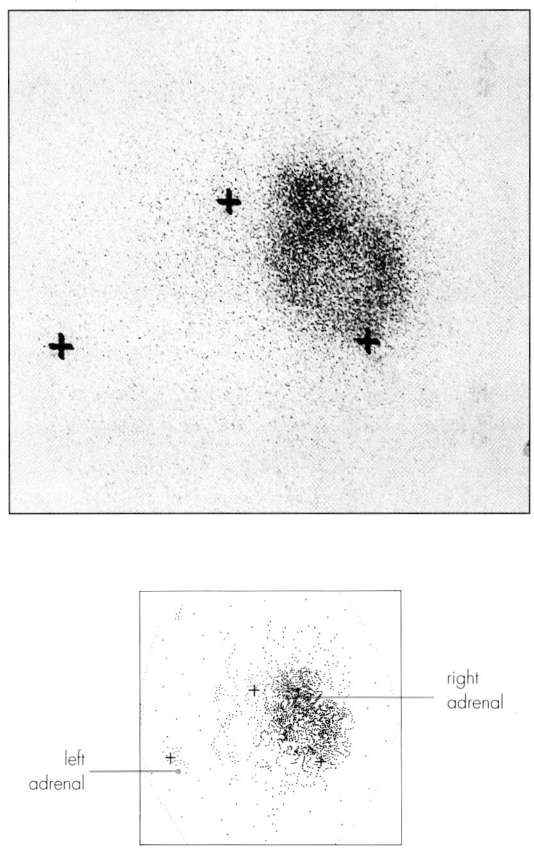

Fig. 8.19 ^{75}Se-cholesterol adrenal scan in a patient with hypertension, low renin, hypokalaemia and hyperaldosteronism. Although both adrenals are shown, there is more activity on the right, suggesting the possibility of an adenoma.

Fig. 8.20 MIBG scan, showing MIBG uptake by a phaeochromocytoma in the right adrenal. MIBG is a noradrenaline analogue.

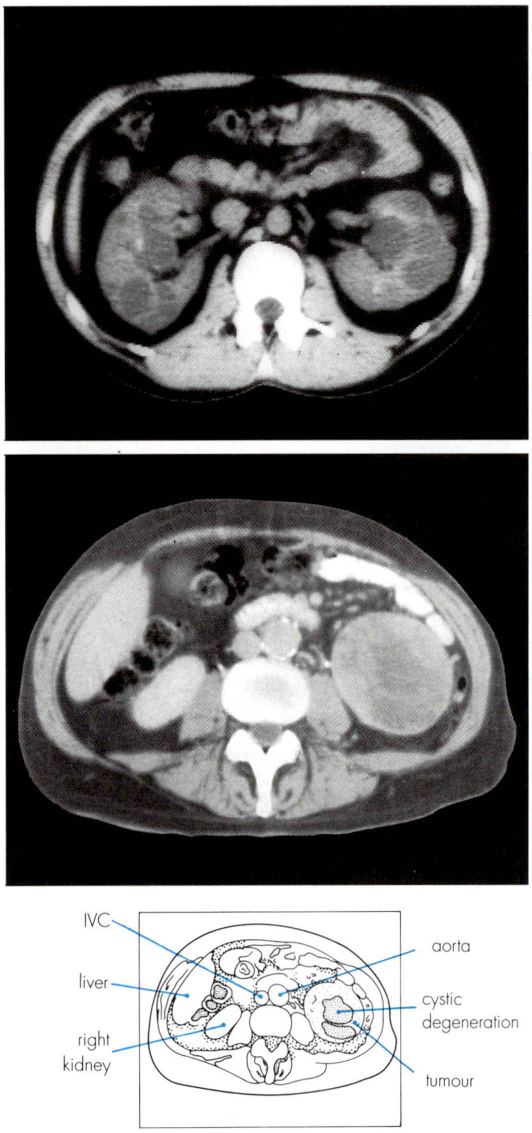

Fig. 8.21 CT scanning. Top: Multiple cysts in both kidneys in a patient presenting with severe hypertension (200/120mmHg). Bottom: A partially cystic renal tumour.

Computerized Axial Tomography (CT)

Tumours of the adrenals (see Fig. 8.51) and cysts or tumours in the kidneys are easily shown by CT scans (Fig. 8.21). When seeking renal causes of hypertension, CT scanning is usually successful in showing very small renal remnants with some flow in the cortical tissue where other techniques (IVP, radioactive isotopes, ultrasound and arteriography) may all fail (Fig. 8.22). Phaeochromocytomas in both usual and unusual sites may also be visualized with CT scans (Fig. 8.23).

Plasma Renin Activity

Renal Artery Stenosis

While the recumbent plasma renin activity (PRA) may be higher than the normal range and rise even further on standing, it is inadequate for screening. The divided renal vein renin (DRVR) assay was introduced to overcome this limitation. This technique presumes that the ischaemic kidney produces more, and the normal kidney less renin, which is usually the case (Fig. 8.24). However, the results were too often misleading in predicting the effects on blood pressure of correction of the stenosis (Fig. 8.25). This led to the introduction of tests designed to improve discrimination by stimulation using diuretics, ACE inhibitors or simple tilting of the patient. They are not sufficiently reliable for general use, but may be used in specialized centres with great experience. Even regional sampling of different veins within one kidney with a suspected renal artery stenosis has occasionally led to confirmation of raised regional renin levels and to partial nephrectomy as the treatment.

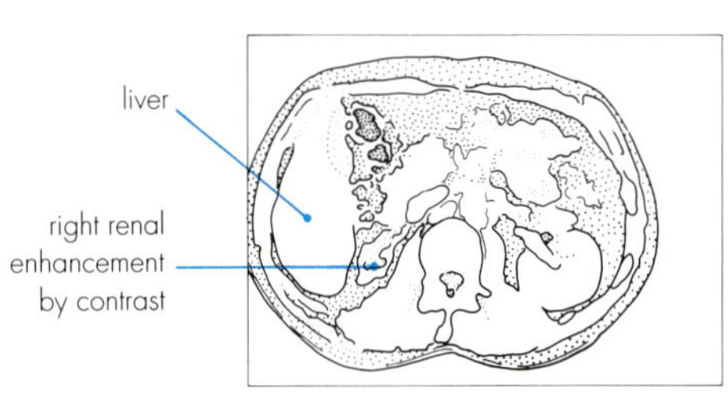

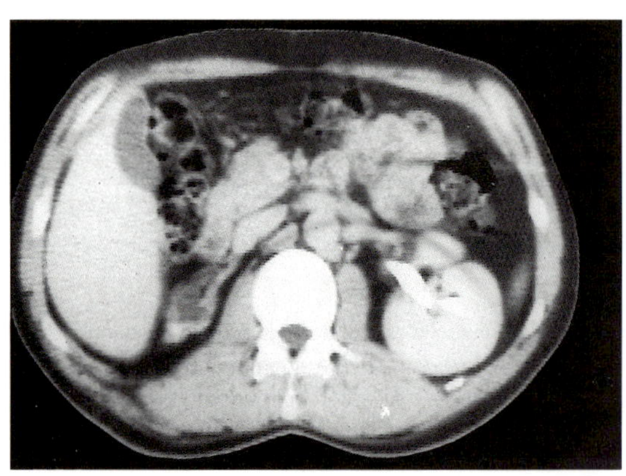

Fig. 8.22 Severe hypertension. CT scan showing small renal remnants, with enhancement showing cortical flow.

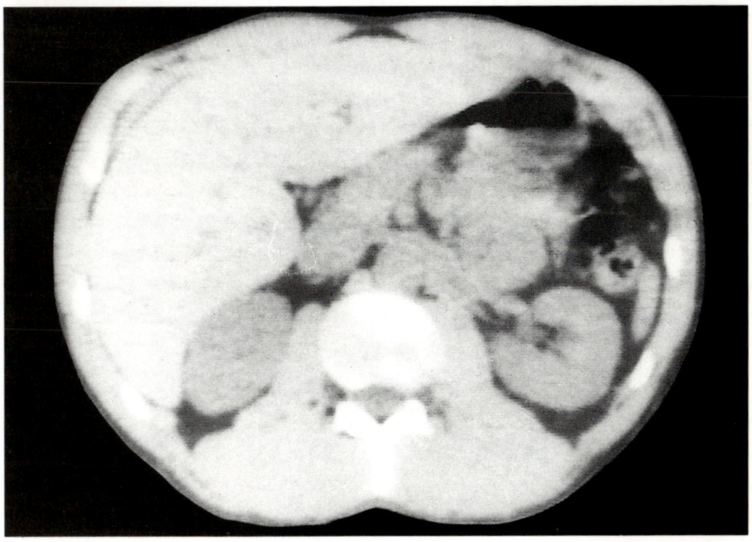

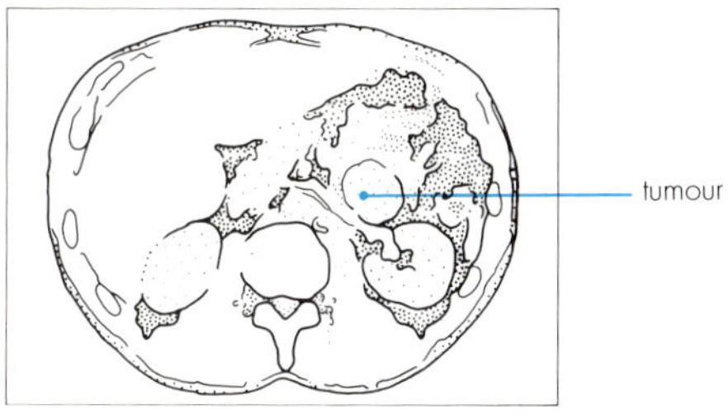

Fig. 8.23 CT scan of phaeochromocytoma resting on the vessels to the left kidney, in a patient with labile hypertension and a high plasma norepinephrine level. It was subsequently removed successfully with cure.

Divided Renal Vein Renin

	preoperative	postoperative
right	187	587
peripheral	163	530
left	1,092	686
peripheral	185	625

Fig. 8.24 Divided renal vein renin activity (pg/ml/hr) in a patient with renal artery stenosis, showing the ratio right:left of over 5:1 before operation, changed to an insignificant difference afterwards.

Renin and Hypertension

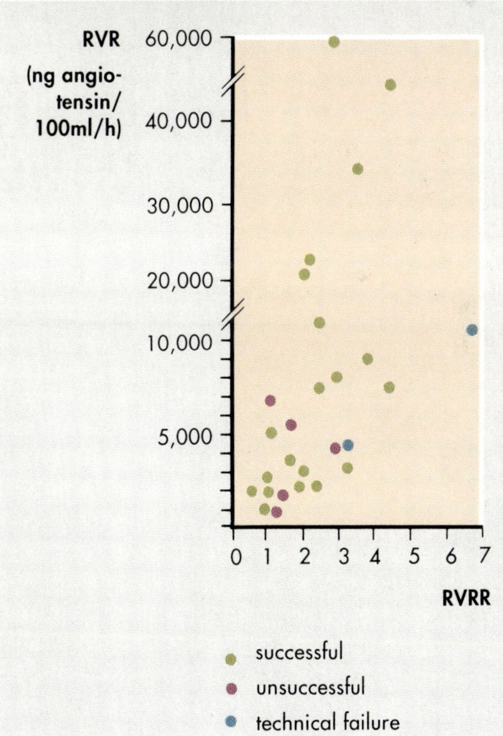

Fig. 8.25 Comparison of absolute renal vein renin (RVR) with renal vein renin ratio (RVRR) in a series of patients with renal artery stenosis. This shows that failure of the operation to relieve hypertension is more common at both lower absolute values and lower ratios, but that success is not precluded. Occasional failure also occurs however, with high absolute value and high ratio.

Conn's Syndrome (Primary Hyperaldosteronism)

Plasma renin levels are very low even in patients on thiazide treatment and can only usually be raised using spironolactone. It should be remembered that many black patients have plasma renin values lying within the low ranges found in white subjects with Conn's tumour (Fig. 8.26), but which are not associated with either a low plasma potassium or a high plasma and urinary aldosterone.

INVESTIGATION OF SPECIFIC CONDITIONS

Renal Artery Stenosis

Renal artery stenosis may be associated with either mild or very severe hypertension: the latter condition may rapidly enter the malignant phase. Fibromuscular hyperplasia of the renal artery is more prevalent in young women than in young men and may present in pregnancy. In severe cases of renal artery stenosis of acute onset, the

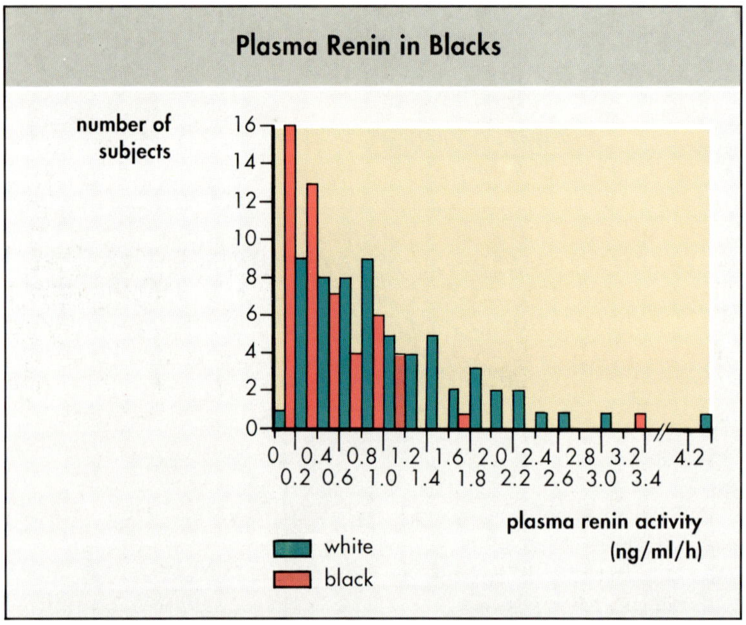

Fig. 8.26 A study of White and Black workers in the same factory with the same age distribution, showing the preponderance of low plasma renin activity in the blacks.

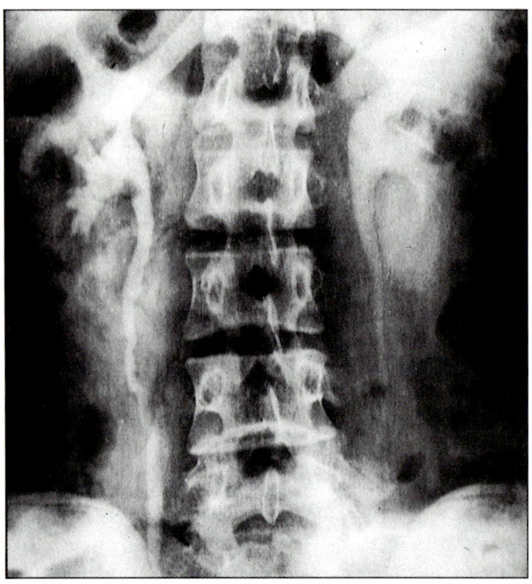

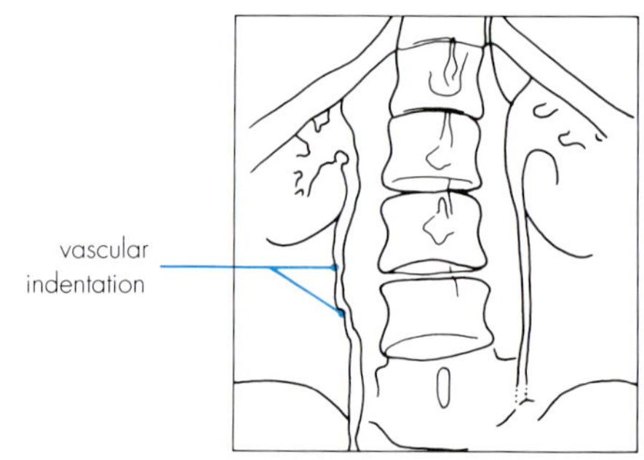

Fig. 8.27 Intravenous pyelogram in patient with renal artery stenosis. The increased density on the right is associated with indentation of the ureter due to collateral vessels running alongside.

hyponatraemic, hypokalaemic, secondary hyperaldosteronism changes associated with very high plasma renin values may be seen. The IVP carried out without lower abdominal compression and with rapid sequence films (one, three and five minutes) may show delayed opacification in the smaller kidney and a small volume collecting system with more intense contrast (Figs 8.27 & 8.28). This increased contrast is the result of a low urine flow on the affected side with high water reabsorption, so that most of the dissolved substances in the urine have an increased concentration, as shown by divided renal function studies (Fig. 8.29). It is for this reason that both creatinine and hippuran increase in concentration but, since sodium reabsorption increases markedly with renal artery stenosis, sodium concentration is less on the affected side. The contrast medium used for pyelography is excreted with the glomerular filtrate and its concentration rises with increased water reabsorption as does the density of the X-ray appearance.

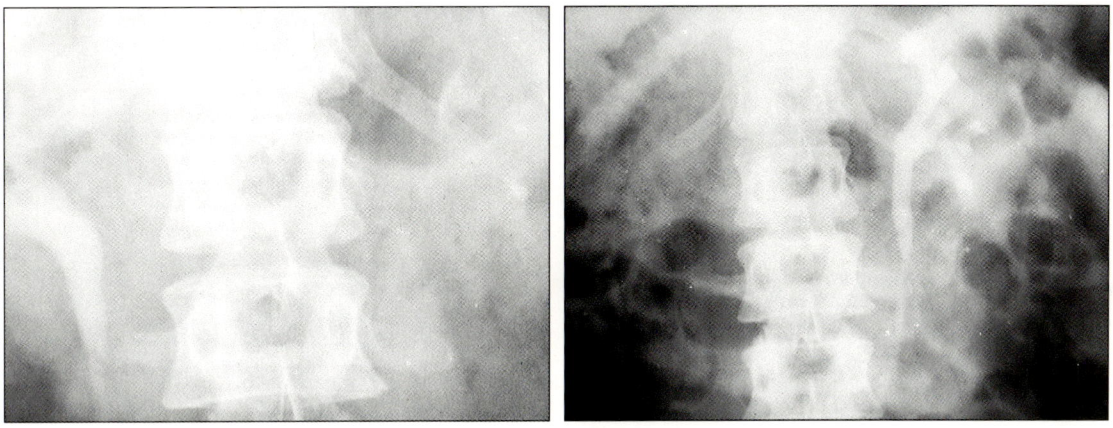

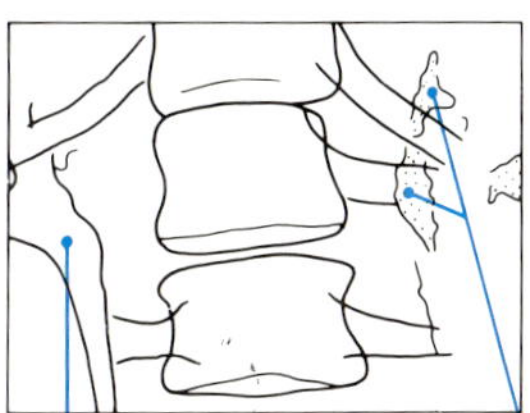

Fig. 8.28 Patient with left renal artery stenosis. Left: An intravenous pyelogram taken under usual conditions, with larger collecting system on the right. Right: An intravenous pyelogram taken after oral water load. The normal right side has been 'washed out', but the left now stands out clearly. This indicates a very tight stenosis.

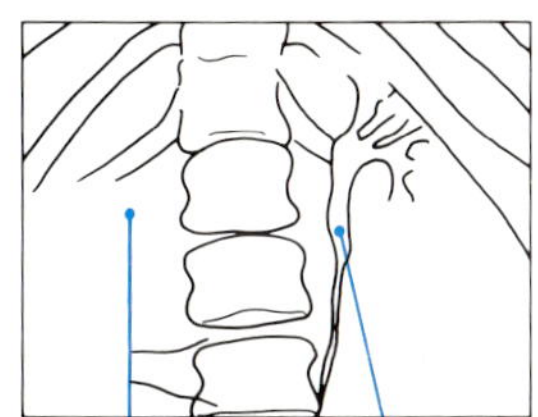

Divided Renal Function Study

	Na+ (mEq/l)	flow (ml/min)	urine concentration		clearance	
			Cr(mg%)	PAH (mg%)	Cr (ml/min)	PAH(ml/min)
preoperative						
left	134	4.4	15	188	83	462
right	90	1.6	32	435	63	387
postoperative						
left	124	2.2	18	240	36	246
right	120	1.9	20	230	35	204

Fig. 8.29 Divided renal function study with separate ureteric collection of urine in a patient with right renal artery stenosis. Note reduced flow with increased concentration of creatine (Cr) and hippuran (PAH) and reduced clearances on the affected side, yet with lowered sodium concentration due to increased reabsorption. This test is no longer used but illustrates the functional principles.

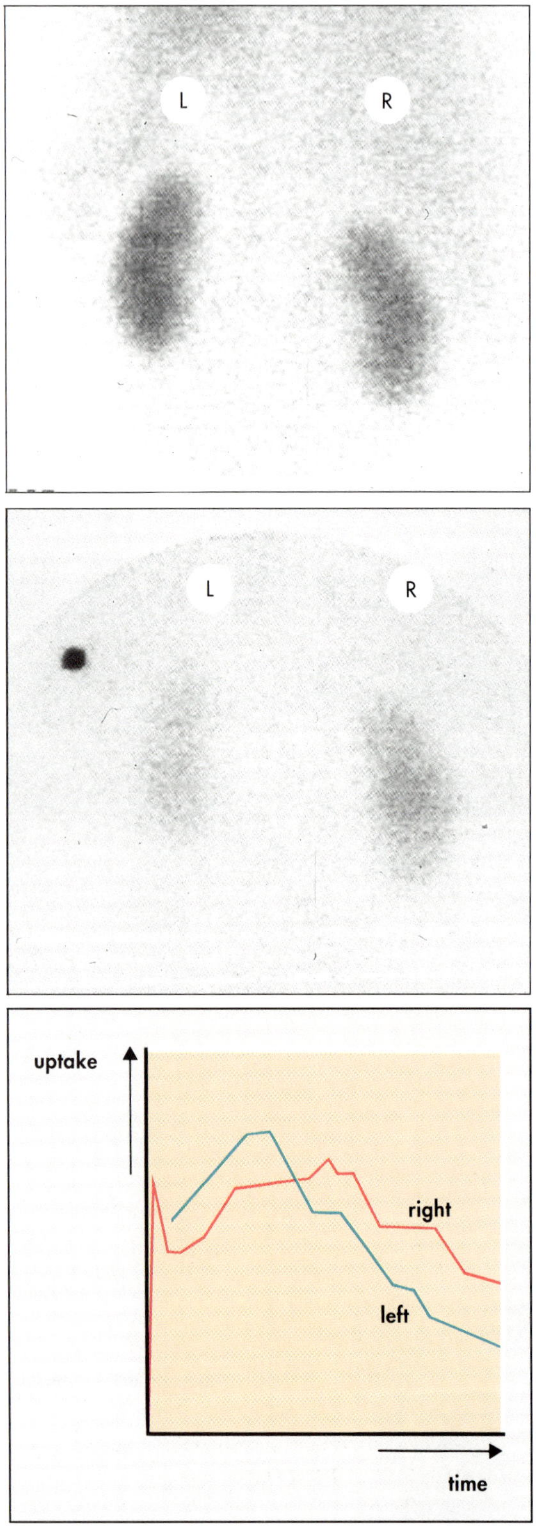

Fig. 8.30 DTPA renal scan showing reduced uptake on the right and delayed clearance, indicating right renal artery stenosis.

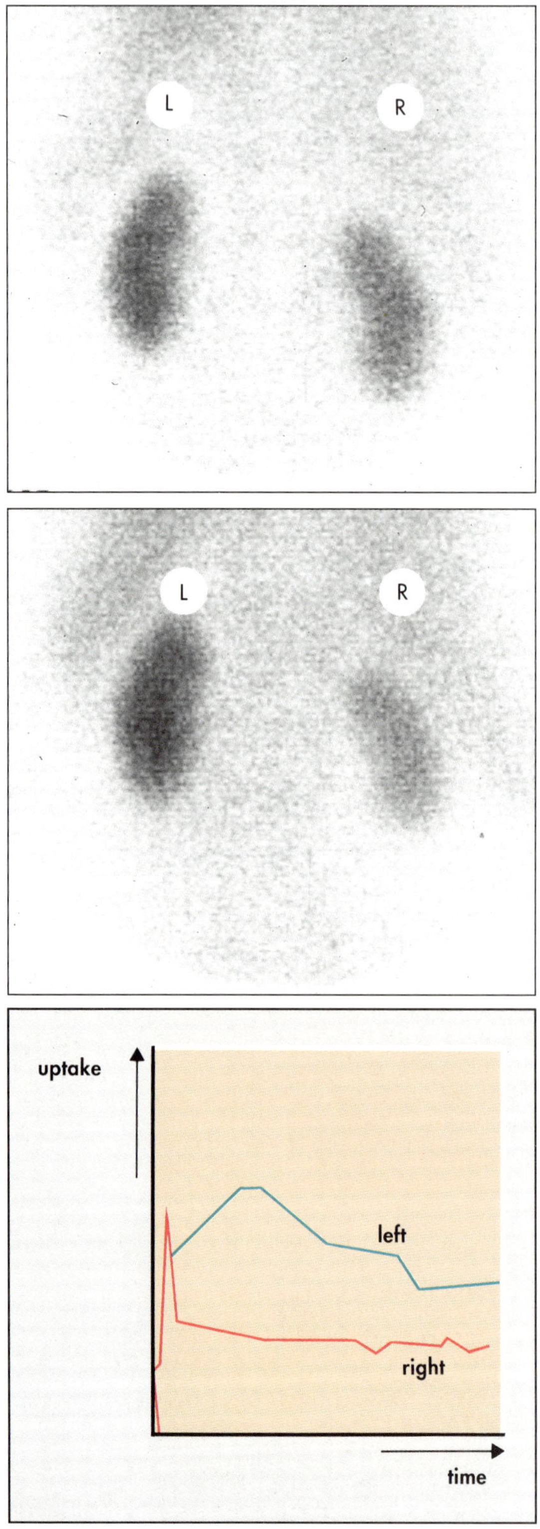

Fig. 8.31 DTPA renal scans before and one hour after 25mg oral captopril showing a marked reduction of function on the right following captopril. This indicates a significant renal artery stenosis.

Gamma Camera Renal Scan

A gamma camera renal scan using ^{99}Tc-DTPA (^{123}I-sodium-O-iodohippurate formerly) shows delayed entry of radioactive tracer into the affected kidney. A slower uptake and delayed clearance of DTPA (which provides a measure of glomerular filtration rate) and sodium O-iodohippurate (which gives an indication of tubular function) also occurs from the affected kidney. However, it is not a very sensitive test.

There have been many attempts to improve the diagnostic reliability of these tests. This has been achieved in part by administering captopril before the DTPA scan. The reduction of GFR in the stenosed kidney (due to blockade of the efferent glomerular resistance by captopril) together with the fall in renal artery pressure differentiates it from the normal kidney (Figs 8.30 & 8.31).

Aortography and, if required, selective renal arteriography can show the different types of renal artery block (Fig. 8.32). Fibromuscular hyperplasia is often seen as beading from the main artery down into the periphery. An atheromatous block often occurs in the proximal segment of the renal artery. Stenosis of any cause may be associated

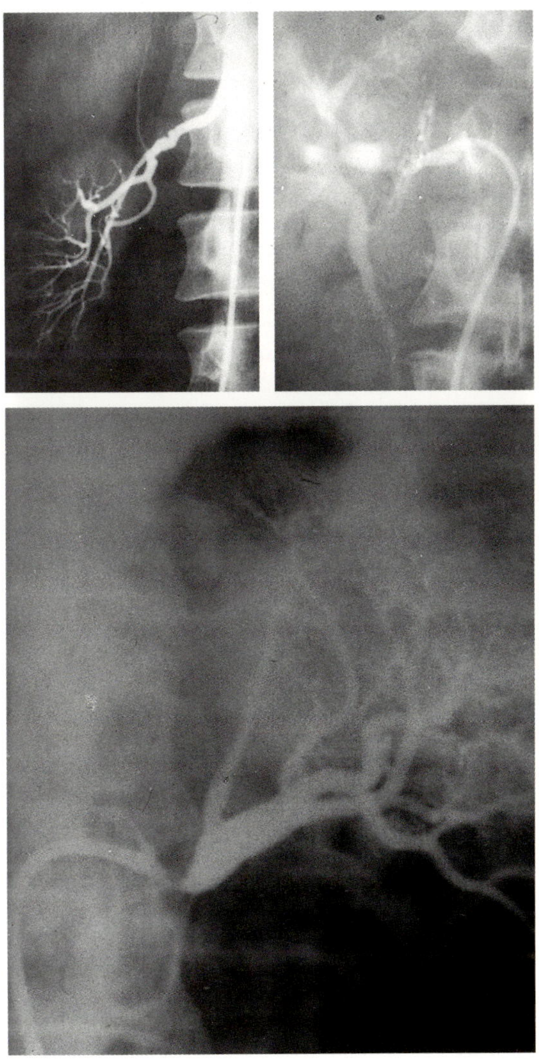

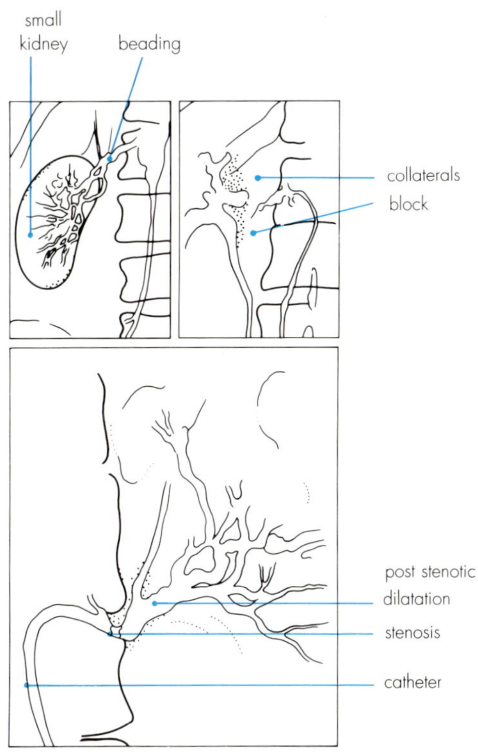

Fig. 8.32 Top left: Arteriogram showing fibromuscular change as beading in the distal part of a long renal artery to a low-set kidney. Top right: A selective renal arteriogram shows almost complete occlusion of the right renal artery in its centre section with post-stenotic dilation and numerous collateral vessels around this area. Left: A selective renal arteriogram shows a tight stenosis at the tip of the catheter with post-stenotic dilation (shown to be atheromatous).

with post-stenotic dilatation and even aneurysm formation (Fig. 8.33). If aortography is associated with measurement of the pressure drop across the stenosis, a direct functional indication is obtained.

Intravenous Digital Subtraction Angiography (IVDSA)

A large intravenous bolus of contrast material is administered. Subsequent pictures of the arterial system from the aorta to the kidneys may, in thin subjects, show the vessels clearly enough for a decision to be made about the presence of a stenosis. Comparisons with aortography show that it is not reliable enough for general use and the patient is not spared very much discomfort.

Pharmacological Tests

Pharmacological tests now centre on captopril or other converting enzyme blockers, which have been used to lower the blood pressure in a prognostic fashion. The results of these tests have been complicated by the different conditions under which they have been carried out. Most seem to require the use of a diuretic and an upright posture to produce a pressure drop; even then the value of the results in prognosis seems to be no better than the renal vein renin ratio (see page 8.15). However, there is no doubt that there is a relationship between the fall of blood pressure produced and the higher levels of plasma renin activity present even without diuretics.

Diagnosis and Treatment

Is there a best approach to the diagnosis and treatment of renal artery stenosis? This is an important question, because although it is the renal condition that most often leads to curable hypertension, it is rare among those hypertensives considered suitable for investigation and treatment. It is therefore important to establish methods that can select patients most likely to have the condition (high sensitivity testing) and then show that the lesion is, with a high degree of probability, the cause of the hypertension (high specificity testing). A number of diagnostic approaches have been used.

Clinical Suspicion

This is raised by

- The presence of diminished or deteriorating renal function even on adequate hypotensive treatment (note the occasional deleterious effects of converting enzyme inhibitor drugs in renal artery stenosis).
- Resistance to treatment or a rise in previously well controlled blood pressure, particularly if associated with any diminution of renal function.

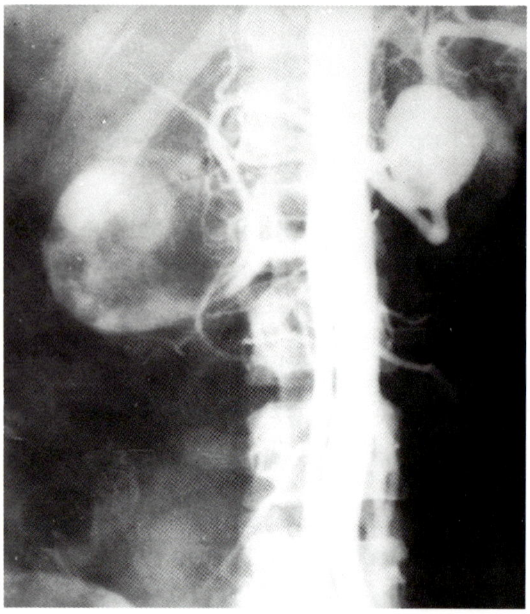

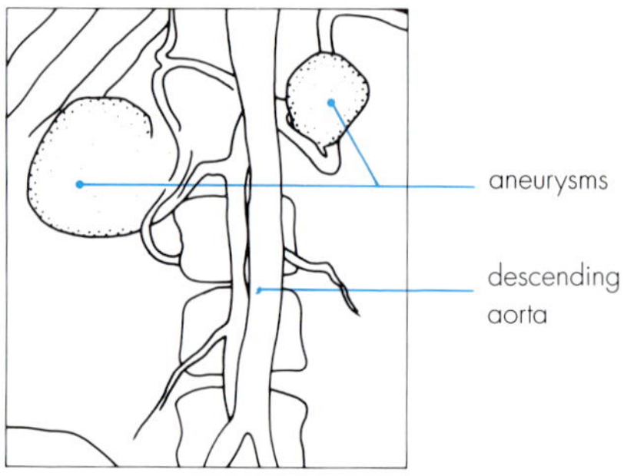

Fig. 8.33 Free aortogram on a patient with bilateral aneurysms which occur particularly in fibromuscular change with severe stenoses.

Indirect Methods

These are based on:

- Individual renal function assessment (glomerular filtration rate and renal plasma flow) and its modification by pharmacological means (e.g. renal scanning with DTPA with and without converting enzyme inhibition).
- Assay methods based on renin measurements in peripheral plasma altered by pharmacological means (e.g. frusemide stimulation; converting enzyme stimulation).

These indirect methods are neither sensitive nor specific.

Direct Methods

Renin Assay in Renal Veins With and Without Pharmacological Stimuli (DRVR)

This can be sensitive and predictive, but requires invasive techniques and a specialized high quality assay service to provide confirmation of the presence of an anatomically functional stenosis.

Aortography With Measurement of Pressure Gradient Across the Stenosis

This can quantitatively define the degree of stenosis in the main renal artery, which is essential to all treatments. Angioplasty can be initiated immediately and the effects on the stenosis measured by the changes in the pressure gradient.

The morbidity of the process must be low to justify a direct attack on all stenoses. It assumes that all stenoses are responsible for the existing hypertension and therefore relies on clinical improvement as the essential criterion and dispenses with all other selection criteria.

In experienced hands it is very successful, but severe atheroma at the origin of the renal artery provides a major technical problem and hazard, with occasional dissection of the renal artery.

The success of surgery or angioplasty depends on numerous factors which are summarized in Figure 8.34. One major influence leading to a variation in these results is the skill of the operator and this should always be considered when deciding upon invasive versus medical treatment.

Factors in the Cure of Renovascular Hypertension
youth and short duration of hypertension
good renal function overall and in opposite kidney
stenosed side – evidence of ischaemia:
• increased water reabsorption ratio 1.5:1 (historical)
• increased renal vein renin concentration ratio >1.5:1
• DTPA renal scan changed by converting enzyme inhibitor
• pressure gradient across stenosis at aortography
hypotensive response to angiotensin or renin blockers (proportional to plasma renin activity)
fibromuscular disease better than atheroma (usually younger patients)
unilateral disease better than bilateral

Fig. 8.34 Major factors associated with a successful outcome in renovascular surgery and angioplasty.

Pyelonephritis

In many patients, the scarred kidney of pyelonephritis has been shown to date from a childhood infection and ureteric reflux (as shown by a micturating cystogram) may still be present with or without chronic urinary infection (Fig. 8.34). Young adults may occasionally present with congenital urethral stenosis, leading to a large bladder and renal impairment. It is sometimes difficult to distinguish chronic pyelonephritis from an agenetic kidney and both may have considerable intimal hyperplasia of major arteries within the kidney (Fig. 8.35). The IVP typically shows clubbing of the calyces (Fig. 8.36). The appearance of 'analgesic abuse kidney' may be similar and asymmetry between the two kidneys may be present (see Fig. 8.36). Excavation around the tip of the papilla is characteristic (the cup and saucer sign – see Fig. 8.36) and, since the tubules are frequently damaged, the urine produced is more dilute and the intensity of contrast less on the IVP. The investigation may reveal more about the use of analgesics, including phloretin and aspirin, than the patient is prepared to admit.

Hydronephrosis is only an accompaniment of pyelonephritis when reflux is marked, or when the passage of stones or the necrotic tip of the papilla (as in diabetics or in analgesic abuse) has blocked the ureter either partially or completely. Infective fibrosis in the wall of the ureter sometimes occurs at the entry into the bladder, and tuberculosis and bilharzia should be remembered and looked for. In most cases, uncomplicated hydronephrosis is not a cause of hypertension, although prostatic obstruction may lead to insidious renal failure and eventual hypertension.

Conn's Syndrome

The first biochemical sign which should arouse suspicion of Conn's syndrome is the presence of low plasma potassium (3mEq/litre) with a normal or slightly raised plasma sodium (146mEq/litre). While hypokalaemia may be associated with a thiazide diuretic, it is then more common to find a plasma sodium at lower levels (138mEq/litre). Many patients with Conn's syndrome are already taking thiazide diuretics to control their hypertension and do not necessarily produce severe symptoms, although an intercurrent illness such as vomiting, diarrhoea, or pneumonia can lead to severe hypokalaemia with paraesthesia, weakness

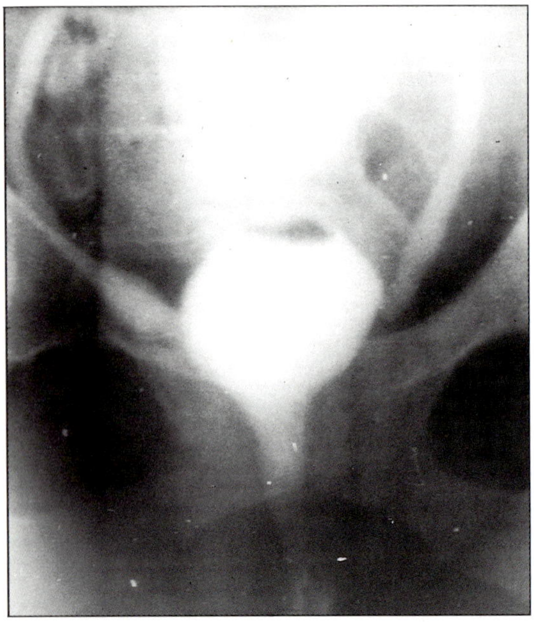

Fig. 8.35 Micturating cystogram. The bladder is filled with contrast and, while passing urine, free reflux can be seen into the ureters: this can sometimes reach the kidneys.

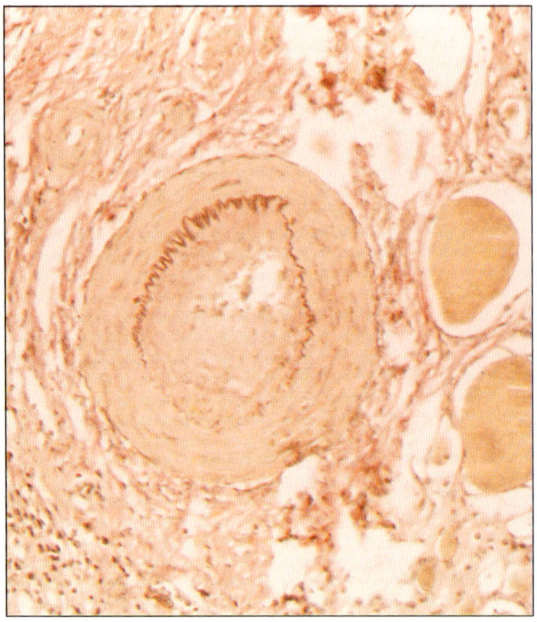

Fig. 8.36 Histological section of a kidney with chronic pyelonephritis showing intimal hyperplasia and perivascular fibrosis seen in pyelonephritis, agenetic kidney and occasionally in hydronephrosis.

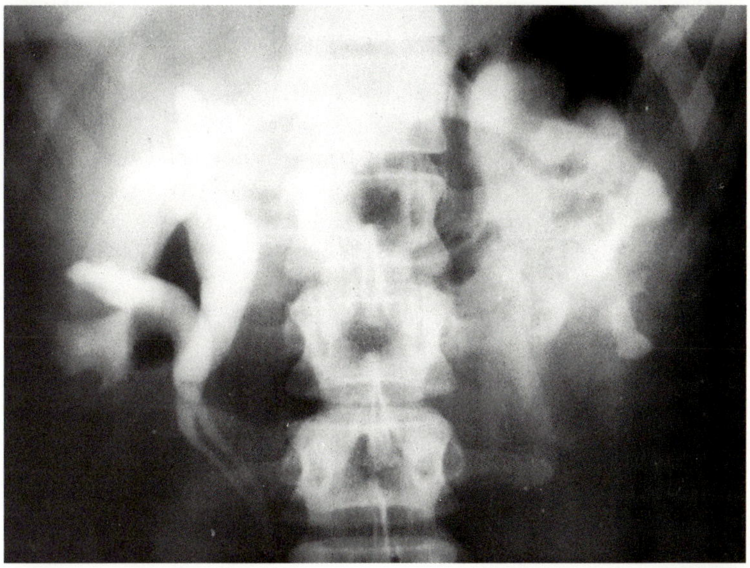

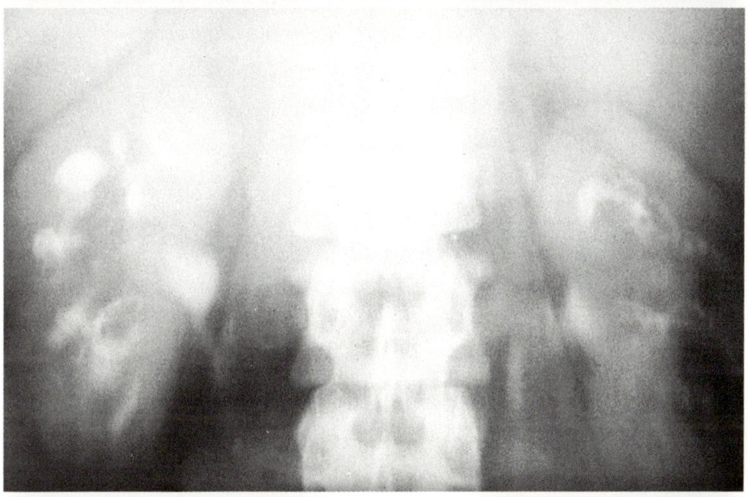

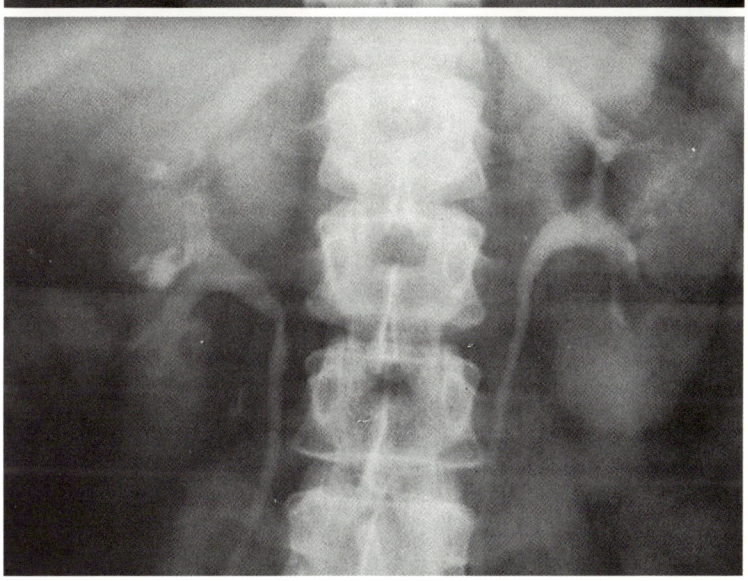

Fig. 8.37 Top: Pyelogram in chronic pyelonephritis with dilated and clubbed calyces and marked thinning of the cortex. This patient had urethral stenosis as a child, corrected by surgery, and presented with malignant hypertension at the age of twenty. Centre: Pyelogram from a case of analgesic abuse illustrates marked clubbing and some excavation of the papillae, particularly in the left kidney. Bottom: A pyelogram from a patient with papillary necrosis of the middle calyx in the right kidney. It has the typical cup and saucer sign due to lateral infiltration around the tip of the papilla, which is often shed, causing secondary obstruction.

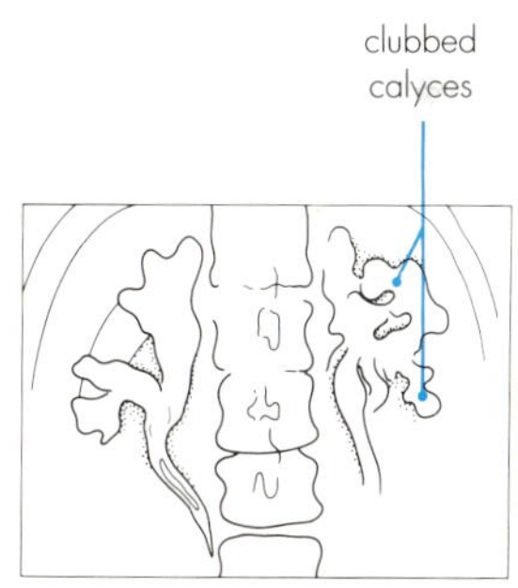

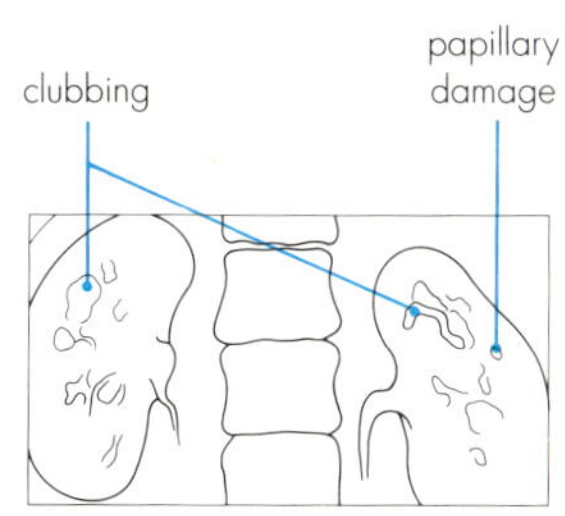

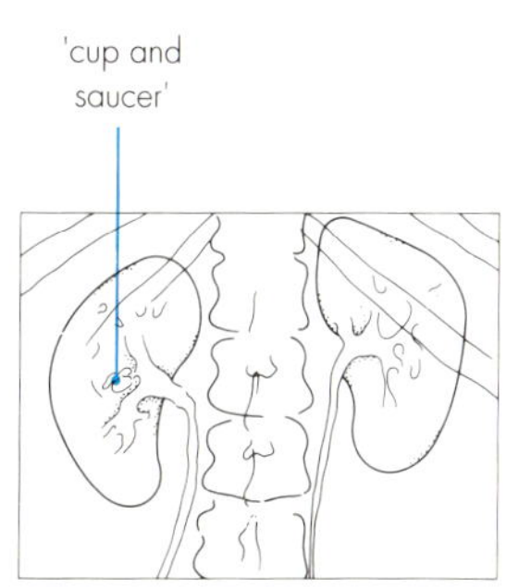

and even paralysis. In recent times, diagnosis of Conn's syndrome has been made much easier. Once the very low plasma renin activity has been shown (it is sometimes necessary to stop diuretics which elevate plasma renin activity), the high resting plasma aldosterone, which does not rise and may even fall on walking about for two hours, provides strong confirmatory evidence and may be contrasted with adrenal hyperplasia (Fig. 8.38). The differentiation of adenoma and hyperplasia depends upon obtaining all of the anatomical and functional information possible (Fig. 8.39). The next two adrenal investigations that should be undertaken are CT scanning (to show immediate anatomy – Fig. 8.40) and radioactive scanning (which demonstrates either two hyperplastic glands or a single adenoma – see Figs 8.18 & 8.41).

The older techniques used to investigate Conn's tumour involved adrenal phlebography (Fig. 8.42) and the separate collection of adrenal vein blood

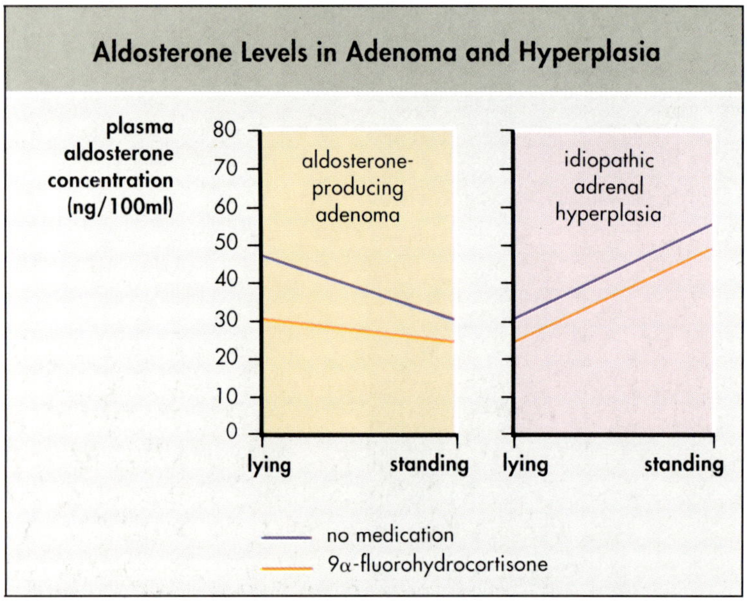

Fig. 8.38 The contrast between the behaviour of plasma aldosterone levels in a patient with an adenoma and one with idiopathic adrenal hyperplasia. Assumption of the upright posture for two hours leads to a fall in plasma aldosterone level with adenoma and a rise with hyperplasia. The depression caused by 9α-fluorohydrocortisone is usually greater with adenoma.

Differences Between Adenoma and Hyperplasia

biochemical	**tumour**	**hyperplasia**
aldosterone (basal)	↑↑	↑
aldosterone (after 4 hours upright)	no change or fall	↑↑
serum K^+	↓↓	normal or ↓
serum Na^+	>142	<140
renin	↓↓	↓
other methods		
adrenal venography venous sample aldosterone : cortisol ratio	++ unilaterally	+ bilaterally
cholesterol scan	++ unilateral	+ bilaterally
cholesterol scan after dexamethasone	++ unilaterally	suppressed bilaterally (unreliable)

Fig. 8.39 Table showing the major differences between adenoma and adrenal hyperplasia.

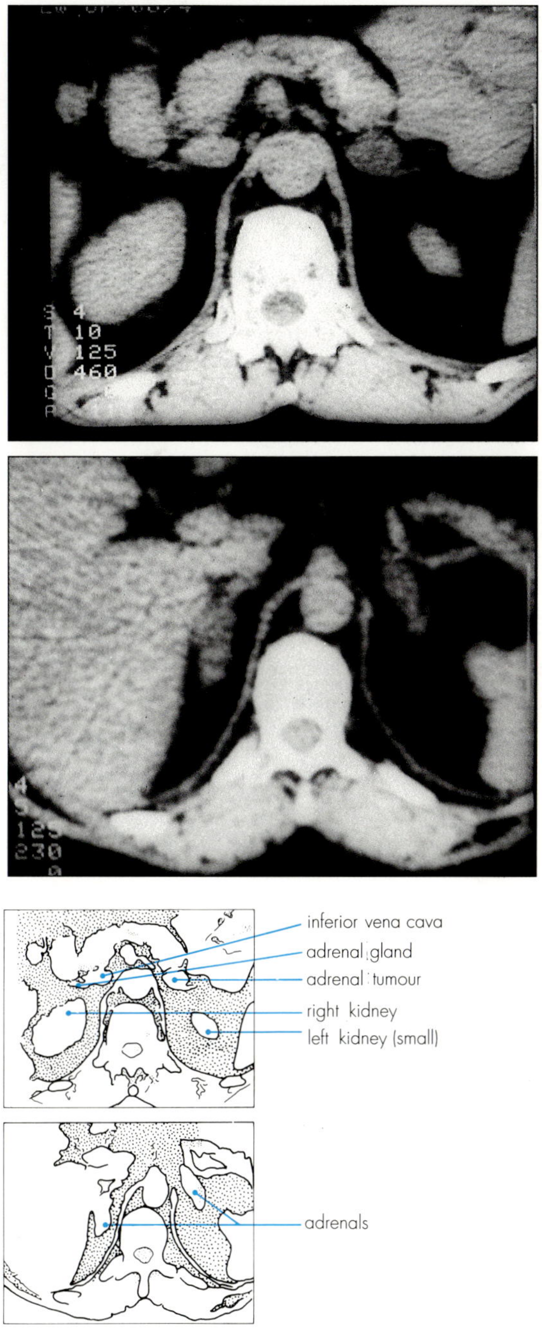

Fig. 8.40 Top: CT scan at the level of the top of the kidneys from a patient with severe hypertension, hypokalaemia, very low plasma renin activity and a high plasma aldosterone level. A large adenoma is seen just lateral to the aorta on the left-hand side and close to the tail of the pancreas. The left kidney in this patient was pathological and small, in contrast to the large normal right kidney. Bottom: CT scan showing a patient with bilateral adrenal hyperplasia.

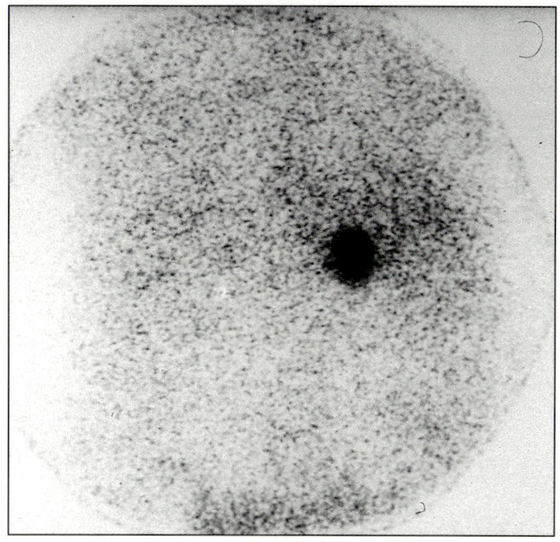

Fig. 8.41 A ^{75}Se-cholesterol adrenal scan showing a single adenoma in the right adrenal gland at seven days following the administration of the isotope. Even in Conn's syndrome, as here, uptake in the opposite normal gland is often negligible.

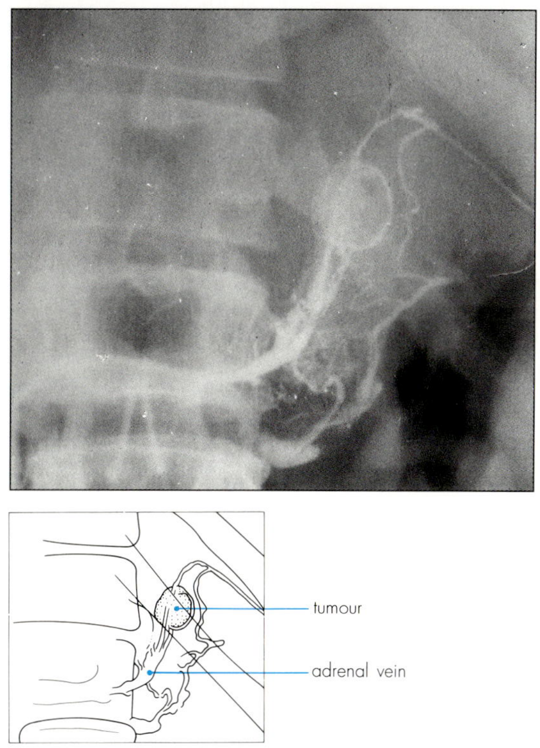

Fig. 8.42 Left adrenal phlebogram in a patient with Conn's syndrome showing a rounded tumour in the middle of the gland around which the veins deviate. This adrenal vein is easier to catheterize since it enters the upper side of the renal vein. This is in contrast to the right, where it enters the inferior vena cava.

from each gland to compare aldosterone–cortisol ratios on the two sides (Fig. 8.43). Phlebography is difficult (especially on the right side) and sometimes dangerous due to adrenal trauma. However, the steroid ratio may be the only definitive test in some cases and should be undertaken where suspicion is strong despite negative preliminary tests, including the scans.

The success of surgery can usually be predicted from the fall in pressure within one month when spironolactone (300mg) is taken daily (Fig. 8.44), although such a fall does not prove the presence of an aldosterone adenoma. There is a high success rate for the operation, but, as with all causes of hypertension, removal does not guarantee a cure even though biochemical improvement is achieved. Failure to cure long-standing hypertension is probably due to secondary vascular damage, especially to the kidney.

Cushing's Syndrome

Biochemical evaluation of Cushing's syndrome may be difficult, since some patients have only

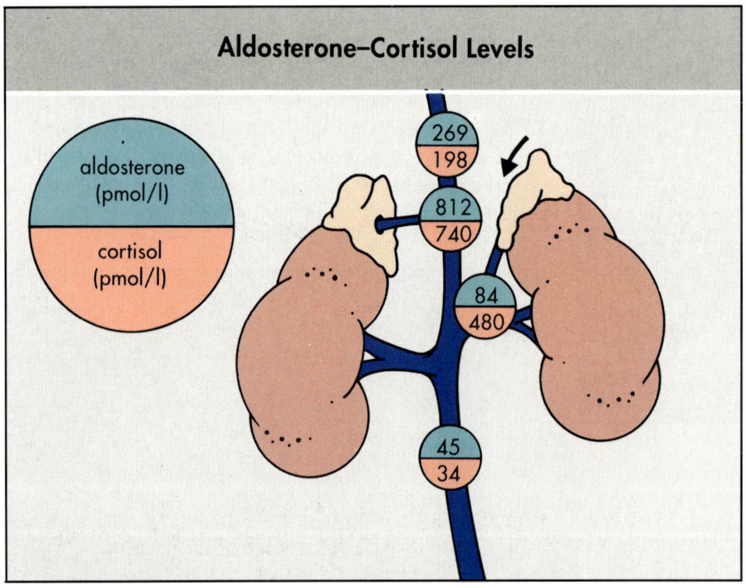

Fig. 8.43 The techniques of catheterization of the separate adrenal veins may be used to show the presence of an adenoma, as in the right adrenal here, where the ratio of aldosterone to cortisol is much higher in the adrenal vein because of the gland containing the adenoma.

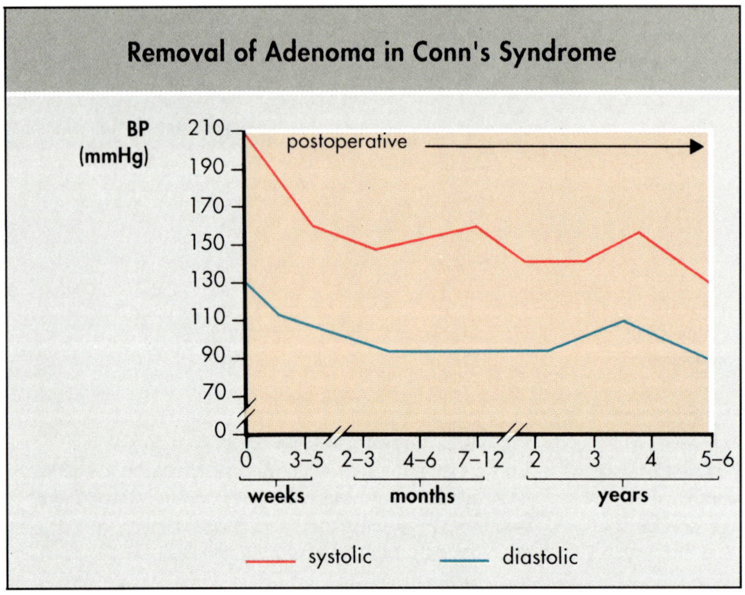

Fig. 8.44 The fall in pressure in a group of patients with Conn's syndrome following removal of the adenoma.

marginally raised levels of plasma cortisol and corticosterone. The lack of circadian rhythm and a failure to suppress plasma cortisol levels with dexamethasone are the two keys to diagnosis. Dexamethasone is usually given either once at night (2–5mg) or as a larger dose over twenty-four hours (2mg three times daily); in both cases the plasma cortisol level is measured at nine o' clock in the morning (Fig. 8.45).

Radiographic investigation to reveal enlargement or a double contour of the pituitary fossa is best shown by tomography and is now reinforced by CT scans which can show any extension upwards (Figs 8.46 & 8.47).

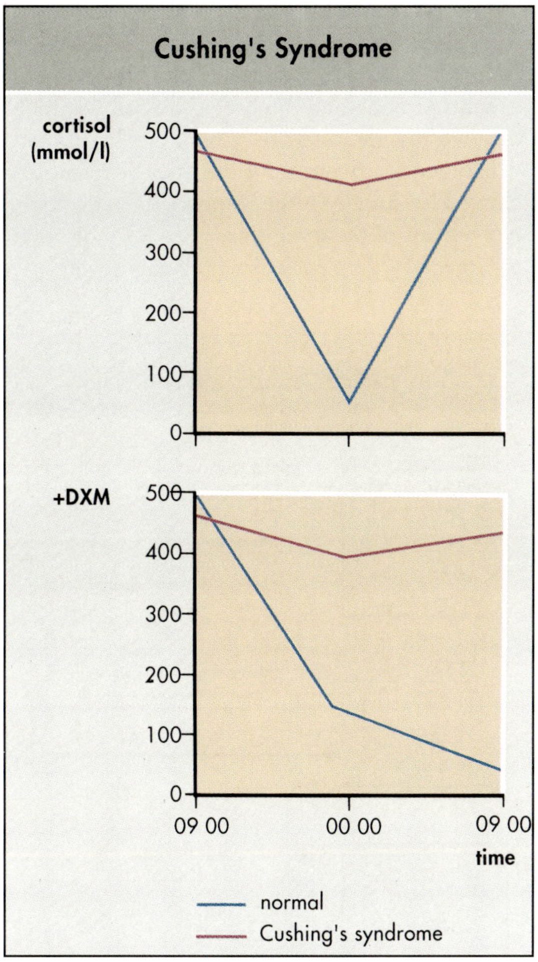

Fig. 8.45 Behaviour of plasma cortisol in a patient with Cushing's syndrome. The normal drop at midnight, followed by a rise in the early morning sample, which usually starts at about 06 00, is absent in Cushing's syndrome, and the usual suppression of the rise in the normal, produced by dexamethasone, which inhibits ACTH, is not present in Cushing's syndrome. DXM = Dexamethasone.

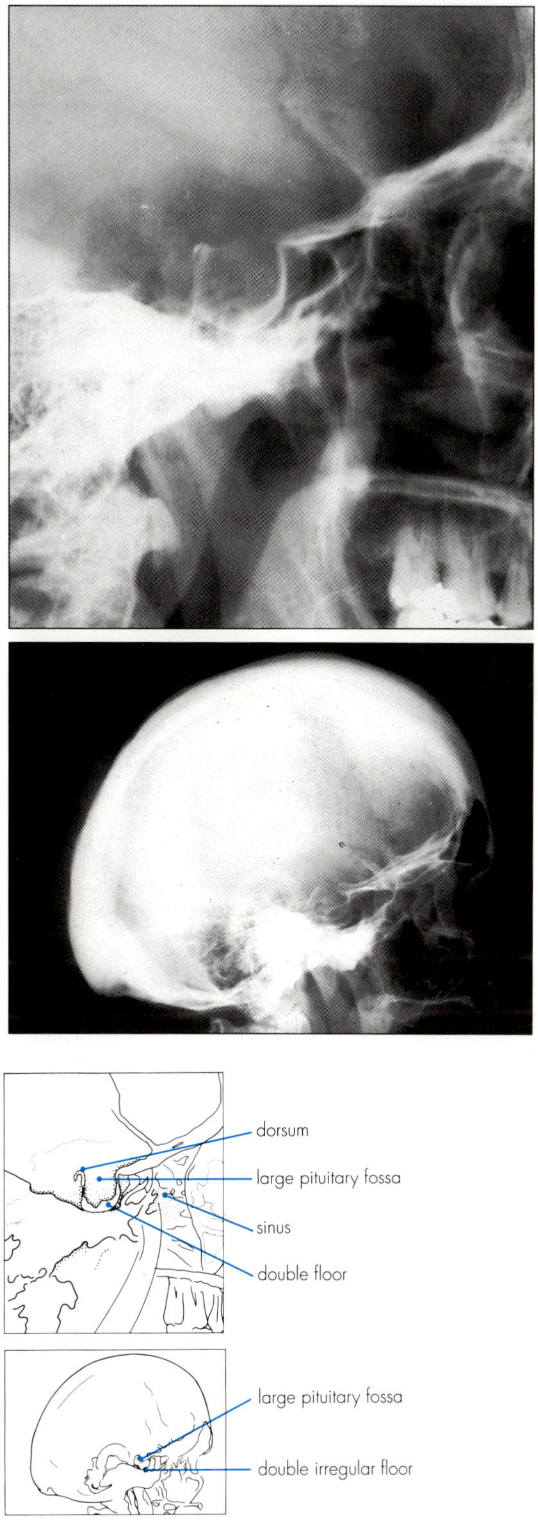

Fig. 8.46 Top: X-ray showing a double floor and large pituitary fossa due to a tumour. Bottom: Similar X-ray at lower magnification.

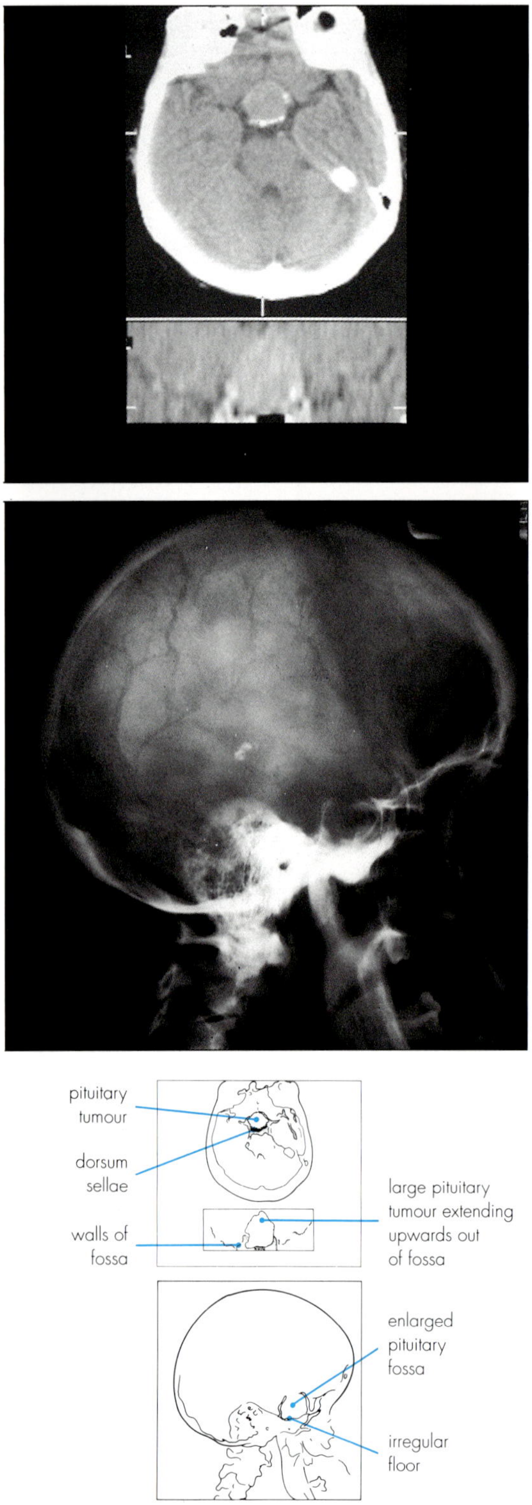

Fig. 8.47 Top: CT scan showing a large pituitary tumour with upward extension. Bottom: X-ray showing large pituitary fossa with an irregular floor.

Despite the lack of uniformity in results, partly due to radioimmunoassay difficulties, a raised plasma ACTH level may point to a pituitary tumour while low levels of ACTH indicate that the adrenals may be the cause, either from hyperplasia or an adenoma providing excess cortisol (Fig. 8.48). Most cases are due to a pituitary tumour, which may be very small, and microsurgery has enabled successful removal in experienced hands.

Acromegaly

The typical appearance (see Fig. 7.13) makes this initially a clinical diagnosis, especially if associated with glycosuria. Investigation demonstrates a large pituitary fossa with similar features to Figures 8.46 & 8.47, increased plasma levels of growth hormone and often of prolactin. As with other organs, the heart may be large. Treatment with bromocriptine may shrink the tumour, followed by surgery if the response is inadequate. Involvement of the optic chiasma is an indication for surgery. Hypertension is not usually severe.

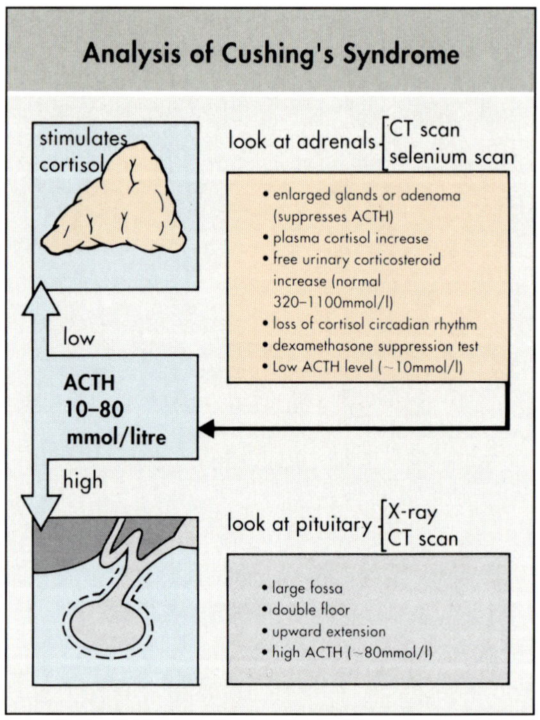

Fig. 8.48 The differentiation of pituitary tumour from adrenal hyperplasia and adenoma in Cushing's syndrome. This is based on changes both in anatomy and function with loss of normal feedback regulation.

Phaeochromocytoma

Many patients with anxiety exhibit signs and symptoms similar to those seen with phaeochromocytoma (Fig. 8.49). Where there is a clinical suspicion of phaeochromocytoma, therefore, the most reliable tests should be used, bearing in mind that this tumour is extremely rare and anxiety is common. Unfortunately the most commonly used screening test, the measurement of urinary vanillylmandelic acid, is also the least reliable. Quantification of free catecholamine metabolites in urine, particularly the metanephrines, is the most reliable and least likely to miss the presence of a tumour (Fig. 8.50). Where accurate measurements of plasma norepinephrine and epinephrine

Symptoms and Signs of Phaeochromocytoma

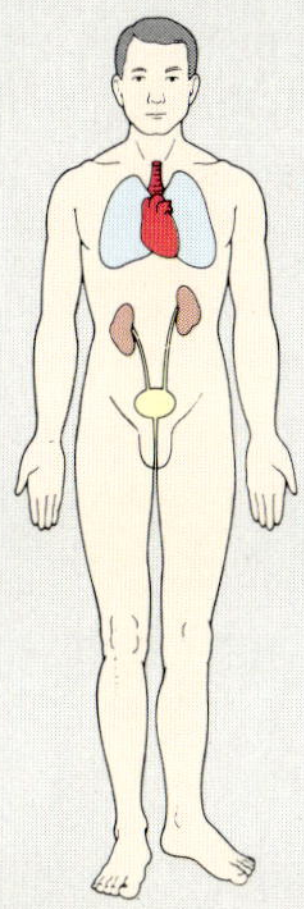

- paroxysmal hypertension
- headache
- pallor/flush
- anxiety
- thyroid swelling
- chest pain
- palpitation
- tachycardia
- nausea/vomiting
- glycosuria
- sweating
- tremor
- weakness

tests for localization		
	venous catheter	VMA/metanephrine/free metanephrine (urine)
	CT scan	epinephrine/norepinephrine (blood)
	arteriogram	
	MIBG radioactive localisation	

Fig. 8.49 The symptoms and signs of phaeochromocytoma. Not all are present but the most common are headache, pallor, sweating, palpitation and nausea. Flushing occurs after the initial pallor, and only rarely is swelling of the thyroid observed. Possible sites for the tumour range from the pelvis to the upper thorax.

Reliability of Urinary Catecholamine Tests

assays performed	patients with both assays normal	patients with both assays elevated	patients with one assay elevated		
			CA only	VMA only	MN only
CA & VMA	20%	60%	12%	8%	
MN & VMA	4%	70%		0%	25%
MN & CA	4%	75%			21%

Fig. 8.50 This table shows the reliability in diagnosis of the measurements of various urinary catecholamine metabolites. Those based on metanephrines are the best. CA = free catecholamines; MN = metanephrine; VMA = vanillylmandelic acid.

can be made, it is found that the vast majority of patients with phaeochromocytoma have plasma levels much higher than patients with other forms of hypertension or with normal blood pressure (Fig. 8.51). False positives are sometimes seen in alcoholic patients (with hypertension complicated by heart failure) and also in myxoedema. Since secretion from some small tumours may be intermittent, a clinical determination to completely exclude a false negative diagnosis requires other techniques. In patients with slightly elevated levels of catecholamines, a clonidine suppression test may be used to differentiate tumour release of catecholamine from other cases of increased sympathetic activity. If a tumour is present, the autonomous release of catecholamine is unaffected by the drug; in other cases of increased sympathetic activity, plasma levels fall after clonidine administration. Most tumours are present either in the adrenals or in the near vicinity and a CT scan of this region may show even a small tumour (1–2cm diameter – Fig. 8.52). Arteriography may show abnormal vessels or a blush, since the tumours are usually very vascular (Fig. 8.53). Finally, sampling blood by catheterization of different branches of the venous system, as well as an arterial sample, may be the ultimate method of locating the tumour when it is combined with accurate measurement of norepinephrine and epinephrine (Fig. 8.54). This is particularly important when the tumour occurs in very unusual sites in the chest or pelvis. The introduction of ^{123}I-metaiodobenzylguanidine as an imaging agent has added to the ease of localization, except in the case of very small tumours (see Fig. 8.8).

Pharmacological tests

While most patients with persistent hypertension due to phaeochromocytoma may have their blood pressure lowered using phentolamine (5mg intravenously), there are both false positives and nega-

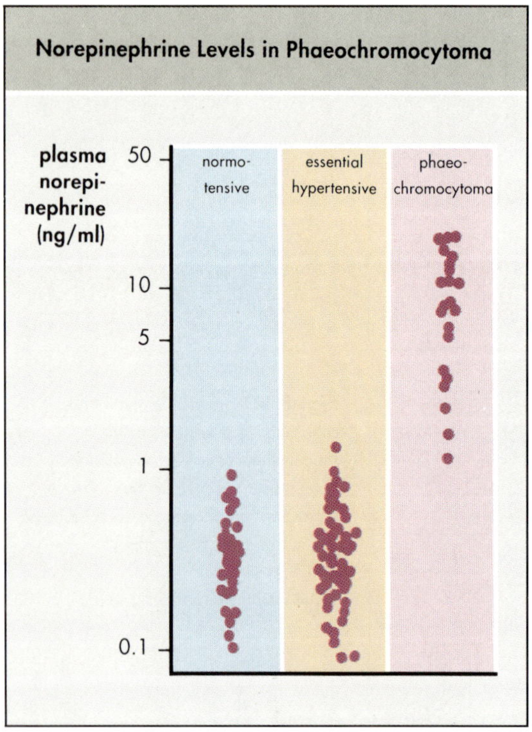

Fig. 8.51 Plasma norepinephrine values in proven phaeochromocytoma. This is the usual picture with practically no overlap of values with normal and essential hypertensive subjects. Some patients have small tumours that secrete intermittently, however, and a strong clinical suspicion should not rule out the diagnosis on an isolated normal laboratory result.

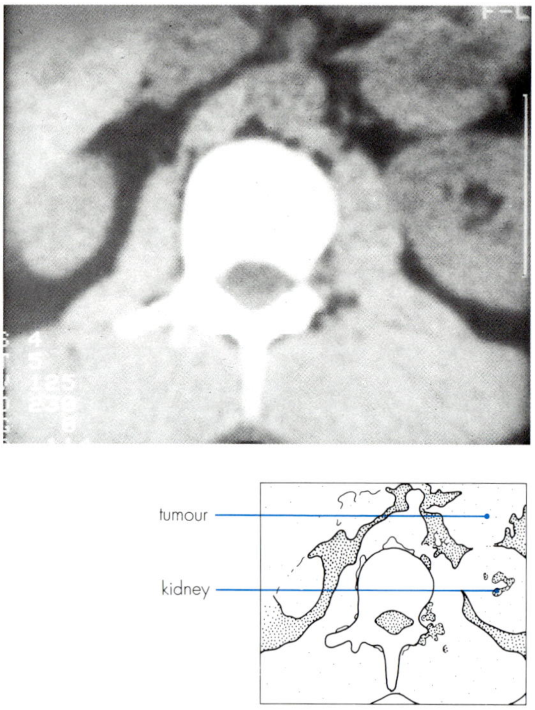

Fig. 8.52 CT scan of phaeochromocytoma anterior to the left kidney. (A different cut and enlarged version from patient in Fig. 8.22).

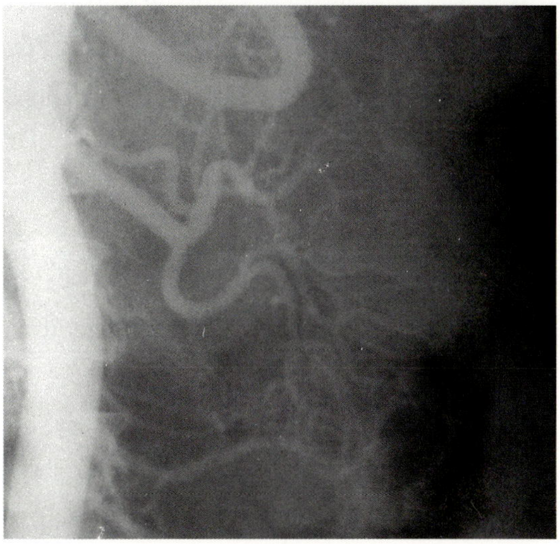

Fig. 8.53 Arteriogram showing a round phaeochromocytoma with abnormal vessels within, a large feeding artery and a 'blush'.

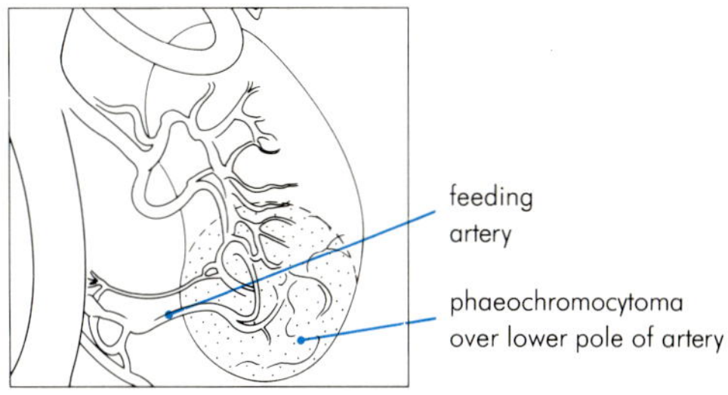

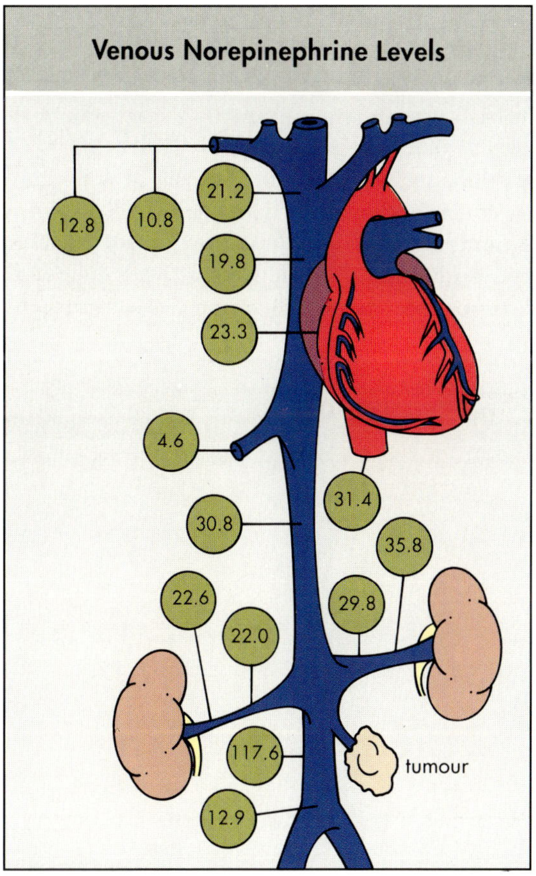

Fig. 8.54 Measurements of norepinephrine levels in blood sampled from different points in the venous system and taken by a catheter. This shows that the level is at its highest point just below the renal veins because of the entry of blood from the tumour which is just to the left of the aorta.

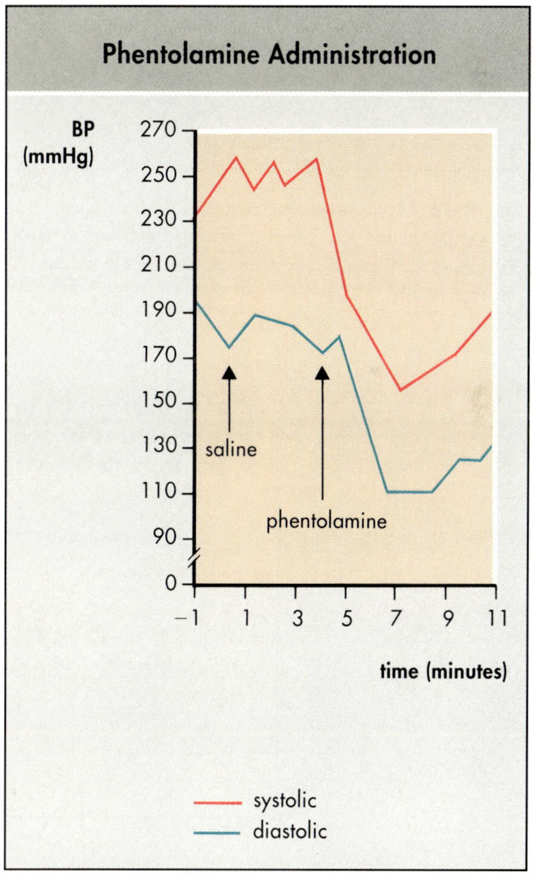

Fig. 8.55 The drop in blood pressure produced by 5mg of phentolamine intravenously in a patient with phaeochromocytoma. The depressor effect usually goes on for five or ten minutes, unlike the transient depressor effect seen in many patients with other forms of hypertension.

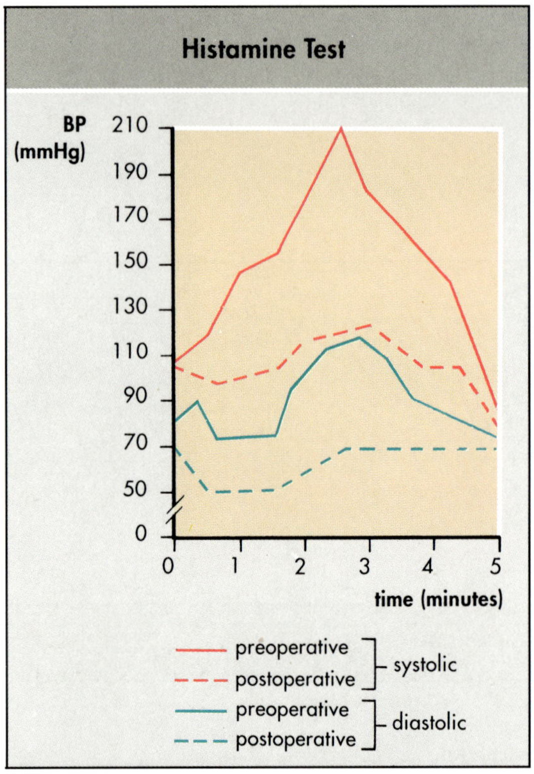

Fig. 8.56 Histamine provocative test (50µg i.v) in a patient before and after removal of a phaeochromocytoma. This shows that the initial pressor response disappeared after operation.

tives (Fig. 8.55). The same applies to provocative tests as with histamine (20, 40, 80µg intravenously – Fig. 8.55) or glucagon. Such tests are only to be given when a syringe containing phentolamine is at hand to block a severe provoked attack, and should only be used in patients with a normal blood pressure and a history of attacks suggestive of the disease and when all the tests are negative. They are largely of historical interest now. Control of blood pressure during spontaneous severe attacks may require large doses of antagonists (Fig. 8.57).

Other Systemic Conditions Affecting the Kidney

When confronted by a patient with unexplained renal disease and hypertension, it is important to determine whether renal involvement is part of a systemic disorder. This requires a broadly based clinical approach which takes account of obvious features of the history and signs of disease; diabetes is an important example. Various possibilities exist, including renal infection and pyelonephritis, papillary necrosis as with analgesic abuse, glomerular and arteriolar change as in Kimmelstiel-Wilson kidney and frank atheromatous obstruction to the main renal arteries (see chapter 5). Some diseases present

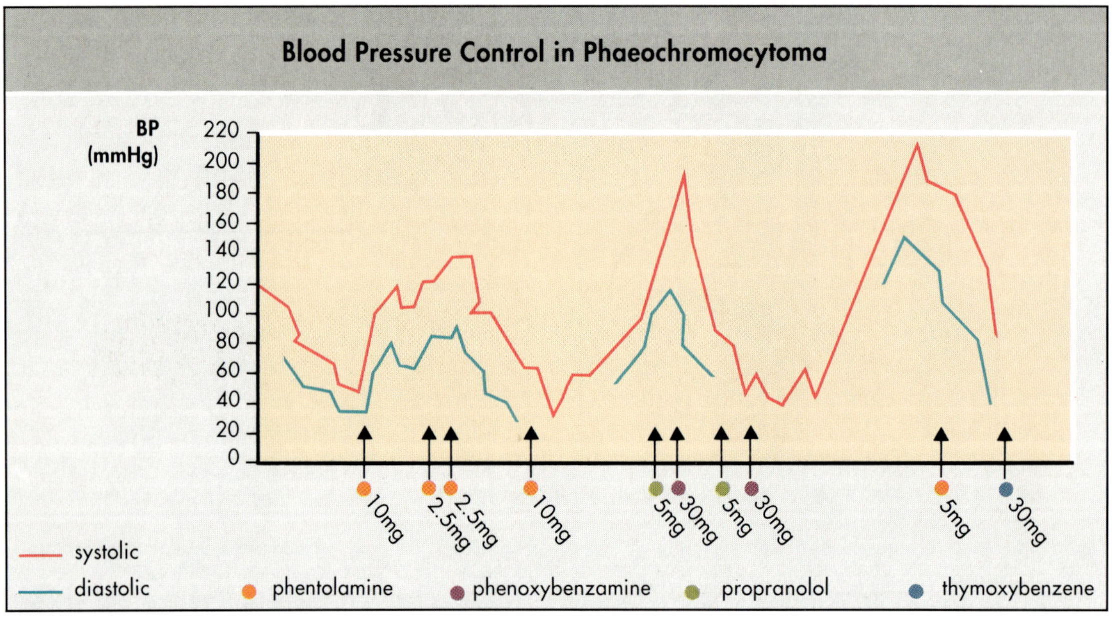

Fig. 8.57 This illustrates the difficulty of controlling the blood pressure in a patient with severe prolonged attacks of hypertension due to a phaeochromocytoma. The use of vasodilators such as sodium nitroprusside should be introduced in such difficult cases.

clinically in other ways; the facial rash of systemic lupus (Fig. 8.58) and the punched out ulcers at the ankle or elbow seen in polyarteritis nodosa (Fig. 8.59), to name but two outstanding signs, indicate the need to look for vasculitis within the kidney. This vasculitis sometimes shows itself only with proteinuria, but occasionally with red cells and red cell casts in the urine.

The appearance of a patient with scleroderma (Fig. 8.60) and hypertension is a reminder that this disorder involves the arteries to the kidney on many occasions.

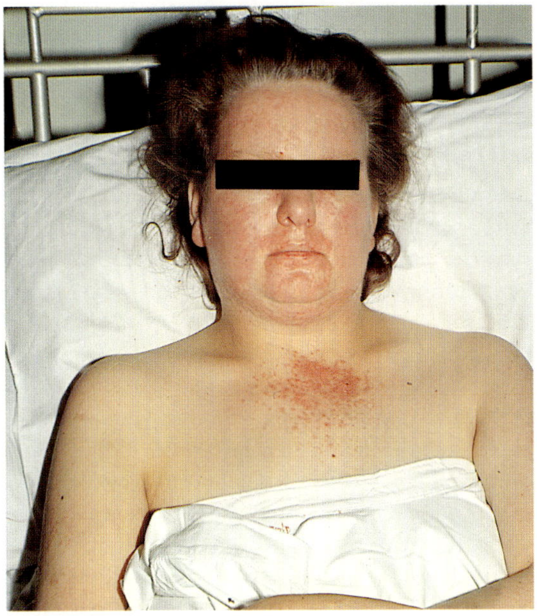

Fig. 8.58 Typical acute erythematous papular rash due to light-sensitivity on the face and chest of a patient with systemic lupus erythematosus.

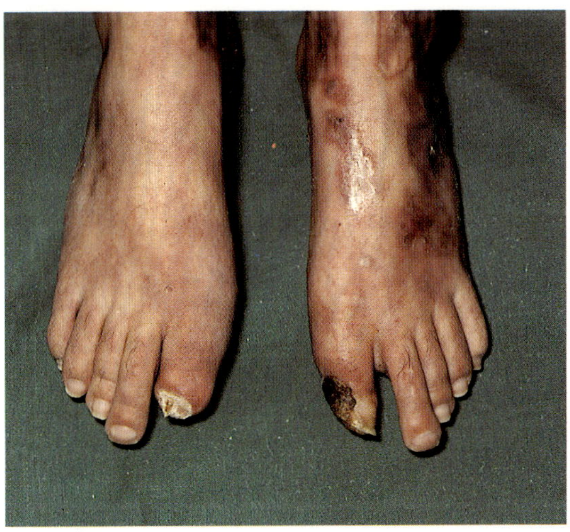

Fig. 8.59 Feet of a patient with a cutaneous vasculitis-like polyarteritis nodosa showing some partially healed ulcers with pigmented edges and an active ulcer on the left big toe. The terminal phalanx on the right big toe has suffered ischaemic necrosis.

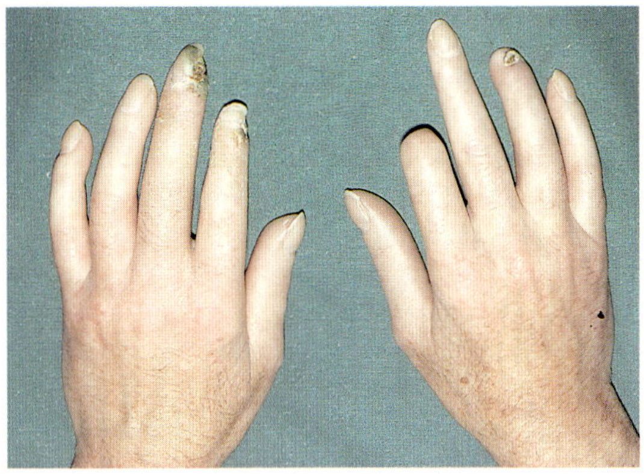

Fig. 8.60 Typical appearance of the hands in a patient with scleroderma shows the smooth, shiny oedematous skin with ischaemic ulceration at the ends of the fingers and loss of the end of the right index finger,

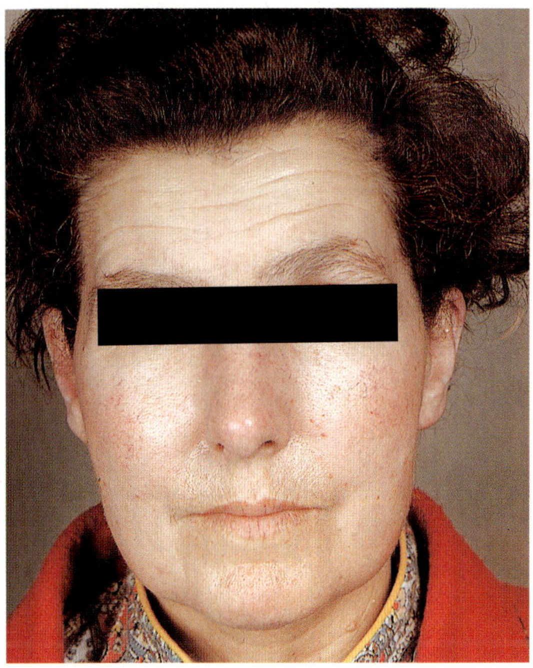

Fig. 8.61 The typical facial appearance of a patient with scleroderma shows telangiectasia over the infiltrated areas of the cheeks, and premature vertical puckering of the lips in a woman of forty-five years.

Of the various conditions which cause infiltration of the glomerulus and are sometimes associated with hypertension, amyloid is an insidious condition that sometimes complicates rheumatoid arthritis.

Finally, glomerulonephritis in its various forms is a condition which commonly requires more precise diagnosis by renal biopsy. This is shown clearly by the findings in Berger's (IgA) nephritis or lupus nephritis; although there is very little functional impairment (the only sign may be microscopic haematuria) glomerular changes may be pronounced. Furthermore, there may be very few signs outside the kidney, and the course may be very protracted, so suspicion of glomerulonephritis should remain high.

Most of the conditions discussed can initially be classified by urine analysis, looking for the presence or absence of infection, protein, pus cells, red cells or red cell casts. The next most useful points are the symmetry and general size of the kidneys. Infective processes with scarring, and major vascular blockage, also with scarring, lead to asymmetry; conditions like glomerulonephritis or microscopic vasculitis lead to symmetrically small, smooth kidneys. Many of these conditions do require renal biopsy for diagnostic and prognostic purposes but this should only be done where there are facilities for electron microscopy and immunochemical histology.

CONCLUSIONS

The most important step in looking at a patient who is thought to have a raised blood pressure is still to be sure that the level of pressure justifies investigation with a view to treatment. Despite injunctions about the importance of treating diastolic pressures at 90mmHg and above, there are two important considerations. The first is that blood pressure is variable and much influenced by the circumstances of its measurement so that one reading may not be truly representative. The second is that treatment of mild hypertension as the only risk factor does not confer much benefit, especially in women. This carries the implication that the presence of other risk factors such as cardiac hypertrophy, ischaemia, obesity, hypercholesterolaemia, lipoprotein levels and a poor family history may affect the decision to treat.

Above all, it should be stressed that time is on the side of the physician, who can take repeated readings, over months if required (including semi-automatic readings at home and at work), before making a decision which, in the case of young people, may expose them to considerable investigation or lifelong treatment. It still remains true that most patients can be classified by simple investigation. Even where more intensive tests are needed, they are steadily becoming less traumatic thanks to modern technology.

CHAPTER 9

Drug Treatment

INTRODUCTION

The first, dramatic response to drug treatment of hypertension was seen in the 1950s, when ganglion blockade was introduced for the therapy of malignant hypertension (Fig. 9.1). Prior to this time, the onset of the malignant phase was inevitably followed by major cardiovascular sequelae, such as heart failure, stroke and progressive renal damage – in nearly every case the patient died. Mortality rates in malignant hypertension were reduced by more than 50% with the introduction of antihypertensive therapy. Over the past 40 years many classes of drugs, with widely differing pharmacological properties, have been introduced. The benefits of treatment can clearly be extended to those patients with the more benign phase of hypertension (see chapter 10).

Irrespective of the underlying cause of blood pressure elevation, drugs lower blood pressure by an effect on one or more of the mechanisms involved in circulatory regulation (see chapter 3 and Fig. 9.2). Arterial pressure is the product of cardiac output and vascular resistance; antihypertensive drugs may act in different ways to reduce either, or in some cases both, haemodynamic indices. In this respect it is of interest to note that, with the probable exception of the early stages of essential hypertension and the much less common volume-dependent hypertension (see Chapter 3), in which cardiac output may be raised, established hypertension is usually associated with an increased total peripheral vascular resistance – the higher the pressure the greater the resistance. It is therefore perhaps surprising that for many years the most widely used antihypertensive drugs (ß-adrenoceptor blockers and diuretics) appeared to exert their primary or initial haemodynamic effects on cardiac output.

Due to the multiplicity of mechanisms involved in blood pressure control, antihypertensive properties are shared by the following classes of drug:

- sympatholytic agents, which may act centrally or peripherally to diminish sympathetic tone;
- drugs reducing cardiac output by competitive inhibition of myocardial ß-adrenoceptors, by calcium entry blockade or by extracellular fluid volume depletion;
- agents which inhibit the activity of the renin–angiotensin system;
- drugs which produce arteriolar dilatation by a variety of mechanisms.

Drugs in the last category may act via direct relaxation of smooth muscle (hydralazine, nitroprusside), by an alteration in the properties of the vessel wall (reducing salt and water content – diuretics) or by alterations in ion flux across vascular smooth muscle cell membranes (calcium channel blockers, potassium channel activators). In recent years it has become evident that the vas-

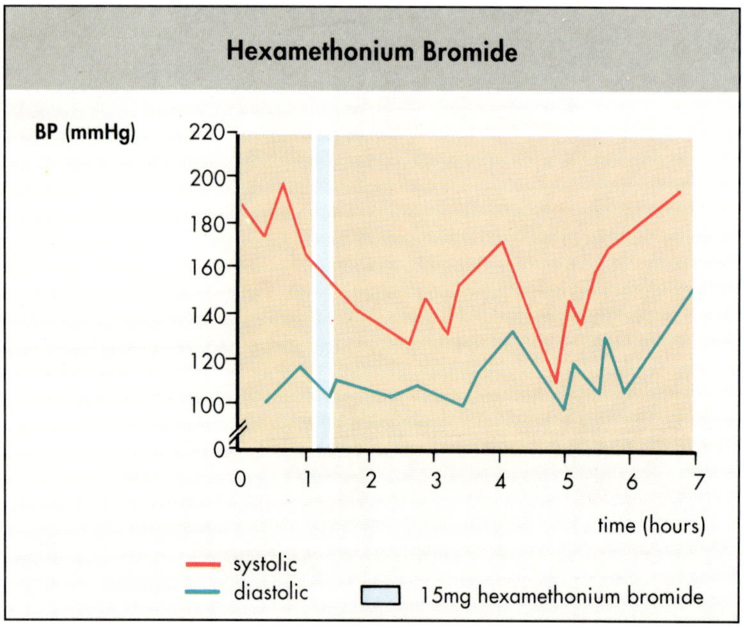

Fig. 9.1 Early experiments with hexamethonium bromide showed that subcutaneous administration of the drug produced a marked hypotensive effect. [Modified from Smirk, F. H. & Alstad, K. S. (1951) *BMJ*, **1**, 1217–1228.]

cular endothelium produces a number of mediators, endothelial derived relaxing factor (EDRF) and prostacyclin for example, which are potent relaxors of the underlying smooth muscle. A number of potent vasodilator compounds, which may eventually find a use in the treatment of hypertension, appear to act by releasing or potentiating endothelial dilator systems (see below).

As a consequence of hypertension an ever increasing afterload is placed on the left ventricle, leading to hypertrophy and failure. Therapy should therefore be directed not only to reducing resistance, but also to reversing the structural changes that occur within the heart and the vasculature. Ideally, underlying causes of pressure elevation would be identified and specific therapy prescribed. Regrettably, this is rarely possible.

Many drugs initiate reflex responses as a consequence of their blood pressure lowering effects, which may not only limit their efficacy in blood pressure control but may also produce adverse effects upon the heart, with an increase in left ventricular hypertrophy. In practice, up to 50% of patients will require more than one drug to control blood pressure (see chapter 10). Combinations of drugs acting at different sites are used because of their complementary actions. This allows rational therapeutic regimes to be tailored to individual patients, enables unwanted reflex responses to certain drugs to be counteracted and, in some cases, prevents the intolerable adverse effects that can be caused by large doses of single drugs.

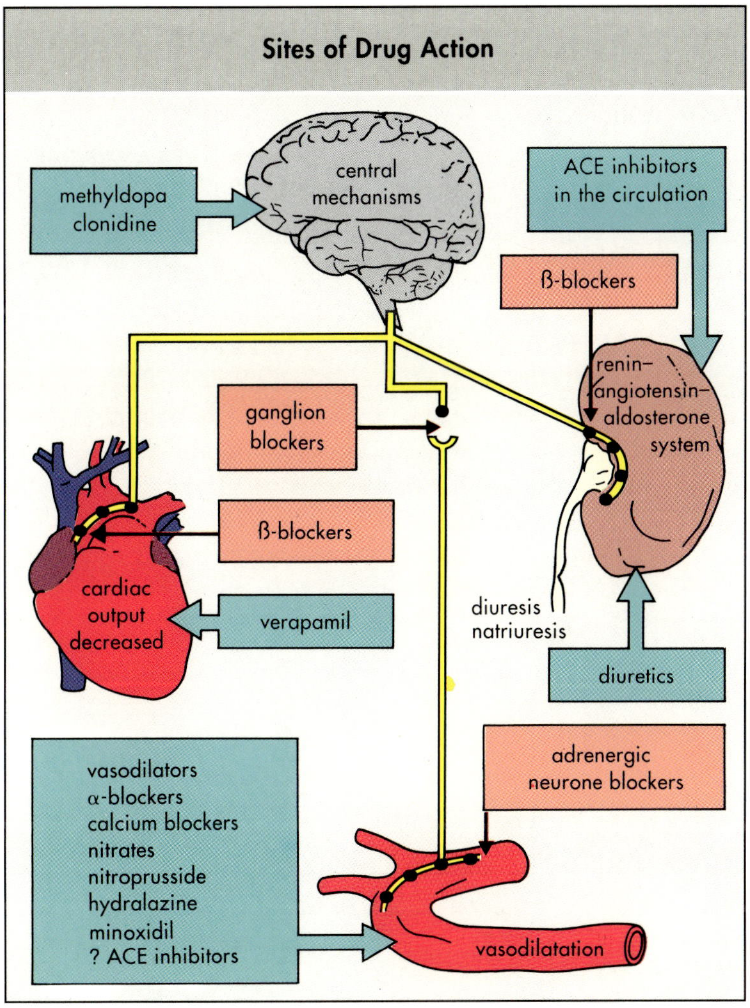

Fig. 9.2 Possible sites of action of antihypertensive drugs.

DIURETICS

Mode of Action

The thiazide diuretics and the closely related phthalimidine derivatives, such as chlorthalidone, have long had a central role in the treatment of hypertension. They are employed either as monotherapy or in combination with other antihypertensive agents, many of which produce significant salt and water retention. The precise mechanism by which the thiazides lower blood pressure is still uncertain; it is unlikely that the initial diuretic effect, which leads to a reduction in extracellular volume, can explain the long-term effects of these agents on arterial pressure.

The immediate effects of thiazide treatment are loss of salt and water from the kidney, a fall in extracellular fluid volume, a reduction in cardiac output and a compensatory rise in peripheral resistance. With chronic therapy plasma volume returns to near pretreatment levels in some patients, whilst in others it remains contracted to differing degrees; the persistence of the antihypertensive effect, which may not become maximal until three months or more of therapy, becomes dependent upon a reduction in peripheral vascular resistance (Fig. 9.3). Nevertheless, it is evident that diuretic-induced sodium loss is a prerequisite for blood pressure reduction. A high dietary sodium intake can reverse the antihypertensive effect; conversely, a low salt intake potentiates the effect of diuretics on blood pressure.

Diazoxide, which is closely related chemically to the thiazide diuretics, lowers blood pressure by direct relaxation of vascular smooth muscle. It therefore seems likely that thiazide diuretics share this, or a similar mechanism (Fig. 9.4). There is experimental evidence to suggest that diuretics mobilize salt and water from blood vessel walls and facilitate muscular relaxation. (some studies have shown a blood pressure lowering effect in bilaterally nephrectomized patients.) There is also evidence that patients on maintenance therapy

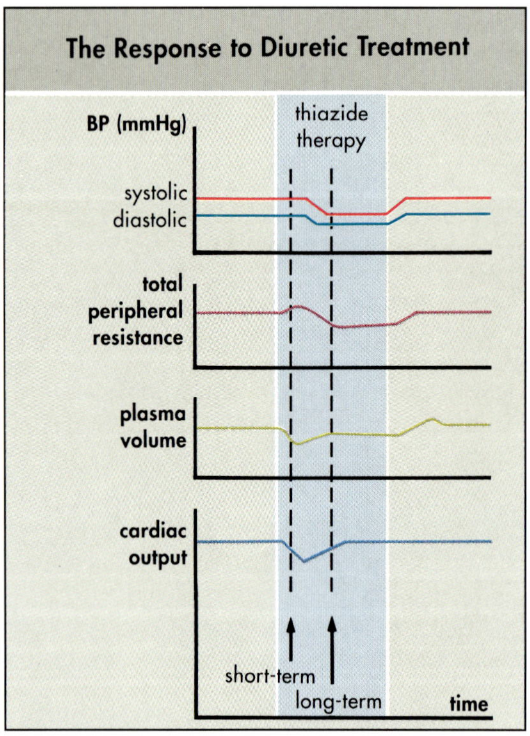

Fig. 9.3 Haemodynamic effects of diuretic treatment to demonstrate differences between short- and longer term response of peripheral resistance, plasma volume and cardiac output.

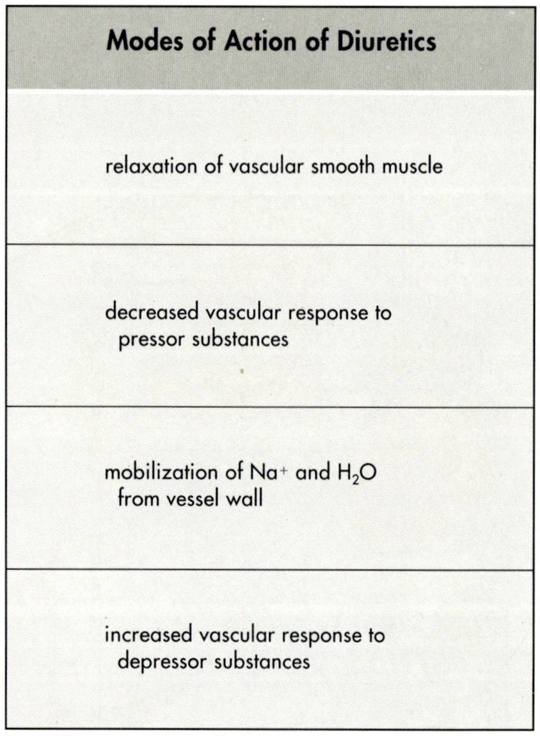

Fig. 9.4 Possible modes of action of diuretics on blood vessels.

with thiazide diuretics have a diminished vascular response to pressor agents such as norepinephrine. This effect could also contribute to the antihypertensive properties of these drugs. The precise mechanisms involved in thiazide-induced vasodilatation remain to be clarified, but it seems likely that effects on sodium transport leading to a reduction in intracellular sodium and calcium are involved. When diuretics are used in combination with other antihypertensives, they probably act principally by reversing salt and water retention (induced by the other drugs) and partly by their direct action on vascular smooth muscle.

All commonly used diuretics inhibit sodium reabsorption in the renal tubules and may be subdivided into three main groups according to the major site or sites of action in the nephron (Fig. 9.5). Despite marked variations in the effectiveness of diuretics in terms of their ability to promote salt and water excretion, all are remarkably similar in potency as antihypertensive agents. The loop diuretics, for example, are no more effective than the thiazides in lowering blood pressure in patients with normal renal function.

The antihypertensive effects of diuretics are of longer duration than the natriuretic effects and occur at lower doses. There is no point in prescribing doses in excess of 25–50mg hydrochlorthiazide (or equivalent) in an attempt to obtain a greater blood pressure lowering effect. Moreover, at higher doses adverse reactions, particularly metabolic effects, are much more common.

Sites of Action of Diuretics

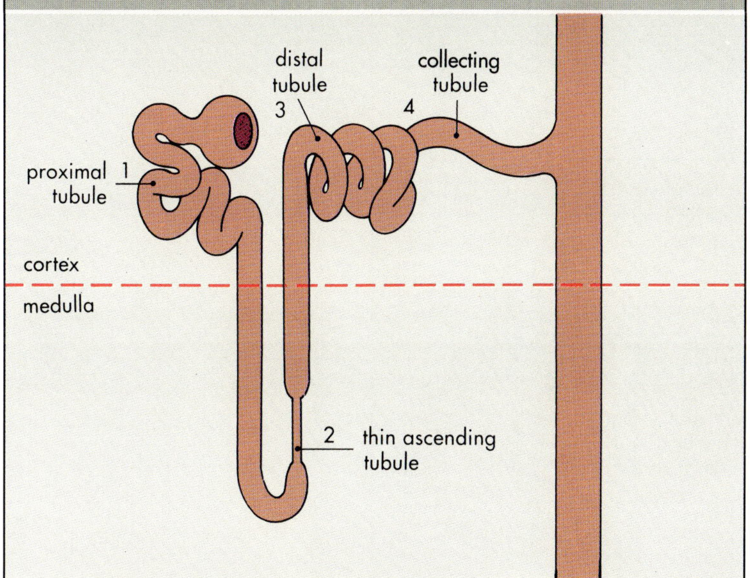

	1	2	3	4
thiazide diuretics chlorthalidone	+		+++	
loop diuretics frusemide bumetanide ethacrynic acid	+	+++	++	
potassium sparing diuretics spironolactone amiloride triamterene				+++

Fig. 9.5 Sites of action of diuretic agents on the renal tubule.

Metabolic and Other Adverse Effects

The initial fall in extracellular fluid volume produced by diuretics leads to the release of renin from the kidney and the stimulation of aldosterone secretion, thus diminishing the diuretic effect (Fig. 9.6). The long-term electrolyte problems encountered with loop diuretics, and to a lesser extent with the thiazides, are consequent upon an inhibition of sodium reabsorption and increased delivery of sodium to the distal tubules, where it is exchanged for potassium and hydrogen ions. Chronic diuretic therapy also predisposes to hypokalaemia, as a result of secondary hyperaldosteronism. Hypokalaemia occurs in approximately 10% of subjects on long-term thiazide treatment, and significantly more frequently when loop diuretics are prescribed. With loop diuretics, potassium-sparing agents or potassium supplements are mandatory. Ventricular extrasystoles are common when the serum potassium falls below 3.5mmol/l. Whether or not these arrhythmias are harmful remains conjectural; many physicians have taken the view that patients on thiazide diuretics should be routinely protected from the effects of hypokalaemia using potassium supplements or potassium-sparing diuretics. However, when smaller doses of thiazides are used (12.5–25mg hydrochlorthiazide or equivalent) it is seldom necessary to add in potassium.

Potassium-sparing diuretics also possess mild antihypertensive properties, although their efficacy is increased when combined with a thiazide. Hyperkalaemia, particularly in the elderly and in patients with impaired renal function, may be a problem and is potentially fatal.

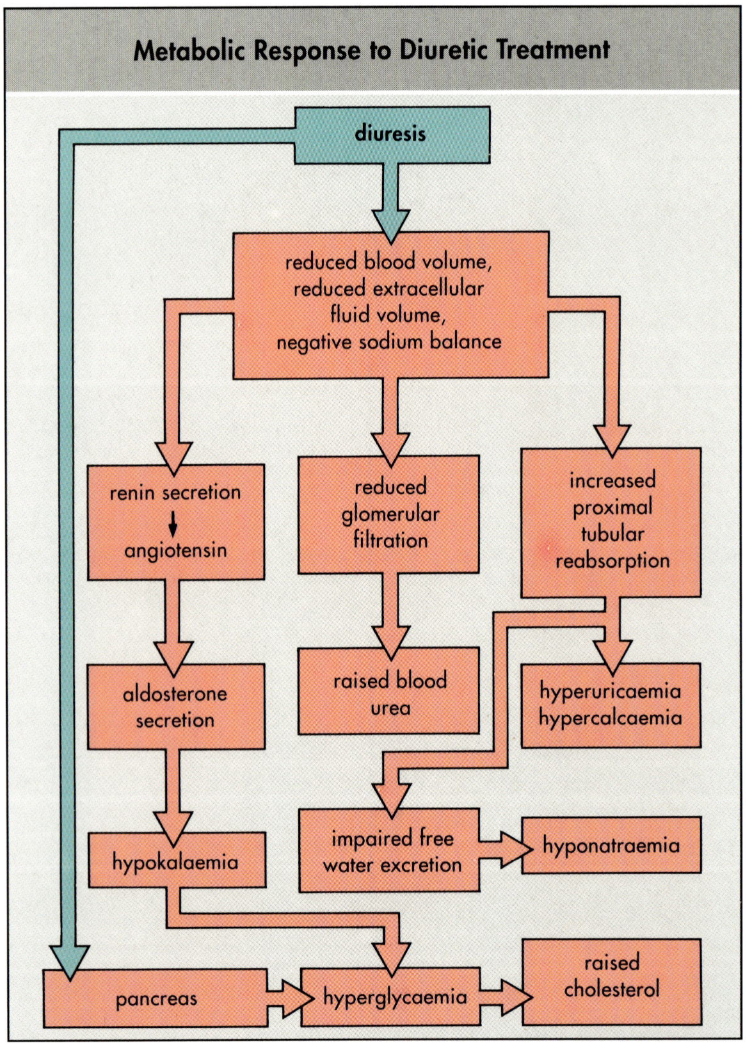

Fig. 9.6 Metabolic response to long-term treatment with diuretics.

Other important metabolic consequences of long-term diuretic therapy include hyperuricaemia and hyperglycaemia. Although elevated levels of serum uric acid are more common in hypertensive subjects than in a normotensive population, hyperuricaemia occurs in over 30% of thiazide-treated hypertensives and may lead to frank gout. While thiazides and loop diuretics may inhibit tubular secretion of uric acid, it is now believed that the hyperuricaemia is secondary to sodium depletion and the reduced clearance of uric acid is the result of a change in the bidirectional flow of urate in the proximal convoluted tubule.

About 30% of patients on thiazides and loop diuretics develop impaired glucose tolerance. Some of the possible mechanisms are indicated in Figure 9.6. However, it has been proposed that this may be related to other actions of the drug on pancreatic islet cells (as with diazoxide), or on the peripheral utilization of glucose.

It is only relatively recently, from good placebo controlled studies (Fig. 9.7), that other common symptomatic complaints have been demonstrated to occur with relatively high frequency in hypertensive patients receiving diuretic treatment. Many of these are undoubtedly dose related, but the effects on quality of life of the patient are important.

A further metabolic consequence of diuretic treatment is their effects on lipids. In several studies chronic therapy has been shown to increase total cholesterol by about 5%, LDL cholesterol by 10% and triglycerides by 10%. Furthermore, levels of the 'protective' HDL cholesterol may fall. These particular features of diuretic therapy in a hypertensive population, already at higher risk of atherogenesis because of their blood pressure, are of some concern.

Thiazides and frusemide rarely cause blood dyscrasias but skin rashes are not uncommon. The loop diuretics may be ototoxic particularly in high dosages and in the presence of renal failure. Other adverse effects may be unique to individual drugs; for example, spironolactone can cause gynaecomastia in men and menstrual irregularities in women; it has also been found to be carcinogenic in animals.

Electrolyte imbalance occurs more commonly in the elderly with thiazides, and the risk of dangerous electrolyte imbalance is much greater with the potent loop diuretics. For long term use, therefore, a thiazide diuretic is preferable to a loop diuretic for all hypertensive patients, apart from those with sodium retention due to renal failure or those receiving potent vasodilators such as minoxidil and diazoxide.

Adverse Effects of Diuretics

	men			women		
	B	P	Pl	B	P	Pl
impaired glucose tolerance	7.7	3.4	3.3	5.9	2.1	-
gout	12.8	1.5	0.9	1.5	-	-
impotence	12.6	6.3	1.3	-	-	-
Raynaud's syndrome	-	5.1	0.2	0.3	4.5	0.3
skin disorder	0.8	1.5	0.3	0.4	1.2	0.1
dyspnoea	0.1	7.1	0.4	0.3	7.1	0.2
lethargy	3.6	5.3	0.5	1.7	8.3	0.3
nausea/dizziness	4.2	4.1	1.4	7.4	9.4	1.8

(red) significant difference from control

Fig. 9.7 A number of unpleasant effects are associated with the use of diuretics. This MRC trial recorded the effects of treatment with bendrofluazide (B), propranolol (P), and a placebo (Pl). The figures show the number of patients who withdrew from the trial as a result of the adverse effect (rate per thousand patient years).

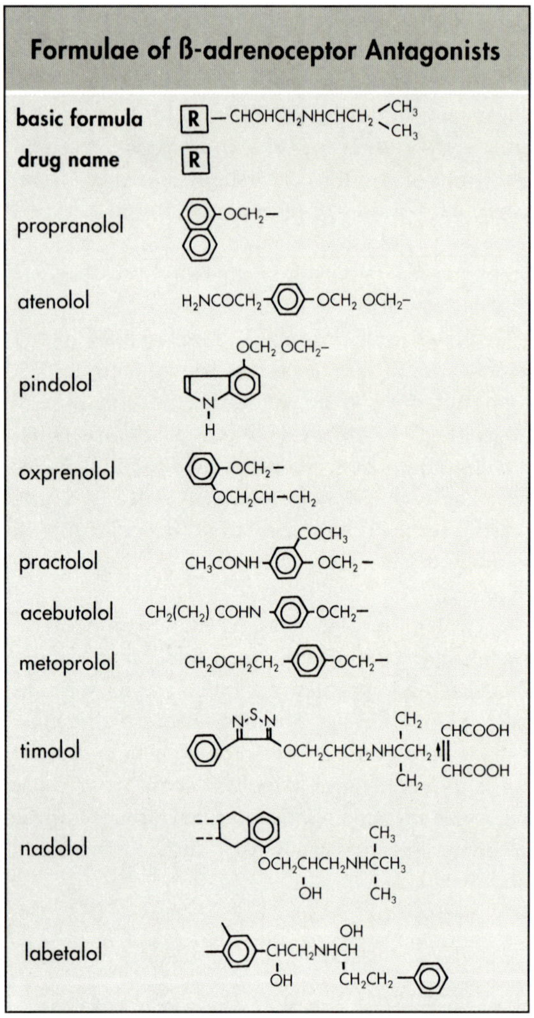

Fig. 9.8 Structural formulae of some ß-adrenoceptor antagonists.

ß-ADRENOCEPTOR ANTAGONISTS

The hypotensive effects of pronethalol and propranolol were first noted in 1964 by Prichard. Over the past quarter-century the ß-adrenoceptor antagonists have established themselves as first line drugs in the management of hypertension.

Modes of action

The ß-adrenoceptor blocking agents are structural analogues of the agonist isoprenaline. A large number of effective antihypertensive compounds are now available (Fig. 9.8). The hydroxyl moeity in the aliphatic side chain is essential for ß-antagonist activity and the laevorotatory isomer is far more potent in this respect.

In addition to their antagonist effects at the ß-adrenoceptor, these drugs possess a number of other pharmacological properties:

- partial agonist or intrinsic sympathomimetic activity (ISA);
- cardioselectivity;
- membrane stabilizing actions
- additional α-adrenoceptor blocking properties (Fig. 9.9), although these are rare.

There is little evidence to suggest that either membrane stabilizing effects or $ß_1$-selectivity confer any significant advantage in terms of the hypotensive response to the drugs. The possession of α-blocking activity markedly alters the haemodynamic profile. The long-term haemodynamic consequences of ß-blockade are to a certain extent determined by the presence or absence of partial

Properties of ß-adrenoceptor Antagonists

drug name	partial agonist	$ß_1$ selectivity	membrane stabilizing	α-blocking activity	lipid solubility
propranolol	–	–	+	–	v. high
atenolol	–	+	–	–	low
pindolol	++	–	–	–	med.
oxprenolol	+	–	+	(weak)	high
acebutolol	+	+	+	–	med.
metoprolol	–	+	(weak)	–	med.
timolol	–	–	–	–	med.
nadolol	–	–	–	–	low
labetalol	–	–	(weak)	+	?

Fig. 9.9 Pharmacological properties of ß-adrenoceptor antagonists.

agonist activity (see below). Lipid solubility is an important property of ß-blockers and directly affects their ability to cross the blood-brain barrier. This property does not apparently influence the blood pressure lowering effects of the drugs. However, the more lipid soluble compounds such as propranolol, commonly induce adverse effects in the central nervous system (CNS), which are less often encountered with the more polar hydrophilic drugs (atenolol for example).

The exact mechanisms by which ß-adrenoceptor antagonists lower blood pressure are complex and still incompletely understood. A number of hypotheses have been proposed to account for their antihypertensive effects (Fig. 9.10), but no single mechanism has been convincingly shown to relate to the fall in pressure.

Most ß-blockers reduce cardiac output and inhibit renin release from the kidney, thereby reducing levels of angiotensin II; this in turn reduces angiotensin-induced stimulation of aldosterone secretion and the facilitatory effects of angiotensin on the activity of the sympathetic nervous system. ß-blockers may also have a peripheral effect, inhibiting prejunctional facilitatory ß-adrenoceptors and reducing noradrenaline overflow at sympathetic nerve endings (Fig. 9.11).

Haemodynamic Effects

ß-blockers which do not possess ISA exert negative inotropic and chronotropic effects on the heart by post-junctional $ß_1$-receptor blockade, thereby reducing cardiac output. The initial fall in cardiac

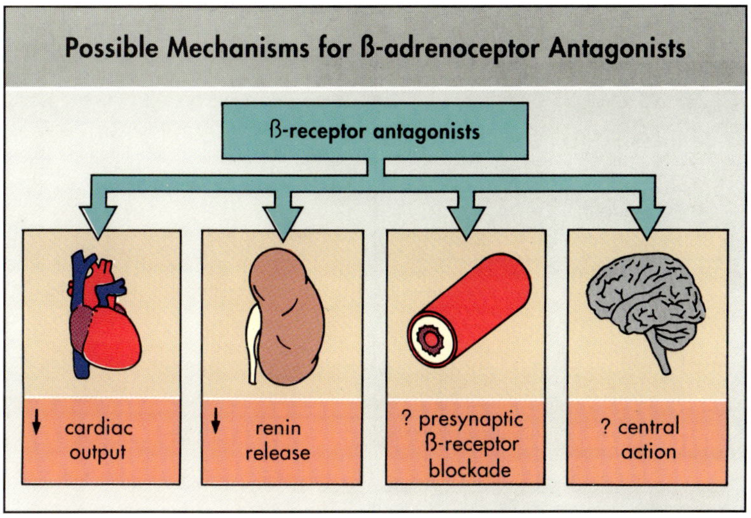

Fig. 9.10 Possible mechanisms involved in the hypotensive action of ß-adrenoceptor antagonists.

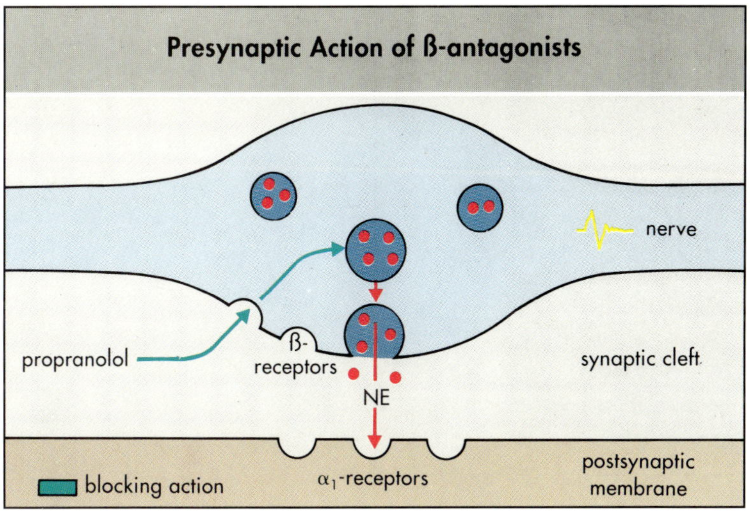

Fig. 9.11 Peripheral sympathetic nerve terminal demonstrating the possible presynaptic ß-blocking action of antagonists, leading to inhibition of norepinephrine (NE) release.

output which follows acute administration is compensated by a baroreflex-mediated increase in efferent vasoconstrictor sympathetic nerve activity; this moderates the fall in blood pressure by increasing peripheral vascular resistance. Blockade of prejunctional facilitatory ß-receptors on peripheral sympathetic noradrenergic neurones abolishes, after a time, the effect of increased sympathetic drive, and vascular resistance falls to pretreatment levels. Blood pressure also falls, primarily as a result of reduced cardiac output (Fig. 9.12).

On the other hand, ß-blockers with ISA sufficiently high to replace basal sympathetic tone (such as pindolol) do not reduce cardiac output, so that reflex changes in vascular resistance do not occur. Eventually prejunctional ß-blockade inhibits norepinephrine overflow and results in a decreased vascular resistance to below pretreatment levels (see Fig. 9.12). Further evidence for this hypothesis comes from studies on plasma norepinephrine levels, which invariably fall with ß-blockers possessing ISA, but remain unchanged or even increase on treatment with pure antagonists.

Renal Effects

The haemodynamic consequences of ß-blockade can affect renal function. The initial rise in vascular resistance that occurs with pure antagonists (such as propranolol) is accompanied by a decline in renal blood flow (RBF) and glomerular filtration rate (GFR) of the order of 15%. This effect is also seen with longer term administration. (Nadolol, which belongs to this group of ß-blockers, is an interesting exception; when nadolol is used RBF and GFR are preserved or, sometimes, increased.) Cardioselective ß-blockers and ß-antagonists with ISA have little or no effect on renal function.

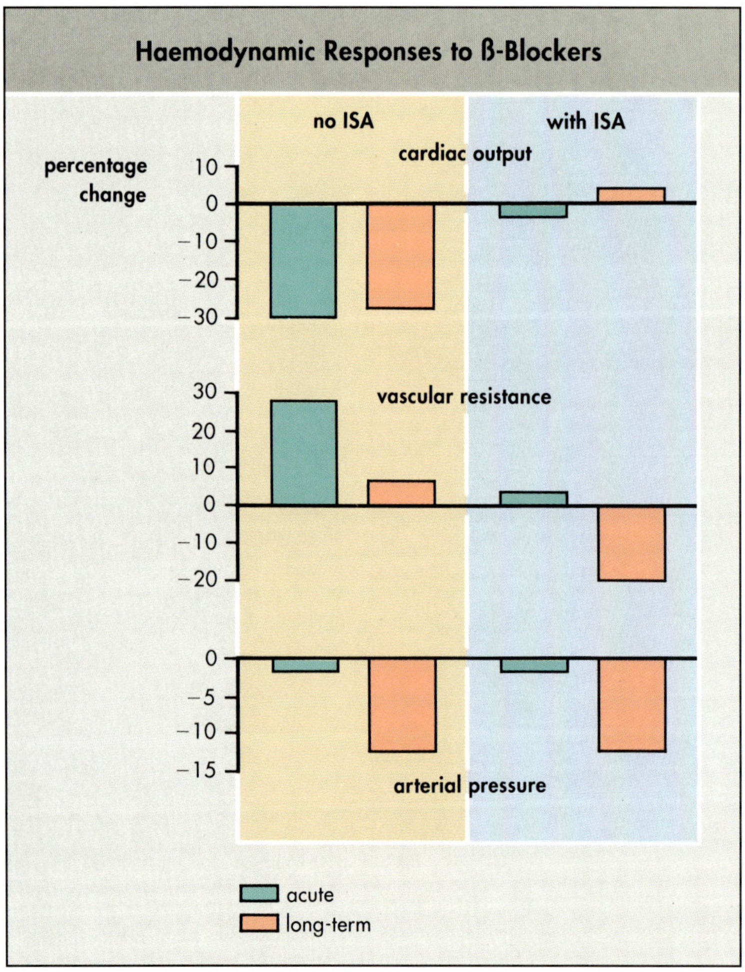

Fig. 9.12 Acute and longer term haemodynamic responses to ß-blockers with and without intrinsic sympathomimetic activity.

The inhibition of renin release from the kidney is an important antihypertensive effect of ß-blockers. It leads to reduced levels of angiotensin I and II and diminishes the effects of angiotensin II on the adrenal gland and on the sympathetic nervous system (see above).
There is evidence that patients with high levels of plasma renin respond better to these drugs than patients with low renins, in whom little or no blood pressure fall may be seen. In some high renin states (such as accelerated phase hypertension) and in patients on vasodilator therapy, the fall in pressure with ß-blockers may be dramatic. Plasma renin levels fall acutely in response to ß-blockade but, apart from the instances cited above, there is often no temporal relationship between the fall in renin and the fall in arterial pressure, partly due to the reflex mechanism operative as already outlined. It must also be pointed out that the influence of ß-blockers on extra-renal renin production in, for example, the vasculature, heart and brain, is unknown.

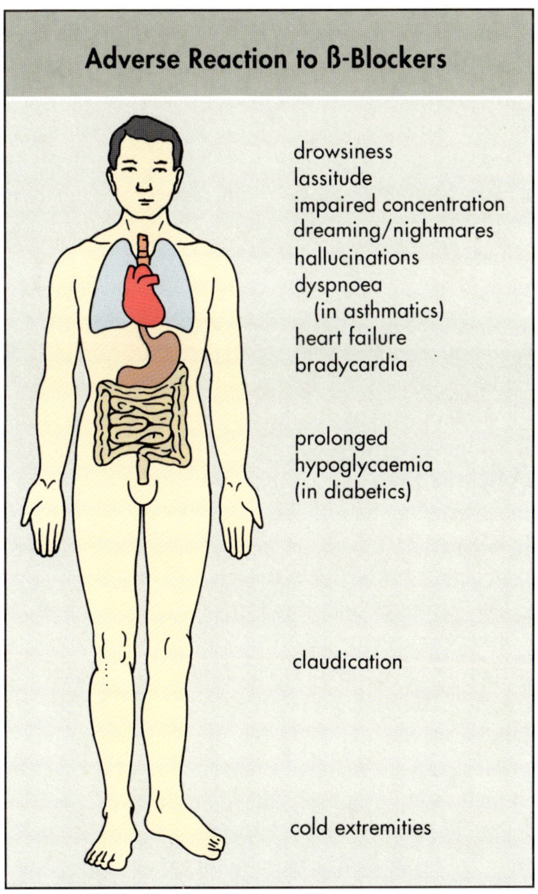

Fig. 9.13 Adverse reactions to ß-adrenoceptor antagonists.

Other Effects

There is some experimental evidence from studies in laboratory animals that ß-blocking drugs produce an antihypertensive effect via an action on the CNS. There is however little or no convincing evidence of a similar action in humans. Furthermore, ß-antagonists that penetrate poorly into the CNS are still effective as antihypertensive agents. Nevertheless, the actions of certain ß-blockers on the CNS are interesting because their central action can produce unwanted, adverse effects in patients.

Unlike the anti-anginal actions of the ß-blocking drugs, which relate to the plasma levels of these compounds, there is no such correlation with the antihypertensive effect. Following oral administration the plasma half-lives of many ß-antagonists are fairly short (approximately 3–10 hours). However, when these drugs are administered in a single daily dose, the fall in blood pressure is maintained for 24 hours or longer.

When ß-blocking agents are used in conjunction with vasodilators in the management of severe hypertension, they act to reduce the effects of reflex sympathetic stimulation of the cardiac ß-receptors and renin release from the kidney.

Adverse Effects

Adverse effects of ß-antagonists are primarily consequent on the effects of ß-adrenoceptor blockade (Fig. 9.13). They are contraindicated in patients with cardiac failure as they antagonize the effects of sympathetic stimulation on the heart and produce marked worsening of the failure. In some patients with incipient cardiac failure, gross failure may be precipitated. These effects may be seen immediately after ß-antagonist therapy is initiated, and are dose-related. They may be mitigated by previous digitalization.

Severe symptomatic bradycardia is observed in a small number of patients and can be avoided by using drugs with partial agonist activity. The fall in cardiac output with these agents is probably the cause of claudication in patients with peripheral vascular disease.

The second contraindication to the use of ß-antagonists is a history of asthma or severe obstruction of the airways. The precipitation of asthmatic attacks by ß-blocking drugs is at times dramatic and potentially lethal. Following the introduction of treatment with ß-antagonists there is sometimes a delay of weeks or even months before asthmatic attacks are precipitated. Although cardioselective antagonists have been advocated as an alternative therapy in the asthmatic hypertensive, they should be used with caution, if at all, since asthmatic attacks can be provoked even with these agents.

Cold extremities and Raynaud's phenomenon are common complaints in patients receiving ß-antagonists, possibly due to unopposed α-mediated constriction of peripheral vessels. Evidence that cardioselective agents are less likely to produce this phenomenon is inconclusive.

Central effects are common with many of these agents. Those most frequently experienced are impaired concentration, sleeplessness and nightmares. Antagonism of the effects of sympathetic stimulation on the bowel may lead to diarrhoea in some patients.

There has been much concern over potentially harmful metabolic effects of ß-antagonists in diabetic subjects. The two most important effects are the delayed recovery from hypoglycaemia, caused by inhibition of ß-receptor mediated glycogenolysis, and the potential masking of warning symptoms of hypoglycaemia. On rare occasions ß-blocking drugs may exacerbate diabetes by interfering with insulin release. Nevertheless, it is generally believed that with careful monitoring of the diabetic patient, ß-adrenoceptor antagonists may be used with caution.

ß-adrenoceptor blockers also affect metabolism through their influence on plasma lipoproteins. Whilst the underlying mechanisms remain to be clarified, reductions in HDL cholesterol and a rise in triglycerides are often seen. Although the magnitude of these lipoprotein changes is not great (about 10%), they are less than desirable in a population of patients in whom cardiovascular risk through atheroma is already increased.

Lastly, there is certainly evidence to support the use of ß-blockers as effective agents for secondary prevention of myocardial infarction. However, there is as yet no evidence for a 'cardioprotective' effect when used in the treatment of hypertension (see Chapter 10).

VASODILATORS

Under normal circumstances vascular smooth muscle tone is maintained by a host of neurohumoral mechanisms, as well as by the mediators derived from the juxtaposed endothelium.

Thus vasodilatation, resulting from relaxation of smooth muscle cells, can theoretically be achieved in a variety of ways (Fig. 9.14); some commonly and less commonly used vasodilators are shown in Figure 9.15. Drugs may act as follows:

- by preventing agonist activation of vascular smooth muscle (angiotensin converting enzyme inhibitors and α-adrenoceptor blockers);
- by blockading voltage-dependent and receptor-operated calcium channels, thus limiting calcium influx into smooth muscle cells (channel entry blockers);
- by exerting direct actions on smooth muscle with the activation of guanylate cyclase (hydralazine, minoxidil and possibly diazoxide).

The active constituent of nitrovasodilators such as the organic nitrates and sodium nitroprusside is nitric oxide (NO), which binds within the vascular smooth muscle cell to thiol groups forming a nitrosothiol intermediate, which then activates soluble guanylate cyclase. In this respect the nitrovasodilators mimic an endogenous vasodilator generated by the vascular endothelium – endothelium derived relaxing factor (EDRF), which has recently been identified as nitric oxide formed metabolically from the precursor L-arginine. A number of peptide hormones, such as calcitonin gene-related peptide and vasoactive polypeptide (analogues of which could potentially be developed as vasodilator drugs), may act primarily on the vascular endothelium by liberating EDRF. Other peptides (such as atrial natriuretic peptide) probably act directly on the smooth muscle.

The vascular endothelium synthesizes another potent vasodilator autacoid, prostacyclin, from its metabolic precursor arachidonic acid. There is clearly potential for elaborating this system to induce vasodilatation in the hypertensive subject; at least one new agent, cicletanine, may operate by facilitating a prostacyclin dependent mechanism.

The haemodynamic properties of vasodilators may be dependent upon whether they act as arteriolar dilators or venodilators or both (see Fig. 9.15). The arterioselective drugs hydralazine and minoxidil and the nonselective drug diazoxide all

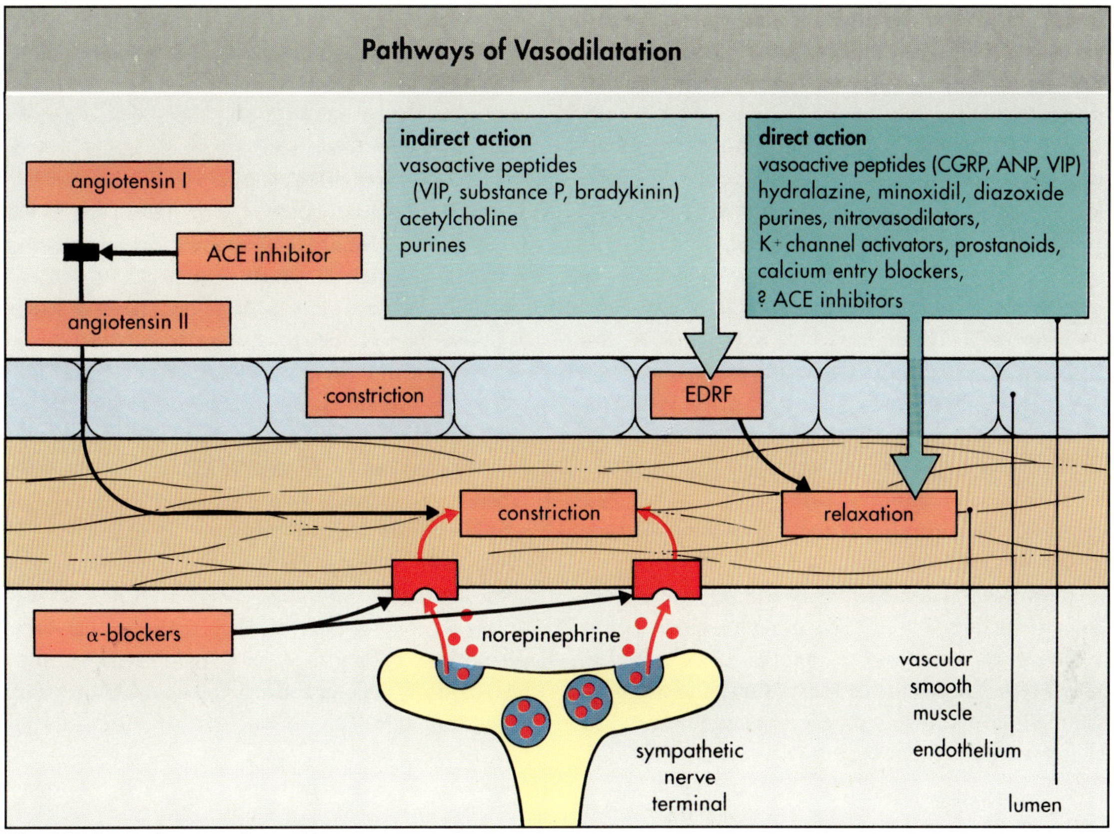

Fig. 9.14 Mechanisms of vasodilatation.

Vasodilators

		vessels dilated		reflex tachycardia
		resistance	capacitance	
nitroprusside		++	++	±
nitrates		++	++	±
hydralazine		++	−	++
diazoxide		++	++	+
minoxidil		++	−	++
α-blockers	non-selective	++	+	++
	selective α_1	++	+	±
converting enzyme inhibitors		++	−	−
calcium channel blockers	nifedipine	++	−	+
	verapamil	++	−	−

Fig. 9.15 Table showing the effects of some vasodilators currently in use.

lower peripheral vascular resistance and arterial pressure. As a consequence of the blood pressure fall there is baroreflex-mediated facilitation of sympathetic outflow from the brain stem, which leads to stimulation of the heart with an increased cardiac output and tachycardia (Fig. 9.16). The kidney releases renin in response to both the fall in pressure and sympathetic stimulation. The consequences of these reflex mechanisms include salt and water retention (mediated partly through aldosterone secretion) and a reduction of the hypotensive effect. (A comparison of the onset and offset of the hypotensive effect of some vasodilators is shown in Fig. 9.17.) An understanding of the physiological responses to arteriolar vasodilation provides a rational basis for the combined administration of a vasodilator, a ß-adrenoceptor antagonist and a diuretic.

Hydralazine was the first of the arteriolar dilators to be introduced. The exact mechanism by which it relaxes arteriolar smooth muscle is uncertain. Hydralazine concentrates in the smooth muscle of the arterial wall; its effects may be related to its chelating properties and to inhibitory effects upon several enzyme systems. It is metabolized by a number of pathways, including N-acetylation; the extent of the metabolism is determined genetically. The hypotensive effect of the drug is little affected by acetylator status when used in the absence of sympathetic blockade. However, in the presence of adequate ß-adrenergic blockade, rapid acetylators, with a more extensive 'first-pass' metabolism than slow acetylators, have a lesser hypotensive response to a given dose.

Other cardiovascular effects of hydralazine include palpitations, the precipitation of angina in some patients, headaches (including migraine) and marked fluid retention. The drug's usefulness when used alone is therefore limited. Prolonged administration of hydralazine (particularly in doses over 200mg/day) may be associated with a clinical picture simulating systemic lupus erythematosus. This occurs mainly in the slow acetylator phenotypes belonging to the HLA-DR4 subgroup. Diazoxide is a potent arteriolar vasodilator and a structural analogue of the thiazide diuretics. It

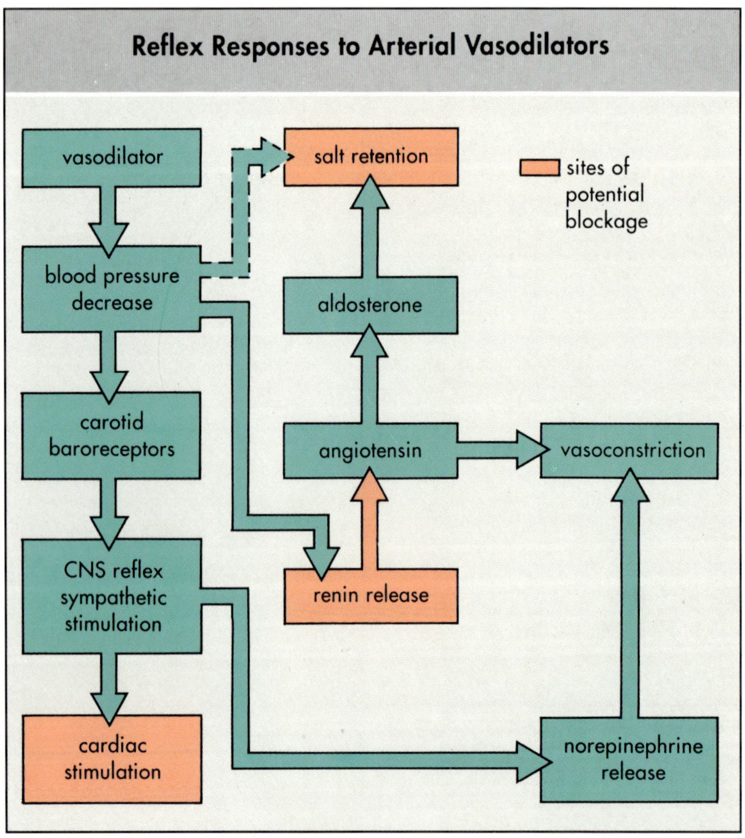

Fig. 9.16 Reflex responses to arterial vasodilator drugs.

possesses no diuretic action, however. Following intravenous injection it becomes strongly bound to plasma proteins and to vascular smooth muscle. Precipitous falls in arterial pressure may occur within minutes of its administration (Fig. 9.18); this seriously limits the drug's use. Cardiovascular reflex responses to the fall in blood pressure are similar to those encountered with hydralazine. Marked fluid retention also occurs. The diabetogenic effect is much more pronounced than it is with some of the thiazide diuretics. Like the thiazides, it gives rise to hyperuricaemia .

Minoxidil is similarly concentrated in the vasculature and is one of the most potent orally-active arteriolar vasodilators. Reflex responses and salt retention occur, in common with other drugs in this group. A curious side effect of prolonged treatment with either minoxidil or diazoxide is the

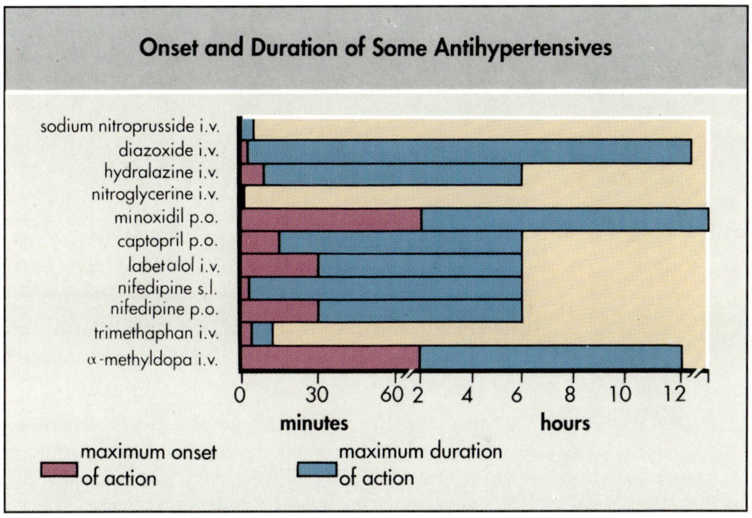

Fig. 9.17 Onset and offset of action of vasodilator and other antihypertensive agents.

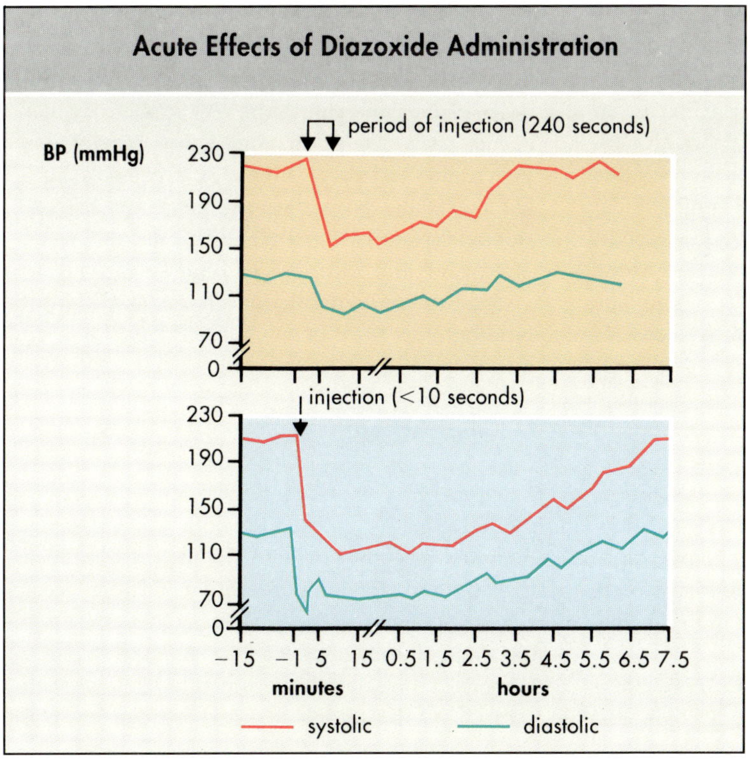

Fig. 9.18 Precipitous fall in blood pressure following the intravenous administration of 300mg diazoxide. Note that the more rapid injection produces a greater fall in blood pressure.

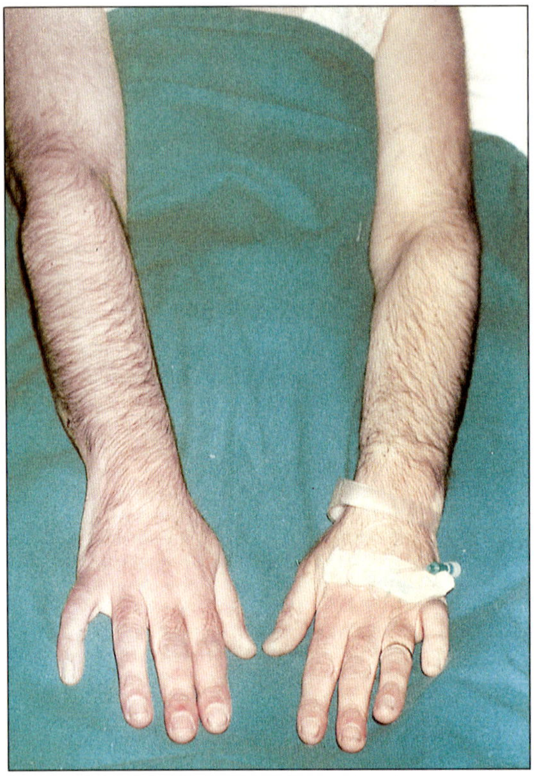

Fig. 9.19 Excessive hair growth in a female patient receiving minoxidil.

promotion of excessive hair growth (Fig. 9.19), perhaps related to cutaneous vasodilatation; this effect limits the use of these agents in women.

Sodium nitroprusside and prazosin have an action on both arterioles and veins. Although both agents have been classified as venoselective, this selectivity may be overridden when conventional doses of the drugs are used. The powerful vasodilatation induced by nitroprusside is related to the active constituent NO, which activates guanylate cyclase. Because of venodilatation, preload is reduced and there is little change in cardiac output; this in contrast with the arteriolar vasodilators (see Fig. 9.15). The action of the compound when given by intravenous infusion is immediate and is reversible within minutes of administration. Sodium nitroprusside is metabolized to thiocyanate and cyanide. Thiocyanate may cause adverse effects when prolonged infusions are given or when patients have renal failure. It may also cause confusion, lassitude, or hypothyroidism. High doses of nitroprusside may cause cyanide toxicity, to which patients with liver disease are particularly prone.

Calcium Entry Blockers
group A verapamil, nifedipine and related dihydropyridines (such as isradipine, nicardipine, nimodipine, nitrendipine amlodipine) diltiazem
group B bepridil, cinnarizine, flunarizine
group C non-specific agents (weak calcium blockers at high doses) chlopromazine

Fig. 9.20 The classification of calcium entry blockers. Group A is the most important.

CALCIUM ENTRY BLOCKERS (CEB)

Fleckenstein attributed the action of verapamil to its ability to block the entry of calcium ions into cells with resultant inhibition of excitation–contraction coupling. Several chemically unrelated groups of drugs have subsequently been shown to block calcium entry into vascular smooth muscle and thereby promote vasodilatation (Fig. 9.20). Those calcium antagonists which now occupy an established place in the treatment of hypertension include verapamil, nifedipine and related dihydropyridines and diltiazem. (A number of other agents, such as bepridil, cinnarizine, flunarazine, trenylamine and perhexiline may possess calcium entry blocking properties; these will not be considered further.) Verapamil, nifedipine, diltiazem, isradipine and nicardipine bind selectively to voltage-dependent calcium channels; different binding sites have been characterized for various agents.

Mode of Action

Calcium entry blockers (CEBs) impede calcium mobilization by blockading both voltage-dependent and receptor-operated channels; this reduces the accumulation of intracellular calcium occurring by either mechanism (Fig. 9.21). However, blockade of voltage-dependent channels in vascular smooth muscle cells occurs at much lower concentrations than those required to interfere with the receptor-mediated mechanism. These agents

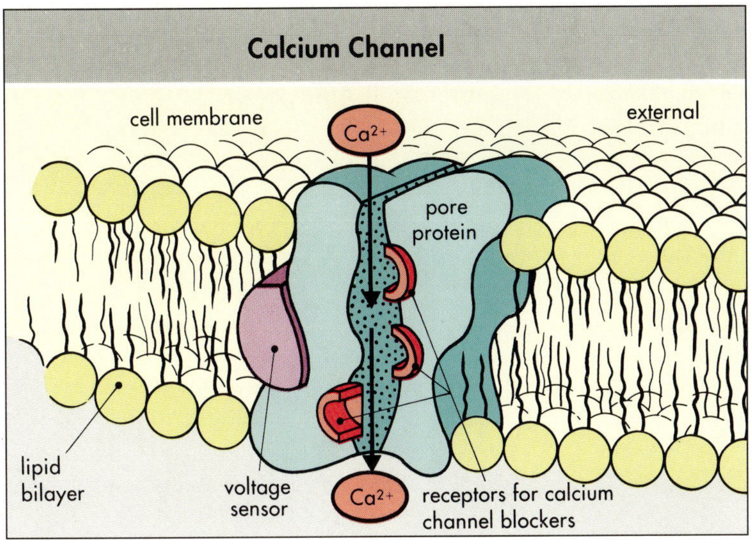

Fig. 9.21 Calcium enters smooth muscle cells via gated calcium channels. The gating of the channel prevents calcium entry and can be induced by drugs acting within the pore, where there are binding sites (such as the dihydropyridine receptor) for calcium channel blockers.

relax arterial smooth muscle but have little effect on most venous beds; this differential action certainly affects the haemodynamic response.

Of the CEBs, the dihydropyridines are the most potent inhibitors of calcium transport and exert most of their effects on the vasculature. Indeed, at doses conventionally used in clinical practice, nifedipine and related drugs exert little or no effect on the heart. In contrast, both verapamil and the less vasoselective diltiazem blockade the slow inward calcium current in myocardial cells of atria, ventricles and conducting tissue, resulting in complex actions on the heart including negative inotropic and chronotropic responses. Verapamil and diltiazem exert these effects on the heart at doses used in clinical practice

The haemodynamic responses obtained when a CEB is used in a hypertensive patient depend upon its selectivity for blood vessels. With the selective agent nifedipine, the dilatation of arterial resistance vessels is accompanied by reflex sympathetic stimulation, tachycardia and a positive inotropic effect (see Fig. 9.16). On the other hand, with verapamil and diltiazem the doses required to produce vasodilatation also produce cardiac effects; the reflexly mediated sympathetic response is offset by the direct negative inotropic and chronotropic effects, with little or no change in heart rate and cardiac output. Acute intravenous administration of diltiazem causes, in some instances, an increase in heart rate which is not seen with longer term oral administration.

Adverse Effects of Calcium Entry Blockers	
headache	hypotension
flushing	peripheral oedema (lower legs and feet)
dizziness	

Fig. 9.22 Adverse effects associated with calcium channel blockers.

Adverse Effects

The major adverse effects of CEBs relate to the vasodilatation that they cause (Fig. 9.22). With nifedipine, headaches, flushing and dizziness are commonly encountered. These effects are more often encountered with short-acting preparations and are probably related to a rapidly rising plasma concentration of the drug. Hypotension may also be precipitated. However, all these effects may diminish with repeated administration. Another fairly common effect is peripheral oedema of the lower legs and feet. This occurs as a consequence of arteriolar and capillary dilatation and is not relieved by diuretics.

With verapamil and diltiazem such vasodilatation-related effects are somewhat less common. However, because of the cardiodepressant effects of these drugs, bradycardia, hypotension and the precipitation of cardiac failure may occur in susceptible individuals.

RENIN–ANGIOTENSIN SYSTEM

A wealth of experimental and clinical data have shown that inhibition of the renin–angiotensin system is accompanied by a lowering of blood pressure. There are a number of ways in which this inhibition can be achieved. Drugs may act in the following ways:

- by suppressing renin release from the kidney (ß-blockers – see above);
- by direct inhibition of renin, the enzyme which converts angiotensinogen to angiotensin I (this new class of drugs is not discussed further in this chapter);
- by inhibiting angiotensin converting enzyme (ACE) which splits angiotensin I to produce angiotensin II;
- by antagonizing the effects of angiotensin II at the angiotensin receptor.

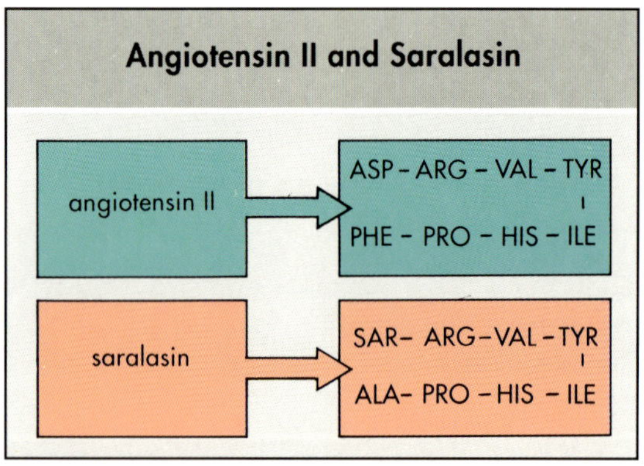

Fig. 9.23 Amino acid sequences of angiotensin II and saralasin.

Angiotensin II Antagonists

The substitution of N-methylglycine (sarcosine) in position 1 and alanine in position 8 of the angiotensin molecule produces a peptide called saralasin (Fig. 9.23); saralasin competitively blocks the action of angiotensin II at the receptor site (Fig. 9.24). Both the pressor and aldosterone responses to angiotensin II are antagonized by saralasin in a dose-dependent fashion. Saralasin also inhibits the pressor response to the central administration of angiotensin II in experimental animals.

Saralasin is not a pure antagonist – it possesses a degree of partial agonist activity (ISA). In hypertensive humans and animals, the blood pressure response to saralasin is largely determined by the angiotensin dependence of the blood pressure. Thus in high-renin states, such as unilateral renal arterial disease, a marked hypotensive response to the infusion of saralasin may be seen (Fig. 9.24); this hypotensive effect is enhanced in the presence of salt depletion. Saralasin has little effect on blood pressure in normal or in low-renin states; indeed, it may manifest its partial agonist activity in this situation by raising blood pressure.

Saralasin and related compounds are peptides and have short half-lives (approximately three to four minutes) and must be administered intravenously. They are not practicable for long-term management of renin-dependent hypertension.

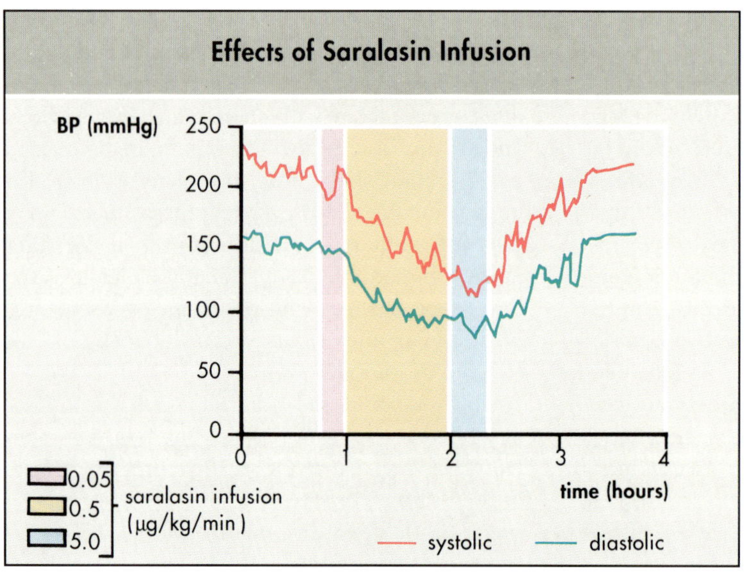

Fig. 9.24 Hypotensive reponse to saralasin infusion in a patient with renin-dependent hypertension (renal artery stenosis).

ACE Inhibitors

It was proposed in the mid-1960s that the enzyme responsible for the conversion of angiotensin I to angiotensin II might be the same enzyme which destroyed the vasodilating peptide bradykinin (Fig. 9.25). A number of peptides were subsequently isolated from the venom of the Brazilian pit viper which contained a substance that potentiated and prolonged the effects of bradykinin. These peptides were found to inhibit converting enzyme in varying degree. Early studies with the nonapeptide teprotide (SQ 20881) showed that the drug was effective at inhibiting the pressor response to exogenous angiotensin I. In hypertensive and salt-depleted normotensive subjects, blood pressure fell in response to the intravenous administration of teprotide and a marked rise in plasma renin was observed.

The use of teprotide was limited owing to the necessity for it to be administered intravenously. A search for an orally active compound led to the development of captopril (by Cushman and colleagues) in 1976, enalapril in 1980 and lisinopril in 1988. Several other ACE inhibitors are currently in development.

These compounds are effective in the majority of hypertensive subjects, whether the raised blood pressure is due to renal or renovascular causes, or to essential hypertension (see later). Although all the drugs currently marketed are structurally similar (Fig. 9.26), only the captopril molecule contains a sulphydryl moeity, which may confer additional pharmacological properties on the drug. Enalapril is a prodrug and is rapidly hydrolysed to the active diacid enalaprilat.

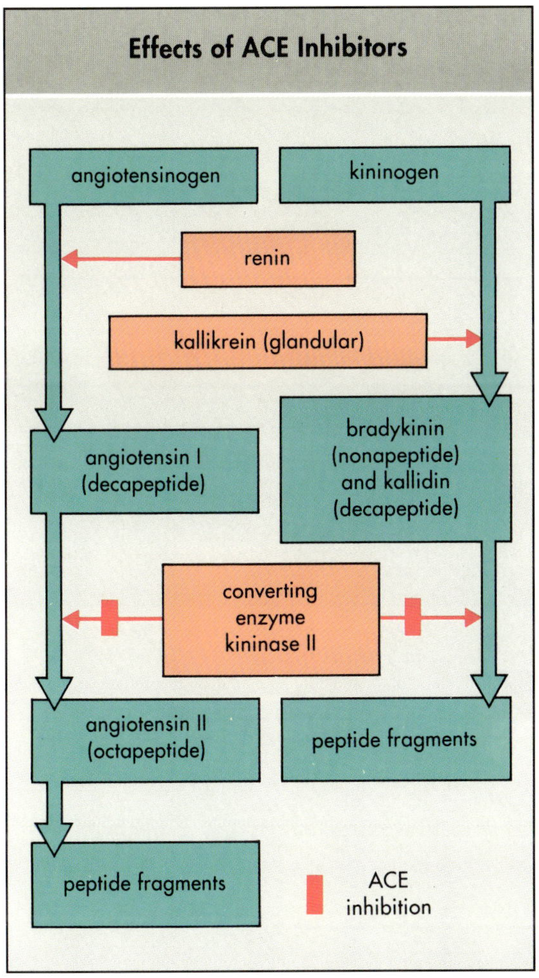

Fig. 9.25 ACE inhibitors also inhibit the breakdown of bradykinin.

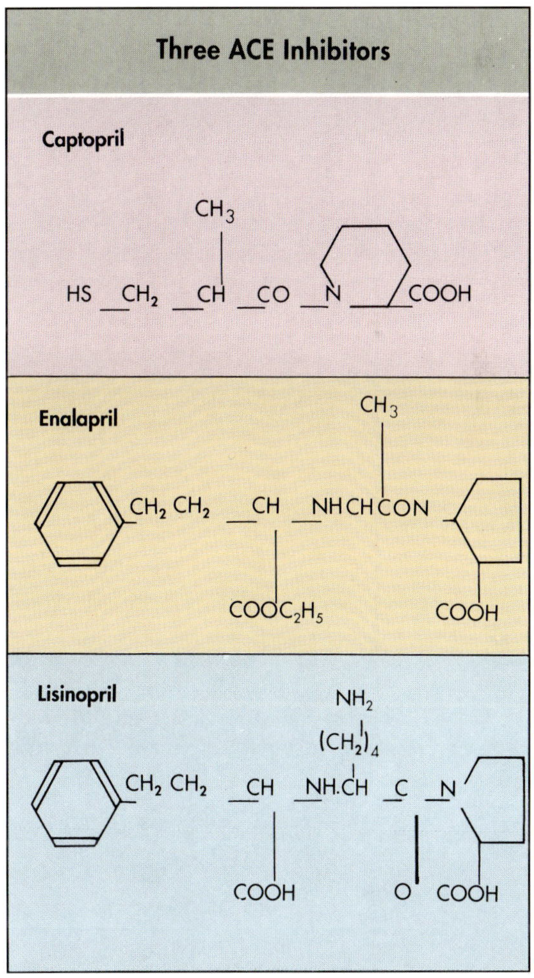

Fig. 9.26 The structures of three ACE inhibitors.

Mode of Action

The duration of activity in the plasma of available ACE inhibitors relates to their differing pharmacokinetic profiles, with the action of captopril considerably shorter than that of either enalapril or lisinopril. Inhibition of plasma enzyme, at least in the short term, seems to relate to the blood pressure lowering effect of these agents, although with longer term therapy the simple relationship is lost. Furthermore the magnitude of the blood pressure fall correlates with pretreatment renin activity in acute studies (Fig. 9.27); again, this simple relationship is not seen with long term therapeutic control of blood pressure.

The pharmacological effect of ACE inhibitors and their mode of action, in terms of short and longer term blood pressure control, are clearly more complicated than was originally assumed. The clinical effects of ACE inhibition may result from inhibition of renin–angiotensin systems in both plasma and in tissues, and from inhibition of kinin degradation. With increased knowledge of the more widespread distribution of components of renin–angiotensin systems in vascular walls, in the heart and in other tissue such as the brain, it seems likely that ACE inhibition has more diverse effects than could simply be accounted for by inhibition of converting enzyme in plasma. The contribution of these tissue renin–angiotensin systems to blood pressure control is as yet unknown, but it is likely that, if it has any influence at all, perturbation of such systems by ACE inhibitors would influence long-term responses to the drug rather than shorter term hypotensive effects.

After oral administration of an ACE inhibitor, levels of plasma angiotensin II and aldosterone fall and there is a rise in levels of renin and angiotensin I, as a result of the removal of the negative feedback inhibition of renin release (Fig.

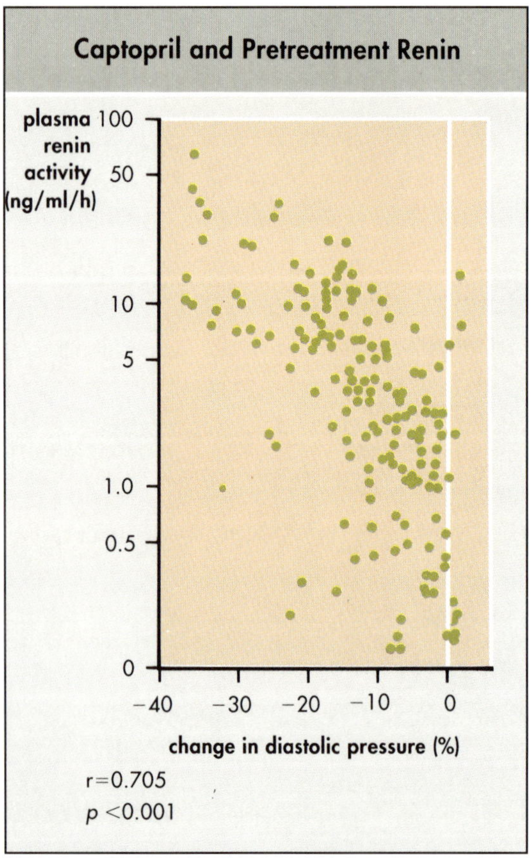

Fig. 9.27 Prediction of an acute fall in blood pressure following 25mg captopril by measurement of pretreatment renin. [Modified from Cody *et al.* (1983) *Hypertension*, **5 (suppl. III)**, 36–42.]

Responses to ACE Inhibition

blood pressure	↓
angiotensin II	↓
aldosterone	↓
renin	↑
angiotensin I	↑
bradykinin	↑
prostaglandin E_2	↑

Fig. 9.28 The humoral and blood pressure responses to ACE inhibition.

9.28). As a consequence of ACE inhibition bradykinin degradation is slowed. This in turn leads to activation of phospholipase with the resultant formation of vasodilator prostaglandins (such as PGE_2) which contribute to the overall hypotensive effects of ACE inhibitors, particularly in patients with low renin.

The multiplicity of sites at which angiotensin acts to produce a pharmacodynamic response (Fig. 9.29) suggests that additional mechanisms may contribute to the blood pressure lowering effect of ACE inhibitors. For example, inhibition of angiotensin II formation may have important sympatholytic effects. The contribution of such an action to blood pressure reduction is not known. It may be beneficial – and therefore of more importance – in the heart, for example preventing reperfusion arrhythmias.

The early haemodynamic effects of ACE inhibition are more pronounced in clinical situations in which the activity of the renin–angiotensin system is activated – sodium depleted individuals, patients on diuretics and patients with renal artery stenosis or accelerated phase hypertension are examples. The decrease in blood pressure is due primarily to a fall in systemic vascular resistance with either no change or a small rise in cardiac output. The absence of marked reflex tachycardia, in common with several other vasodilators (such as hydralazine) may be explained by resetting of the baroreflex, by a facilitation of vagal influences on the heart or by blockade of angiotensin's facilitatory effect on sympathetic outflow.

With longer term treatment with ACE inhibitors there is evidence, both from experimental animals and from humans with hypertension, that therapy causes regression of left ventricular hypertrophy. Although the associated blood pressure reduction may be important in this respect, it is possible that the ACE inhibitors reverse the trophic influence of

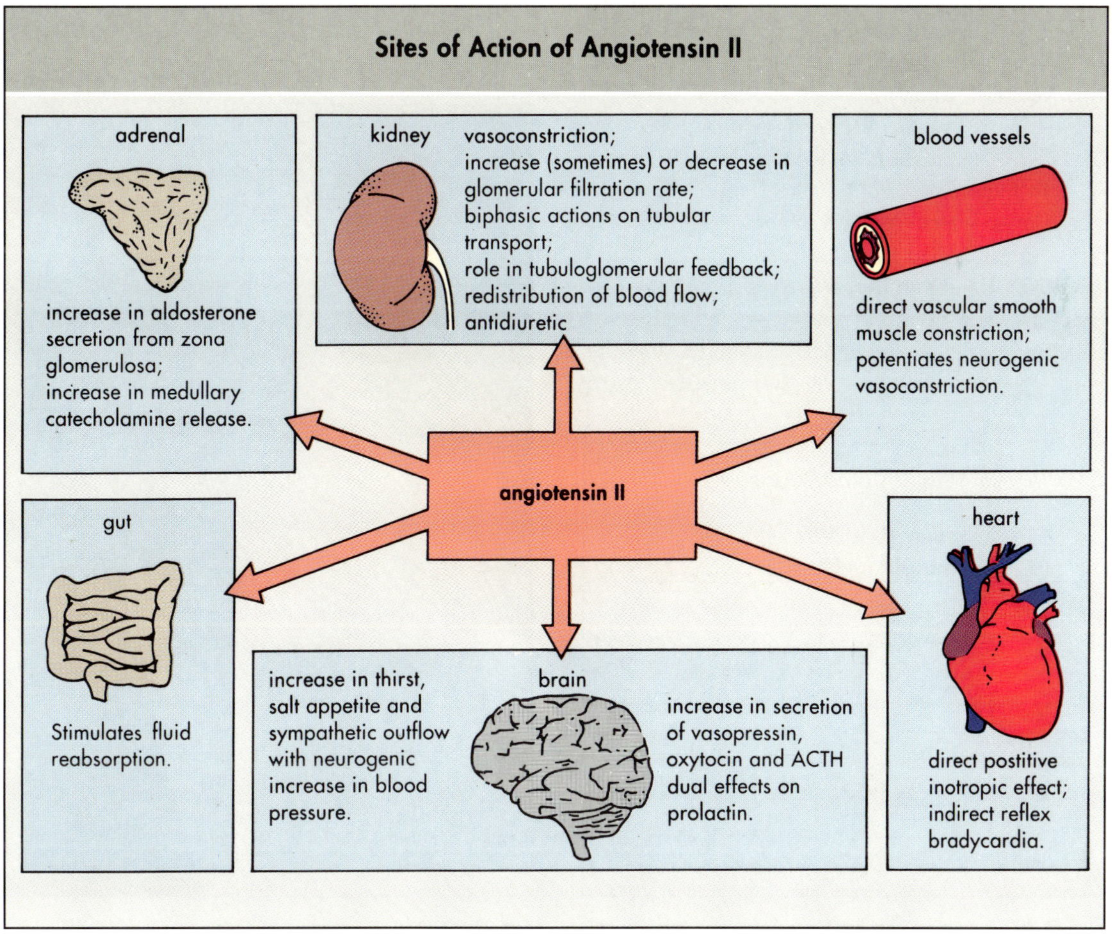

Fig. 9.29 The multiple sites of action of angiotensin II.

angiotensin (and conceivably norepinephrine) on cardiac myocytes.

In the kidney, despite a reduction in blood pressure, there is an increase in renal plasma flow, a decrease in renal vascular resistance and little change in GFR. Sodium loss with mild potassium retention occurs as a consequence of the associated reduction in aldosterone. There is considerable interest in the effects of ACE inhibitors in patients with impaired renal function, as glomerular filtration may be improved and renal function preserved. In hypertensives (and in diabetics) proteinuria may be diminished.

In some patients with renal artery stenosis renal failure may, however, be precipitated by the introduction of therapy with ACE inhibitors. Usually seen in patients with bilateral renovascular disease, the removal of angiotensin II-dependent vasoconstrictor tone from the efferent arteriole leads to a dramatic fall in GFR and ultimately to renal failure. Fortunately in most cases these effects are reversible on withdrawal of the drug. This observation has been exploited in the development of the captopril–DTPA test for renal artery stenosis (see chapter 8).

The haemodynamic effects of ACE inhibitors on the cerebral circulation are also potentially important. In hypertensive subjects the blood pressure range over which cerebral blood flow is maintained is shifted to the right (Fig. 9.30). With the administration of antihypertensive drugs, particularly in emergencies such as hypertensive encephalopathy, there is a real danger that the blood pressure fall will be accompanied by a reduction in cerebral blood flow, usually with disastrous consequences. However, ACE inhibitors, although often producing large falls in blood pressure, appear to preserve cerebral blood flow as they do so. This clearly is a major advantage in certain clinical situations.

Adverse Effects

In contrast to many other classes of antihypertensive drugs, adverse metabolic effects of ACE inhibitors are few. Hyponatraemia may occur, particularly in individuals who are sodium-depleted or on diuretics, and potassium retention may be exaggerated if potassium-sparing diuretics are given (these should of course be avoided). No changes in blood glucose or blood lipids are encountered with ACE inhibitors.

In the early days following the introduction of captopril a number of potentially serious adverse reactions were reported, including neutrapenia and proteinuria. It is now recognised that these reactions were dose related and associated with

Vasodilator Drugs

	arterio-selective	non-selective	venoselective
drug types	hydralazine minoxidil	diazoxide	glyceryl trinitrate sodium nitroprusside prazosin
cardiac output	↑↑	↑	supine: little change upright: ± ↑
arterial pressure	↓	↓	supine: ↓ upright: ↓↓

Fig. 9.30 Selectivity of vasodilator drugs and their effect on cardiac output and arterial pressure.

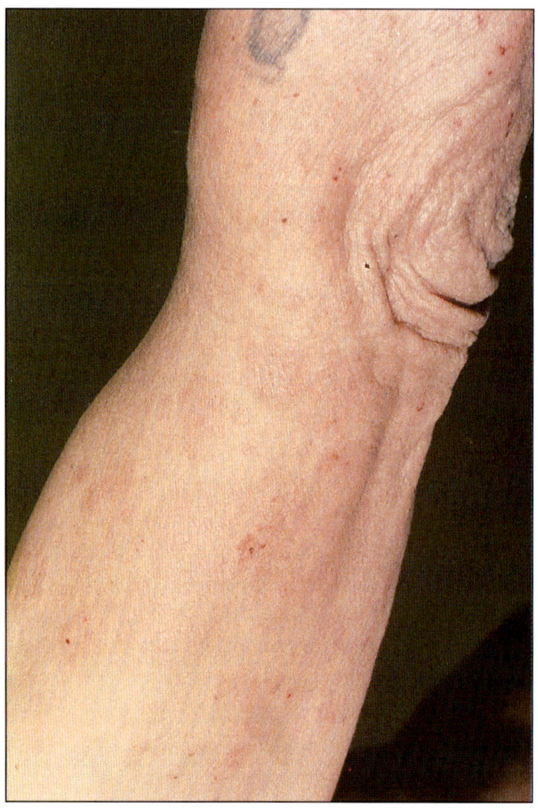

Fig. 9.31 Skin rash in a patient receiving captopril.

much higher doses of the drug than are now conventionally used. Present dosage regimes (up to 150mg/day captopril) are seldom associated with serious adverse reactions. An altered appreciation of taste, a dry cough and a transient rash (Fig. 9.31) are not uncommonly seen.

Several studies have compared ACE inhibitor and other drug therapies for their effects on various aspects of quality of life (Fig. 9.32). Overall, it appears from these studies that ACE inhibitors are less likely to compromise lifestyle and quality of life than other groups of agents.

Quality of Life During Drug Therapy

	captopril	methyldopa	propranolol
well being	↑	–	–
physical symptoms	–	↓	↓
sexual performance	–	↓	↓
work performance	↑	↓	–
sleep	–	–	–
cognition	↑	↑	↑
life satisfaction	–	↓	↓
social interaction	–	–	↑

Fig. 9.32 Changes in the quality of life following the onset of drug therapy. The consistent improvement in measures of cognition seen with all drugs is probably accounted for by an increasing familiarity with the questionnaire as the tests are repeated.

α-BLOCKING DRUGS

The α-blocking properties of the competitive α-adrenoceptor antagonist phentolamine and the noncompetitive inhibitor phenoxybenzamine have been widely utilized in, respectively, the diagnosis and management of phaeochromocytoma.

Phentolamine is a nonselective antagonist at both presynaptic (α_2) and postsynaptic (α_1) adrenoceptors (Fig. 9.33) and, following intravenous administration, rapidly antagonizes the α-mediated pressor effects of norepinephrine and epinephrine released from catecholamine-secreting tumours. The short half-life of this compound (three minutes) prevents its more widespread use in the management of this condition.

Phenoxybenzamine has a much longer action by reason of its irreversible blockade. Although it is more effective as an α_1-antagonist, it also inhibits the presynaptic α_2-receptors that modulate neurotransmitter release.

Vasodilatation resulting from postsynaptic α_1-blockade with these agents has not been acceptable in the management of non-catecholamine mediated hypertension because the non-selectivity of these compounds is associated with severe postural hypotension, increased cardiac output and tachycardia. The increases in cardiac output and tachycardia, probably the result of presynaptic α_2-receptor blockade, tend to negate the hypotensive action of the drug.

Prazosin is a selective competitive postsynaptic α_1-receptor blocking drug. The vasodilatation which it induces is associated with a minimal increment in heart rate, unlike non-selective α-

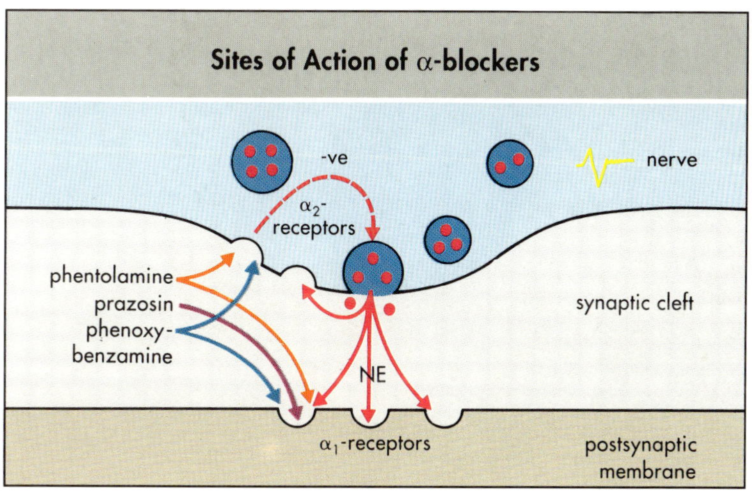

Fig. 9.33 Site of action of α-blocking drugs on pre- and postsynaptic receptors. NE = norepinephrine.

blocking agents whose action is accompanied by a marked tachycardia. Prazosin reduces vascular tone in both resistance vessels and capacitance vessels and there is little change in cardiac output associated with the fall in arterial pressure. A postural fall occurs but is not as severe or as disabling as that observed with non-selective α-blockers. Providing a low starting dose of 1mg prazosin is administered, the severe orthostatic hypotension seen with a high first dose (2mg) does not occur (Fig. 9.34).

Two new selective α_1-adrenoceptor antagonists have recently been introduced, namely doxazosin and terazosin. Their main advantage appears to lie in their longer duration of action and the reduced tendency to first dose hypotension. An interesting additional property of this class of drugs, which contrasts with other commonly used agents, is the tendency for treatment to be associated with a modest fall (5–10%) in total and LDL cholesterol (Fig. 9.35). The significance of this is as yet unknown.

Labetalol is a ß-receptor antagonist which can block α-receptors at the same time. It is used not only in hypertensive states associated with excessive catecholamine secretion, such as phaeochromocytoma and clonidine withdrawal, but also in essential hypertension.

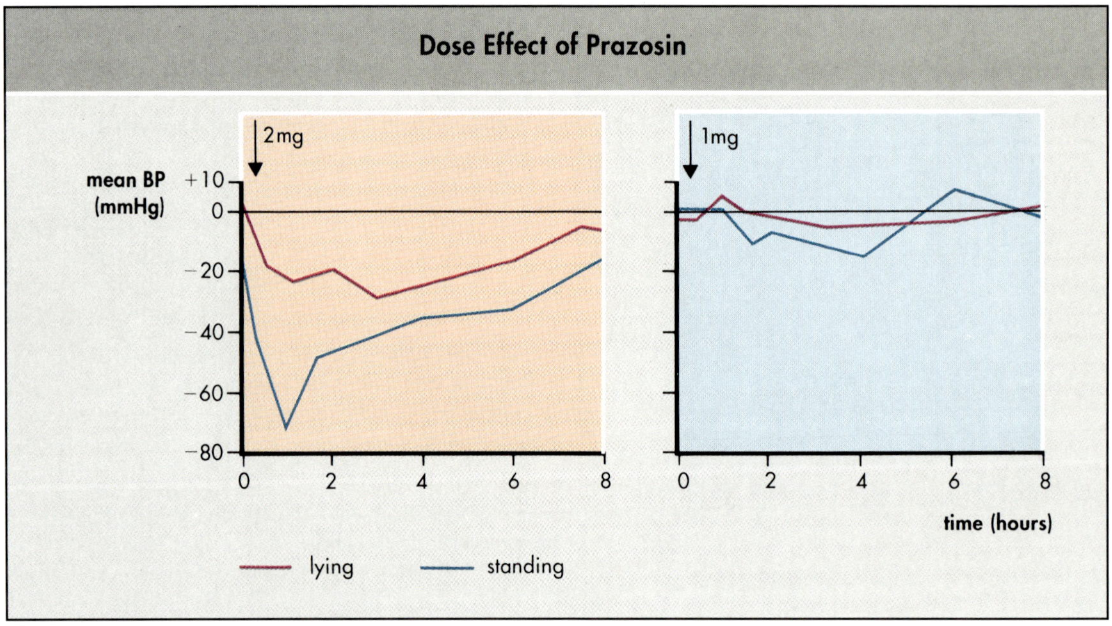

Fig. 9.34 First-dose hypotensive effect of prazosin.

The Effects of Antihypertensive Drugs on the Lipid Profile

drugs	total cholesterol	LDL cholesterol	HDL cholesterol	triglycerides
thiazides	↑	↑	↔ ↓	↑
ß-blockers	↔	↔ ↑	↓	↔ ↑
α_1-inhibitors	↔ ↓	↔ ↓	↔ ↑	↓
ACE inhibitors	↔	↔	↔	↔
Ca^{2+} antagonists	↔	↔	↔	↔

Fig. 9.35 The effects of antihypertensive drugs on the lipid profile.

CENTRALLY ACTING DRUGS

α-Methyldopa

Mode of Action

It was initially proposed that the action of methyldopa in lowering blood pressure was due to competitive inhibition of L-aromatic amino acid decarboxylase (Fig. 9.36), with a consequent decrease in peripheral norepinephrine stores. It was, however, subsequently demonstrated that decarboxylation of methyldopa is a prerequisite for the hypotensive effect of the drug. A second hypothesis put forward to explain the action of methyldopa was that the hypotensive effect was due to the replacement of norepinephrine in peripheral nerve stores by α-methylnorepinephrine, which acted as a 'false' neurotransmitter. However, the potency of α-methylnorepinephrine as a vasopressor amine approximates to that of norepinephrine. Furthermore, agents which inhibit peripheral decarboxylation of methyldopa fail to prevent the hypotensive effect of the drug. That conversion of methyldopa to α-methylnorepinephrine in the brain is necessary for the hypotensive action is shown by experiments in which inhibition of both peripheral and central

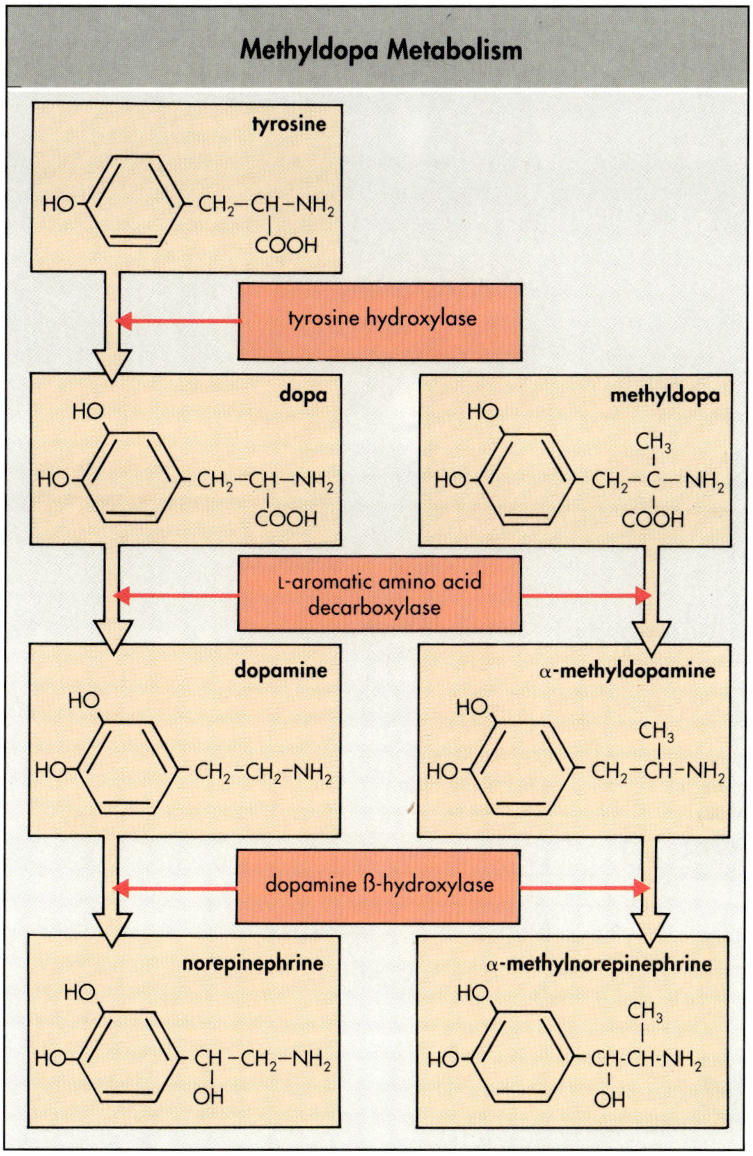

Fig. 9.36 Metabolism of methyldopa showing interrelationship with the biosynthetic pathway for norepinephrine and the formation of the false neurotransmitter, α-methylnorepinephrine.

decarboxylation of methyldopa block the effect of the drug on blood pressure (Fig. 9.37).

The prolonged duration methyldopa's action (up to 24 hours after oral administration) and the failure to demonstrate any correlation between blood levels of methyldopa and hypotensive action, both lend further support to the hypothesis that the agent responsible for the antihypertensive action is a metabolite of the parent compound. Thus the stimulation of central α-receptors (probably α_2-receptors) by α-methylnorepinephrine and the consequent reduction in sympathetic outflow from the brain stem accounts for the major component of the hypotensive property of methyldopa. However, a peripheral mechanism cannot be completely ruled out; a part of the hypotensive effect may be secondary to the stimulation of inhibitory presynaptic α_2-receptors.

The fall in pressure produced by methyldopa is largely associated with a fall in peripheral vascular resistance. In most series, cardiac output is slightly reduced. The effect on the vasculature is predominantly in the arterioles and significant orthostatic hypotension is rarely a problem. Renal blood flow is hardly altered and renin secretion is reduced.

Other Effects

Methyldopa, in common with certain other antihypertensive drugs, reverses left ventricular hypertrophy in the spontaneously hypertensive rat. There is apparently no such reversal in these animals, however, when blood pressure is controlled with some vasodilators – in the case of minoxidil, hypertrophy is actually increased. The mechanism underlying the effect of methyldopa on cardiac muscle remains unclear, but is probably related to a reduction in the trophic influence of adrenergic drive to the heart. These direct studies in animals have led to many investigations using echocardiography to assess the response of left ventricular hypertrophy to antihypertensive therapy in man. The results seem to suggest the following:

- sympatholytics have been associated with a reversal of hypertrophy in most reports;
- although there is still some controversy surrounding the effects of ß-blockers, a majority of reports indicate a reduction in ventricular mass;
- converting enzyme inhibition appears to lead to a regression in left ventricular wall thickness and wall mass;

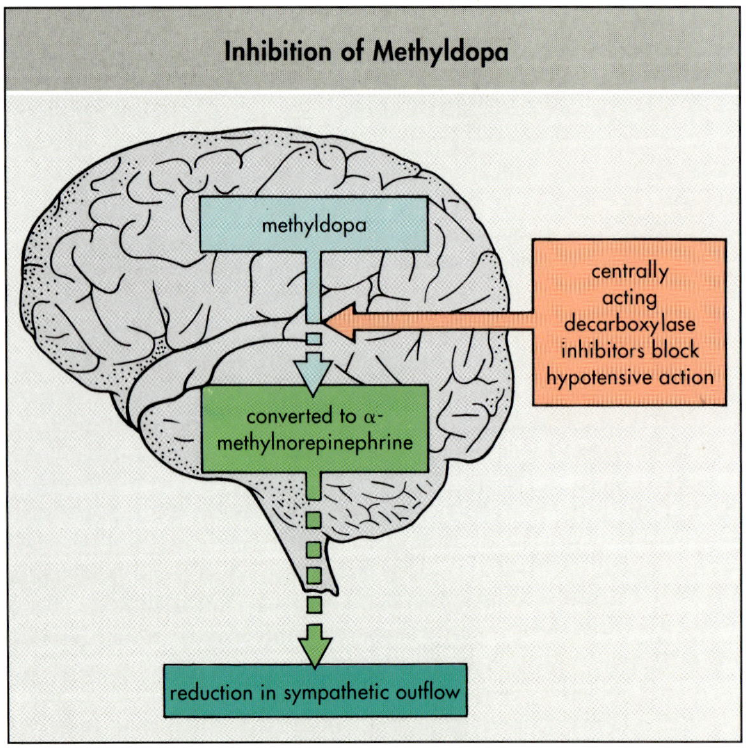

Fig. 9.37 The hypotensive action of methyldopa is blocked by centrally acting dopa decarboxylase inhibitors.

- while diuretics and vasodilators reduce blood pressure, neither type of drug has been shown consistently to reverse hypertrophy or reduce ventricular mass when used alone.

Methyldopa has a number of adverse effects (Fig. 9.38). The relatively common problem of drowsiness, particularly during initiation of therapy, is due to the central locus of action of the drug. The more serious problems, although infrequently encountered, include the development of an autoimmune haemolytic anaemia, drug fever and drug-induced hepatitis. 20% of patients on methyldopa develop a Coomb's positive antiglobulin test, but only rarely do patients develop haemolysis. In the male, impotence is probably mediated through central stimulation of prolactin release. (Impotence is also a common problem with other antihypertensive drugs, including the diuretics, but with other agents the mechanisms of the effect are less clear.)

Clonidine

Mode of Action

During the investigation of a possible mucosal vasoconstrictor drug, the observation was made that the imidazoline clonidine lowered arterial pressure and heart rate. Considerable attention has since been focused on the possible role of central α-adrenoceptors in blood pressure regulation.

As discussed previously, there are two types of α-adrenoceptors. The α_1 subtype corresponds to those postsynaptic adrenoceptors in the peripheral and central nervous systems that are blocked by prazosin and stimulated by phenylephrine. α_2-adrenoceptors, which are antagonized by yohimbine, are located on the prejunctional membrane and their stimulation has an inhibitory effect upon norepinephrine release. There is also good evidence for the existence of postsynaptic α_2-adrenoceptors.

When clonidine is administered intravenously an initial rise in blood pressure precedes a more prolonged hypotensive effect as well as bradycardia and a reduction in cardiac output. It is believed that the initial hypertensive effect is due to stimulation of peripheral postsynaptic vascular α_1-adrenoceptors. The cardiovascular depressant effects of clonidine are mediated through an action on the central nervous system. The probable locus of clonidine's central action is in the region of the nucleus tractus solitarius. This central effect leads to a reduction in sympathetic outflow from the brain stem. It is thought that activation of postsynaptic α_2-adrenoceptors is responsible for this response. This has been concluded from experiments in which depletion of central endogenous catecholamines has had little effect on the reduction in sympathetic outflow induced by clonidine. There is other evidence, however, that clonidine acts centrally through presynaptic α_2-adrenoceptors to reduce norepinephrine and/or epinephrine turnover. It is also possible that stimulation of

Adverse Effects of Methyldopa	
central nervous system lethargy lack of concentration depression dry mouth nasal congestion impotence	**fever** **hepatitis**
	cardiovascular system postural or exercise hypotension sodium and water retention (less than adrenergic neurone blockers)
blood positive direct Coomb's test autoimmune haemolytic anaemia	**others** Parkinsonism gynaecomastia (and lactation)

Fig. 9.38 Adverse effects of methyldopa.

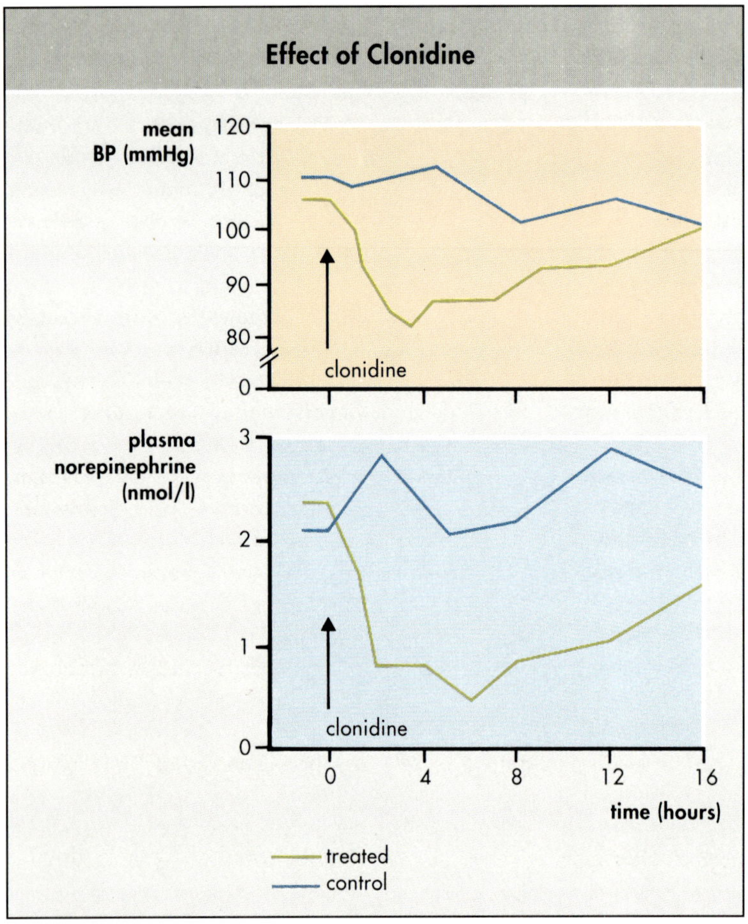

Fig. 9.39 Mean blood pressure and plasma norepinephrine response to a single oral dose of 300μg clonidine in normal subjects compared with a placebo (control).

peripheral presynaptic α_2-adrenoceptors may contribute to the reduction in sympathetic tone.

In man, a single oral dose of clonidine produces a marked fall in blood pressure (Fig. 9.39). Evidence that this is mediated by a reduction in sympathetic activity can be inferred from the associated reduction in circulating levels of norepinephrine. With single doses of clonidine there may be a rise in plasma renin, but repeated administration of the drug induces renin suppression. Both central and peripheral mechanisms may be involved in this action.

Other Effects

The adverse effects of clonidine are troublesome and include sedation and dry mouth. Sedation is linked to the stimulation of central α_2-adrenoceptors and possibly to a reduction in the turnover of norepinephrine in the brain. The reduction in salivary flow is mediated through activation of presynaptic α_2-adrenoceptors leading to a reduction in cholinergic transmission.

A potentially dangerous effect of clonidine is the rebound (withdrawal) hypertension that occurs when therapy with the drug is stopped abruptly (Fig. 9.40). It has been proposed that chronic administration of the drug leads not only to desensitization of presynaptic α_2-adrenoceptors but also to supersensitivity of peripheral postsynaptic α_1- and β_1-receptors, a consequence of reduced noradrenergic transmission. On withdrawal of the drug there is an increase in norepinephrine release, hypertension and tachycardia. This is the result of subsensitivity of presynaptic inhibitory α_2-receptors and supersensitivity of postsynaptic α_1- and β_1-receptors in the vascular smooth muscle and in the heart respectively. As with other antihypertensives, impotence has been reported in some patients taking this drug.

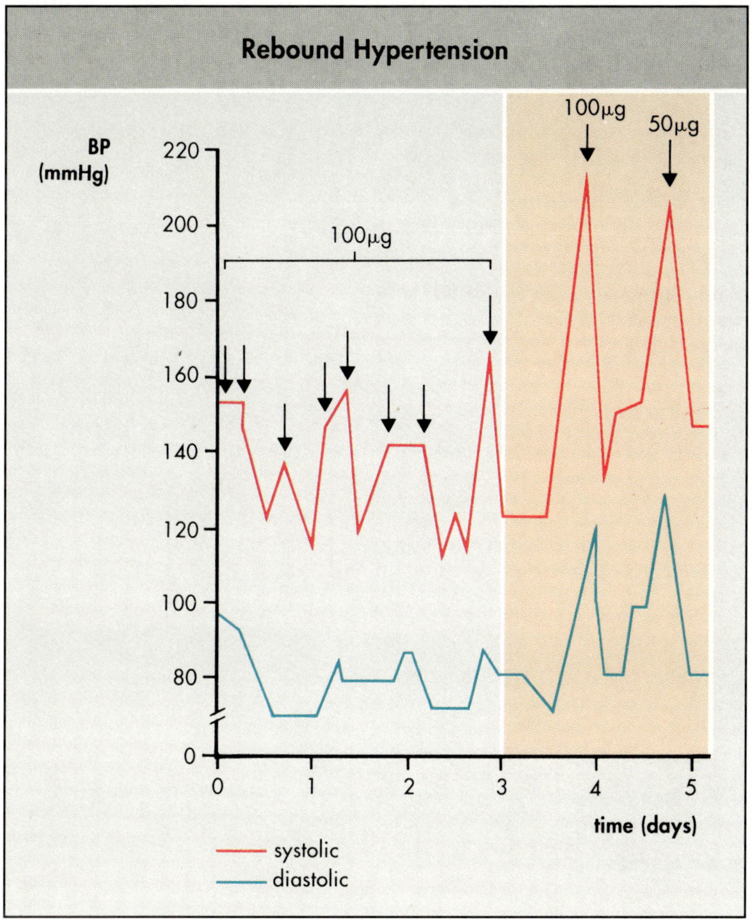

Fig. 9.40 Rebound hypertension occurring approximately 24 hours after the dose of clonidine given on day three.

Other Sympatholytics

Reserpine

The rauwolfia alkaloids have been used for centuries in the treatment of psychotic illness and their hypotensive effects were noted more than fifty years ago. Reserpine causes marked depletion of catecholamines from storage granules in the peripheral sympathetic neurones, the brain and, to a lesser extent, the adrenal medulla. The initial effect of the drug is to release granular stores of norepinephrine. This may be accompanied by transient hypertension when the drug is given parenterally. The prolonged hypotensive effect is secondary to the prevention of an $MgATP^{2-}$-dependent uptake of dopamine into storage granules and the consequent depletion of stores of norepinephrine. The antihypertensive effect is believed to be primarily peripheral, although a central component to reserpine's action cannot be ruled out.

The major disadvantage of reserpine is the profound depression induced in many subjects by the central depletion of monoamines. Reserpine should only be administered in low dosages (0.05–0.1mg) and in combination with diuretic agents, which increase the antihypertensive effect.

α-Methylparatyrosine

This sympatholytic was discovered during the search for an inhibitor of the rate-limiting step in catecholamine biosynthesis. It is a potent inhibitor of tyrosine hydroxylase and, when administered to patients with catecholamine-secreting tumours, causes a marked reduction in tumour synthesis of amines and a fall in blood pressure. Its clinical use ie restricted to patients with malignant phaeochromocytomas for whom surgery is impractical.

GANGLION-BLOCKING DRUGS

Mode of Action

Several quaternary ammonium compounds have been found to interrupt transmission at autonomic ganglia by competitive antagonism of acetylcholine receptor sites on the postsynaptic membrane. A number of related drugs were subsequently introduced, including pentolinium, chlorisondamine and the triethylsulphonium salt trimetaphan. The secondary amine mecamylamine and the tertiary amine pempidine were also shown to have ganglion-blocking properties. When introduced into clinical medicine in the early 1950s they were the first effective antihypertensive agents, and for this reason they will be discussed briefly here.

The magnitude of the blood pressure reduction induced depends upon the existing level of sympathetic activity. Thus, there is little change in pressure in recumbent normotensive subjects but a dramatic fall in the semi-recumbent or upright posture when arterial pressure is maintained by sympathetically mediated vasoconstriction. In hypertensive subjects the fall in pressure is most marked in the sitting or standing position (Fig. 9.41). Cardiac output is reduced due to venous pooling of blood. Heart rate changes little in the recumbent state, but may rise with hypotension.

Other Effects

Because of the non-selective properties of these agents at all automatic ganglia, widespread physiological actions of the ganglion-blocking drugs are evident and depend upon the predominant tone of the various organs (Figs 9.42 and 9.43). The severity of the adverse effects (particularly orthostatic hypo-tension) has led to the replacement of these drugs by more modern agents, except for occasional use during anaesthesia and (in some centres) in the management of hypertensive emergencies.

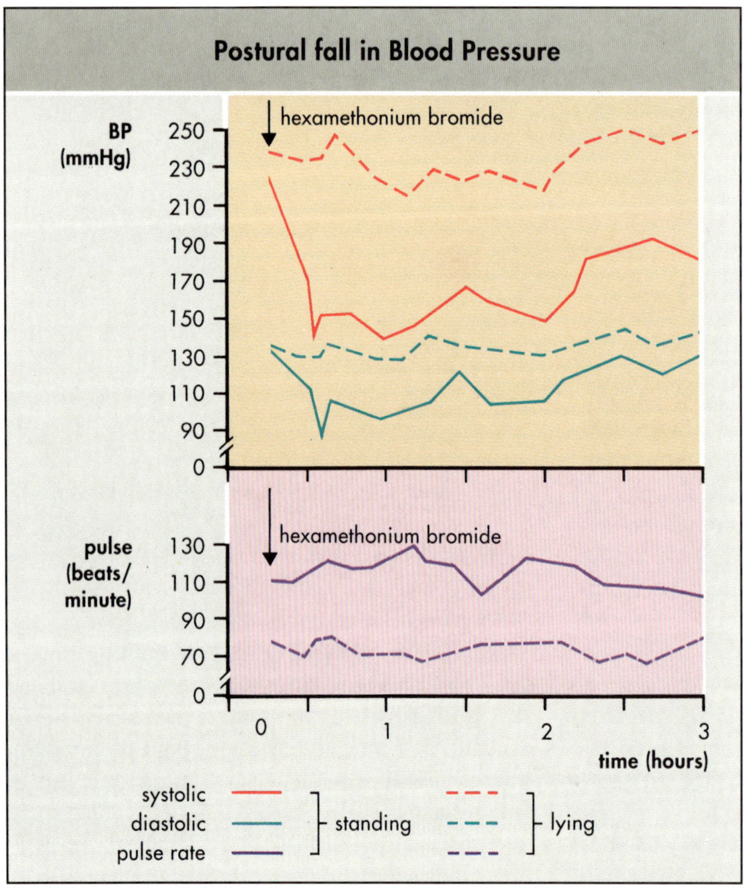

Fig. 9.41 Postural fall in blood pressure produced by the ganglion blocking drug hexamethonium bromide.

Effects of Ganglionic and Adrenergic Blockade			
site	predominant tone	effect of ganglionic blockade	effect of adrenergic blockade
arterioles and veins	sympathetic (adrenergic)	vasodilatation; hypotension: postural hypotension	vasodilatation; hypotension postural hypotension; nasal stuffiness
heart	parasympathetic (cholinergic)	tachycardia	bradycardia
gastrointestinal tract	parasympathetic (cholinergic)	reduced tone and motility; constipation	increased motility; diarrhoea
urinary tract	parasympathetic (cholinergic)	urinary retention	-
salivary glands	parasympathetic (cholinergic)	xerostomia	-
sweat glands	sympathetic (adrenergic)	anhydrosis	-
organs	sympathetic and parasympathetic	impotence and impaired ejaculation	impaired ejaculation
central nervous system	-	-	sedation or depression

Fig. 9.42 The multiple effects of ganglionic and adrenergic neurone blockade.

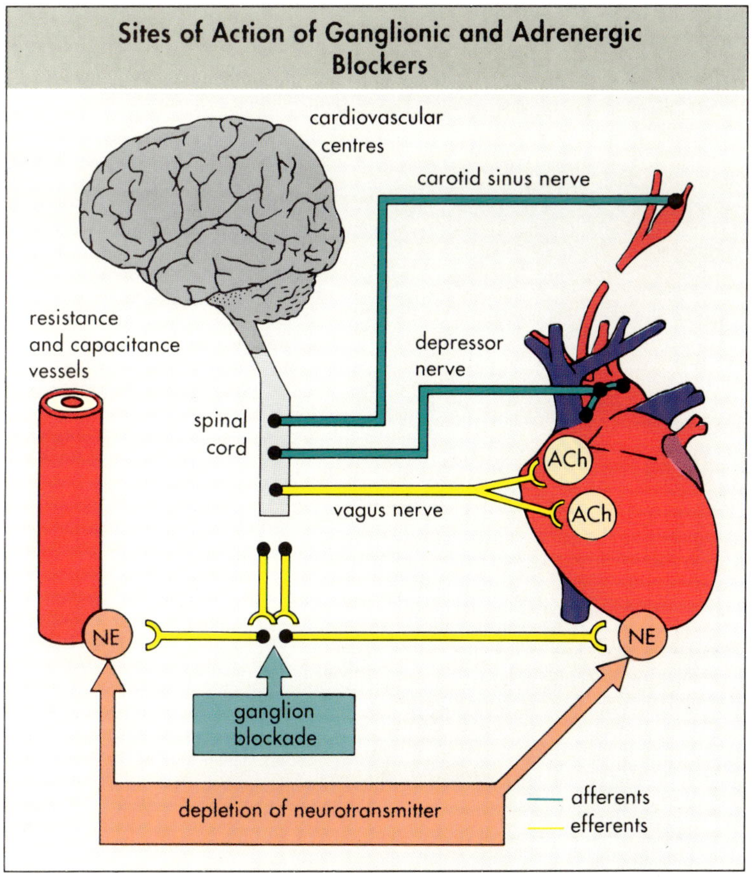

Fig. 9.43 The site of action of ganglion blocking and adrenergic neurone blocking drugs in the abolition of normal cardiovascular orthostatic reflexes.
NE = norepinephrine.
ACh = acetylcholine.

ADRENERGIC-NEURONE-BLOCKING DRUGS

Mode of Action

The antihypertensive effects of the adrenergic-neurone-blocking drugs are due to their ability to inhibit the function of postganglionic sympathetic neurones. Guanethidine (Fig. 9.44), bethanidine and debrisoquine are actively transported into the nerve terminals by the same mechanism (uptake$_1$) responsible for the reuptake of norepinephrine. Guanethidine is stored in the amine-containing storage vesicles, where it depletes the granular store of norepinephrine and thus reduces the amount of neurotransmitter released by exocytosis. Although both bethanidine and debrisoquine are taken up into the nerve terminals and reduce the overflow of norepinephrine into the synaptic cleft, the extent of granular depletion of norepinephrine stores may be rather less than that produced by guanethidine. There is evidence that the antihypertensive effect is related more to the inhibition of neurotransmitter release than to the depletion of norepinephrine stores.

The intravenous administration of all three drugs causes an immediate rise in arterial pressure due to the initial release of norepinephrine from neuronal stores. In the case of debrisoquine administered both orally and intravenously, this hypertensive response may last for two to three hours. Debrisoquine is an inhibitor of monoamine oxidase and this property may account in part for the prolonged pressor response. Bethanidine may also inhibit monoamine oxidase.

Haemodynamic studies indicate that the fall in blood pressure caused by these drugs is associated with reductions in both cardiac output and peripheral vascular resistance as a consequence of sympathetic inhibition. Because reflex-mediated vasoconstriction is blocked by these drugs, a much greater antihypertensive effect occurs in the upright posture (see Fig. 9.43) and postural hypotension is common. Although more selective than the ganglion-blocking agents, the use of this group of drugs is associated with the occurrence of many unwanted side effects as a consequence of widespread sympathetic blockade and salt and water retention.

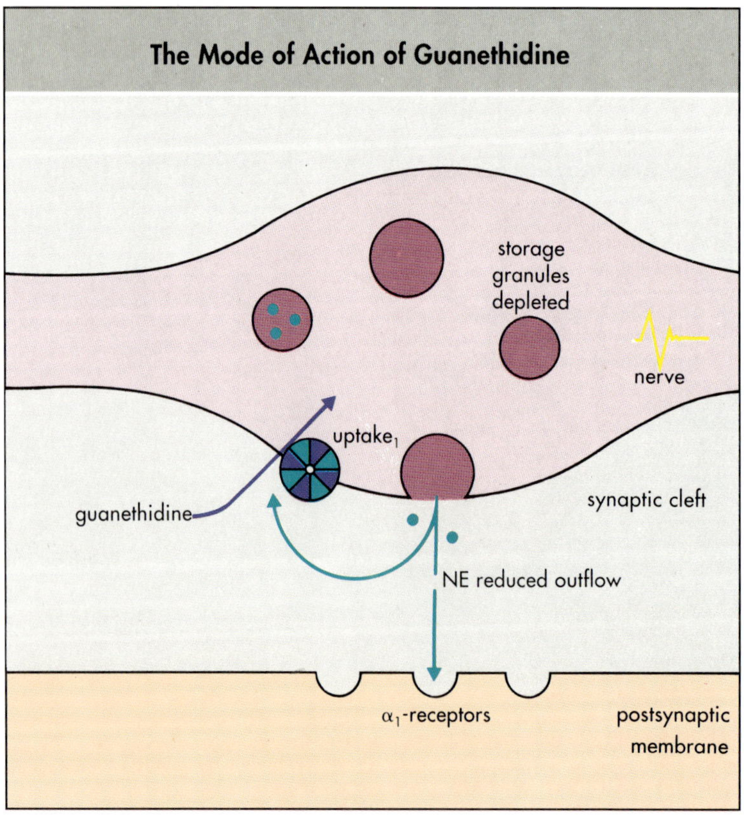

Fig. 9.44 The site of action of the adrenergic neurone blocking drug guanethidine at the sympathetic nerve terminal.

Other Effects

Because long-term neurotransmitter depletion leads to postsynaptic receptor supersensitivity, drugs that compete with the adrenergic-neurone-blockers for uptake into the nerve terminals (such as tricyclic antidepressants) and sympathomimetics (both mixed and direct acting), may occasionally provoke acute severe hypertensive episodes (Figs. 9.45 and 9.46).

The important clinical differences between the three drugs are in the onset and duration of their actions. Guanethidine may take two to three days after initiation of therapy to produce its antihypertensive effect. This effect will last for several days after the drug has been discontinued. With the other drugs the antihypertensive onset is earlier (after three to four hours), and the duration of action much shorter (up to eight hours). The response to debrisoquine is partly genetically determined. The poor metabolizer of the drug responds with a more severe and prolonged hypotension compared with the rapid metabolizer phenotype.

All three drugs are also concentrated in postganglionic nerve cell bodies. If large doses of guanethidine are administered to young experimental animals, cytotoxic effects may be observed which lead to chemical sympathectomy.

The high rate of adverse reactions encountered with the use of these drugs, particularly in the elderly, has resulted in a marked decline in their use in most countries.

NEW AGENTS

The past decade has seen an explosion in research and development of new agents which have the potential for lowering blood pressure in hypertensive subjects. Within the existing classes of drugs, molecular modification and alterations in formulation of compounds are being undertaken in order to alter pharmacokinetic profiles with a view to increasing duration of action. Pharmacodynamic differences appear within each class of agent which may be of importance in relation to sites of

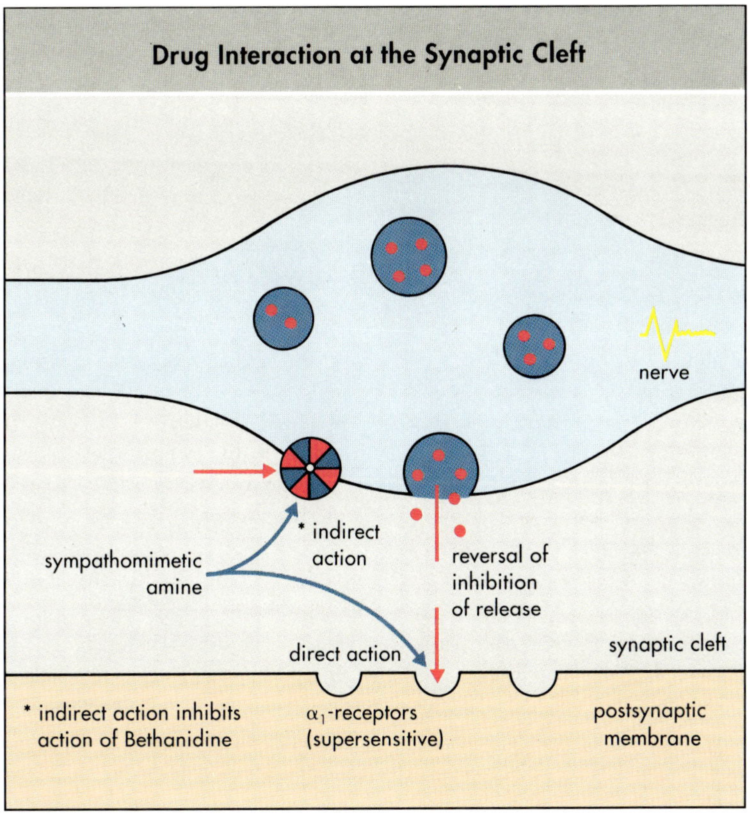

Fig. 9.45 The interaction of sympathomimetic amines and the adrenergic neurone blocking drug bethanidine at peripheral sympathetic nerve terminals.

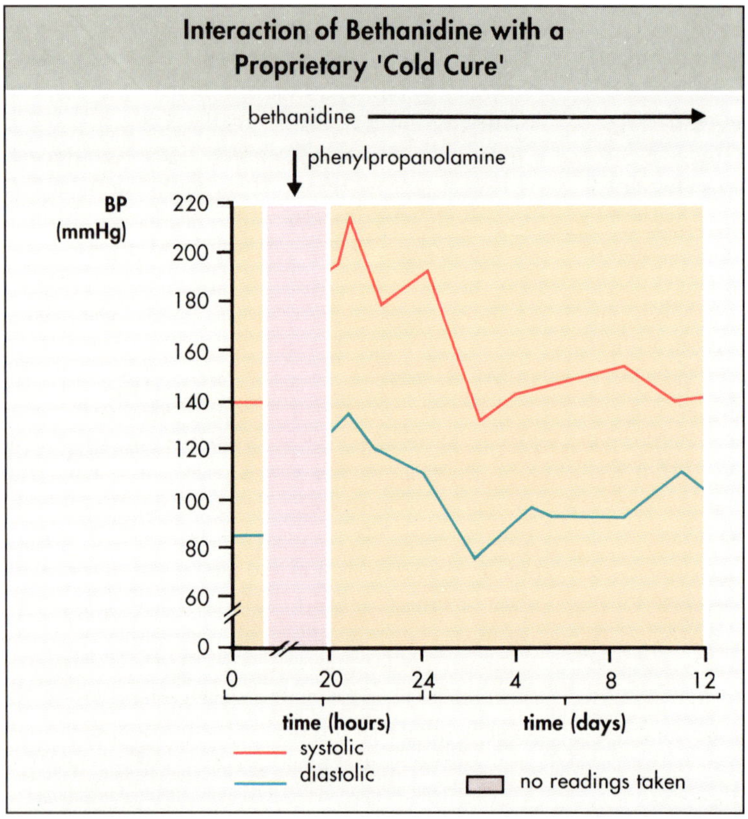

Fig. 9.46 Acute hypertensive response to a proprietary cold cure containing a mixed-acting sympathomimetic amine (phenylpropranolamine) and bethanidine.

action and selectivity for different vascular tissues. We have seen the emergence of longer acting ACE inhibitors and dihydropyridine calcium channel blockers. Within the diuretic field there are continued attempts to promote diuresis without potentially harmful concomitant metabolic effects.

A number of newer agents in the adrenoceptor blocking group of drugs are under investigation, for example, optical isomers of labetolol, such as dilevalol, appear to have rather different properties to those of labetolol itself, in that partial agonist effects at β_2-adrenoceptors are combined with β_1-adrenoceptor blockade within the same molecule. Other ß-blockers may possess vasodilator properties conferred by as yet unknown mechanisms, and there is clearly much interest in compounds which do not induce bronchoconstriction. There has been considerable interest in $5HT_2$ antagonists such as ketanserin, which undoubtedly has vasodilator properties, but the consensus opinion appears to be that this may be largely explained by the drug's α_1-blocking action.

The DA_1 agonist fenoldopam is a particularly interesting compound. Early clinical investigations revealed that the vasodilatation induced by fenoldopam was far more extensive than would have been predicted from previous knowledge on the distribution of vascular dopamine receptors. Although the drug has a predilection for the renal vasculature, it has potent effects on other vascular beds. Regrettably the catechol nucleus accounts for very high first pass elimination; its use as an orally administered drug is therefore limited.

The potent vasodilator properties of atrial natriuretic peptide have been exploited, with much effort devoted to the search for analogues that would be active when taken orally. To date, attempts have been largely unsuccessful. An alternative approach has been the development of inhibitors of the degradative enzyme atriopeptidase; early clinical trials with one such inhibitor have shown considerable promise, not only because of the vasodilatation conferred but also because of the associated natriuresis.

With an increase in the understanding of the complexity of the vascular endothelium and the local synthesis of endothelial derived mediators, it is not surprising that attempts are being made to facilitate vasorelaxation by pharmacological manipulation of these endothelial systems. To date vasodilator prostanoids have not emerged as real candidates for antihypertensive drug therapy, although some may occupy a useful role in the treatment of some peripheral vascular diseases. One compound, cicletanine, lowers blood pressure by a complex mechanism, which may be in part be due to an increased synthesis of prostacyclin. Other agents, for example, thromboxane A_2 antagonists, are still at an early stage of development. Obviously, with increasing knowledge of the mechanisms leading up to the release of EDRF (nitric oxide) and details regarding its metabolic precursor (L-arginine), potential mechanisms exist for the development of new agents targetted at the endothelium. The physiological or pathophysiological role of endothelial derived constrictor substances is far from clear, but here again there may be potential for pharmacological intervention to facilitate vasodilatation.

An alternative approach to inhibition of the renin–angiotensin–aldosterone system by converting enzyme inhibition is to inhibit the enzyme renin itself. Studies are already being undertaken with prototype renin inhibitors in man. Such compounds lower blood pressure by vasodilatation in hypertensive subjects, but their ultimate role in relation to ACE inhibitors is far from clear.

Another new group of agents under intense scrutiny are drugs which cause relaxation of vascular smooth muscle through hyperpolarization, probably due to the opening of smooth muscle membrane potassium channels (potassium channel activators, such as pinacidil). Studies confirming the blood pressure lowering effects of these agents are convincing, but early trials in human hypertensive subjects suggest that unwanted effects commonly encountered with potent vasodilators, such as headache, flushing and oedema, are a considerable problem.

There are other novel potential areas for new drug development which have come about as a consequence of increased awareness of mechanisms controlling the heart and, particularly, the vasculature. For example, it is probable that agents modelled on the cotransmitter adenosine and analogues of the potent vasoactive peptides (vasoactive intestinal polypeptide or calcitonin gene related peptide) will be developed. However, despite their attraction, few appear on the horizon at the present time.

CONCLUSION

With a wealth of new opportunities emerging for pharmacological intervention in hypertension, the future looks promising. However, the developer, the researcher and the clinician must not lose sight of their therapeutic goals, namely to lower blood pressure and to reverse hypertension-related cardiovascular morbidity and mortality using drugs whose use is not associated with adverse effects, either metabolic or symptomatic. Today we are far from achieving these goals; coronary heart disease is still largely unaffected by treatment, at least in the short term, and the use of the currently available drugs still causes undesirable effects in many of those who take them.

FURTHER READING

Ganten, D. & Mulrow, P. J. (eds) (1990) *Pharmacology of Antihypertensive Therapeutics (Handbook of Experimental Pharmacology, Volume 93).* Berlin–Heidelberg: Springer Verlag.

Doyle, A. E. (ed) (1984) Clinical Pharmacology of Antihypertensive Drugs. In *Handbook of Hypertension, Volume 5.* Amsterdam: Elsevier.

Goodman Gilman, A., Goodman, L. S., Rall, T. W. & Murad, F. (eds) (1985) *Goodman and Gilman's The Pharmacological Basis of Therapeutics*. New York: Macmillan.

Laragh, J. H. & Brenner, B. M. (eds) (1990) *Hypertension: Pathophysiology, Diagnosis and Management*. New York: Raven Press.

CHAPTER 10

Treatment

INTRODUCTION

The consequences of a sustained elevation of blood pressure are increased cardiovascular morbidity and mortality from a variety of causes (see chapter 4). The main objectives of treatment are, therefore:

- stroke prevention;
- reduction in the incidence of coronary heart disease and myocardial infarction;
- reversal of cardiovascular structural changes that occur as a consequence of hypertension;
- prevention of cardiac failure;
- prevention of progressive renal damage;
- prevention of more severe forms of hypertension, such as accelerated phase or malignant hypertension.

Data from several prospective epidemiological studies have shown that cardiovascular risk increases in a linear fashion with increments in blood pressure and there is no obvious threshold level of blood pressure beyond which risk becomes apparent (Figs 10.1 & 10.2).

Prior to therapeutic intervention it is necessary to consider evidence from controlled clinical trials of antihypertensive regimes (pharmacological and non-pharmacological) to confirm that overall benefit is achieved by active treatment and that such benefit, in terms of reduction in cardiovascular risk, is not offset by harmful or adverse effects.

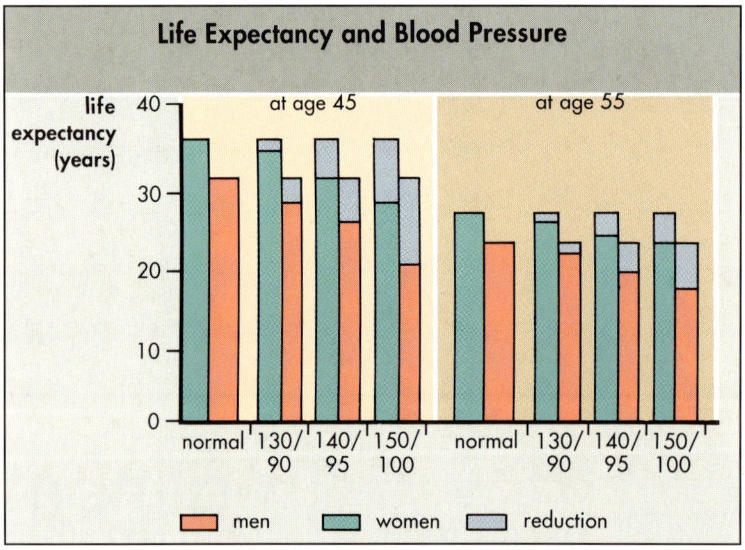

Fig 10.1 Reduction in life expectancy produced by mild blood pressure elevation.

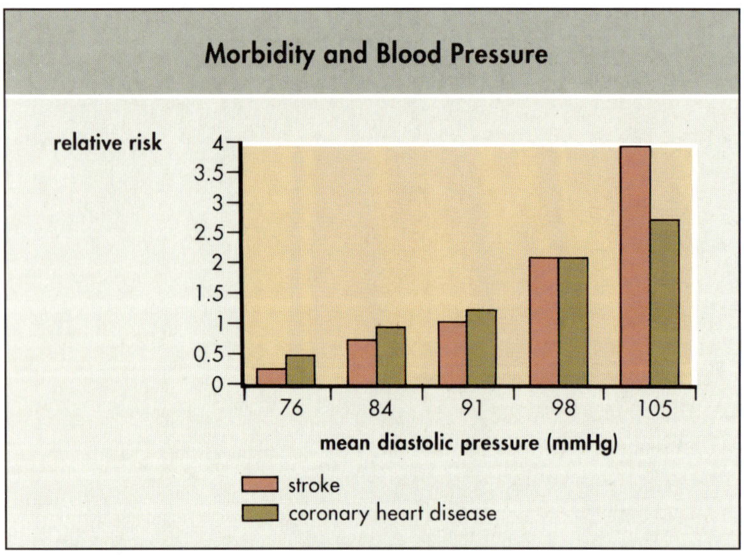

Fig. 10.2 Relative risk of stroke and coronary heart disease, defined by baseline diastolic blood pressure, estimated from the combined results of prospective observational studies. [Modified from McMahon *et al.* (1990) *Lancet*, **335**, 768.]

EVIDENCE FROM THE TRIALS

Before the introduction of drug therapy for severe hypertension, morbidity and mortality was high. In the Mayo Clinic reports of 1939, 80% of hypertensive patients who developed papilloedema died within a year, 90% were dead within two years and few remained alive after three years.

With the introduction of drug therapy, survival was dramatically improved; in the early study from the Hammersmith Hospital, 50% of treated patients survived two years (Fig. 10.3).

The benefits of treating mild–moderate hypertension (benign phase) have been demonstrated in controlled clinical trials. The results of the Veterans Administration Study, for example, were separated into two groups by inclusion diastolic blood pressure criteria (90–114mmHg and 115–129mmHg, phase V). Drug treatment reduced strokes, heart failure, other cardiovascular and renal end points, but not myocardial infarction (Fig. 10.4). From this and other early trials, the following generalizations could be made:

- a greater reduction in morbid events was seen in the higher blood pressure groups at entry;
- men fared better than women;
- the incidence of accelerated phase hypertension was greatly reduced by treatment.

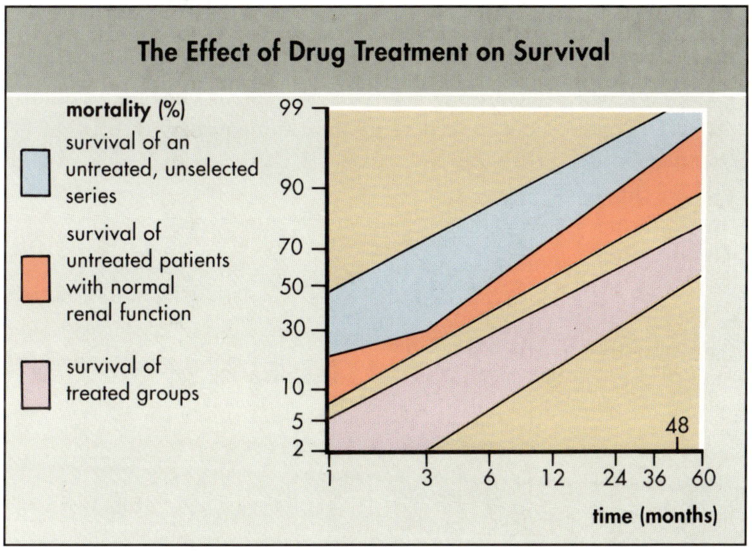

Fig. 10.3 The impact of drug treatment on the survival rate in malignant hypertension. [Modified from Pickering, Cranston and Pears (1961) The Treatment of Hypertension. Springfield: Charles C. Thomas.]

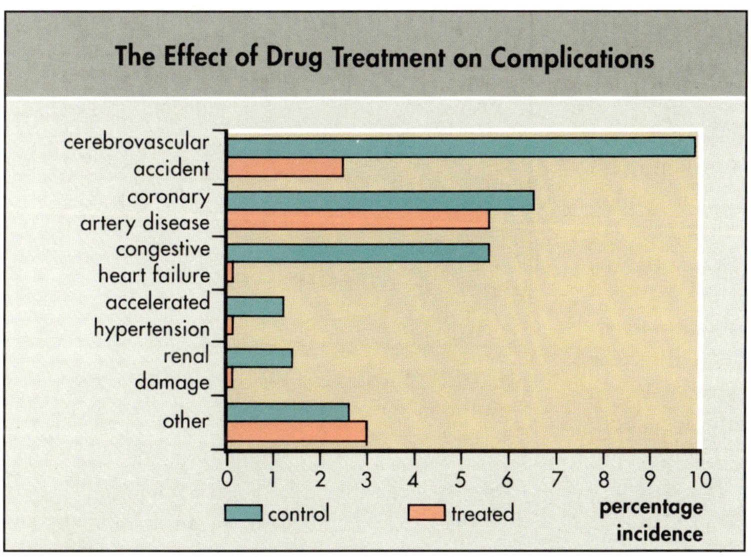

Fig. 10.4 The effect of drug treatment on the incidence of complications of hypertension. [Modified from Veterans Study (1970) *J Am Med Assoc*, **213**, 1143–1152.]

On the whole, the limited numbers of participants reduced the power of the trials to specifically answer the question as to whether treating blood pressure reduced coronary events.

The benefits of treating hypertension can be extended to the larger population at risk from mild hypertension; this has been confirmed in several studies. In these patients it was particularly important to demonstrate that the advantages of blood pressure reduction are not counteracted by long-term adverse responses to the antihypertensive drugs. This assessment of the risk–benefit ratio is particularly important in a group of patients for whom the individual attributable risk (from mildly raised blood pressure) is relatively small.

In all the trials that have involved patients with mild hypertension, active treatment has conferred benefit when compared with placebo or, in the cases of the Hypertension Detection and Follow-up Programme (HDFP) and the Multiple Risk Factor Intervention Trial (MRFIT), the outcome in the special care group was better than those patients who continued with 'usual' medical care. Outcome varied for many reasons, the principal ones being:

- individual trial designs;
- patient selection and number of trial participants;
- duration of trial, choice of drug(s);
- methods of data analysis.

In the Australian Trial (entry diastolic pressures 95–109mmHg) active treatment reduced the incidence of strokes. Although fewer cases of fatal ischaemic heart disease occurred in the active treatment group, the numbers were small and the difference just failed to achieve statistical significance (Fig. 10.5).

In the Medical Research Council Trial of mild hypertension (diastolic pressure 90–109mmHg) stroke rate was again reduced by active treatment but there was no overall reduction in coronary events (Fig. 10.6) The results of subgroup analysis from this trial (Figs 10.7 & 10.8) require cautious interpretation. Comparing the two active treatment regimes, the diuretic (bendrofluazide) was more effective than the ß-blocker (propranolol) in reducing stroke rate. Strokes were reduced in both smokers and non-smokers by the diuretic, but only in non-smokers by propranolol. With the exception of non-smoking males in whom a modest reduction in coronary events was associated with the ß-blocker, there was no effect of either treatment on coronary morbidity. When overall morbidity was assessed (including silent infarcts diagnosed electrocardiographically) the ß-blocker group fared significantly better than the diuretic or placebo group. In the HDFP, which also included patients in the mild hypertension category, special treatment conferred added benefits to usual care, both with respect to stroke prevention and to coronary morbidity. However, because neither this study nor the MRFIT were placebo controlled, no conclusive statement can be made about the definitive benefits of antihypertensive treatment.

The International Prospective Primary Prevention Study in Hypertension (IPPPSH) addressed the question of whether the incidence of cardiac and cerebrovascular events could be influenced by the inclusion in an antihypertensive regime of a ß-adrenoceptor blocker (oxprenolol), compared with treatment not containing a ß-blocker. No overall differences were found

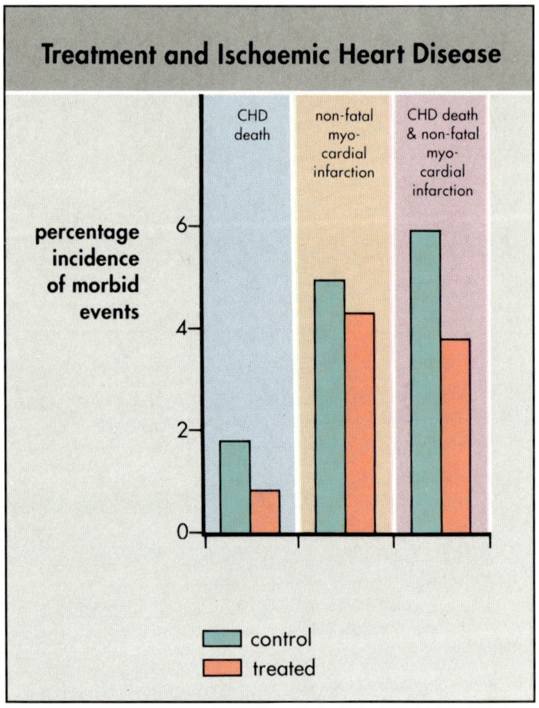

Fig. 10.5 The effect of treatment on ischaemic heart disease in the Australian Therapeutic trial. There was a significant reduction in the incidence of ischaemic heart disease in patients with diastolic blood pressures of 100mmHg or more. [Modified from the Australian Therapeutic Trial (1979) *Clin Sci*, **57**, 449s–452s.]

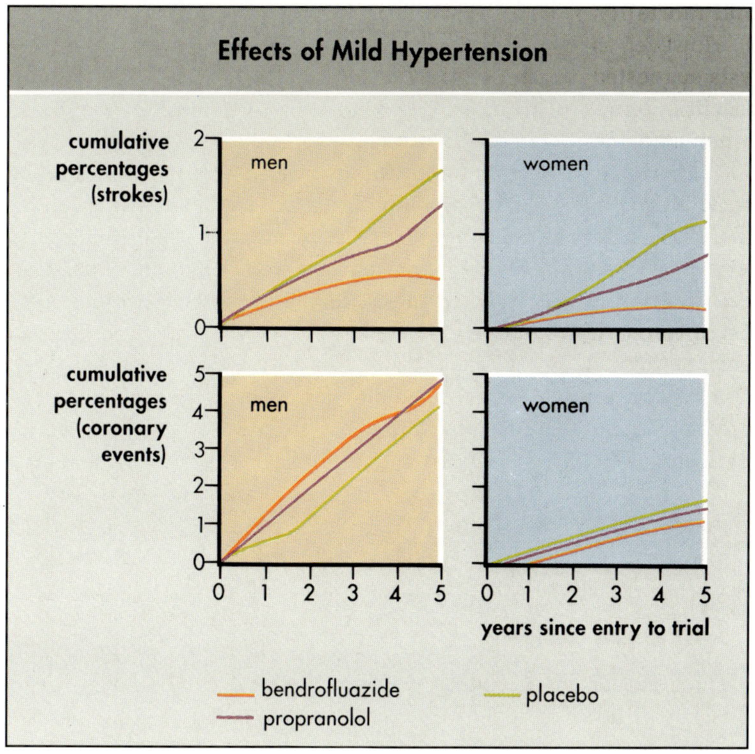

Fig. 10.6 Graphs showing the cumulative percentages of strokes and coronary events in the five year follow-up period in the MRC trial of treatment of mild hypertension.

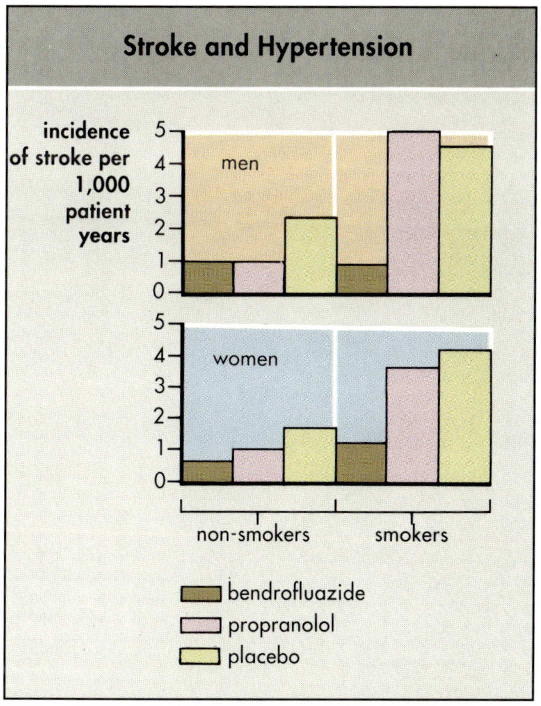

Fig. 10.7 Incidence of stroke per 1,000 person years of observation according to randomized treatment regime and cigarette-smoking status in the MRC trial of mild hypertension. [Modified from The MRC Working Party (1985) *Brit Med J*, **291**, 102.]

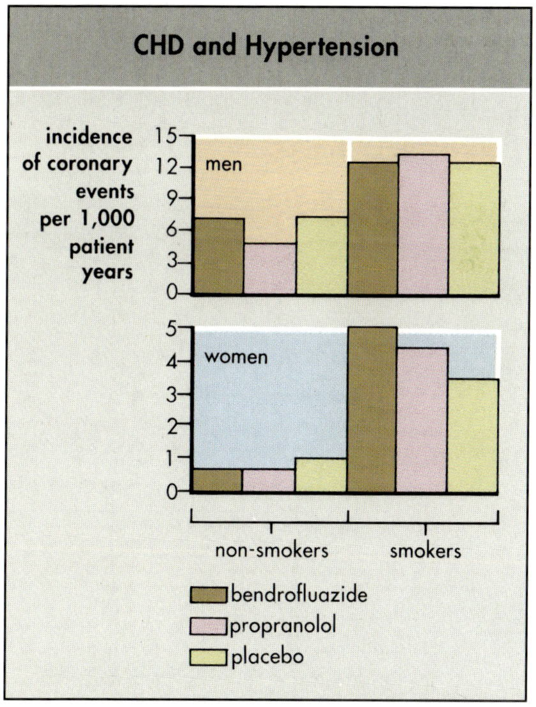

Fig. 10.8 Incidence of coronary heart disease per 1,000 person years of observation according to randomized treatment regime and cigarette-smoking status in the MRC trial of mild hypertension. [Modified from The MRC Working Party (1985) *Brit Med J*, **291**, 102.]

between treatment groups in total mortality, cardiac events or strokes (Fig. 10.9). However, as in the MRC Trial, subgroup analysis suggested that ß-blockers may confer some benefit in terms of a reduction in cardiac events in non smoking men.

Another trial, the Heart Attack Primary Prevention trial in Hypertension (HAPPHY), also addressed the question of whether a ß-blocker based regime differed from a diuretic based regime with regard to the prevention of coronary artery disease in men with mild–moderate hypertension. The outcome of the trial was similar for the two groups and neither regime preferentially reduced the incidence of hypertensive complications, including CHD (Fig. 10.10). Further analyses failed to confirm the observations (from the MRC and IPPPSH studies) that non-smokers benefited from ß-blockers compared with diuretics with respect to coronary morbidity.

Patients in the HAPPHY trial received one of two ß-blockers, atenolol or metoprolol. Those receiving metoprolol were followed for a slightly longer period and the data were analyzed separately. In the metoprolol treated group overall mortality was lower than in the thiazide group because of fewer deaths from CHD and stroke. However, the number of end points was small in this subgroup analysis, so these data should be interpreted with caution.

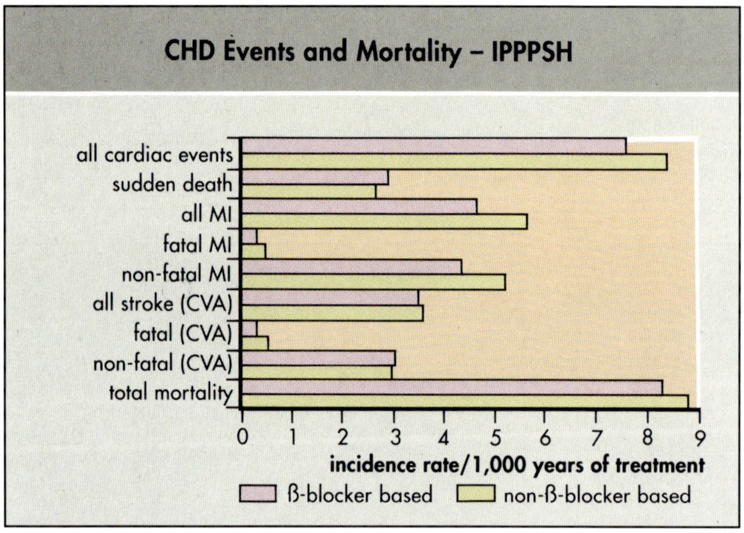

Fig. 10.9 Critical cardiovascular events and mortality according to treatment regimes (ß-blocker based and non-ß-blocker based) in the IPPPSH trial. [Modified from The IPPPSH Collaborative Group (1988) *J Hypertension*, **3**, 386.]

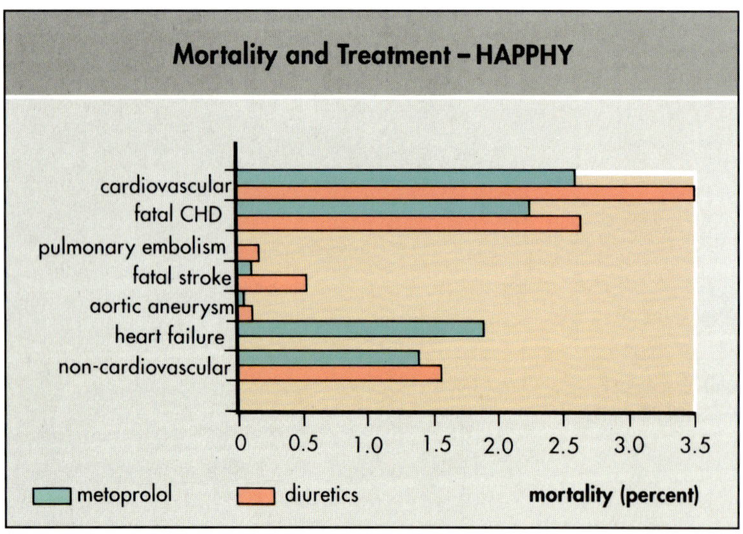

Fig. 10.10 Cause-specific mortality according to treatment regime in the HAPPHY trial. [Modified from Wikstrand *et al.* (1988) JAMA, **259**, 1980.]

Meta-analysis

In evaluating the potential benefits from drug treatment of hypertension, it is important to remember that individual trials rarely have sufficient power to reliably detect differences between drug and placebo, or between one drug and another in overall cardiovascular morbidity and mortality. With the exception of stroke, for which the benefits of treatment are consistent, an apparently negative outcome (particularly with respect to CHD) may be explained by this lack of sensitivity, giving insufficient power to detect a real difference if one exists.

Blood Pressure Reduction		
	stroke	CHD
predicted decrease (observational studies)	35–40%	20–25%
observed decrease (clinical trals)	42±6%	14±5%

Fig. 10.11 Incidence of stroke and CHD predicted for a reduction in diastolic blood pressure of 6mmHg maintained over five years from prospective observational studies and actually observed reduction seen in intervention trials. (For source see Fig. 10.2).

MacMahon has pooled data from a number of prospective observational studies. His analysis suggests that a prolonged reduction of 6mmHg in diastolic pressure would lead to 35%–40% fewer strokes and 20%–25% fewer coronary events. When the results of the intervention trials were analysed, treatment was found to have reduced the risk of stroke by 42% and that of non-fatal myocardial infarction and CHD death by 14% (Fig. 10.11). There is therefore a shortfall in benefit from drug treatment on coronary disease (see below).

Trials in the Elderly

The results of trials of drug treatment in elderly patients with hypertension are generally consistent with those undertaken in younger subjects. However, because the absolute risks of stroke and heart failure associated with high blood pressure are much greater in older subjects, the potential benefits from treatment are considerable.

The percentage reduction in the incidence of strokes in the elderly hypertensive receiving drug treatment is similar to that seen in the young. In the European Working Party on Hypertension in the Elderly (EWPHE) a significant reduction in cardiac mortality was also observed (Fig. 10.12).

In these trials no benefits were seen in patients over 80 years of age.

Mortality and Treatment - EWPHET			
	intention to treat	on randomized treatment	significance level
total mortality	−9	−26	-
cardiovascular mortality	−27	−38	<0.05
cardiac mortality	−38	−47	-
stroke mortality	−32	−43	-
cardiovascular events	-	−36	<0.01
non-fatal MI	-	−14	NS
non-fatal stroke	-	−38	-

Fig. 10.12 Percentage reduction in cardiovascular and other end-points attributable to drug treatment in the European Working Party on Hypertension in the Elderly Trial.

Conclusions from the Trials

The following conclusions regarding drug treatment can be drawn from the trials:

- drug treatment is beneficial for those with diastolic blood pressures greater than 100mmHg (phase V);
- drug treatment is beneficial up to the age of 80 years;
- the higher the initial pressure the greater the potential benefit;
- men benefit more than women;
- benefits from lowering pressure are greater in patients with target organ damage (for example, left ventricular hypertrophy);
- the better the control during treatment, the better the outcome (but note the 'J' shaped curve below).

The absolute benefits of active treatment in reducing the incidence of stroke in individuals with mild hypertension are difficult to determine from the trials. The methods of data analysis, losses from the placebo group and the fact that the overall blood pressures were lower than originally planned would all tend to underestimate the benefits. Thus, figures for reduction in stroke rate of 1.2 per 1,000 patient years of treatment (MRC) and reduction in rate of end points of 4.8 per 1,000 patient years (Australian trial) are likely to be underestimates of the true benefits of blood pressure reduction. However, as will be considered later, the price paid for the benefits (a reduction in cardiovascular end points) was a high incidence of adverse effects from drug treatment leading to drug withdrawal, for example, in up to 25% of subjects over the 5 year period of the MRC trial (Fig. 10.13).

What is the reason for the apparent failure to achieve the expected reduction in coronary risk by drug treatment of hypertension? Several explanations have been proposed:

- the trials were initiated too late in the natural history of hypertensive vascular disease;
- the trials were too short in duration to reverse the atheromatous process;
- the trials were not specifically designed to answer this question;
- the potential benefits of blood pressure reduction on coronary disease were mitigated by the harmful metabolic effects of the most commonly used antihypertensives (for example the effect of diuretics and ß-blockers on serum lipids (see chapter 9);
- the overiding influence of other risk factors for coronary disease in hypertensive patients masked the effects of the antihypertensive drugs.

Some or all of the above may well have influenced trial outcome with respect to coronary disease. For example, despite the fact that the drug induced changes in serum lipids are small, for every 1% increase in serum cholesterol a 2–3% increase in CHD mortality could be anticipated over a 5–10 year period of treatment.

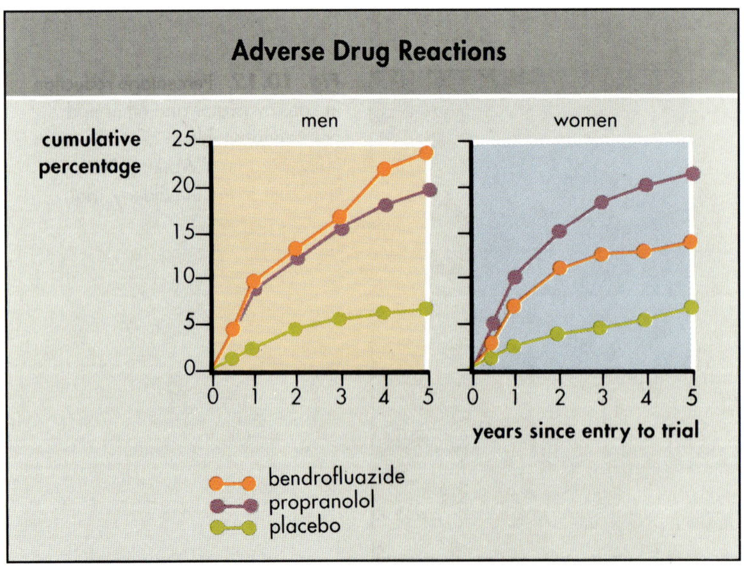

Fig. 10.13 Cumulative percentage of patients withdrawing because of suspected adverse reactions to drugs in the MRC trial of mild hypertension. [Modified from MRC Working Party (1985) *Brit Med J*, **291**, 100.]

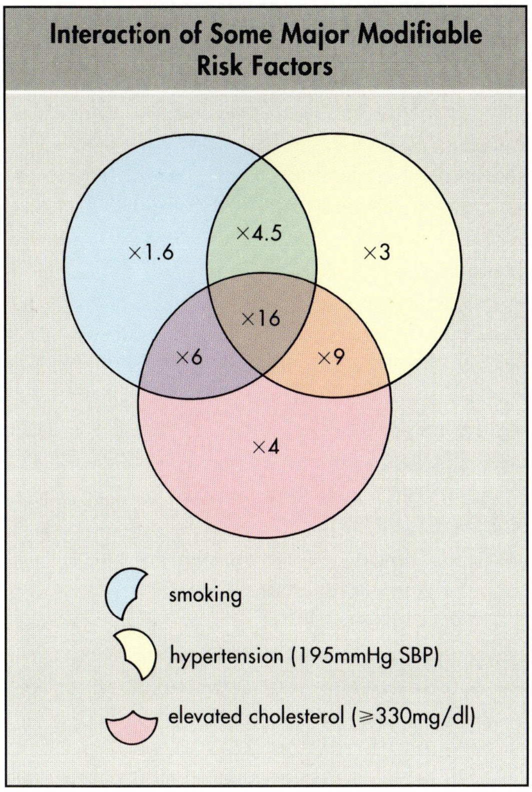

Fig. 10.14 Increase in the risk of coronary heart disease as a result of smoking, hypertension and hypercholesterolaemia, relative to a 45 year old non-smoking man with a systolic blood pressure of 110mmHg and total cholesterol of 185mg. Data from the Framingham Study. [Modified from Kannel, W. B. (1977) Importance of hypertension as a major risk factor in cardiovascular disease. In: Hypertension: physiopathology and treatment. pp 888–910. New York: McGraw Hill.]

Given the multifactorial aetiology of coronary heart disease (Fig. 10.14), it is inevitable that attention to a single risk factor produces limited benefits. The prevalence of some potentially modifiable risk factors for CHD in hypertensive patients is shown in Figure 10.15. High serum cholesterol is found to occur more frequently in a hypertensive population (Fig. 10.16).

CHD Risk Factors	
elevated total serum cholesterol	70%
smoking	35%
low HDL–cholesterol	25%
low exercise output	>50%
diabetes	>5%
synthetic oestrogens	3%
left ventricular hypertrophy	30%

Fig. 10.15 Prevalence of CHD risk factors in hypertensive subjects. Most hypertensives have at least two other risk factors.

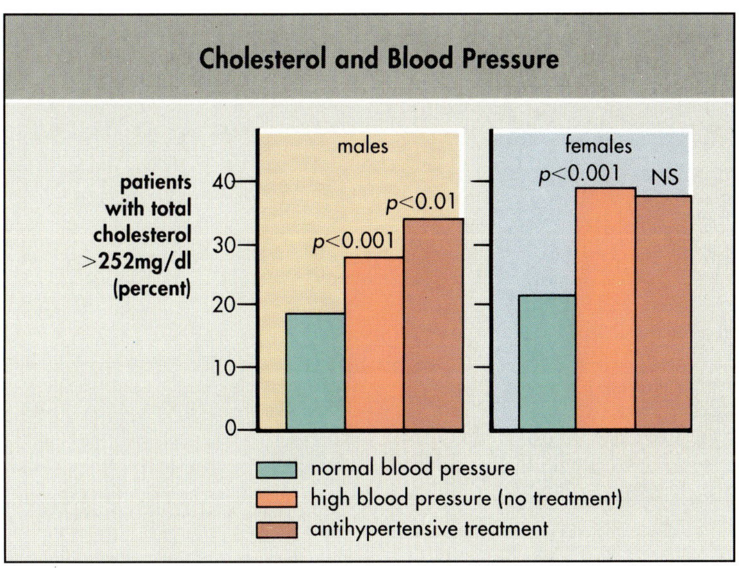

Fig. 10.16 Raised cholesterol levels in three groups of subjects; normal blood pressure, high blood pressure without treatment and high blood pressure on treatment.

That cholesterol exerts an overiding effect on CHD in the hypertensive subjects may be inferred from the Gothenberg primary prevention trial in hypertension. In this study, when both serum cholesterol and systolic blood pressure were reduced, coronary events occurred less frequently than in those subjects with similar blood pressure reduction but little or no change in blood lipids (Fig. 10.17).

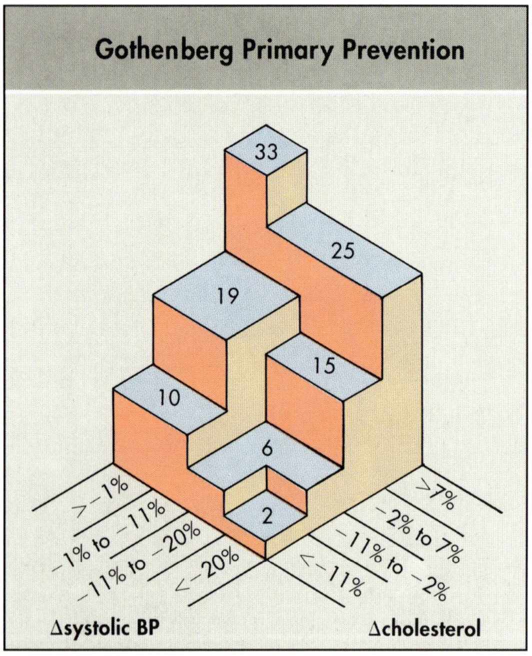

Fig. 10.17 Reduction in CHD events in the Gothenburg primary prevention trial.

BLOOD PRESSURE ASSESSMENT

The various techniques and pitfalls of blood pressure measurement are discussed in chapter 1. In usual clinical practise, blood pressure is measured by conventional sphygmomanometer. If electronic or automated instruments are used, it is vital that they are routinely validated against a standard sphygmomanometer.

Repeated measurements of blood pressure should be obtained before making any decisions about treatment. Particularly in patients with mild hypertension, for whom there is no urgency to initiate therapy, these measurements may be obtained weekly over a 2–3 month period. There is a tendency for blood pressure to fall with repeated measurements (Fig. 10.18); drug treatment should be initiated only in those patients with diastolic pressures consistently in excess of 100mmHg.

The phenomenon of 'white coat' hypertension may be observed in a number of patients. Often of a nervous disposition and suspected at the time of examination (tachycardia accompanying a raised blood pressure), their blood pressure is usually found to be much lower when taken in different circumstances (by a person with whom the patient is more familiar, or at home by the patient him/herself or a relative). Where there is a major discrepancy between the clinic and home values (>15mmHg), and particularly with patients in whom no evidence of target organ damage can be found, clinicians should probably be more cautious in basing decisions to treat on clinic

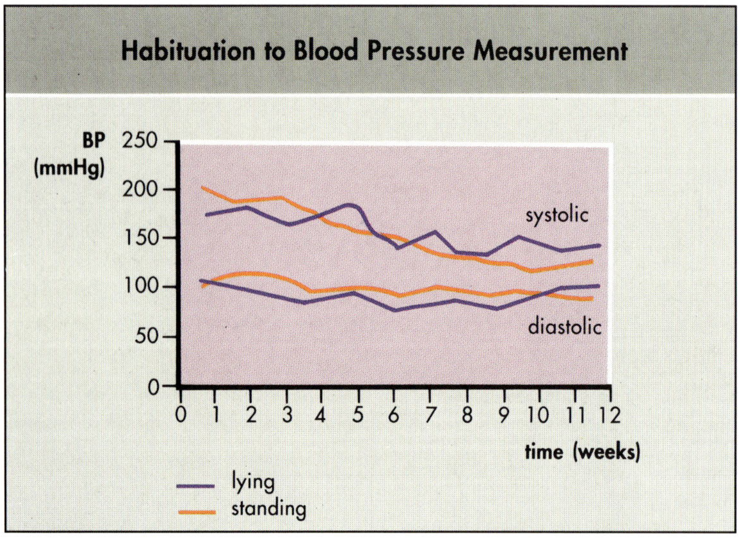

Fig. 10.18 Fall in blood pressure with repeated measurement of blood pressure over a twelve week period. Increasing familiarity with the procedure may result in observed blood pressures falling from the levels at which treatment would be seriously considered, to borderline or apparently normal values.

blood pressures. In such patients, 24-hour non-invasive ambulatory blood pressure monitoring may be helpful (Fig. 10.19).

During the period of blood pressure assessment, detailed information should be obtained about modifiable risk factors for both high blood pressure and CHD. Where there is target organ damage (including left ventricular hypertrophy), hypercholesterolaemia, diabetes, a history of smoking or a strong history of heart disease, then the risk from hypertension is substantially increased and there is a greater urgency and need for treatment. Patients should be counselled and active measures taken where appropriate to modify lifestyle (diet, alcohol consumption, smoking and exercise – see below). Figure 10.20 outlines a management plan for intervention in hypertensive subjects.

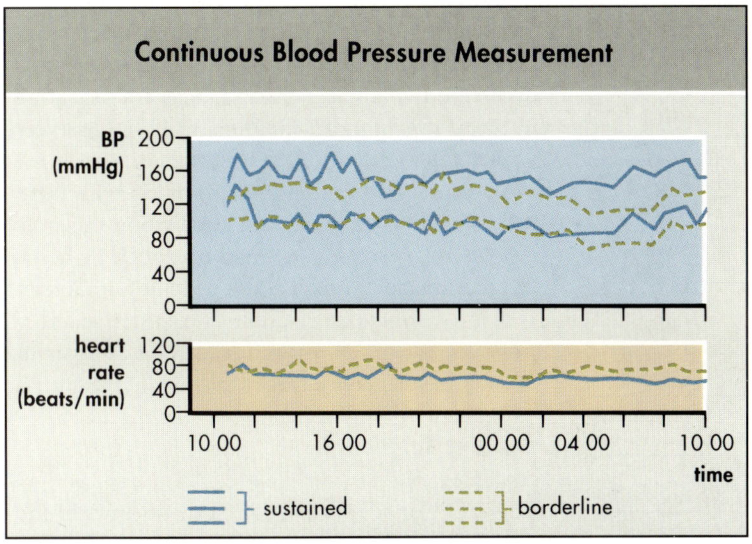

Fig. 10.19 24-hour ambulatory blood pressure recording using a non-invasive monitor in borderline and sustained hypertension.

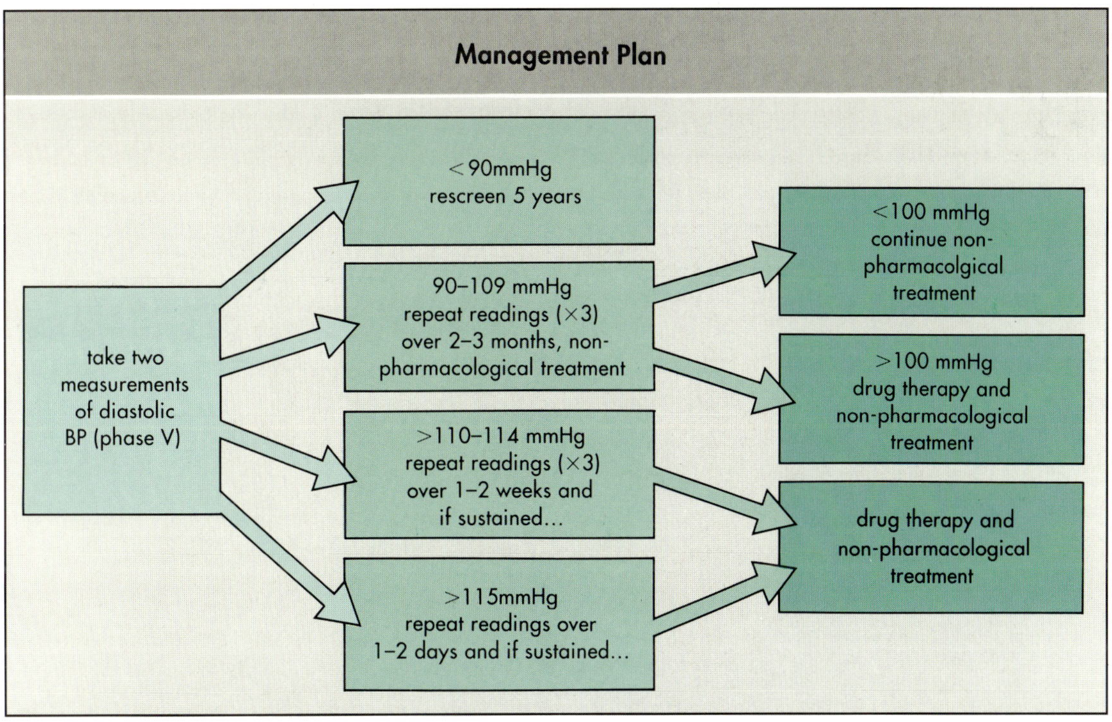

Fig. 10.20 Management plan determined by screening.

NON-PHARMACOLOGICAL TREATMENT

If blood pressure can be lowered to 'normal' or acceptable levels by non-pharmacological methods then drug therapy may be avoided. Non-pharmacological treatment constitutes an important part of any management scheme for the hypertensive patient, since even if such methods are insufficient alone to control blood pressure in a patient, they may reduce the drug requirement and the number and/or frequency of unwanted effects. Non-pharmacological methods are outlined in Figure 10.21.

Non-pharmacological Control

	effectiveness
↓ weight	•••••••
↓ alcohol	•••••
↓ sodium intake	•••
↑ physical exercise	•••
↑ potassium intake	•
↓ saturated fat intake	•
relaxation techniques	•

Fig. 10.21 Non-pharmacological methods for control of blood pressure.

Weight Reduction

The importance of weight or body mass as a determinant of blood pressure was discussed in chapter 3. Weight restriction leads to a fall in blood pressure in both hypertensive and normotensive subjects (Fig. 10.22). Several intervention studies have confirmed the benefits of this approach in hypertensive subjects (Fig. 10.23) with greater blood pressure reduction in those with higher initial pressures. In one study, normotensive levels of blood pressure were achieved in most hypertensive subjects when they lost only half of their excess body weight. For each kilogram lost a fall in blood pressure of 3/2mmHg may be observed, with greater effects seen in men than in women.

Weight reduction may be associated with other potential benefits, including a reduction in serum cholesterol, blood glucose and uric acid. It should be recommended for all obese patients with hypertension. However, it must be recognised that pressure is not always reduced in such patients even if they achieve a reasonable loss of weight.

Sodium Restriction

The relationship between sodium and blood pressure has been considered in chapter 3. Few dispute the historical evidence demonstrating the benefit of Kempner's low-sodium rice diet in malignant hypertension and in some less severe hypertensive patients. However, the role of dietary

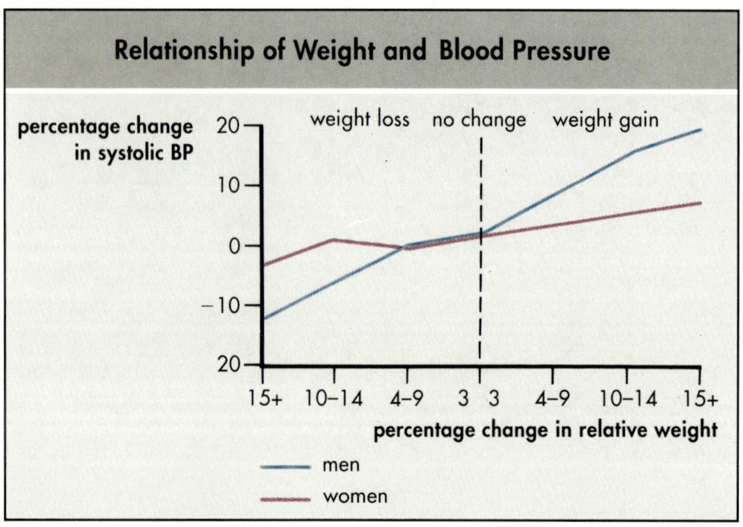

Fig. 10.22 Increase of weight in underweight individuals and loss of weight in the obese both tend to restore blood pressure levels to the population mean.

sodium restriction in mild–moderate benign phase hypertension has been the subject of much controversy. This has largely resulted from the paucity of well-controlled studies, using large numbers of patients and carried out for long periods of time. Many studies reported considerable heterogeneity in blood pressure responses to sodium restriction; this has led to attempts to segregate patients into 'salt-sensitive' and 'salt-resistant' groups. Such typing of patients is arbitrary and inappropriate, since there is no evidence that discrete subpopulations of subjects or patients exist. Many hold the view that dietary sodium needs to be reduced to less than 70mmol/day to achieve blood pressure reduction. Such levels of sodium intake are more difficult to achieve and are, for many patients, less palatable.

The difficulties in reaching a uniform conclusion on the benefits of salt restriction are illustrated by the inconsistent results of intervention studies (Fig. 10.24). Reviewing results from studies in hypertensive patients, it would seem that a fall in blood pressure of 5–8mmHg might be achieved by reducing sodium intake from 160mmol/day to 80mmol/day. It has also been claimed that the level of pretreatment blood pressure determines

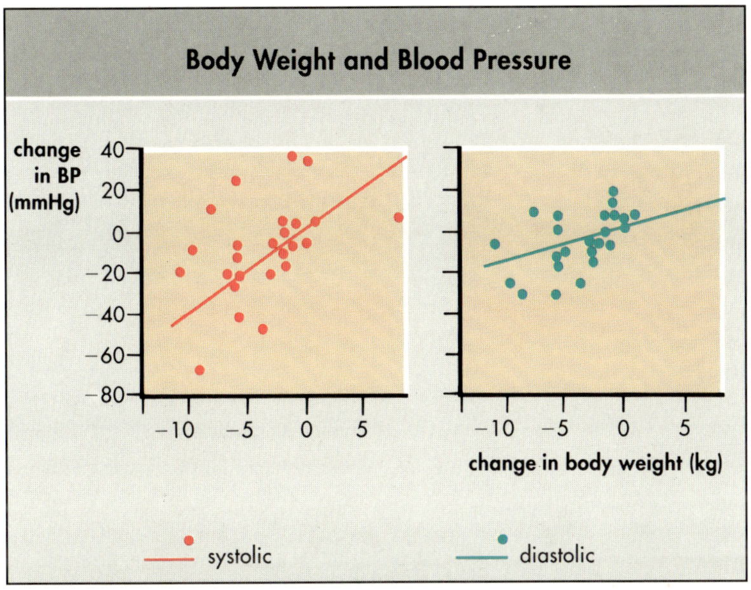

Fig. 10.23 Changes in blood pressure in relation to changes in body weight over one year in untreated hypertension patients. [Modified from Ramsay *et al.* (1978) *Brit Med J*, **2**, 244–245.]

Salt Restriction and Hypertension

	blood pressure (mmHg)		sodium (mmol/day)		
	baseline	change	initial	final	change
Parijs *et al.*	147/98	−9.1/−5.8	191	93	−98
MacGregor *et al.*	117	−7.1	191	83	−108
Morgan *et al.*	160/97	−7.3	191	157	−34
Ewrteman *et al.*	143/94	−1.9/−0.5	130	72	−58
Watt *et al.*	136/82	0.5/−0.3	143	87	−56
Silman *et al.*	165/98	−8.7/−6.3	151	117	−34
Puska *et al.*	138/86	−0.7/+0.8	192	77	−115
Richards *et al.*	137/86	−4.0/−3.0	180	80	−100
Longworth *et al.*	121	−1.7	197	70	−127
Grobbee *et al.*	141/76	−0.8/−0.8	129	57	−72

Fig. 10.24 Controlled trials on the efficacy of salt restriction in hypertension.

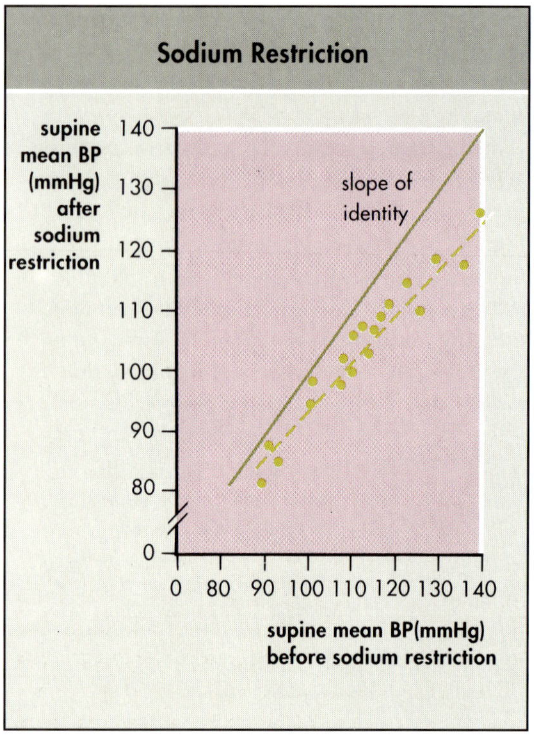

Fig. 10.25 Pretreatment mean blood pressure plotted against mean blood pressure following sodium restriction. Each point represents the results of an entire study.

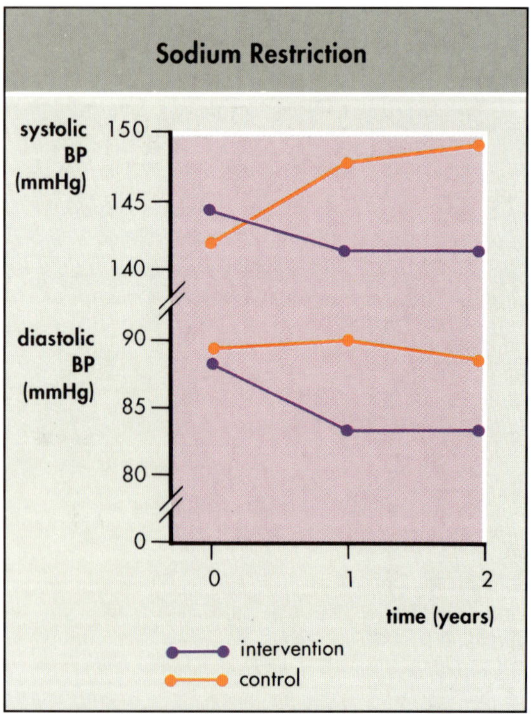

Fig. 10.26 Effects of sodium restriction on blood pressure. [Modified from Rose, G. *et al.* (1989) In *Concepts in Hypertension.* Matthias, C. T. and Sever, P. S. (Eds).]

the magnitude of the fall with sodium restriction (Fig. 10.25). In this context one should mention a population-based intervention study in which a high dietary sodium intake (360mmol/day) was reduced by, on average, 160 mmols/day. This resulted in a fall in the population's mean blood pressure of 5/5mmHg, compared with a rise in blood pressure in a control population in which no intervention took place (Fig. 10.26)

A more consistent observation has been the apparent benefit of salt restriction when implemented together with pharmacological treatment of hypertension. With the exception of the calcium antagonists, salt restriction complements the reduction in blood pressure produced by all classes of antihypertensive agents. In many cases satisfactory control of pressure can be obtained with lower doses of individual drugs.

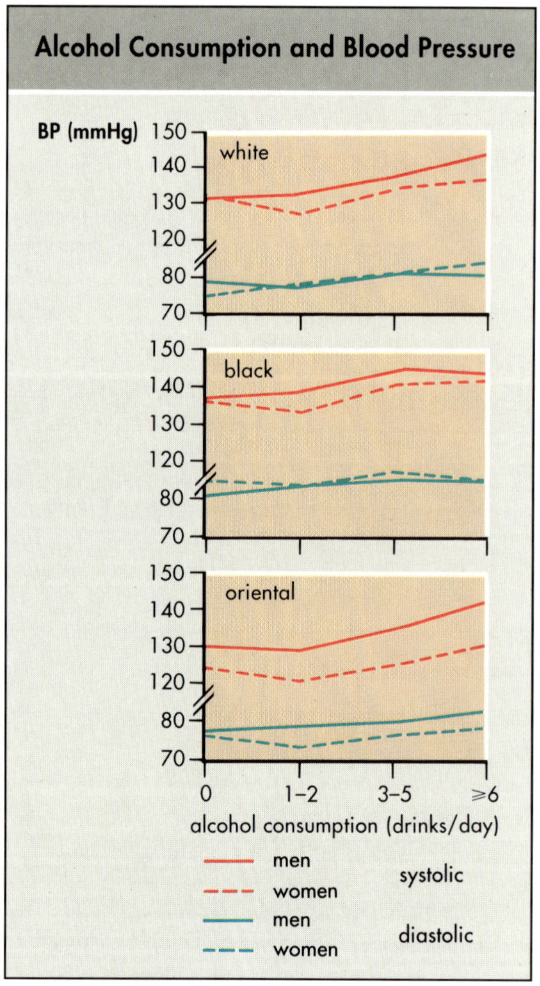

Fig. 10.27 Heavy alcohol consumption is associated with a high mean blood pressure in most populations.

Potassium

There are fewer studies of dietary potassium supplementation in hypertensive subjects than of sodium restriction, and the results are again inconsistent. Some report a modest blood pressure reduction (a few millimetres of mercury) when dietary potassium is increased by about 60mmol/day to around 120mmol/day. Long-term trials have not been undertaken and the potential risks from potassium supplements administered over prolonged periods probably preclude any specific recommendations to increase potassium intake as an antihypertensive measure. There is evidence from studies in experimental models of hypertension and also from epidemiological studies in man that higher potassium intakes may confer a protective effect against stroke. Thus, any potential benefits from dietary potassium supplementation may not be related simply to blood pressure lowering.

Calcium and Other Minerals

Some doubtful epidemiological data has suggested an inverse relationship between dietary calcium and blood pressure. This has led to proposals that dietary calcium supplements may lower blood pressure in hypertensive subjects. At present the results of such intervention studies have been inconsistent and, on the balance of the available evidence no recommendations can be made on calcium intake in hypertensive subjects. With reference to other minerals, including magnesium, at present there is no basis to support dietary manipulation.

Alcohol

The importance of excessive alcohol consumption as a cause of raised blood pressure has been discussed in chapter 1. From epidemiological studies, consumption of three or more units of alcohol per day is associated with higher blood pressures than moderate (less than three units per day) or non-drinkers (Fig. 10.27). Up to 10% of hypertension in men may be alcohol related. Careful assessment of alcohol intake, although frequently inaccurate, is important in all hypertensive patients and the curbing of excessive alcohol intake is an important constituent of any antihypertensive regime. In prospective studies of heavy drinkers, abstention from alcohol has been associated with a marked fall in arterial pressure over the ensuing months, compared with little or no change in those who continue to drink (Fig. 10.28).

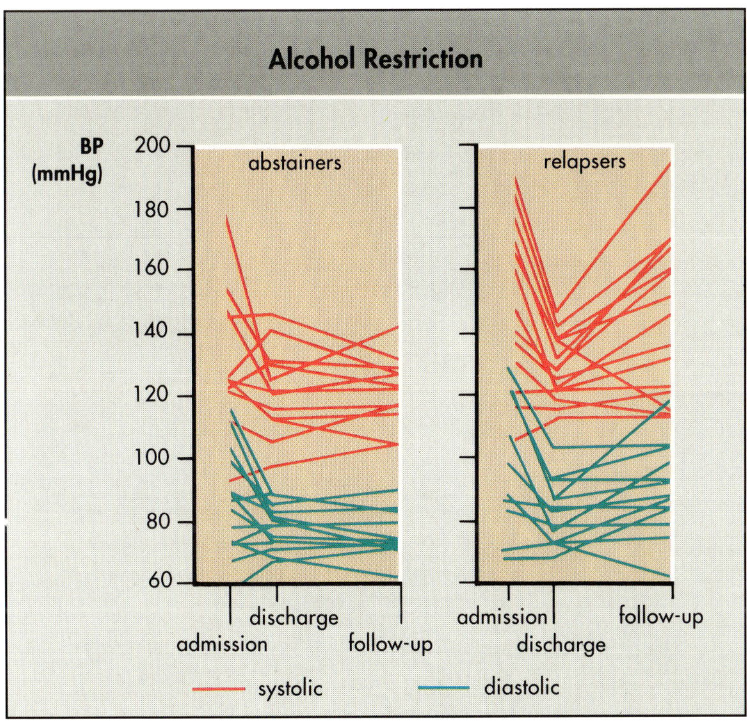

Fig. 10.28 Changes in systolic and diastolic pressure following detoxification and either continued abstention or relapse. (Courtesy of Dr G. Beevers.)

Other Dietary Constituents

Isolated studies have indicated that a wide variety of other dietary constituents may influence blood pressure. Vegetarian diets, for example, are associated with a fall in systolic and diastolic pressure when compared with omnivorous diets. Low-fat diets (particularly those with a high ratio of polyunsaturated to saturated fats) may also induce lower blood pressures. In this context there have been some encouraging studies with ω3 unsaturated fatty acids derived from fish oil. Studies of this kind are, however, difficult to design. Only two definitive dietary recommendations can be made: total calorie intake must be controlled; animal fat intake should be reduced, not to lower blood pressure but to reduce the risk of coronary artery disease (see Fig.10.2).

There is much interest in the syndrome complex of hypertension, carbohydrate intolerance, obesity, hyperlipidaemia and insulin resistance. In certain experimental studies high glucose or sucrose intake has been shown to raise blood pressure. Clearly in the obese subject with glucose intolerance, dietary carbohydrate intake must be reduced together with a general plan for overall weight reduction. More relevant information on the non-obese hypertensive is required; there is at present little evidence to support the recommendation of a reduction in dietary carbohydrates.

Physical Exercise

Investigations of the longer term effects of (dynamic) physical exercise and blood pressure have been difficult to undertake. Nevertheless, in studies which have taken into account associated changes in other potentially confounding factors such as weight reduction, it does appear that regular physical exercise (for example, jogging for 30 minutes, three times a week) and overall improvements in the level of fitness do have beneficial blood pressure lowering effects that are independent of weight reduction (Fig. 10.29). Other forms of physical training, particularly those involving isometric efforts, should not be encouraged as part of a general exercise programme because of the very high levels of pressure that can be generated during static exercise and the potential hazards associated with such activities.

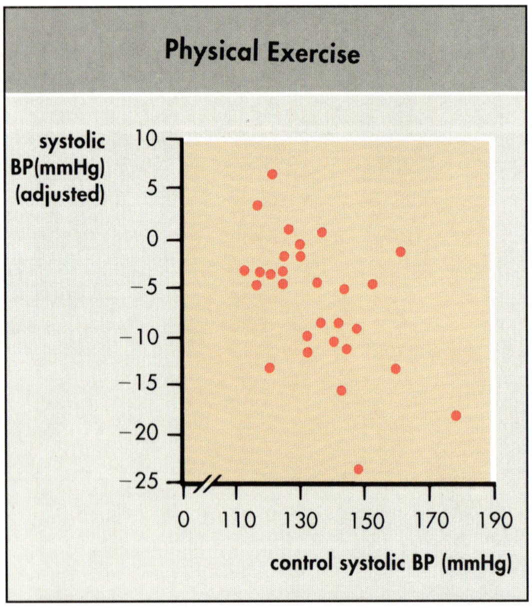

Fig. 10.29 The effect of regular physical exercise on blood pressure. Subjects undertook three training sessions per week for a period of 1–8 months. Average reductions in blood pressure were 4/4mmHg in normotensives and 11/6mmHg in hypertensives. [Modified from Fagard *et al.* (1990). In *Hypertension: Pathophysiology, Diagnosis and Management.* New York: Raven Press.]

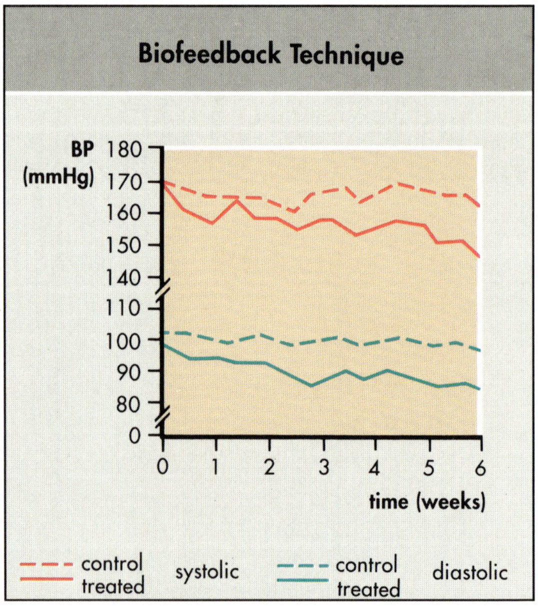

Fig. 10.30 In some studies, training and relaxation and/or biofeedback have produced significant falls in blood pressure in hypertensive subjects.

Yoga, Relaxation and Biofeedback

Whether or not environmental stress has a role in the aetiology and/or pathogenesis of high blood pressure in some patients with essential hypertension, there is certainly accumulating evidence that a variety of relaxation techniques, including yoga, meditation, and biofeedback-assisted relaxation treatment, may induce variable falls in blood pressure. Many studies utilizing such techniques have been poorly controlled and it has been hard to distinguish genuine benefits of the technique from simple familiarization to the process of blood pressure measurement. In one well controlled study (Fig. 10.30) blood pressure reduction was maintained for a least six months after completion of a short course of biofeedback. A major problem with the widespread use of such an approach is that it is costly and labour intensive.

Overview of Non-pharmacological Treatment

Non-pharmacological measures play an important part in any blood pressure control programme. In mild hypertension such treatment may be used from the outset in an attempt to eliminate the need for drug therapy. In the Trial of Mild Hypertension Study (TOMHS) the reduction of pressure using a combination of non-pharmacological measures reduced blood pressure by 10.5/8.2mmHg, compared with drug regimes (Fig. 10.31) which produced falls of 18.2/12.8mmHg. In patients with higher levels of pressure, non-pharmacological measures may facilitate blood pressure reduction with lower doses of drugs or, in some patients, reduce the need for multiple drug regimes.

Weight loss and reduced alcohol intake are of proven efficacy. A reduction in salt intake to around 80mmol/day is unlikely to do harm and may well benefit some hypertensive patients, although such a view is not universally accepted. As part of a general non-pharmacological programme, measures should also be taken in the hypertensive patient to reduce the long-term risks of coronary disease. Thus patient counselling to stop smoking is mandatory and dietary saturated fat intake should be reduced in all subjects with cholesterol levels in excess of 5.2mmol/litre (200mg%).

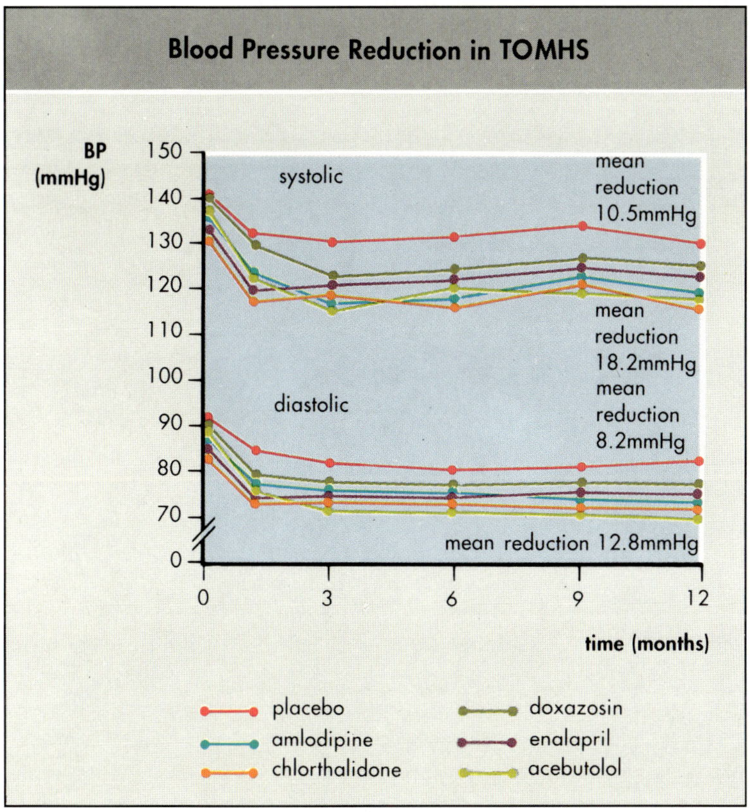

Fig. 10.31 Blood pressure reduction in the trial of mild hypertension study in TOMHS. Courtesy of Grimm, R. *et al.* The mean reduction was, for placebos, 10.5/12.8 mmHg. While for all drug treatments it was 18.2/12.8 mmHg.

PHARMACOLOGICAL TREATMENT

Non-pharmacological and pharmacological methods for lowering blood pressure should not be considered in isolation and, in the design of any treatment regime, a combination of methods will frequently be necessary. For example, when non pharmacological treatment fails to reduce blood pressure to predetermined goals, drugs are introduced as an adjunct to rather than a substitute for non drug therapy.

The level of blood pressure at which drug therapy is indicated has already been discussed and the individual drugs have been dealt with in chapter 9. The initial choice of drug and the subsequent management of the patient should no longer be based on the traditional step care approach outlined in Figure 10.32. Using this management scheme, 50–60% of patients were controlled on the initial drug, 80–95% on two drugs and the remainder required three or more agents. Such a regime ignores the heterogeneity of the hypertensive population with respect to aetiology, pathogenesis and therapeutic response. Using step care, many patients initially receive drugs which elicit little or no hypertensive response; instead of being withdrawn, these agents are incorporated into a multiple drug regime with its inevitable attendant unwanted effects. An alternative management scheme is outline in Fig. 10.33. In this plan the initial choice of therapy is dependent upon patient profiling.

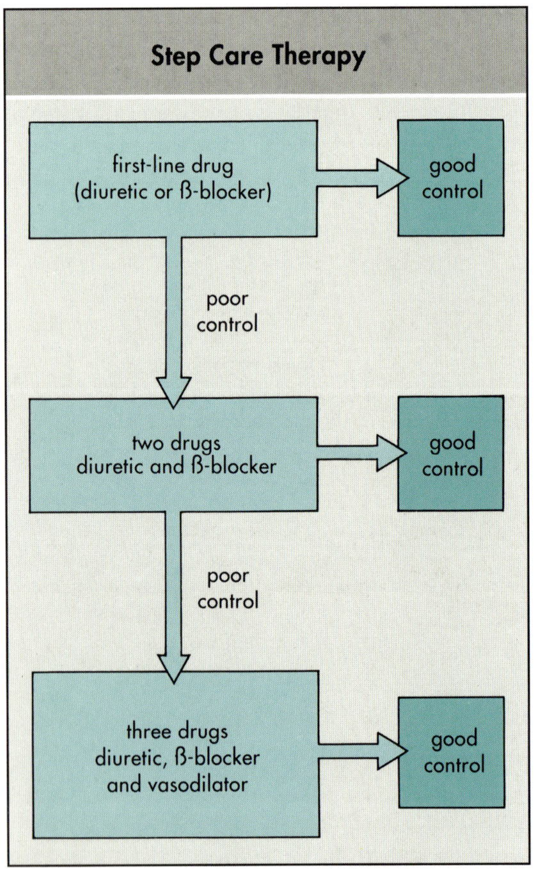

Fig. 10.32 Step care therapy. The physician initially selects one, conventional, 'first-line' drug (either a diuretic or a ß-blocker). If, after a period of time with or without dosage adjustment, blood pressure is not adequately controlled another drug is added. After a further period a third drug can be incorporated into the regime in an attempt to normalize blood pressure.

It is clear from a number of studies that efficacy is not the major factor which determines the initial choice of drug. In TOMHS, for example, drugs representing each of the major classes of agent were compared in a parallel group study. Blood pressure reduction was similar with all the agents, as indeed was the incidence of adverse effects, although the latter differed qualitatively according to drug class.

Factors taken into consideration in the initial choice of drug include coexistent conditions (such as gout, asthma, glucose intolerance, angina, hyperlipidaemia), race, occupation and lifestyle. Examples of possible first choice agents in a number of individual patients are shown in Figure 10.34. Details of individual drugs and drug classes are discussed in chapter 9. Irrespective of the agent chosen, the initial dosage should always be low in an attempt to lower blood pressure without inducing unwanted adverse effects. It is noteworthy that much lower doses of thiazides and ß-blockers can be shown to lower blood pressure effectively than those traditionally recommended.

If blood pressure fails to respond to the initial drug, an alternative agent should be substituted in the first instance. If blood pressure cannot be controlled with low or conventional doses of a single drug, then rational combinations of drugs should be employed. The number of blood pressure recordings and the duration of observation prior to dosage adjustment or substitution of therapy will vary according to the severity of the hypertension. For asymptomatic patients with diastolic pressures less than 115mmHg, two or three readings taken at weekly or two–weekly intervals over a 3–6 week period would be appropriate.

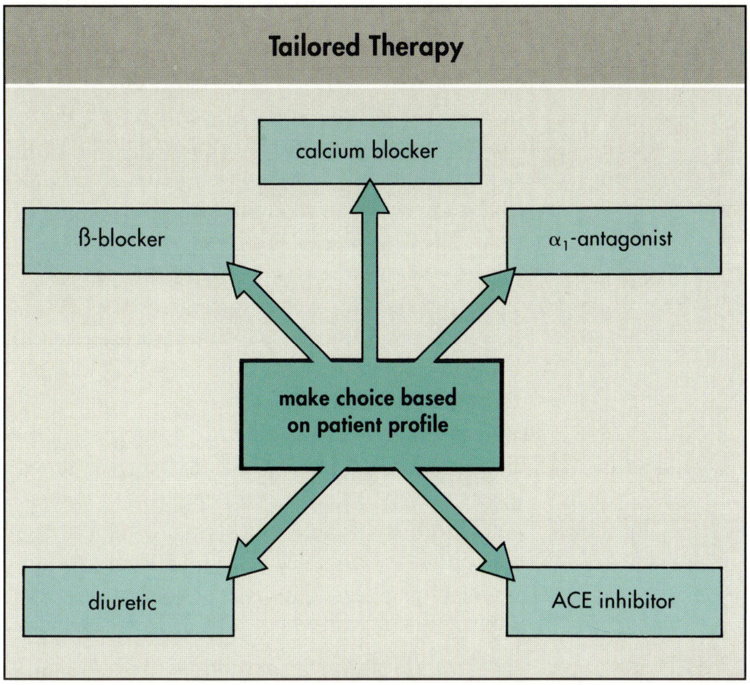

Fig. 10.33 Tailored therapy.

Patient Profiling

	D	BB	Ca^{2+}	ACE	α_1B
male business executive (40) sportsman (squash) sexually active			●	●	●
West Indian carpenter (50) sexually active			●		●
housewife (45), ++anxious normal lipids		●		●	●
female asthmatic (55) ↑ cholesterol			●	●	●
male (60) previous myocardial infarct and gout		●	●	●	●
black male (65) normal lipids	●		●		
diabetic (NIDDM) (55) abnormal lipids			●	●	●
diabetes, heart failure (60)	?		?	●	?
uncomplicated HT (55) normal lipids no specific complications	●	●	●	●	●

Fig. 10.34 Example of patient profiling in hypertension using diuretics (D), ß blockers (BB), calcium antagonists (Ca^{2+}), ACE inhibitors (ACE) and α_1 blockers (α_1B). Dots show preferred options. Blanks should be avoided.

Drug Combinations

diuretic and ß-blocker

ACE inhibitor and diuretic

calcium entry blocker and ß-blocker (not verapamil)

calcium entry blocker and ACE inhibitor

α-blocker and ß-blocker

Fig. 10.35 Some logical combinations of drugs.

Drug Combinations

Many patients require more than one drug to control arterial pressure. Depending upon the hypertensive population (in primary health care or in specialist referral centres) up to 40% of patients will need two or more agents. Combinations of drugs (Fig. 10.35) should be selected rationally and choice based on the following principles.

- Where possible, use combinations of drugs which act on different physiological systems to achieve control of blood pressure e.g. sympatholytics and diuretics;
- where reflex responses mitigate the blood pressure lowering effect of a drug, a second agent may be used to counteract that response e.g. vasodilators and ß-blockers;
- two different drugs which act on the same or different physiological systems should be given at subuptimal doses, to avoid the adverse effects of higher doses of a single agent.

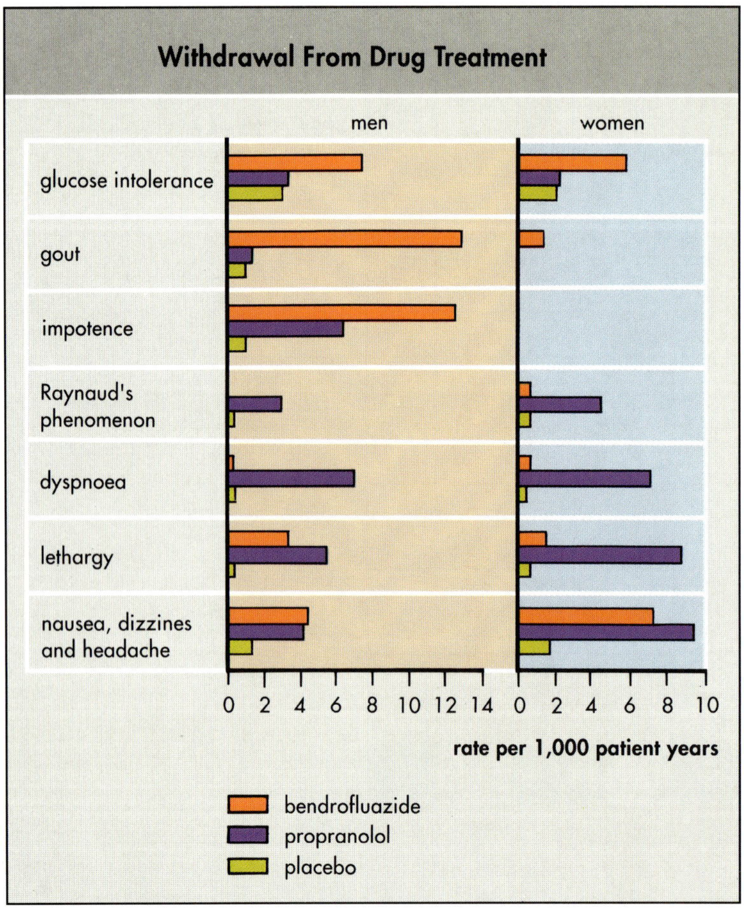

Fig. 10.36 Reasons for withdrawals of randomized treatment in the MRC trial of mild hypertension.

Adverse Effects and Quality of Life

Fortunately, currently available antihypertensive drugs are much better tolerated than older agents. However, when more detailed information is recorded on effects of treatment and, in particular, when more sophisticated methods of assessment are used, the impact of drug therapy on the hypertensive population is seen to cause a multitude of problems. Adverse effects of particular drugs are outlined in chapter 9. Adverse drug reactions led to the withdrawal of up to 25% of male and 20% of female patients over 5 years in the MRC trial of mild hypertension (see Fig. 10.13) and the principal reasons for withdrawal (compared with placebo) are shown in Figure 10.36. It is particularly important when evaluating apparent drug-related effects to compare with placebo, since symptomatic complaints occur with relatively high frequency in this latter group.

Several claims have been made for improvements in 'quality of life' with certain agents such as the converting enzyme inhibitors, (see Fig. 9.31). Caution must be exercised in overinterpreting such data and more detailed studies comparing examples of currently used drugs (such as the TOMHS study) are needed.

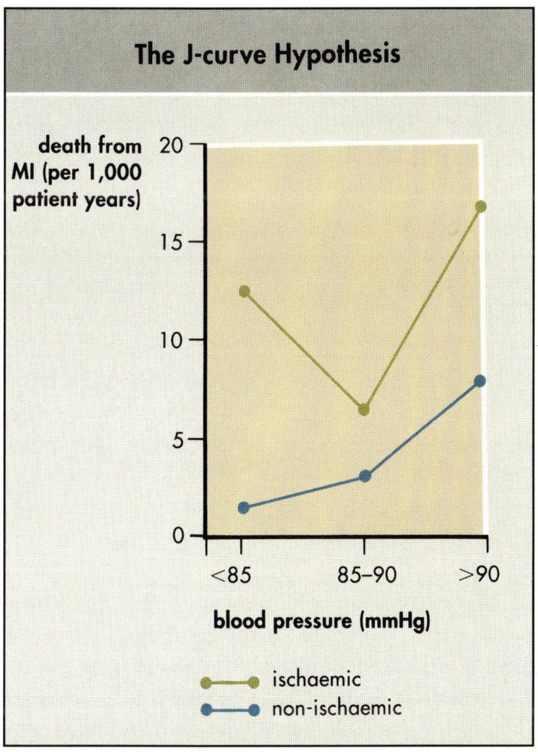

Fig. 10.37 Apparent J-shaped curve demonstrating the relationship between mortality rate from myocardial infarction in ischaemic and non-ischaemic patients and treated diastolic blood pressure. [Modified from Cruikshank, J. M. *et al.* (1987) *Lancet*, **i**, 581–584.]

Goal Blood Pressures

Prospective studies have shown a clear linear positive relationship between levels of blood pressure and the incidence of stroke and coronary heart disease with no evdence for a threshold effect (see Fig 10.2). Lowering blood pressure reduces the risk of stroke and, to a lesser extent, coronary artery disease (see above). Some recent studies have suggested that there is a 'J' shaped relationship between deaths from myocardial infarction and treated diastolic pressure, with mortality at its nadir at 85–90mmHg diastolic (Fig. 10.37). However, in other studies no such 'J' curve has been observed. The 'J' curve hypothesis has been criticized on the grounds that bias due to selection of unrepresentative results and random errors in the estimates of the associations between pressure levels and the incidence of CHD could produce an spurious 'J' relationship. A plausible explanation for an apparent increase in CHD mortality at low levels of diastolic blood pressure (less than 80mmHg) is that patients in this subgroup have low pressures due to pre-existing disease, rather than disease (impaired coronary perfusion and mortality from coronary ischaemia) due to pre-existing low blood pressure.

Although this debate is not yet resolved, in clinical practice it seems reasonable in most hypertensive patients to aim to lower diastolic pressure to between 80 and 90mmHg.

Follow-up of Patients

The frequency of blood pressure assessment and the interval between visits obviously depends on the severity of the hypertension, the presence of associated cardiovascular problems and, therefore, the urgency to lower the pressure. For most patients who are asymptomatic with blood pressures less than 220/120mmHg, initial fortnightly visits followed by monthly visits as blood pressure stabilizes would be appropriate. When goal blood pressures have been achieved three monthly intervals between visits are often all that is required.

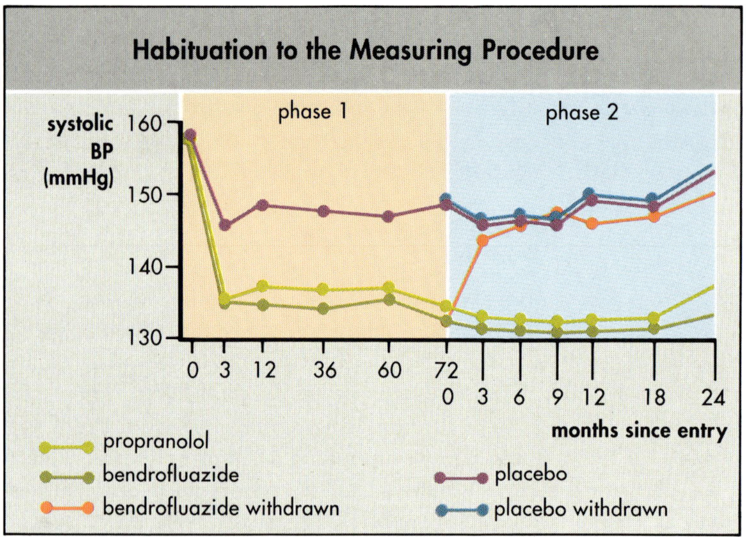

Fig. 10.38 Habituation to the measuring procedure produces a drop in blood pressure, as can be seen here. Note also that where treatment was withdrawn (in phase 2), blood pressure rose to join that of subjects in the placebo group. [Modified from MRC Trial Group (1986) *BMJ*, **293**, 990.]

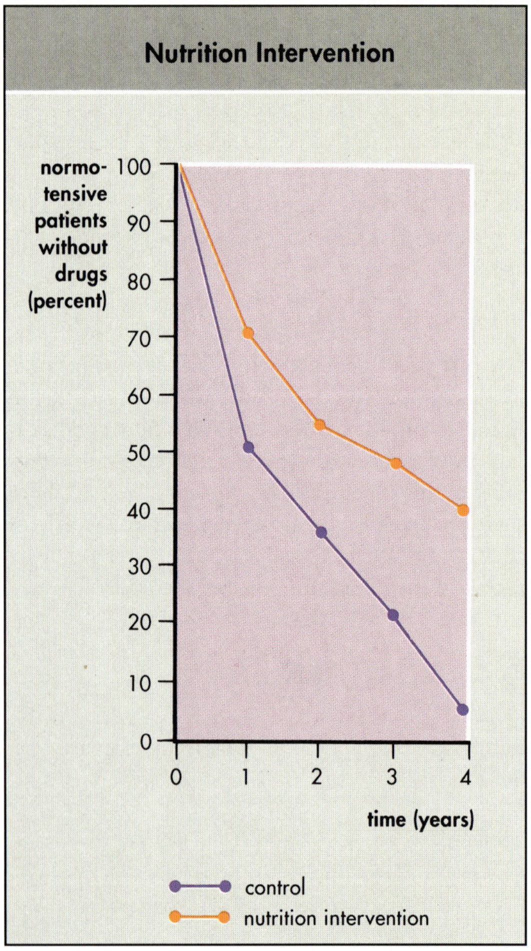

Fig. 10.39 Percentage of patients remaining normotensive after withdrawal of antihypertensive drug therapy. [Modified from Stamler *et al.* (1987) *JAMA*, **257**, 1488.]

At each visit the opportunity should be taken to assess modifiable risk factors for both hypertension and coronary artery disease (see above). Time should be devoted to educating the patient towards a more healthy lifestyle. Drug effects should be noted and adjustments to therapy made if untoward responses materially affect the patient's quality of life (for instance work performance and leisure activities) or if drug related problems such as gout, dyspnoea or glucose intolerance are precipitated.

Higher levels of pressure demand more careful observation with frequent measurements of pressure at weekly or twice weekly intervals. Severe hypertension with symptoms and/or cardiovascular complications including those with accelerated phase hypertension, should be admitted to hospital for monitoring and close supervision.

Stopping Therapy

Is drug treatment for hypertension lifelong? It is a widely held view that although blood pressure may be lowered to normal levels for months or years by treatment, withdrawal leads to a return of pressure to hypertensive pressure levels over a variable period of time. In the MRC trial of mild hypertension, treatment was followed by a return to pretreatment pressure levels over a period of several months; the period varied according to the treatment regime (about three months for the ß-blocker based regime and four to six months for the diuretic based regime – Fig. 10.38). Clearly, these findings indicate that the long-term effects of drugs on a patient's blood pressure are not simply related to their primary pharmacological properties, which are related to the presence of the drug in the body.

The resetting of a number of homeostatic mechanisms for blood pressure control, together with reversal of cardiovascular structural change (which is consequent upon hypertension, yet also responsible for maintaining it) may account for the slow return of blood pressure to hypertensive levels in many patients.

In the Hypertension Control Programme (HPC), patients whose blood pressure had previously been controlled on drug therapy were randomized to one of three groups:

- group 1 – no drugs; reduce weight, excess salt intake and alcohol intake;
- group 2 – no drugs; no nutritional programme;
- group 3 – continue drugs.

After four years 40% of group 1, but only 5% of group 2 remained normotensive without drug therapy (Fig. 10.39) Thus substituting non-pharmacological therapy may obviate the need for drugs in some patients. In others the return to hypertensive levels may be very slow.

SPECIAL CATEGORIES

The Elderly

The elderly patient (more than 65 years old) clearly benefits from antihypertensive therapy; this has been confirmed in several hypertension trials. In general, the approach to management in the elderly is similar to that for younger patients with the proviso that patients over 80 years of age will probably not benefit from drug treatment. It is widely believed that the elderly tolerate drugs less well than the young, but the evidence is not always convincing.

Associated diseases such as chronic obstructive airways disease, heart failure, gout and diabetes will obviously limit the choice of therapy. Adverse reactions to drugs frequently occur in elderly patients because attention is not paid to these important factors.

Cardiovascular reflexes and homeostatic responses to blood pressure lowering agents are blunted in elderly subjects and postural effects of antihypertensive drugs including the diuretics are not uncommonly encountered.

There is little evidence to support the notion that age *per se* influences the response to different antihypertensive drugs and the initial choice of agent is similar to that for younger patients, as long as contraindications to individual drugs have been considered.

Therapy should commence with low doses of agents. Frequent, careful monitoring should be undertaken to facilitate a gradual reduction in blood pressure, avoiding dramatic falls which may impair cerebral perfusion (see chapter 4).

Systolic Hypertension

The possible benefits of treating systolic hypertension remain uncertain. In the elderly, high isolated systolic pressures arise from increasing rigidity of the large arteries (Windkessel vessels). Despite the evidence from prospective studies that this phenomenon is associated with increased cardiovascular morbidity and mortality, no firm recommendations on therapeutic intervention can be made until the results of trials currently under way are reported.

Hypertension in Children

The management of hypertension in children in most cases involves a search for the underlying cause, which will require specific treatment. When drug therapy is necessary the principles of treatment are similar to those applied to adults, with appropriate dosage adjustment. Attention should be directed to simple drug regimes whenever possible, to facilitate compliance.

Hypertension in Pregnancy

Pre-eclampsia (see chapter 6) is one of the most common causes of reversible hypertension. It is invariably 'cured' by delivery of the infant. However, it is a common cause of fetal and maternal morbidity and occasional deaths, both fetal and (rarely) maternal, do occur. When blood pressure rises during the last trimester several measures (often controversial) may be employed in an attempt to improve fetal and maternal outcome. Bedrest is commonly imposed upon women whose diastolic pressure exceeds 90mmHg, although the evidence for any benefit from such action is unreliable. Likewise, sedatives have no place in the management of hypertension of pregnancy.

Whether or not mild–moderate pre-eclamptic hypertension (140–170/90–110mmHg) should be treated remains the subject of much controversy. One view is that maternal hypertension and perinatal morbidity and mortality are causally related, and the higher the pressure, the greater the perinatal risk. Therefore it is logical to intervene pharmacologically at lower pressures in the hope of improving perinatal outcome. The alternative view is that blood pressure and perinatal mortality are not causally related and that because moderate hypertension (less than 170/110mmHg) is unlikely to be associated with maternal morbidity in the short term, then treatment should be reserved for more severe hypertension (greater than 170/110mmHg).

The former view is supported by evidence from intervention trials which have led to improved fetal outcome when drug therapy has been introduced for blood pressure elevations in the mild–moderate range.

Drugs which have been extensively used in pregnancy include methyldopa, ß blockers and hydralazine. In controlled studies (Fig. 10.40) both methyldopa and atenolol have been shown to be preferable to placebo with respect to fetal outcome. Experience with the ß-blocker labetolol suggests that this may be a useful alternative to methyldopa. From this pooled data it is evident that the drug's effect with respect to mortality (fetal, perinatal and neonatal) is beneficial.

Treatment in Pregnancy

authors	entry criteria (mmHg)	active treatment	relative risks treatment vs no treatment (95% CI)
Leather *et al.*	⩾90 diastolic	methyldopa and bendrofluazide methyldopa	0.61 (0.19–1.98)
Redman *et al.*	140–170 systolic or 90–110 diastolic	methyldopa	0.13 (0.02–0.99)
Walker *et al.*	95–109 diastolic	labetolol	no deaths
Rubin *et al.*	⩾140/110, <170 systolic or 110 diastolic	atenolol	0.50 (0.05-5.53)
Winchman *et al.*	140–170 systolic 90–110 diastolic ↑ 30 systolic or ↑ 15 diastolic	metoprolol	0.0

Fig. 10.40 Table summarizing the results of randomized control trials comparing the effects of antihypertensive treatment and non-treatment.

There is clearly concern that lowering blood pressure will lead to further impairment of placental perfusion. However, until safe, non-invasive methods to study individual drug effects on placental flow, become more widely used, no specific recommendations can be made regarding drugs which maintain (or increase) placental flow.

Although diuretics may facilitate the relief of oedema, they should in general be avoided in pre-eclampsia, since they aggravate the hypovolaemia and may further reduce placental perfusion. Furthermore, their metabolic effects, particularly the rise in uric acid, are undesirable. In the case of the latter, this obscures an important prognostic index of the severity of the pre-eclampsia.

Severe pre-eclampsia and eclampsia are treated with vasodilator drugs and anticonvulsants are administered to prevent and control fits. Hydralazine together with ß blockade to inhibit reflex sympathetic discharge, has been widely used. Intravenous diazoxide in conventional doses (300mg) should be avoided because of the danger of precipitous falls in pressure (see later).

Drug Treatment	
recommended	
methyldopa	
hydralazine	
ß-blockers	atenolol
	propranolol
labetolol	
avoid	
diuretics	
ACE inhibitors	
use not established: calcium channel blockers	

Fig. 10.41 Drug treatment of hypertension in pregnancy.

Sublingual or oral (capsule) nifedipine have been shown to be rapidly effective. In the eclamptic crisis an intravenous infusion of nitroprusside or nitroglycerine may be necessary to prevent maternal intracerebal catastrophe.

Essential Hypertension in Pregnancy

As with pre-eclampsia, there remains controversy over the need to maintain treatment of established mild–moderate hypertension during pregnancy. Because the aims of treatment are, in general, to prevent long term morbidity and mortality in the mother, in the short term (of pregnancy) some would take the view that drug treatment should be avoided in patients with pressures under 170/110mmHg. Consistent with this view is the observation that treatment of essential hypertension in pregnancy does not prevent the subsequent superimposition of pre-eclampsia. However, other evidence suggests that fetal outcome is improved by maintaining good blood pressure control throughout pregnancy in patients with mild–moderate essential hypertension. If such a course is taken then, of the currently available agents, only those with an established record of safety in pregnancy should be used. Diuretics are best avoided, unless required in combination with other drugs to antagonise drug induced salt and water retention. ACE inhibitors should not be administered to pregnant women because of the potential hazards of teratogenesis. Figure 10.41 outlines drugs that can and cannot be administered to pregnant women.

Conn's Syndrome

The definitive management of Conn's Syndrome with unilateral adenoma is adrenalectomy, or adrenal ablation, following the retrograde instillation into the adrenal vein of ethanolamine as a sclerosant. The latter procedure is successful in approximately 50% of cases with unilateral disease. For those patients with bilateral adrenal hyperplasia, or for those in whom surgical or radiological intervention is delayed or not possible, medical therapy with the aldosterone antagonist spironolactone is most appropriate. Combinations of drugs are necessary in many patients and alternative agents, particularly the calcium channel blockers, may be effective at lowering blood pressure in this syndrome

Renal Artery Stenosis

Surgical reconstruction of the renal artery or percutaneous transluminal angioplasty have been the preferred treatment for renovascular disease due to both fibromuscular hyperplasia and atheromatous disease of the renal artery. In the former case, often detected in younger patients who fail to respond adequately to antihypertensive drugs, the results of intervention are good (Fig. 10.42) with 50% or more being 'cured' of their hypertension and a further 40% improved (a diminished requirement for drug therapy – Fig. 10.43).

The results of surgical or radiological intervention in atheromatous renal artery stenosis are much less impressive, with a 'cure' rate of around 20% and improvement in a further 50% (see Fig. 10.43). These patients are, however, generally older and many have widespread hypertensive vascular disease which presumably contributes to the maintenance of high blood pressure despite removal of the atheromatous renal artery stricture. In many cases restenosis occurs. With newer radiological techniques, including intravenous digital subtraction angiography, many more patients with occult atheromatous renovascular disease are being identified during the course of investigation of other vascular territories, such as the coronary and peripheral arteries. Up to 40% of patients with peripheral vascular disease show some renal artery narrowing. The benefits of intervention (whether by surgery or angioplasty) in these patients and also in older patients (more than 55 years old) with atheromatous renovascular disease have been questioned. There are no good trial data comparing intervention versus pharmacological treatment in such patients. Attempts to predict outcome prior to intervention using a number of tests, including plasma renin estimations, divided renal vein renins and pharmacological blockade of the renin–angiotensin system, have been inconsistent. In addition to blood pressure control, surgery or angioplasty may be undertaken to improve renal function and protect the kidney from thrombotic occlusion of the stenosed renal artery.

In those patients for whom surgery or angioplasty cannot be performed, pharmacological therapy is required. Drugs that inhibit the renin–angiotensin system (ß-blockers for example) are logical choices but great care is required with converting enzyme inhibitors, which may lead to a rapid deterioration in renal function and the pre-

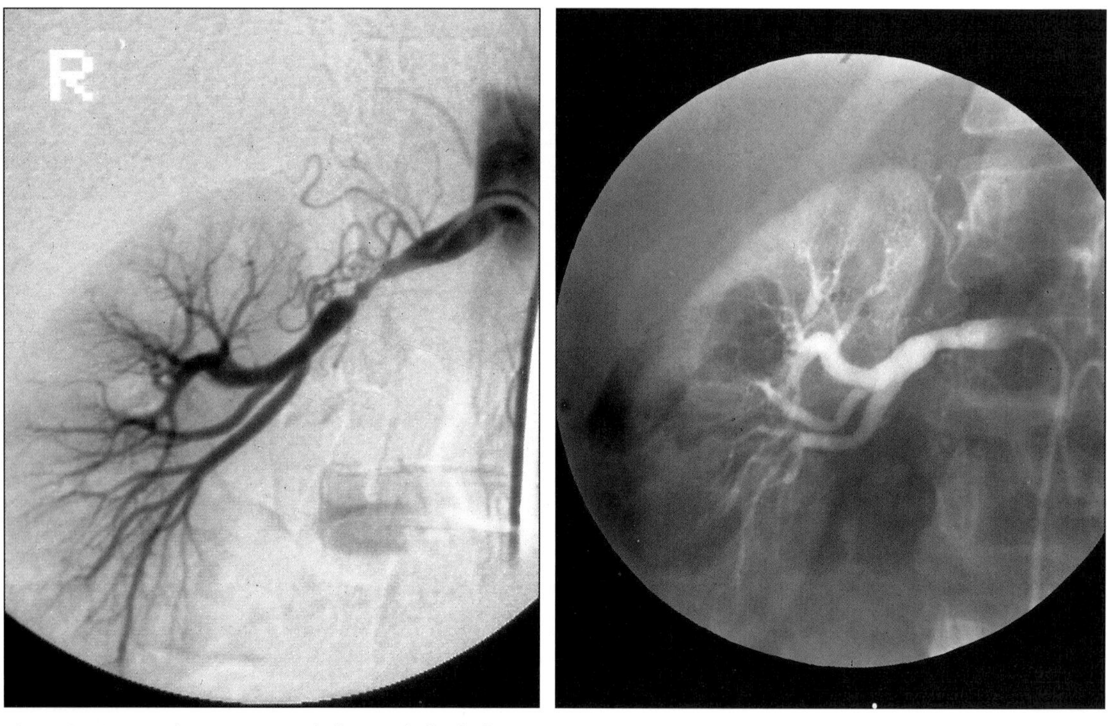

Fig. 10.42 Renal artery stenosis before and after balloon dilatation of the renal artery.

cipitation of renal failure in patients with bilateral renovascular disease (see chapter 9). Renal function should be carefully monitored before and immediately following the introduction of converting enzyme inhibitors in any patients with suspected renal artery stenosis.

Phaeochromocytoma

The treatment of phaeochromocytoma is surgical excision of the tumour(s), the only exception being disseminated malignant disease. The purpose of drug therapy is to control blood pressure prior to surgery (during the period of investigation to localize the tumours) and intraoperatively. The aim is to block the actions of the catecholamines (noradrenaline and adrenaline) released from chromaffin tissue at the α_1 and α_2 (vascular) and ß (cardiac) receptors. A combination of α- and ß-blockade is necessary with, for example, phenoxybenzamine and a ß-blocker or, in some cases, the combined α- and ß- blocker labetolol. The nonselective blocker phenoxybenzamine is preferable to the selective α_1-blockers e.g. prazosin in phaeochromocytoma, because circulating catecholamines exert their vasoconstrictor actions through both α_1-and α_2-adrenoceptors. ß-blockers should not be administered in the absence of α-blockade to such patients because of the hazards of intense peripheral vasoconstriction.

Intraoperative blood pressure control can be very difficult owing to dramatic swings in pressure (Fig. 10.44) particularly when the tumour is manipulated. Intravenous labetolol, or preferably an intravenous infusion of phentolamine titrated against the pressure, should be used. Nitroprusside or nitroglycerine may also be administered. All patients should be ß-blocked prior to induction of anaesthesia.

Precipitous falls in pressure may occur following removal of the tumour or at the time when the venous drainage of the tumour is clamped. In anticipation of this, blood pressure must be maintained and occasionally pressor agents (noradrenaline or angiotensin II) may be required.

In patients with disseminated malignant phaeochromocytoma, α-methylparatyrosine, the inhibitor of the rate-limiting enzyme of catecholamine biosynthesis, may be used (see chapter 9).

Results of Angioplasty

	blood pressure		
	cured	improved	failed
all patients	24	43	33
fibromuscular hyperplasia	50	42	9
atheromatous disease	19	52	30

Fig. 10.43 Outcome (percent) following angioplasty for renal artery stenosis. [Modified from Ramsey & Waller (1990) *Brit Med J*, **300**, 569–572.]

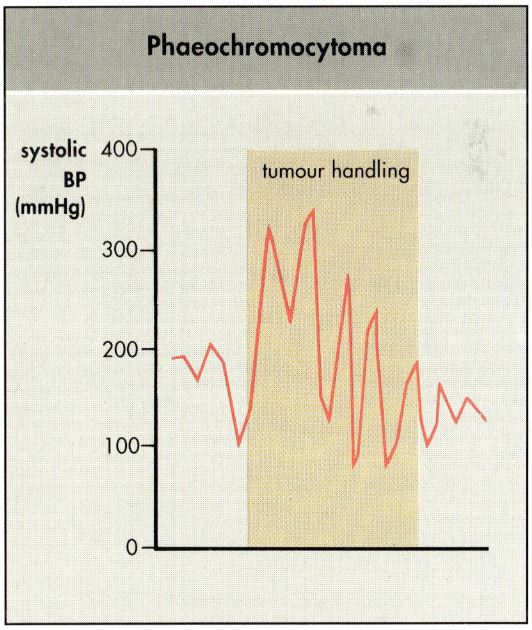

Fig. 10.44 Blood pressure changes occurring during tumour handling at operation on a patient with phaeochromocytoma who had received inadequate α- and ß-receptor blockade. Wild fluctuations in blood pressure were only eliminated when the adrenal blood supply was occluded.

Hypertensive Emergencies

The more severe the hypertension, the greater the urgency to lower pressure to prevent progressive vascular damage (haemorrhage and thrombosis), cardiac failure and deterioration of renal function. In symptomatic patients with a very high pressure (greater than 220/130mmHg) who have not yet developed signs of accelerated or malignant phase hypertension, the pressure may be reduced using conventional orally administered drug therapy, with frequent monitoring of blood pressure, aiming to lower the diastolic pressure to about 100mmHg over a period of several days. There are, however, circumstances in which more rapid reductions in arterial pressure are required (Fig. 10.45). The factors to be taken into consideration prior to initiation of treatment for accelerated phase or malignant hypertension are:

- the time course of vascular damage if blood pressure is not reduced;
- cerebral autoregulation;
- renal function;
- the role of the renin–angiotensin system;
- the reflex mechanisms induced by vasodilators;
- the onset and duration of action of the drugs.

Patients with encephalopathy will need rapid reduction of pressure, with sodium nitroprusside for example, to an initial diastolic pressure of about 110mmHg. This should be undertaken with continuous blood pressure recording and dosage adjustment as appropriate. Precipitous falls in pressure must be avoided to prevent impairment of cerebral blood flow. In such patients, as blood pressure falls there may be a temporary deterioration in renal function. This should not deter the physician from aiming to maintain pressures of about 110mmHg, since the progressive vascular damage associated with the malignant phase can only be prevented by lowering the pressure.

Hypertensive Emergencies
hypertensive encephalopathy
hypertension and pulmonary oedema
accelerated phase hypertension
eclampsia
dissecting aortic aneurysm
catecholaminergic crises (phaeochromocytoma or drug-induced)
hypertension and intracranial haemorrhage

Fig. 10.45 Hypertensive emergencies.

Agents such as diazoxide given by intravenous bolus injection may be dangerous (see Fig. 9.18). In other patients, where there is a less urgent need for dramatic blood pressure reduction the aim should be to reduce diastolic pressure over a period of hours to approximately 110mmHg. This may be achieved in most cases with conventional oral drug therapy. The onset and duration of drug action is discussed in chapter 9. Great care is needed when ß-blockers are administered to a patient with renin-dependent hypertension (as is the case with malignant hypertension and patients who have been treated with vasodilators such as hydralazine). Very small doses of ß-blockers should be used initially (12.5–25mg atenolol or equivalent) to avoid precipitous falls in arterial pressure. Examples of agents that may be used in other hypertensive emergencies are outlined in Figure 9.17.

Index